Dynamic Treatment Regimes

MONOGRAPHS ON STATISTICS AND APPLIED PROBABILITY

Editors: F. Bunea, R. Henderson, N. Keiding, L. Levina, R. Smith, W. Wong

Recently Published Titles

For more information about this series please visit: *http://crcpress.com/go/monographs*

Dynamic Treatment Regimes

Statistical Methods for Precision Medicine

Anastasios A. Tsiatis
Marie Davidian
Shannon T. Holloway
Eric B. Laber

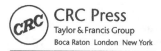

CRC Press
Taylor & Francis Group
Boca Raton London New York

CRC Press is an imprint of the
Taylor & Francis Group, an **informa** business

CRC Press
Taylor & Francis Group
6000 Broken Sound Parkway NW, Suite 300
Boca Raton, FL 33487-2742

Library of Congress Cataloging-in-Publication Data

Names: Tsiatis, Anastasios A. (Anastasios Athanasios), author.
Title: Dynamic treatment regimes : statistical methods for precision
medicine / Anastasios A. Tsiatis, Marie Davidian, Shannon T. Holloway,
and Eric B. Laber.
Description: Boca Raton : Chapman and Hall/CRC, 2020. | Series: Chapman &
Hall/CRC monographs on statistics and applied probability | Includes
bibliographical references and index. | Summary: "Precision medicine
seeks to use data to construct principled, i.e., evidence-based,
treatment strategies that dictate where, when, and to whom treatment
should be applied. This book provides an accessible yet comprehensive
introduction to statistical methodology for dynamic treatment regimes"--
Provided by publisher.
Identifiers: LCCN 2019038384 (print) | LCCN 2019038385 (ebook) | ISBN
9781498769778 (hardback) | ISBN 9780429192692 (ebook)
Subjects: LCSH: Medical statistics. | Medical records--Data processing.
Classification: LCC RA409 .T75 2020 (print) | LCC RA409 (ebook) | DDC
610.2/1--dc23
LC record available at https://lccn.loc.gov/2019038384
LC ebook record available at https://lccn.loc.gov/2019038385

Visit the Taylor & Francis Web site at
http://www.taylorandfrancis.com

and the CRC Press Web site at
http://www.crcpress.com

To my mother, Anna, and my son, Greg
        – A.A.T.

To my mother, Dorothea, and my brother, John
        – M.D.

To my mother, Carin, my husband, Jim, and my grandson, Lukas
        – S.T.H.

To my wife, Sheela, and our stochastic processes, Madeline and Juliet
        – E.B.L.

Contents

Preface

Treatment of a chronic disease or disorder almost always involves a series of decisions. For example, treatment of cancer involves a succession of decisions at key milestones in the disease progression; for example, selection of a first-line chemotherapy at the time of diagnosis, of a maintenance regimen for a patient who responds to first-line therapy or of a second-line/salvage chemotherapy for a patient who does not, and of additional intervention in the event of recurrence. Similarly, management of a behavioral or mental health disorder such as substance abuse or depression requires a series of decisions in which the clinician may start, stop, maintain, modify, or adjust interventions on the basis of a patient's response and other characteristics.

A dynamic treatment regime is a set of sequential decision rules, each corresponding to a key decision point in the disease or disorder process. Each rule maps information on a patient accrued to that point to a set of feasible treatment options, so basing selection of treatment at each decision point on a patient's baseline and evolving characteristics. Thus, a dynamic treatment regime formalizes the process by which a clinician synthesizes patient information to select treatment options in practice.

The emphasis on precision medicine, which involves tailoring treatment to a patient's characteristics in an evidence-based manner, has led to an increasing focus on statistical methodology for the discovery of dynamic treatment regimes from data. In particular, there is considerable interest in estimation, from suitable data, of an optimal dynamic treatment regime, one that, if used to select treatment for the patient population, would lead to the most beneficial outcome on average. The foundations of statistical methodology for this enterprise were pioneered by James Robins through several seminal publications starting in the mid-1980s, and fundamental advances on characterization and estimation of an optimal treatment regime by Susan Murphy and Robins in the mid-2000s formed the basis for a growing subsequent body of work by these researchers and others in the late 2000s and early 2010s.

Since that time, the literature on statistical methodology for dynamic treatment regimes has experienced a veritable explosion as the goal of precision medicine has become a central pillar of health sciences research. In addition, there are parallel developments on methodology for sequential decision making in different contexts in computer science and other disciplines. As a consequence, there is a vast and expanding literature relevant to discovery of dynamic treatment regimes from data, in which different terminology, notation, and perspectives abound, making this topic difficult to approach for the first time.

Our goal in writing this monograph is to address this challenge by presenting a unified and systematic introduction to methodology for dynamic treatment regimes. We do not intend for the book to be an exhaustive account of methodology in this area, however. Rather, we hope that the book will provide readers with foundational knowledge and a strong basis for studying the broader literature, including advances that post-date the book's publication. Accordingly, we present fundamental statistical frameworks along with selected methods that lay the groundwork for further study of this topic. Our ultimate objective is to enhance awareness of and appreciation for this body of work and its critical importance in the treatment of chronic diseases and disorders.

Our target audience is researchers and graduate students in statistics and related quantitative disciplines who are familiar with probability and statistical inference and popular statistical modeling approaches but have no prior exposure to dynamic treatment regimes or other relevant topics, such as causal inference. As discussed in the outline given in Section 1.5, the book includes both foundational and more advanced material. Thus, a reader can study selected portions of the book or the book in its entirety depending on his or her goals and background. Reading plans suited to those who seek a broad introduction to the foundations and key methods in this area and to those who desire in addition a deep, comprehensive understanding of the theoretical underpinnings are presented in Section 1.5.

As the focus of this book is on statistical methodology and its theoretical foundations for this audience, the book is likely not suitable for domain science investigators and other practitioners whose primary goal is to understand the methods at an applied level with an eye toward implementation in practice. We refer such readers to articles specifically designed for this purpose, such as Collins et al. (2004), Murphy et al. (2007a), Murphy et al. (2007b), Lei et al. (2011), Nahum-Shani et al. (2012b), Almirall et al. (2012a), Nahum-Shani et al. (2012a), Almirall et al. (2014), Kidwell (2014), and Kelleher et al. (2017).

The book is an outgrowth of notes developed by one of us (Tsiatis) for a PhD-level special topics course taught in the North Carolina State University (NC State) Department of Statistics over the past decade. We started with these notes as a foundation and have refined, expanded, and added to them to develop the book in its current form. As reviewed in Section 1.5, a subset of the material in the book is suitable as the basis for an introductory PhD-level course on this topic. We are indebted to the Statistical and Applied Mathematical Sciences Institute (SAMSI) in Research Triangle Park, North Carolina, for hosting a PhD course taught by three of us (Davidian, Holloway, Laber) in spring 2019 as part of its Program on Statistical, Mathematical, and Computational Methods for Precision Medicine, which provided us with invaluable feedback from students at NC State, Duke University, and the University of North Carolina at Chapel Hill (UNC-CH).

One of us (Holloway) is the developer of a comprehensive R package, DynTxRegime, that implements a number of the methods for estimation of optimal dynamic treatment regimes from data reviewed in this book. The package is meant to be a "one-stop-shop" for methodology for dynamic treatment regimes and is available from the Comprehensive R Archive Network (CRAN). We gratefully acknowledge National Cancer Institute program project grant P01 CA142538, awarded to a consortium of NC State, Duke University, and UNC-CH, which has supported not only the development of this package but the efforts of the authors to conceive and complete this monograph.

We deliberately do not include in the book static accounts of application of methods covered in each chapter. Instead, detailed demonstrations of application of selected methods are presented on a dedicated, publicly accessible website, http://dtr-book.com. Most of these applications make use of the DynTxRegime package and are meant to assist a reader who has studied the methods in detail with their implementation and with gaining proficiency with the package. We intend for the website to be "dynamic," with periodic updates and modifications as the package and methods evolve. We also hope to post supplemental materials and other resources and encourage readers to check the website often.

We offer our profound thanks to John Kimmel, Executive Editor, Statistics, at Chapman & Hall/CRC Press of Taylor & Francis for encouraging us to take on this project and for his infinite patience with our frequent failure to meet our own self-imposed deadlines. Two of us (Tsiatis and Davidian) have had the privilege of working with John on previous books and are delighted to have had the opportunity to benefit from his extensive experience and guidance again. We also thank the several reviewers of the book-in-progress for their suggestions and feedback. We are grateful to Lisa Wong for creating the cover art. Finally, we thank our families, friends, and colleagues for their support.

Anastasios A. (Butch) Tsiatis, Marie Davidian,
Shannon T. Holloway, Eric B. Laber

Raleigh, North Carolina
September 2019

Chapter 1

Introduction

1.1   What Is a Dynamic Treatment Regime?

In the context of treatment of a chronic disease or disorder, a *dynamic treatment regime* is a set of sequential decision rules, each corresponding to a key point in the disease or disorder progression at which a decision on the next treatment action for a patient must be made. Each rule takes as input information on the patient to that point and returns the treatment he/she should receive from among the available, feasible options. A dynamic treatment regime thus formalizes the process by which a clinician treating a patient synthesizes information and selects treatments in practice. Dynamic treatment regimes are also referred to as *adaptive treatment strategies* or *adaptive interventions*, notably in the literature on treatment of mental health and behavioral disorders.

Precision medicine focuses on tailoring treatment decisions to a patient's characteristics and the incorporation of evidence in guiding these decisions. Dynamic treatment regimes thus provide a formal, principled framework for this enterprise. An *optimal dynamic treatment regime* can be defined as one that, if used to select treatment actions for the patient population, would lead to the *most favorable outcome on average*. Accordingly, formulation of dynamic treatment regimes and methodology for their development and evaluation based on data are of considerable interest to a growing community of clinical and intervention scientists wishing to develop optimal regimes for precision medicine and quantitative researchers seeking tools to support them in these efforts.

Accounts of methodological developments for dynamic treatment regimes are scattered across a vast literature in *statistics*, computer science, and *medical decision-making*. The resulting differences in notation and terminology and the complex concepts involved can make this important topic difficult to approach. The purpose of this monograph is to provide a unified, systematic introduction to statistical methods for dynamic treatment regimes. Our focus is on their use in the *health sciences*; namely, for guiding treatment, prevention, and diagnosis of a disease or disorder. However, the ideas and concepts are relevant in other settings in which sequential decisions on interventions or *policies* must be made,

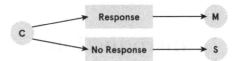

Figure 1.1 *Schematic depiction of two key decision points in treatment of a acute leukemia. At Decision 1, an induction chemotherapy* C *is selected. At Decision 2, for a patient for whom a response is induced, a maintenance therapy* M *is selected; for a patient for whom no response is induced, a salvage therapy* S *is selected.*

as in education, engineering systems, economics and finance, marketing, and resource management.

1.2   Motivating Examples

We begin by considering three applications that illustrate and motivate subsequent developments and to which we refer in later chapters.

1.2.1   Treatment of Acute Leukemias

Figure 1.1 presents schematically two key decision points in the treatment of acute leukemias, a setting to which we refer in subsequent chapters as a running example. When a patient diagnosed with a particular type and stage of the disease presents, the first decision a clinician faces is to select a chemotherapeutic regimen meant to induce a positive response, such a partial or complete remission. Assume that at Decision 1 there are two available induction therapy options, denoted as C_1 and C_2. Typically, following a cycle of induction therapy, a bone marrow biopsy is performed to assess whether or not the patient has achieved the desired response. If so, the patient is deemed a responder at that point; if not, the patient receives a second cycle of induction therapy, after which response status is again assessed. Thus, the desired response might be achieved sooner for some patients than others or not at all. The second key decision confronting the clinician is to determine the next step of treatment, which is dictated by the patient's response status. If the patient has achieved a satisfactory response, Decision 2 involves selecting a maintenance treatment, the goal of which is to sustain the response. If not, at Decision 2, a second line or salvage therapy must be chosen. Suppose there are two maintenance options, M_1 and M_2, and two salvage options, S_1 and S_2.

The goal of the clinician is thus to select an induction therapy from the set of available treatment options $\{C_1, C_2\}$ at Decision 1 and then a maintenance or salvage option from the set of all available treatment options $\{M_1, M_2, S_1, S_2\}$ at Decision 2, where, clearly, only maintenance options are feasible for patients who respond and only salvage options are feasible for those who do not. The clinician seeks to make these decisions so as to maximize the expected benefit to the patient with respect to a health outcome such as disease-free or overall survival time. In making these decisions in practice, the clinician uses his or her expert judgment to take account of accrued information on the patient available at each decision point, where this information may include demographics, prior medical history, genetic and genomic characteristics, initial and evolving physiologic and clinical variables, occurrence and timing of adverse reactions to induction therapy, and so on.

If attention is restricted to these two decision points, then a corresponding dynamic treatment regime comprises two _decision rules_. The first rule, associated with Decision 1, takes as input all information available on the patient at the time he or she presents (baseline) and returns an induction option selected from $\{C_1, C_2\}$. The second rule, corresponding to Decision 2, takes as input all of the information available at Decision 1 plus additional information evolving in the intervening period between Decisions 1 and 2, including response status, and returns a maintenance or salvage option as appropriate from $\{M_1, M_2, S_1, S_2\}$. Shortly, we introduce a mathematical representation of such rules and regimes and in subsequent chapters use it to characterize formally the clinician's goal of maximizing expected benefit to the patient as the problem of seeking an _optimal set_ of such rules; that is, an optimal dynamic treatment regime.

Single and Multiple Decision Regimes

This situation exemplifies what is referred to as a _multiple decision_ or _multistage_ problem, where several, in this case two, sequential decision points can be identified; and selection of treatment over the entire sequence is of interest. In a multiple decision problem, dynamic treatment regimes thus comprise multiple decision rules, and the focus is on an outcome, in this case, survival time, that may be ascertained subsequent to the final decision.

In a _single decision_ or _single stage_ problem, a single decision point is identified. In this example, if the focus is on the role of induction chemotherapy in inducing remission (the desired response), then it is natural to restrict attention to Decision 1, where response is now the outcome of interest. Here, a dynamic treatment regime consists of a

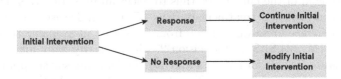

Figure 1.2 *Schematic depiction of two key decision points in treatment of attention deficit hyperactivity disorder. At Decision 1, an initial intervention is selected. At Decision 2, for a child who responds to his initial intervention, there is a single option, to continue the initial intervention. For a child who does not respond, the initial intervention either can be augmented by adding the other intervention or intensified by increasing the dose.*

single rule taking all information available at the time a patient presents as input and returning an option in $\{C_1, C_2\}$.

It is conventional in much of clinical chronic disease research, and from a regulatory perspective, to focus on a single decision point in isolation, even if it is recognized that subsequent decisions are required in the intervening period between that decision point and ascertainment of the outcome. For example, interest may be in the choice of induction therapy at Decision 1 as it relates to survival outcome. It is of course possible to conceive of single decision dynamic treatment regimes in this situation, as above. The outcome that results from treatment selection according to the single, Decision 1 rule will also be affected by the inevitable subsequent decisions that will be made (without reference to further, formal decision rules). We defer discussion of this point to later chapters; for now, we emphasize only that, depending on the setting, single or multiple decision dynamic treatment regimes may be of interest.

1.2.2 Interventions for Children with ADHD

Figure 1.2 depicts two decision points in the treatment of children with attention deficit hyperactivity disorder (ADHD). For a child diagnosed with ADHD, Decision 1 involves selection of an initial intervention, where here we consider two options, low dose medication M or low intensity behavioral modification therapy B, which will be administered ideally for twelve weeks. During the next twelve weeks, the child is evaluated periodically for response status, which is based on a clinical assessment of ADHD severity. A child who shows satisfactory response over the entire period can be considered a responder to the initial treatment, and there is no reason to alter that treatment at the end of the twelve weeks. Thus, the second decision for the clinician, at twelve weeks, involves choosing the single option C, continue the child on the initial intervention. Alternatively, if at any assessment during the twelve weeks the child does not or ceases to show a response, it is not beneficial to continue the initial treatment, so a second decision must be made by the clinician at that point, which involves two options. If the child is on medication, the clinician can choose to increase the dose, thereby intensifying the treatment; or she can maintain the dose but also place the child in behavior modification therapy, so augmenting the initial intervention. Likewise, for a child initially receiving behavioral therapy, the clinician can increase the intensity of the behavioral therapy or continue the low intensity therapy but augment it by prescribing medication. Thus, for a child with negative response status, the two options at Decision 2 are to intensify, I, or augment, A, the initial intervention. As in the leukemia example, the timing of Decision 2 can be different for different children, with all children reaching Decision 2 by twelve weeks.

Here, then, the clinician's objective is to select an initial intervention from the set of available options {M, B} at Decision 1 and, following ascertainment of response status, to select at Decision 2 an option from {C, I, A}, where C is feasible only for children who are responding to their current interventions and {I, A} are appropriate for children who are not. As in the acute leukemia setting, the clinician would like to make these decisions to maximize the expected benefit to the child, where benefit is reflected in a longer-term outcome such as a parent or teacher reported assessment or an academic achievement measure. With attention restricted to these two decision points, a dynamic treatment regime involves a decision rule at Decision 1 (baseline) that takes as input all information on the child, including demographic, socioeconomic, achievement, and clinical assessment variables, and outputs an initial intervention selected from {M, B}. The Decision 2 rule takes this information plus additional, intervening information ascertained up until the time of the decision, including response status, and returns an option from {C, I, A}. As in the acute leukemia setting, of obvious interest is development of an optimal regime.

One can envision extension of this scenario to additional decision points, where, following Decision 1, at each subsequent decision point children who continue to respond to the initial intervention receive C, and the clinician can choose I or A for those who cease to respond to the initial intervention. For children who fail to respond to both their initial and either augmented or intensified subsequent interventions, further options could be established and corresponding rules devised.

This exemplifies a common situation, particularly in behavioral and mental health contexts, where, for individuals who respond to initial treatment, there is one option, to continue that treatment on the grounds that it would be pointless to alter an apparently efficacious intervention. For individuals for whom initial treatment does not induce the desired response, there may be multiple follow-up options. In some applications, the roles of response and nonresponse are reversed.

1.2.3   Treatment of HIV Infection

As a final example, consider treatment for infection with the human immunodeficiency virus (HIV). After a patient is diagnosed with HIV infection, it is typical for the patient to be evaluated at regular, for example, monthly, clinic visits and for decisions on administration of antiretroviral therapy to be made at each visit. Initially and at each subsequent clinic visit, measures of the immunologic and virologic status of the patient are obtained to monitor the progression of the disease. A standard measure of immunologic status is CD4 T cell count (cells/mm^3), where lower counts reflect compromised immunologic status; and virologic status is indicated by viral load, the amount of HIV genetic material (RNA) present in a blood sample (viral RNA copies/ml), where smaller viral loads reflect better control of the virus.

On the basis of current and past measures of CD4 count and viral load, as well as other accrued information on the patient, the goal of the clinician at these clinic visits is to make decisions on therapy with the goal of maximizing the expected benefit to the patient after some period, say one year. Benefit may be reflected in the binary outcome of whether or not, after one year, viral load is below the level that can be detected by the assay used to ascertain viral load measurements. For simplicity, suppose that the clinician can choose either to administer antiretroviral therapy for the next month, coded as 1, or not, coded as 0. Then a dynamic treatment regime comprises a decision rule at Decision 1, the time a patient presents with HIV infection; and decision rules at Decisions $2, \ldots, 12$, say, corresponding to the monthly visits. The rule at Decision 1 takes as input baseline CD4 count, viral load, and other information and selects an option from the set of possible options $\{0, 1\}$; those at Decisions $2, \ldots, 12$ take as input previous and current CD4 counts, viral load measures, and any other baseline and evolving information on the patient and recommend an option from $\{0, 1\}$. A complication is that the virus can become resistant to antiretroviral therapies over time, in which case administration of such a therapy henceforth is of no benefit to the patient. In this simple example, for a patient whose accrued information at the time of a decision includes an indication that resistance has developed, the only feasible option from among those coded as 0 and 1 at this and all future decision points is option 0, do not administer therapy.

Here, in contrast to the previous two examples, the timing of the decisions is predetermined and fixed according to the clinic visit schedule. As before, development of an optimal treatment regime is of interest.

1.3 The Meaning of "Dynamic"

One of the first uses of the term "dynamic treatment regime" is by Murphy et al. (2001), who define dynamic treatment regimes as comprising "rules for how the treatment level and type should vary with time," where "these rules are based on time-varying measurements of subject-specific need for treatment." These authors go on to highlight the distinction between a dynamic and *nondynamic* treatment regime, stating that the latter "is a special case of a dynamic treatment regime in which the treatment assignments do not vary by posttreatment observations." An interpretation of this is that a nondynamic regime involves rules that do not take into account patient information in assigning treatment. Such regimes have been called "static" rather than nondynamic in later literature.

For instance, consider again treatment of HIV-infected patients with antiretroviral therapy as in Section 1.2.3. Using this definition in this context, an example of a nondynamic or static treatment regime is one for which the rule at each monthly decision point dictates that therapy always be administered, so that a patient following this regime would always receive therapy regardless of his evolving virologic and immunologic status, side effects, or possible development of resistance of the virus to the antiretroviral agents. Another nondynamic regime might dictate that therapy should be administered for the first six months after the patient is diagnosed and then withdrawn for the next six months, again regardless of the progression of her disease. In contrast, a dynamic treatment regime involves rules that incorporate virologic, immunologic, and other information, so that the resulting treatment options administered vary according to values of the input information and are thus "dynamic," allowing treatment decisions to be responsive to the progression of the patient's disease. Clearly, the foregoing static/nondynamic regimes are of little relevance in practice, as it is unlikely that a clinician would be willing to, for example, withdraw therapy from a patient whose viral levels are not under control or to continue therapy for a patient whose virus has become resistant to it.

More recently, some authors have used "dynamic treatment regime" to refer to the fact that a regime involves multiple decision points, without regard to the nature of its rules, thus tacitly implying that a single decision regime is "nondynamic." In their definition above, Murphy et al. (2001) do allow a nondynamic regime with any number of decision points to involve rules that incorporate baseline information, so that "dynamic" refers to the additional dependence of the rules following the initial decision point in a multistage situation on evolving information. This definition is thus consistent with the view of any single stage regime as "nondynamic."

Other authors have used "dynamic treatment regime" to refer to any regime, single or multistage, whose rules dictate treatment decisions that vary according to the values of the accrued patient information the rule takes as input, including at Decision 1, where the accrued information is that available at baseline.

A reader who is confused at this point has every right to be so. The convention we adopt in this book is that a dynamic treatment regime is as defined in the last paragraph; that is, a regime involving one or more decision points for which the decision rules potentially incorporate baseline and evolving patient information and thus lead to treatment selections that vary according to this information, including at Decision 1. A "static" regime is a special case of a dynamic treatment regime with one or more decision points whose rules do not incorporate such information. This definition of a dynamic treatment regime is aligned with the goal of precision medicine, even if attention is focused on a single decision point only.

As illustrated by the HIV example, static regimes are of limited interest in and are inconsistent with clinical practice and precision medicine. Consequently, we often refer to dynamic treatment regimes simply as "treatment regimes," without qualification.

1.4   Basic Framework

1.4.1   Definition of a Dynamic Treatment Regime

We now define more precisely the notion of a dynamic treatment regime and present the basic notational framework and conventions we adopt throughout this book.

In most of this book, we consider the situation where we can identify a finite number $K \geq 1$ decision points at which a treatment must be selected from among a set of available, feasible options. Indexing the decision points by $k = 1, \ldots, K$, we let $\mathcal{A}_k$ denote the set of available treatment options at Decision k, and let a_k represent an option in $\mathcal{A}_k$. We restrict attention mainly to the case where the number of options in $\mathcal{A}_k$ for each $k = 1, \ldots, K$ is finite and possibly different for different k. It is also possible for $\mathcal{A}_k$ to be an infinite set, as would be the case when the treatment options are doses of a drug in a continuous range of possible doses, which we mention at some points later in the book.

For definiteness, consider the setting of acute leukemia in Section 1.2.1, which involves $K = 2$ decision points. At Decision 1, $\mathcal{A}_1 = \{C_1, C_2\}$, so comprises the two induction chemotherapy options available when an individual is diagnosed. At Decision 2, $\mathcal{A}_2 = \{M_1, M_2, S_1, S_2\}$, so contains the two maintenance and two salvage therapies. As noted previously, only the maintenance options are feasible for individuals who respond to the induction therapy initiated at Decision 1, and only the salvage options are appropriate for nonresponders to induction therapy. In general, $\mathcal{A}_k$ includes all available options, where of necessity some options may not be feasible for some individuals because of their past histories; we formalize this consideration later in the book.

Let x_1 denote the collection of information available on an individual at Decision 1, so at baseline. Let $a_1 \in \mathcal{A}_1$ be a treatment option at Decision 1, and let x_2 be additional information arising between Decisions 1 and 2. Let $a_2 \in \mathcal{A}_2$ be a treatment option at Decision 2, and let x_3 be additional information ascertained between Decisions 2 and 3. Continuing in this fashion, letting x_k be additional information collected between Decisions $k-1$ and k after receipt of option $a_{k-1} \in \mathcal{A}_{k-1}$ at Decision $k-1$, at Decision k, we denote by h_k the accrued information, or history, available on an individual. At Decision 1, the accrued information or history is simply the baseline information x_1; at subsequent decisions, the history consists of the additional information arising between previous decisions and the treatment options administered at those decisions. Thus, we define the history h_k formally as

$$
\begin{aligned}
h_1 &= x_1, \\
h_k &= (x_1, a_1, \ldots, x_{k-1}, a_{k-1}, x_k), \quad k = 2, \ldots, K,
\end{aligned}
\tag{1.1}
$$

where $a_1, \ldots, a_{k-1}$ are the treatment options administered at Decisions 1 to $k-1$. Let $\mathcal{H}_k$ denote the support of h_k, $k = 1, \ldots, K$.

Thus, from (1.1), in the leukemia example, the history $h_1 = x_1$ available at Decision 1 might include baseline demographic, physiologic, and clinical variables; prior medical history; and genetic and genomic information, and $a_1 \in \mathcal{A}_1$ is the induction therapy option administered at Decision 1. The information x_2 collected intermediate to Decisions 1 and 2 might include updated measures of clinical variables, evolving marker values, indicators of occurrence of and timing of adverse events, and response status. Then the history available at Decision 2 is $h_2 = (x_1, a_1, x_2)$. The option $a_2 \in \mathcal{A}_2$ is the maintenance or salvage therapy administered at Decision 2, which clearly depends on the value of response status contained in x_2 and thus in h_2.

It proves convenient later in the book to define

$$
\overline{x}_k = (x_1, \ldots, x_k), \quad \overline{a}_k = (a_1, \ldots, a_k), \quad \text{so that} \quad h_k = (\overline{x}_k, \overline{a}_{k-1}).
\tag{1.2}
$$

The "overbar" notation in (1.2) is standard and allows us to reference the components of the history, namely, all information ascertained on an individual and the treatment options administered to an individual up to the current decision, separately when we discuss multiple decision problems. If we define $\overline{\mathcal{A}}_k = \mathcal{A}_1 \times \cdots \times \mathcal{A}_k$, $k = 1, \ldots, K$, to be the set of all possible combinations of treatment options that could be administered through Decision k, then clearly $\overline{a}_k \in \overline{\mathcal{A}}_k$.

Armed with this notation, we now define formally a dynamic treatment regime. At Decision k, a *decision rule* $d_k(h_k)$ is a function that maps an individual's history to a treatment option in $\mathcal{A}_k$, that is, $d_k : \mathcal{H}_k \to \mathcal{A}_k$, $k = 1, \ldots, K$. This definition makes precise that, at Decision k, a decision rule is a function that takes as input the accrued information or history for an individual and returns a treatment option from among the available options. Then a dynamic treatment regime d is defined to be a collection of such rules; that is, with K decision points,

$$d = \{d_1(h_1), \ldots, d_K(h_K)\}. \tag{1.3}$$

When $K = 1$, corresponding to a single stage setting, a dynamic treatment regime is a single rule, so that $d = \{d_1(h_1)\}$. For brevity, we often suppress the arguments of the rules and refer to a regime with K decision points as

$$d = (d_1, \ldots, d_K).$$

Corresponding to the convention set forth in Section 1.3, a dynamic treatment regime is one for which the rules $d_k(h_k)$ return different treatment options $a_k \in \mathcal{A}_k$ depending on the value of h_k for at least one of $k = 1, \ldots, K$. A static regime is then one for which each rule $d_k(h_k)$ returns the same treatment option in $\mathcal{A}_k$ regardless of the value of the history h_k. For example, if we restrict attention to the single stage problem involving Decision 1 in the leukemia context, so that all dynamic treatment regimes involve a single rule $d_1(h_1)$, and $h_1 = x_1$ comprises baseline information, an example of a static regime is one with rule

$$d_1(h_1) = \mathsf{C}_1 \qquad \text{for all } h_1.$$

That is, the rule is of the form "give C_1 regardless of the baseline information on an individual." Note that, if we consider both decisions, $K = 2$, it is impossible to conceive of a plausible static regime for this problem, because any reasonable decision rule at Decision 2 must take into account response status, as, for example, a rule that assigns salvage therapy to all individuals regardless of whether or not they responded to induction therapy would contradict acceptable clinical practice and indeed be unethical.

These definitions of decision rules and treatment regimes are formulated in terms of information that would be realized by an individual over the course of the K decisions. Given a set of rules, treatment decisions for an individual can be made according to them as information accrues. We emphasize that nowhere in these definitions do we refer to observed data, for example, from a clinical trial or observational study. A dynamic treatment regime can be defined independently of any data, as it is certainly possible to conceive of decision rules purely on the basis of knowledge of the information that would be available at each decision, subject matter expertise, and practical considerations.

In the foregoing formulation of a treatment regime, the decision rules can be viewed as deterministic or *nonrandom* in the sense that, at Decision k, given history h_k, the rule $d_k(h_k)$ assigns one and only one treatment option from among those in $\mathcal{A}_k$, $k = 1, \ldots, K$. It is also possible to define the notion of a *random dynamic treatment* regime, which is a regime for which the rule $d_k(h_k)$ assigns treatment options in $\mathcal{A}_k$ according to some prespecified probabilities depending on h_k. In the vast majority of applications, interest focuses on nonrandom regimes. Accordingly, in this book, we restrict attention to methodology for nonrandom dynamic treatment regimes. See Murphy et al. (2001) for discussion of random regimes.

1.4.2 *Data for Development and Evaluation of Dynamic Treatment Regimes*

In the classical study of the effect of a specific treatment option, a fundamental goal is to deduce the expected outcome if it were to be used in a population of interest and how that expected outcome compares to that for a competing option. This is based on estimation of the expected outcome for each option from data, where it is widely accepted that data from a clinical trial in which participants are assigned at random to receive the treatment options under consideration are most suitable for this purpose. As reviewed in detail in Chapter 2, data from randomized studies allow apparent differences in expected outcome to be attributed to the treatments under study. In contrast, data from observational studies in which the treatments received by participants are at their and their physicians' discretion can lead to biased inferences. This is due to the possibility that the effects of treatments are *confounded* with individual characteristics; for example, such that sicker individuals are more likely to receive one treatment option over another.

Given a particular dynamic treatment regime involving $K \geq 1$ decision points, it is of similar interest to estimate the expected outcome if the population were to receive treatment according to its rules and to compare the expected outcome to that associated with another regime. Data appropriate for this purpose are thus required. More generally, it is clear that an infinitude of possible regimes can be conceived, depending on different choices of rules. As we have noted, a fundamental objective is to identify an optimal set of rules; that is, an optimal regime, from among all possible regimes that can be conceived. Estimation of an optimal regime thus must be based on suitable data. For these objectives, when $K = 1$, the issues are the same as in the classical setting.

When $K > 1$, estimation of the expected outcome if the population were to receive treatment according to the rules in a particular treatment regime and of an optimal regime involves additional considerations. As discussed in detail in Chapter 5, it is not possible to "piece together" analyses of data from K separate randomized or observational studies, each focused on a single decision point in isolation and each involving different sets of subjects, for this purpose. A major reason for the failure of this approach is that treatments administered at earlier decisions may have effects that do not manifest immediately and thus have implications for selection of treatments at later decision points. Accounting appropriately for such "delayed effects" requires that data be available on the same set of subjects through all K decisions. Data from a longitudinal, observational study in which the same patients are followed through all K decisions are one possible such resource, but could be subject to significant potential for confounding, now in a time-dependent fashion as detailed in Chapter 5, leading to biased inferences. Intuitively, data from a study in which individuals are randomly assigned to the treatment options at each decision point should be preferable to data from a such a longitudinal, observational study.

These considerations have led to great interest in the sequential multiple assignment randomized trial (SMART) design (e.g., Lavori and Dawson, 2004; Murphy, 2005). Given a set of $K > 1$ decision points, in a SMART, participants are randomized repeatedly to the available, feasible options at each decision point. Accordingly, discussion of methodology for dynamic treatment regimes of necessity must include a discussion of this study design, which is the topic of Chapter 9. In Chapters 5 and 6, a formal statistical framework for multiple decision problems is presented in which the conditions under which observed data are appropriate for estimation of dynamic treatment regimes can be clarified. This framework demonstrates that the SMART design yields a "gold standard" data source for this purpose.

1.5 Outline of this Book

The goal of this book is to present detailed, systematic overview of methodology for dynamic treatment regimes. With efforts to collect and curate patient-level data that can be used to inform estimation of treatment regimes rapidly evolving, we hope to make the foundations of the area and both fundamental techniques and newer advances accessible to statisticians and other researchers, who can use them to exploit these rich data resources.

The book is appropriate for graduate students and researchers in statistics and related quantitative fields and assumes no prior exposure to dynamic treatment regimes, causal inference, or associated topics. Chapters 1–7 and 9 present foundational material that could comprise an introductory PhD-level course on this topic. Familiarity with probability and statistical inference and popular statistical modeling approaches at a graduate (PhD) level should provide adequate background for much of this material, although parts of Chapters 6, 7, and 9 are at a somewhat higher mathematical level. On a first reading, technical arguments in these chapters can be omitted without loss of continuity. Chapters 8 and 10 cover more specialized material, which we recommend be approached after the reader feels comfortable with Chapters 1–7.

Central to this area is *causal inference*, particularly in the setting of time-dependent treatment assignment. In Chapter 2, we review the fundamentals of causal inference in a situation analogous to the setting of a single decision point. This chapter also reviews standard statistical modeling strategies and associated large sample theory, as these play an essential role in methodology for dynamic treatment regimes. Chapters 3 and 4 focus on treatment regimes in the single decision setting. Chapter 3 presents a causal inference framework in which an optimal single decision regime can be defined precisely, which provides the groundwork for methodology for estimation of optimal regimes from data. Several key approaches are presented in which a decision rule can be represented through a finite set of parameters that are estimated from data. Chapter 4 covers additional approaches, including those motivated by viewing estimation of an optimal regime as a classification problem, allowing techniques from machine learning to be exploited.

Chapters 5–7 cover the fundamentals of multiple decision dynamic treatment regimes. Because a formal account is rather involved, Chapter 5 presents a high level, less technical introduction to the multiple decision problem, which serves as a "roadmap" to the detailed, precise treatment in the next two chapters. Chapter 6 begins with a rigorous account of an appropriate statistical framework and of key assumptions that are required to deduce multiple decision regimes from observed data based on causal inference concepts in a time-dependent setting. Methodology for estimating the expected outcome of a given, specified, multistage treatment regime from data is reviewed. Chapter 7 presents a formal characterization of an optimal, multiple decision treatment regime and an overview of methodology for estimation of an optimal regime. This includes methods based on viewing the problem from a classification perspective. Chapter 8 extends the framework and methods to the setting where the outcome is a time to an event, which involves additional challenges owing to the fact that individuals may experience the event before reaching all K decision points and that the outcome may be censored for some individuals in the observed data.

Chapter 9 provides an overview of SMARTs, including methods for sample size determination for these studies. Statistical inference on quantities associated with optimal dynamic treatment regimes is challenging. This is because this is an inherently nonsmooth statistical problem, so that standard asymptotic theory does not apply. Chapter 10 starts with an explicit demonstration of this problem and then presents an account of approaches to achieving valid large sample inference in single and multiple decision settings. Of necessity, this chapter is technical in nature.

Research on methodology for dynamic treatment regimes is still undergoing vigorous development. Chapter 11 provides a brief account of some additional topics. Supplemental material on these topics is available on the website dedicated to this book, which is noted in the Preface.

Many of the methods presented in this book involve quantities such as regression relationships between an observed outcome and patient characteristics and treatment options received and probabilities of receiving treatment options at a decision point given an individual's history. In most of the book, we focus on methods based on specification of parametric models for these relationships. This is consistent with how the methods are most often implemented in practice and in some cases leads to consideration of regimes whose rules are of a relatively straightforward form. Although this supports presentation of the methods in terms of approaches and theory that are likely to be familiar to most readers, it is not a requirement. As is noted in later chapters, in most cases it is possible to use instead more flexible modeling approaches, and, indeed, some methods are predicated on flexible representation of relationships.

Readers seeking a broad introduction to the foundations of and key methods in this area should read Chapters 1–5, the first two sections of Chapter 6, and Chapters 9 and 11. Those interested in a deeper, more comprehensive review should also read the remainder of Chapter 6, Chapter 7, and the first two sections of Chapter 10. Those familiar with survival analysis may also wish to read Chapter 8; the material on single decision problems is more accessible than that on multiple decisions, which is rather involved. Readers interested in the theoretical underpinnings of inference should cover Chapter 10, recognizing that this chapter is rather technical, as noted above.

Detailed accounts of application of some methods reviewed in Chapters 2–4, 5–7, and 8, are available on the dedicated website for this book given in the Preface. Many of these analyses are demonstrated using the R package DynTxRegime, developed by the authors, which is available on the website and at the Comprehensive R Archive Network (CRAN).

Remark. In this book, we use the term *fixed treatment regime* to refer to a given, specified treatment regime. That is, we refer to a particular regime d with a given set of rules as a fixed regime. In the context of the HIV infection example in Section 1.2.3, where the history h_k at Decision k contains current CD4 count $CD4_k$, say, an example of a fixed regime is the regime d with rules d_k such that $d_k(h_k) = 0$, do not administer antiretrovial therapy for the next month, if $CD4_k > 200$ cells/mm^3; and $d_k(h_k) = 1$, do administer antiretroviral therapy for the next month, if $CD4_k \leq 200$ cells/mm^3, $k = 1, \ldots, K$. Here, the rules characterizing d are given, specified functions of h_k. Another example of a fixed regime might involve different CD4 thresholds at different decision points; e.g., if there are $K = 12$ monthly visits, $d_k(h_k) = 0(1)$ if $CD4_k > (\leq) 200$ for $k = 1, \ldots, 6$ and $d_k(h_k) = 0(1)$ if $CD4_k > (\leq) 400$ for $k = 7, \ldots, 12$.

A fixed regime as defined here should not be confused with a static regime. As defined in Section 1.3, a static regime is such that all of its rules do not use any patient information to select treatment. As the examples in the previous paragraph demonstrate, a fixed regime need not involve static rules. Our use of the term "fixed" also should not be construed to imply that the timing of the decision points is according to a predetermined, or "fixed," schedule. In the acute leukemia and ADHD examples in Sections 1.2.1 and 1.2.2, the timing of the second decision point in any particular regime in these contexts is not predetermined but rather depends on a patient's response status.

Remark. Throughout the book, we present formal arguments justifying theoretical and methodological developments. To avoid having measure-theoretic considerations distract from appreciation of the conceptual foundations embodied in some of these arguments, particularly in early chapters, we often treat random variables that may be continuous or discrete as discrete without comment. The arguments of course can be generalized under appropriate conditions.

Chapter 2

Preliminaries

2.1 Introduction

The statistical framework underlying the study of dynamic treatment regimes relies on fundamental concepts for *causal inference*, and methodology for estimation of dynamic treatment regimes from observed data depends on that for estimation of parameters of interest in statistical models that may be involved. In this chapter, we review these key topics as a prelude to the discussion of the characterization, formulation, and estimation of dynamic treatment regimes in the rest of the book.

In general, statistical inference is concerned with associational relationships among variables in a population of interest. This problem is ordinarily formulated within a *statistical model* in which the variables are represented as a random vector Z. The observed data upon which inference on these associations is based are denoted as $Z_1, \ldots, Z_n$, arising from a sample from the population. Formally, a statistical model is a class of probability distributions that is thought to contain the distribution generating the data. Often, the statistical model embeds the assumption that $Z_1, \ldots, Z_n$ are independent and identically distributed (i.i.d.) random vectors, where Z has distribution with probability density or mass function $p_Z(z; \theta)$, and θ denotes a vector of parameters indexing the model whose elements represent relationships of interest regarding the distribution of Z in the population.

For example, let $Z = (X, Y)$, where Y is a scalar outcome variable, and $X = (X_1, \ldots, X_k)^T$ is a vector of covariates. A ubiquitous statistical (associational) model is the linear regression model

$$Y = \beta_1 + \beta_2^T X + \epsilon,$$

where $\beta_2 = (\beta_{21}, \ldots, \beta_{2k})^T$, so that

$$\beta_2^T X = \beta_{21} X_1 + \cdots + \beta_{2k} X_k;$$

ϵ is distributed as $\mathcal{N}(0, \sigma^2)$; and ϵ is independent of X, denoted as $\epsilon \perp\!\!\!\perp X$. For this statistical model, the parameter $\beta = (\beta_1, \beta_2^T)^T$ describes the form of the conditional mean of Y given X, $E(Y|X)$ (the regression of Y on X), and thus the association between Y and X, in a meaningful way.

Consider two individuals in the population: one individual with covariates $(x_1, \ldots, x_j, \ldots, x_k)^T$ and the other with $(x_1, \ldots, x_j + 1, \ldots, x_k)^T$. According to this model, if β_j is positive, the average outcome among individuals like the second is β_j units greater than the average outcome for individuals with the same covariate values as the first, so that larger values of x_j are associated with larger average outcomes in the population. However, we cannot necessarily infer from the model alone that increasing x_j by one unit for individuals like the first, assuming that we could even intervene in such a way, would result in, or cause, an increase in the average outcome of β_j units for such individuals.

Across the spectrum of scientific research, interest is more often in causal rather than associational relationships (even if the investigators involved do not admit it explicitly). That is, does action A cause effect B? This is certainly true in the evaluation of treatments, where, for example, investigators wish to attribute improvement in health outcome to administration of treatment. It is thus natural that establishing and estimating causal relationships between treatment actions or interventions and subsequent outcome is essential to the development of dynamic treatment regimes.

Although the study of causality has been considered from different perspectives within different disciplines, a particular point of view advocated by Neyman (1923), Rubin (1974, 2005), Robins (1986, 1997), and others using *potential outcomes* (or counterfactual random variables) is fruitful for this purpose. In this chapter, we adopt this perspective and demonstrate the use of potential outcomes to formalize under what conditions and how causal interpretations on the effects of treatments can be made from observed data.

We begin by discussing *point exposure studies*, where we are interested in the causal effects that treatments have on outcome when they are given at a specific decision point and the outcome is ascertained at some later time. This setting is thus relevant to dynamic treatment regimes involving a single decision point. In subsequent chapters, we consider the more complicated setting of time-dependent causal inference, which focuses on causal relationships among a series of treatment actions over time and outcome. This is the foundation for developments for dynamic treatment regimes involving multiple decision points.

As is evident in this and the chapters that follow, statistical modeling, and in particular regression-type modeling, plays a central role in the estimation of dynamic treatment regimes. As noted in Section 1.5, we focus on the use of popular parametric models in this chapter, for which fitting methods can be characterized as specific cases of the general technique referred to as M-estimation. We thus review the basic approach and theory of M-estimation, which figures prominently in this and subsequent chapters.

2.2 Point Exposure Studies

In the typical point exposure study, each individual in a sample of individuals from a specified population is exposed to one of several agents or interventions, and an outcome is ascertained at some later time. In our context, the exposures studied comprise the (finite) set of treatment actions of interest. Analogous to Section 1.4, we denote this set of possible treatment action options under study as $\mathcal{A}$ and denote an option in $\mathcal{A}$ by a; we suppress subscripting here, as we focus solely on a single exposure. In the simplest case, $\mathcal{A}$ contains two treatment options, which are usually coded as 0 or 1, so that $\mathcal{A} = \{0, 1\}$, and a takes on values 0 or 1. We consider this situation in this chapter; the development can be generalized to a finite number of more than two options.

As an example, interest may be in whether or not an antihypertensive drug reduces systolic blood pressure after six months of treatment relative to not taking the drug in individuals with moderate to high hypertension. The set of treatment options to be studied is thus $\mathcal{A} = \{0, 1\}$, where $a = 1$ corresponds to receiving the drug (active treatment) and $a = 0$ to not (control), and we might define the population of interest precisely to be individuals with systolic blood pressure greater than 140 mmHg. A sample from this population is then obtained, where some individuals begin receiving the drug when they enter the study (baseline) and others do not, and the outcome, change in systolic blood pressure from baseline, is recorded after six months. This can take place in different ways. If the study is conducted as a controlled clinical trial, then each individual in the sample is randomly assigned to receive the drug or not by the study investigators. In contrast, if the study is observational, each individual may or may not receive the drug according to the preference of his or her physician, and the study investigators simply record the option chosen. In either case, systolic blood pressure is measured at baseline, prior to treatment, for each individual and then again at six months, and the observed change in blood pressure, Y, is recorded.

The data that would be available from such a study can be summarized as

$$Z_i = (X_i, A_i, Y_i), \ i = 1, \ldots, n, \tag{2.1}$$

where, for the ith individual, Y_i denotes the observed outcome, change in blood pressure; A_i denotes the treatment received; and X_i comprises covariates collected on individual i prior to the intervention (at baseline), such as age, race, gender, health history variables, and so on.

The ultimate goal of such a study is to use these data to infer a causal relationship between the antihypertensive drug and the outcome. That is, does the drug have an effect on systolic blood pressure after six months? More precisely, is the reduction in blood pressure achieved after six months greater than that achieved (if at all) if it were not used?

As in Section 2.1, the usual statistical paradigm is to view the data $Z_1, \ldots, Z_n$, as i.i.d. random vectors and posit a statistical model for Z in terms of parameters θ indexing the model. For example, one might assume that the conditional distribution of Y given A is normal with mean that depends on A and common variance,

$$Y | A = 0 \sim \mathcal{N}(\mu_0, \sigma^2), \qquad Y | A = 1 \sim \mathcal{N}(\mu_1, \sigma^2),$$

where θ contains $\mu_0, \mu_1 \in \mathbb{R}$ and $\sigma^2 > 0$.

In this model, the parameter

$$\delta = E(Y|A = 1) - E(Y|A = 0) = \mu_1 - \mu_0 \qquad (2.2)$$

represents the difference in mean outcome (change in systolic blood pressure) between individuals who are observed to receive the antihypertensive drug and those who do not receive it. As in the linear model in Section 2.1, the conditional mean of Y given A reflects the association between Y, observed outcome, and A, treatment received, in the population. That is, in a population where some individuals receive the drug and others do not, δ represents the difference in the mean outcome for these two groups and thus has to do with the difference in the associational relationship between outcome and treatment received.

In the observational study above, where individuals in the population of interest receive the drug or not according to the preferences of their physicians, this associational relationship does not necessarily reflect the causal relationship in which we are interested. Intuitively, individuals who receive the drug may be inherently different from those who do not. For instance, individuals who do not receive the drug may be younger, tend to smoke less, have better diets, or be more conscious of their health in general than those who do. Consequently, the associational parameter, δ, may reflect inherent differences among individuals as well as any effect of the drug. Factors that are thought to be related both to the observed outcome and to which individuals receive treatment are referred to as confounding variables or confounders, as they may distort, or confound, the apparent effect of the drug on the outcome.

In the clinical trial, in contrast, individuals in the sample are randomly assigned to receive drug or not; accordingly, they can be thought to reflect a population in which individuals receive drug or not in a way that has nothing to do with, and is thus independent of, any of their inherent characteristics. Thus, it is widely accepted that there are no confounding variables, so that δ reflects purely the effect of the drug.

In the next section, we formalize these ideas through the framework of potential outcomes.

2.3 Potential Outcomes and Causal Inference

We have argued heuristically that statistical associations, which are represented through statistical models for observed data, may not be adequate to describe causal relationships. Given this, how can we represent and deduce causal effects?

Philosophically, the meaning of causation itself is not necessarily clear because an intervention may trigger a number of events that ultimately affect outcome. The point along this sequence of events that we attribute to causality may be difficult to establish. Thus, the study of causality can involve considerable abstract challenges. Luckily, a somewhat simplified yet important point of view on causality can be taken that is useful for conceptualizing casual effects and for drawing causal inferences from observed data.

2.3.1 Potential Outcomes

The concept of potential outcomes, or counterfactual random variables, is widely attributed to Neyman (1923) and Rubin (1974, 2005). Consider a set of possible treatment options $\mathcal{A}$. It is assumed that there exists a random variable $Y^*(a)$ that represents the outcome that would be achieved by a randomly chosen individual in the population of interest if he or she were to receive treatment option $a \in \mathcal{A}$. Such a random variable is referred to as a potential outcome for obvious reasons. Potential outcomes are thus a hypothetical construct: at a specific decision point in an individual's disease or disorder progression, he or she can receive only one of the options in $\mathcal{A}$, so we observe his or her outcome only for that option. However, we can conceive of what the outcome potentially would have been had he or she received a different treatment option.

The random variable $Y^*(a)$ has also been referred to as a counterfactual because it represents a hypothetical outcome that is contrary to fact if an individual actually is observed to receive a treatment option different from a. We use the term potential outcome in this book.

For simplicity, we discuss in detail the situation in which the set of possible treatment options $\mathcal{A} = \{0, 1\}$; the principles generalize to more than two options. Here, with two possible treatments, there are two corresponding potential outcomes, $Y^*(0)$ and $Y^*(1)$. For a single individual from the population, if the difference in outcomes the individual would achieve on each treatment, $\{Y^*(1) - Y^*(0)\}$, is not equal to zero, then, intuitively, this non-zero difference must be attributable to the treatments. Thus, the *causal treatment effect* at the individual level is defined as

$$\{Y^*(1) - Y^*(0)\}.$$

Remark. This definition of causal treatment effect may not address the actual mechanism of causality, especially if, as noted above, treatment triggers a series of events prior to outcome. Nevertheless, there is some appeal to the notion of "what the difference in outcome would be for the same individual under two different treatments," regardless of the underlying processes that lead to the difference.

This definition of causal treatment effect is individual-specific. Thus, because only one of $Y^*(1)$ or $Y^*(0)$ can be observed for any given individual, it is not possible in general to measure $\{Y^*(1) - Y^*(0)\}$. This has led to focus on another measure of causal treatment effect at the level of the population, referred to as the *average causal treatment effect,* given by

$$\delta^* = E\{Y^*(1) - Y^*(0)\} = E\{Y^*(1)\} - E\{Y^*(0)\}. \qquad (2.3)$$

From (2.3), the average causal treatment effect δ^* represents the difference between the average outcome that would be achieved if all individuals in the population were to receive option 1 and that if all were to receive option 0.

Suppose we have carried out a point exposure study and have observed data (X_i, A_i, Y_i), $i = 1, \ldots, n$, i.i.d. across i, as in (2.1). We now discuss under what conditions and how the average causal treatment effect (2.3) can be estimated using these data.

Underlying this causal problem is the conceptualization that there exist random variables $\{X, A, Y^*(1), Y^*(0), Y\}$ with some joint distribution. We wish to estimate $E\{Y^*(1)\}$ and $E\{Y^*(0)\}$, which must be done using the observable (X, A, Y). We thus must deduce the distribution of $Y^*(1)$ and $Y^*(0)$ from the distribution of (X, A, Y). We first state a fundamental assumption that is required.

Stable Unit Treatment Value Assumption

The *stable unit treatment value assumption,* coined SUTVA by Rubin (1980), is usually stated as

$$Y_i = Y_i^*(1)A_i + Y_i^*(0)(1 - A_i), \quad i = 1, \ldots, n. \qquad (2.4)$$

That is, the outcome that is observed for the ith individual in the sample, Y_i, who received treatment A_i, is the same as his or her potential outcome for that treatment regardless of the conditions under which he or she received that treatment.

SUTVA (2.4) thus states that a treatment option is consistent regardless of how it is administered; that is, there are no "versions" of a treatment option. For example, under SUTVA, if individual i received treatment 1 as the result of randomized assignment in a clinical trial in which some individuals received treatment 1 and others received treatment 0, her observed outcome would be identical to the observed outcome she would achieve if she instead received treatment 1 in an observational study where some individuals received treatment 1 and others received treatment 0 according to the discretion of their physicians. Likewise, her observed outcome would also be the same if the entire population were to receive treatment 1. In all of these scenarios, then, SUTVA states that the observed outcome for i would be the same and equal to $Y_i^*(1)$ regardless of how the decision to administer treatment 1 was made.

Also implicit in SUTVA is that the potential outcomes for any one individual are unaffected by the treatment assignments or potential outcomes of other individuals, which is referred to as the notion of no interference. Although no interference may be reasonable in many settings, it is clearly suspect when the treatment options are vaccine interventions for prevention of an infectious disease, where the outcome of one individual can be affected by the interventions received by and outcomes of others. A formal framework for this situation is available (e.g., Hudgens and Halloran, 2008; Tchetgen Tchetgen and VanderWeele, 2012). We do not dwell on this issue except to caution that the plausibility of SUTVA should be critically evaluated on a case by case basis.

SUTVA has also been referred to as the consistency or stability assumption by some authors.

Review of Conditional Independence

We close this section by reviewing the definition of conditional independence. In the rest of the book, we make considerable use of relationships (2.8)–(2.10) below.

Two random variables or vectors Z_1 and Z_2 are statistically independent, written as $Z_1 \perp\!\!\!\perp Z_2$, if

$$p_{Z_1,Z_2}(z_1, z_2) = p_{Z_1}(z_1)p_{Z_2}(z_2), \tag{2.5}$$

or

$$p_{Z_1|Z_2}(z_1|z_2) = p_{Z_1}(z_1), \text{ if } p_{Z_2}(z_2) > 0, \tag{2.6}$$

or

$$p_{Z_2|Z_1}(z_2|z_1) = p_{Z_2}(z_2), \text{ if } p_{Z_1}(z_1) > 0 \tag{2.7}$$

for all realizations z_1, z_2, where $p_Z(z)$ denotes either the probability mass function $P(Z = z)$ if Z is a discrete random variable or vector or the probability density if Z is continuous. Similarly, $p_{Z_1|Z_2}(z_1|z_2)$ denotes the conditional probability or conditional density of Z_1 given Z_2.

For random variables or vectors (Z_1, Z_2, Z_3), Z_1 is conditionally independent of Z_2 given Z_3, written as $Z_1 \perp\!\!\!\perp Z_2|Z_3$, if

$$p_{Z_1,Z_2|Z_3}(z_1, z_2|z_3) = p_{Z_1|Z_3}(z_1|z_3)p_{Z_2|Z_3}(z_2|z_3), \text{ if } p_{Z_3}(z_3) > 0, \tag{2.8}$$

or

$$p_{Z_1|Z_2,Z_3}(z_1|z_2,z_3) = p_{Z_1|Z_3}(z_1|z_3), \text{ if } p_{Z_2,Z_3}(z_2,z_3) > 0, \qquad (2.9)$$

or

$$p_{Z_2|Z_1,Z_3}(z_2|z_1,z_3) = p_{Z_2|Z_3}(z_2|z_3), \text{ if } p_{Z_1,Z_3}(z_1,z_3) > 0 \qquad (2.10)$$

for all realizations z_1, z_2, z_3. That is, all definitions of independence given in (2.5)–(2.7) hold conditionally at all levels of z_3.

2.3.2 Randomized Studies

Within the foregoing potential outcome framework, we now examine the widely accepted and intuitive premise that the data from a randomized study can be used to estimate a treatment effect that has a causal interpretation. This is based on the fact that, because individuals receive the treatment options under study according to a random mechanism, the treatments they receive are assigned independently of all other factors. This is usually expressed as saying that the individuals in the study receiving different treatments are "similar" on average with respect to all characteristics except for the treatments to which they are assigned, so that a difference in average observed outcome among treatment groups can be reasonably attributed solely to the treatments. That is, as noted in Section 2.2, there is no confounding of treatment effects.

Specifically, we demonstrate formally that the usual estimator for treatment effect in a randomized study, the difference of sample averages, is a consistent estimator for the average causal treatment effect and thus indeed has the desired causal interpretation.

For each individual i in a randomized study, there are potential and observed data, which we denote collectively as

$$\{A_i, Y_i^*(1), Y_i^*(0), Y_i\}, \quad i = 1, \ldots, n;$$

for now, we do not consider additional baseline covariates X_i. Assume that SUTVA (2.4) holds.

As above, the role of randomization is to ensure that treatment assignment is independent of all other factors, which of course includes the outcome an individual would achieve under any of the treatment options under study. Thus, randomization ensures that, for each individual i, treatment assignment, A_i, is independent of the potential outcomes, $\{Y_i^*(1), Y_i^*(0)\}$. The assumption that randomization imposes this independence can be expressed formally as

$$\{Y^*(1), Y^*(0)\} \perp\!\!\!\perp A. \qquad (2.11)$$

Remark. In interpreting (2.11), it is fruitful to think of the potential outcomes $\{Y^*(1), Y^*(0)\}$ as inherent, baseline characteristics of an individual that are unobserved. It is well-accepted that randomization ensures that treatment assignment is independent of baseline characteristics.

The independence result (2.11) should not be confused with treatment assignment being independent of observed outcome, which is expressed as $Y \perp\!\!\!\perp A$. That is, using SUTVA (2.4), $Y \perp\!\!\!\perp A$ is equivalent to

$$\{Y^*(1)A + Y^*(0)(1-A)\} \perp\!\!\!\perp A,$$

which clearly is not true, as the left-hand side depends on and is thus not independent of A. Intuitively, the observed outcome Y is the consequence of the assigned treatment A, as this demonstrates, whereas $\{Y^*(1), Y^*(0)\}$, are inherent characteristics of individual i that are not affected by treatment assignment. Indeed, if $Y \perp\!\!\!\perp A$, then assigned treatment has no effect on outcome, so that $Y \perp\!\!\!\perp A$ corresponds to the null hypothesis of no treatment effect of interest in a clinical trial. If there is a treatment effect, then clearly $Y \not\perp\!\!\!\perp A$.

We now show that, under SUTVA and (2.11), the average (associational) treatment difference (2.2),

$$\delta = E(Y|A=1) - E(Y|A=0),$$

is the same as the average causal treatment effect (2.3),

$$\delta^* = E\{Y^*(1)\} - E\{Y^*(0)\}.$$

Consider $E(Y|A=1)$. Because of SUTVA,

$$E(Y|A=1) = E\{Y^*(1)A + Y^*(0)(1-A)|A=1\}$$
$$= E\{Y^*(1)|A=1\}.$$

But, because of the randomization assumption (2.11),

$$E\{Y^*(1)|A=1\} = E\{Y^*(1)\},$$

so that $E(Y|A=1) = E\{Y^*(1)\}$. Similarly, $E(Y|A=0) = E\{Y^*(0)\}$. It follows that

$$\delta = E(Y|A=1) - E(Y|A=0) = \delta^* = E\{Y^*(1)\} - E\{Y^*(0)\}. \quad (2.12)$$

Result (2.12) demonstrates that the average causal treatment effect δ^* can be estimated from the observed data (A_i, Y_i), $i = 1, \ldots, n$, from a randomized study. Because $E(Y|A=1)$ is the mean outcome among those observed to receive treatment 1, it can be estimated consistently (for $n \to \infty$) by the sample average outcome among those receiving treatment 1, and similarly for $E(Y|A = 0)$. Thus, the difference in treatment-specific sample averages, $\widehat{\delta} = \overline{Y}_1 - \overline{Y}_0$, where

$$\overline{Y}_1 = \frac{\sum\limits_{i=1}^{n} A_i Y_i}{\sum\limits_{i=1}^{n} A_i}, \quad \text{and} \quad \overline{Y}_0 = \frac{\sum\limits_{i=1}^{n} (1 - A_i) Y_i}{\sum\limits_{i=1}^{n} (1 - A_i)},$$

is a consistent, asymptotically normal estimator for δ and thus, by (2.12), for δ^*. This argument justifies formally the accepted use of $\widehat{\delta}$ as an estimator for treatment effect with a causal interpretation in the analysis of clinical trials.

2.3.3   Observational Studies

In an observational study, individuals are not assigned treatment via randomization according to some experimental design, but rather receive treatment according to physician discretion or their own choice. In some situations, it may be unethical to conduct a randomized study; for example, it would be unacceptable to undertake a study randomizing participants to smoking or not. Thus, it is of interest to consider whether or not it is possible to estimate the average causal treatment effect δ^* from the data from such a study and under what conditions.

Because individuals in an observational study who receive treatment 1 may have different characteristics from those who receive treatment 0, they may not be prognostically similar to those receiving treatment 0. Formally, because the potential outcomes $\{Y^*(1), Y^*(0)\}$ are inherent characteristics that reflect prognosis, that is, how an individual would fare on either treatment, it may not be reasonable to assume that (2.11), $\{Y^*(1), Y^*(0)\} \perp\!\!\!\perp A$, holds. Accordingly, the arguments in the last section leading to (2.12) do not hold, and it is not necessarily the case that $\widehat{\delta}$ will consistently estimate the average causal treatment effect.

However, if individual characteristics (covariates) X^* ascertained prior to initiation of treatment can be identified that are believed to be associated with both prognosis and how treatment is selected, so that the elements of X^* are confounders, it may be reasonable to assume that treatment assignment is otherwise at random. That is, among individuals sharing the same value of X^*, all factors that might have been associated with treatment selection and that are associated with outcome are taken into account, so that the fact that some may receive treatment 1 and others treatment 0 is effectively at random. This can be expressed formally as

$$\{Y^*(1), Y^*(0)\} \perp\!\!\!\perp A | X^*, \tag{2.13}$$

where this notation indicates conditional independence of the potential outcomes and treatment received given X^*.

Remark. When a clinician makes a decision on which treatment to give to an individual patient, she does not know the patient's potential outcomes. The choice must be made based on the information on the patient that is available to the clinician. The difficulty is that, in an observational study, some of the information available to the clinician that affects treatment choice and is associated with outcome (the information in X^*) may not have been captured in the observed data that are available to the analyst; that is, $X^* \not\subset X$ (X^* is not fully contained in X). There may be variables U, often referred to as *unmeasured confounders,* that are associated with both treatment choice and outcome and that are thus part of X^* but are not contained in X.

If we are willing to believe that X contains all of X^*, so that all of the information that clinicians use to make treatment decisions is captured in the data, then, from (2.13), we may be willing to make the assumption that

$$\{Y^*(1), Y^*(0)\} \perp\!\!\!\perp A|X. \tag{2.14}$$

Rubin (1978) refers to (2.14) as the *strong ignorability assumption;* (2.14) has also been referred to as the assumption of *no unmeasured confounders.* We generally use the latter term in this book.

The difficulty with the no unmeasured confounders assumption (2.14) is that it cannot be verified directly from the observed data. That is, we cannot determine from the data we do get to see that there are additional variables that are not recorded in those data that are associated with both prognosis and treatment choice. Consequently, whether we are willing to adopt (2.14) or not depends on the specific situation and subject matter expertise.

As we have discussed, in a randomized study, the fact that treatment is assigned at random makes the assumption (2.11), $\{Y^*(1), Y^*(0)\} \perp\!\!\!\perp A$, tenable. In contrast, one can never have the same level of confidence in assumption (2.14) holding in an observational study. This formalizes the reason that randomized clinical trials are considered to provide a much higher standard of evidence than observational studies (and is why many clinical trialists and others are skeptical of observational analyses).

In the rest of this book, we assume that the analyst is willing to adopt the no unmeasured confounders assumption (2.14) in an observational study. However, we emphasize again that, in practice, one must critically evaluate its plausibility on a case by case basis.

We demonstrate in the next section that the no unmeasured confounders assumption (2.14) together with SUTVA (2.4) allows identification of the average causal effect $\delta^* = E\{Y^*(1)\} - E\{Y^*(0)\}$ from the distribution of the observed data (X,A,Y). This result is the basis for two general classes of techniques for estimation of δ^* from observed data $(X_i, A_i, Y_i), i = 1, \ldots, n$: outcome regression methods, presented in Section 2.4, and methods using the so-called propensity score, discussed in Section 2.6.

2.4   Estimation of Causal Effects via Outcome Regression

The basis for the use of outcome regression modeling to estimate the average causal treatment effect δ^* from observed data is the following fundamental calculation. Consider $E\{Y^*(1)\}$. Using SUTVA (2.4) and the no unmeasured confounders assumption (2.14), we have

$$E\{Y^*(1)\} = E[E\{Y^*(1)|X\}] \qquad\qquad (2.15)$$

$$= E[E\{Y^*(1)|X, A = 1\}] \qquad\qquad (2.16)$$

$$= E\{E(Y|X, A = 1)\}. \qquad\qquad (2.17)$$

We emphasize that the outer expectations in these expressions are with respect to the marginal distribution of X, so that, for example, the right-hand side of (2.15) is given by

$$\int_{\mathcal{X}} E\{Y^*(1)|X = x\}\, p_X(x)\, d\nu(x), \qquad\qquad (2.18)$$

where X takes values in $\mathcal{X}$; $p_X(x)$ is the marginal density or mass function of X; and $\nu(\cdot)$ is a dominating measure, which is Lebesgue measure for continuous random variables and the counting measure for discrete random variables. This technicality allows us to write expectations as integrals for both continuous and discrete random variables. The equality in (2.16) follows from the assumption of no unmeasured confounders and the definition of conditional independence given in (2.9) with Z_1 identified with $Y^*(1)$, Z_2 identified with A, and Z_3 identified with X; and that in (2.17) follows from SUTVA.

It is important to recognize that the expectation in (2.17) is with respect to the marginal distribution of X as in (2.18) and not the conditional distribution of X given $A = 1$. Specifically, (2.17) is given by

$$\int_{\mathcal{X}} E(Y|X = x, A = 1)\, p_X(x)\, d\nu(x),$$

and not by

$$\int_{\mathcal{X}} E(Y|X = x, A = 1)p_{X|A}(x|A = 1)d\nu(x), \qquad\qquad (2.19)$$

because (2.19) is $E(Y|A = 1)$. By analogous calculations,

$$E\{Y^*(0)\} = E\{E(Y|X, A = 0)\}.$$

Thus, under the no unmeasured confounders assumption and SUTVA, the average causal treatment effect can be written as

$$\delta^* = E\{E(Y|X, A = 1)\} - E\{E(Y|X, A = 0)\}. \tag{2.20}$$

The result in (2.20) demonstrates that δ^* can be expressed in terms of the observable data (X,A,Y) if both SUTVA and the no unmeasured confounders assumption hold. In particular, (2.20) shows that δ^* depends on the regression of observed outcome on covariates and treatment received, $E(Y|X, A)$.

Remark. For the conditional expectations $E\{Y^*(1)|X, A = 1\}$ and $E(Y|X, A = 1)$ in (2.16) and (2.17) and the analogous expressions with $A = 0$ to be well defined, it must be that $p_{X,A}(x, a) > 0$ for $a = 0, 1$. As in the remark at the end of Chapter 1, to avoid measure theoretic distractions in arguments in the sequel, we usually treat all random variables as discrete and write this condition as $P(X = x, A = a) > 0$ for $a = 0, 1$, which can be regarded as an abuse of notation for the density $p_{X,A}(x, a)$ when X is not discrete. For all x such that $p_X(x) = P(X = x) > 0$, this will hold if $P(A = a|X = x) > 0$. Later in this chapter, we refer to this last condition as the *positivity assumption.* Thus, the positivity assumption is required to justify the argument leading to (2.20).

Denote the true regression relationship as

$$E(Y|X = x, A = a) = Q(x, a), \tag{2.21}$$

where we use the symbol Q for consistency with the conventional notation for the multiple decision case in later chapters. In (2.21), $Q(x, a)$ is the true function of x and a relating observed outcome to covariates and treatment received, so that we can write (2.20) equivalently as

$$\delta^* = E\{Y^*(1)\} - E\{Y^*(0)\} = E\{Q(X, 1)\} - E\{Q(X, 0)\}. \tag{2.22}$$

The true function $Q(x, a)$ is ordinarily unknown in practice. It is thus natural to posit a model for $Q(x, a)$; here, we consider parametric regression models of the form

$$Q(x, a; \beta), \tag{2.23}$$

where (2.23) is a linear or nonlinear function of x, a, and a finite-dimensional parameter β. The parameter β can be estimated from the observed data (X_i, A_i, Y_i), $i = 1, \ldots, n$, using statistical methods relevant to the form of the model.

For example, if Y is a continuous outcome, we might consider a linear model with main effects of covariates,

$$Q(x, a; \beta) = \beta_1 + \beta_2 a + \beta_3^T x, \qquad (2.24)$$

or a linear model with treatment-covariate interaction term,

$$Q(x, a; \beta) = \beta_1 + \beta_2 a + \beta_3^T x + \beta_4^T xa. \qquad (2.25)$$

Ordinary or weighted least squares methods can then be used to fit models like (2.24) and (2.25) as appropriate. More elaborate linear models in which x is replaced by a vector $\tilde{x}$ comprising known functions, or features, of the components of x, including polynomial, other nonlinear, and interaction terms, are of course possible.

If Y is binary (e.g., success or failure), then $E(Y|X = x, A = a) = P(Y = 1|X = x, A = a)$, and a popular model is the logistic regression model

$$\text{logit}\{Q(x, a; \beta)\} = \beta_1 + \beta_2 a + \beta_3^T x, \qquad (2.26)$$

or a version including a treatment-covariate interaction,

$$\text{logit}\{Q(x, a; \beta\} = \beta_1 + \beta_2 a + \beta_3^T x + \beta_4^T xa, \qquad (2.27)$$

where $\text{logit}(p) = \log\{p/(1 - p)\}$; that is,

$$Q(x, a; \beta) = \frac{\exp(\beta_1 + \beta_2 a + \beta_3^T x + \beta_4^T xa)}{1 + \exp(\beta_1 + \beta_2 a + \beta_3^T x + \beta_4^T xa)}.$$

Models such as (2.26) and (2.27) can be fitted via maximum likelihood, which is ordinarily implemented via an iteratively reweighted least squares algorithm. As above, x can be replaced by a vector $\tilde{x}$ of known functions of x.

Remark. As in any regression modeling context, the posited model $Q(x, a; \beta)$ may or may not be correctly specified. Formally, if the model is correctly specified, then there exists a value β_0, referred to as the true value of the parameter β, such that $Q(x, a; \beta)$ evaluated at β_0 yields the true function $Q(x, a)$. If no such β_0 exists, then the model is not correctly specified.

If the true function $Q(x, a)$ were known, given observed data (X_i, A_i, Y_i), $i = 1, \ldots, n$, and under the assumption of no unmeasured confounders and SUTVA, it is natural to replace the expectations in (2.22) by empirical averages and estimate δ^* by

$$n^{-1} \sum_{i=1}^{n} \{Q(X_i, 1) - Q(X_i, 0)\}. \qquad (2.28)$$

Thus, under the assumption that the posited model $Q(x, a; \beta)$ is correctly specified, it is reasonable to obtain an estimator $\widehat{\beta}$ for β and to substitute the model evaluated at $\widehat{\beta}$ into (2.28), which yields the so-called _outcome regression estimator_ for the average causal treatment effect given by

$$\widehat{\delta}^*_{OR} = n^{-1} \sum_{i=1}^{n} \{Q(X_i, 1; \widehat{\beta}) - Q(X_i, 0; \widehat{\beta})\}. \qquad (2.29)$$

Marginalization

In the case of a linear regression model as in (2.24), the estimator (2.29) takes a simple form. Note that in this case *No interaction*

$$\{Q(X, 1; \beta) - Q(X, 0; \beta)\} = (\beta_1 + \beta_2 + \beta_3^T X) - (\beta_1 + \beta_3^T X) = \beta_2.$$

Thus, under the assumption that this model is correctly specified, the coefficient of the treatment indicator, β_2, corresponds to the average causal treatment effect δ^*. In fact, any model of the form

identity

$$Q(x, a; \beta) = \phi(x; \beta_1) + \beta_2 a, \quad \text{*No interaction*}$$

where $\phi(x; \beta_1)$ is an arbitrary function of x and parameter β_1, leads to the same result that $\delta^* = \beta_2$. Thus, in such models with no treatment-covariate interaction terms and under the assumption of no unmeasured confounders and SUTVA, the estimator for the average causal treatment effect can be obtained directly from the fit of the model, and there is no need to use (2.29). However, for more complex models, such as those in (2.25), (2.26), and (2.27), which are nonlinear in β and/or contain interaction terms, the fitted model must be substituted into (2.29) to estimate δ^*.

Of course, in addition to $\widehat{\delta}^*_{OR}$ itself, a formal estimate of the uncertainty associated with the estimator is required. To obtain a standard error; test statistics, for example, for testing the null hypothesis $\delta^* = 0$; and for constructing confidence intervals for the true average causal treatment effect, we must be able to derive the sampling distribution of the estimator $\widehat{\delta}^*_{OR}$. Clearly, the properties of $\widehat{\delta}^*_{OR}$ will depend on those of $\widehat{\beta}$. For all but the simplest statistical models, this will be accomplished via large sample approximation. In the next section, we take a brief detour to review the derivation of large sample properties of estimators in a broad class of statistical models.

2.5   Review of M-estimation

Consider a generic statistical model for which we have i.i.d. random vectors $Z_1, \ldots, Z_n$, where $Z \sim p_Z(z)$. Suppose interest focuses on a p-dimensional parameter θ. Here, θ may fully characterize the distribution of Z, in which case we can write $p_Z(z; \theta)$; or θ may characterize aspects of the distribution of Z, such as first and second moments. Let θ_0 denote the true value of θ; that is, the value of θ corresponding to the true distribution generating the data. If, for example, θ fully characterizes the density, then this implies that $p_Z(z; \theta_0)$ is the true density.

The statistical problem is to derive an estimator for θ and establish its large sample properties. In many common models, natural and popular estimators for θ are M-estimators. An M-estimator for θ can be characterized as the solution $\widehat{\theta}$ (assuming it exists and is well defined) to the $(p \times 1)$ system of estimating equations

$$\sum_{i=1}^{n} M(Z_i; \widehat{\theta}) = 0. \tag{2.30}$$

In (2.30), $M(z; \theta) = \{M_1(z; \theta), \ldots, M_p(z; \theta)\}^T$ is a $(p \times 1)$ unbiased estimating function satisfying

$$E_\theta\{M(Z; \theta)\} = 0 \quad \text{for all } \theta, \tag{2.31}$$

where this notation implies that the expectation is taken with respect to the distribution of Z evaluated at θ. For example, with a fully parametric model $p_Z(z; \theta)$, (2.31) is stated precisely as

$$E_\theta\{M(Z; \theta)\} = \int M(z; \theta)\, p_Z(z; \theta)\, d\nu(z) = 0 \quad \text{for all } \theta.$$

When (2.31) is evaluated at the true value θ_0, we suppress the subscript, and expectation is with respect to the true distribution of Z.

Note that with a fully parametric model $p_Z(z; \theta)$, taking

$$M(z; \theta) = \frac{\partial \log\{p_Z(z; \theta)\}}{\partial \theta},$$

MLE as M-estimator

where the right-hand side is the $(p \times 1)$ vector of derivatives of the logarithm of $p_Z(z; \theta)$ with respect to the elements of θ (the score), yields the maximum likelihood estimator for θ under this model. Thus, the maximum likelihood estimator is an M-estimator, and the corresponding unbiased estimating function is the score.

Under suitable regularity conditions, the M-estimator $\widehat{\theta}$ satisfying (2.30) is a consistent and asymptotically normal estimator for θ; that is,

$$\widehat{\theta} \xrightarrow{p} \theta_0$$

and

$$n^{1/2}(\widehat{\theta} - \theta_0) \xrightarrow{\mathcal{D}} \mathcal{N}(0, \Sigma), \tag{2.32}$$

where $\xrightarrow{p}$ denotes convergence in probability. The expression (2.32) is shorthand notation representing the fact that the expression on the left-hand side converges in distribution to a normal random vector with mean zero and covariance matrix Σ.

We now present a sketch of the argument demonstrating the asymptotic normality result (2.32) and the form of the matrix Σ. A first-order Taylor series expansion of each row of (2.30) in $\widehat{\theta}$ about θ_0 yields

$$0 = \sum_{i=1}^{n} M(Z_i; \theta_0) + \left\{ \sum_{i=1}^{n} \frac{\partial M(Z_i; \theta^*)}{\partial \theta^T} \right\} (\widehat{\theta} - \theta_0), \tag{2.33}$$

where, in (2.33), $\partial M(z; \theta^*)/\partial \theta^T$ is shorthand for the $(p \times p)$ matrix

$$\begin{pmatrix} \dfrac{\partial M_1(z; \theta)}{\partial \theta_1} \bigg|_{\theta=\theta^{(1)*}}, & \cdots, & \dfrac{\partial M_1(z; \theta)}{\partial \theta_p} \bigg|_{\theta=\theta^{(1)*}} \\ \vdots & \ddots & \vdots \\ \dfrac{\partial M_p(z; \theta)}{\partial \theta_1} \bigg|_{\theta=\theta^{(p)*}}, & \cdots, & \dfrac{\partial M_p(z; \theta)}{\partial \theta_p} \bigg|_{\theta=\theta^{(p)*}} \end{pmatrix};$$

and, for each $j = 1, \ldots, p$, $\theta^{(j)*}$ is a value between $\widehat{\theta}$ and θ_0. Expression (2.33) yields

$$\left\{ -n^{-1} \sum_{i=1}^{n} \frac{\partial M(Z_i; \theta^*)}{\partial \theta^T} \right\} n^{1/2}(\widehat{\theta} - \theta_0) = n^{-1/2} \sum_{i=1}^{n} M(Z_i; \theta_0). \tag{2.34}$$

Because $\widehat{\theta}$ is a consistent estimator for θ and because $\theta^{(j)*}$, $j = 1, \ldots, p$, is between $\widehat{\theta}$ and θ_0, each $\theta^{(j)*}$ also converges in probability to θ_0. Thus, under sufficient smoothness conditions and using the law of large numbers, we can conclude that

$$-n^{-1} \sum_{i=1}^{n} \frac{\partial M(Z_i; \theta^*)}{\partial \theta^T} \xrightarrow{p} -E \left\{ \frac{\partial M(Z_i; \theta_0)}{\partial \theta^T} \right\}, \tag{2.35}$$

where $\partial M(z; \theta_0)/\partial \theta^T$ is shorthand for evaluation of each element of the $(p \times p)$ matrix $\partial M(z; \theta)/\partial \theta^T$ at θ_0. Moreover, assuming that the $(p \times p)$ matrix $E\{\partial M(Z, \theta^*)/\partial \theta^T\}$ is nonsingular, then, with increasingly high probability as $n \to \infty$, the left-hand side of (2.35) is also nonsingular, and

$$\left\{ -n^{-1} \sum_{i=1}^{n} \frac{\partial M(Z_i; \theta^*)}{\partial \theta^T} \right\}^{-1} \xrightarrow{p} \left[-E \left\{ \frac{\partial M(Z_i; \theta_0)}{\partial \theta^T} \right\} \right]^{-1}. \tag{2.36}$$

Thus, we can rewrite (2.34) as

$$n^{1/2}(\widehat{\theta} - \theta_0) = \left\{ -n^{-1} \sum_{i=1}^{n} \frac{\partial M(Z_i; \theta^*)}{\partial \theta^T} \right\}^{-1} n^{-1/2} \sum_{i=1}^{n} M(Z_i; \theta_0). \quad (2.37)$$

By the central limit theorem,

$$n^{1/2} \sum_{i=1}^{n} M(Z_i; \theta_0) \xrightarrow{\mathcal{D}} \mathcal{N}\left[0, E\{M(Z; \theta_0)M^T(Z; \theta_0)\}\right]. \quad (2.38)$$

Thus, using (2.36) and (2.38) and applying Slutsky's theorem, it follows from (2.37) that

$$n^{1/2}(\widehat{\theta} - \theta_0) \xrightarrow{\mathcal{D}} \mathcal{N}(0, \Sigma), \quad (2.39)$$

where Σ is given by

$$\left[E\left\{ \frac{\partial M(Z; \theta_0)}{\partial \theta^T} \right\} \right]^{-1} E\{M(Z; \theta_0)M^T(Z; \theta_0)\} \left[E\left\{ \frac{\partial M(Z; \theta_0)}{\partial \theta^T} \right\} \right]^{-T}, \quad (2.40)$$

and $A^{-T} = (A^{-1})^T$ for matrix A; (2.40) is referred to as the *sandwich formula*.

An estimator for Σ can be obtained in the obvious way by substitution of sample averages for expectations and $\widehat{\theta}$ for θ_0 in (2.40). Specifically,

$$\left[E\left\{ \frac{\partial M(Z; \theta_0)}{\partial \theta^T} \right\} \right]^{-1}$$

can be estimated by

$$\left[n^{-1} \sum_{i=1}^{n} \frac{\partial M(Z_i; \widehat{\theta})}{\partial \theta^T} \right]^{-1}, \quad (2.41)$$

and an obvious estimator for $E\{M(Z; \theta_0)M^T(Z; \theta_0)\}$ is

$$n^{-1} \sum_{i=1}^{n} M(Z_i; \widehat{\theta})M^T(Z_i; \widehat{\theta}). \quad (2.42)$$

The estimator $\widehat{\Sigma}$ is then obtained by substitution of (2.41) and (2.42) into the expression for Σ in (2.40). The estimator $\widehat{\Sigma}$ is popularly referred to as the *sandwich variance estimator*. The approximate sampling distribution

$$\widehat{\theta} \overset{\cdot}{\sim} \mathcal{N}(\theta_0, n^{-1}\widehat{\Sigma}),$$

where "$\overset{\cdot}{\sim}$" means "approximately distributed as," follows from (2.39).

Standard errors for the elements of $\widehat{\theta}$ can be obtained as the square roots of the diagonal elements of $n^{-1}\widehat{\Sigma}$, and this result can be used to construct test statistics and confidence sets in the usual way.

Example: Least Squares

Given an outcome regression model $Q(x, a; \beta)$ for $E(Y|X = x, A = a)$, as in (2.23), the ordinary least squares (OLS) estimator for β is obtained from the observed data $Z_i = (X_i, A_i, Y_i)$, $i = 1, \ldots, n$, by minimizing

$$\sum_{i=1}^{n} \{Y_i - Q(X_i, A_i; \beta)\}^2,$$

which leads to the estimating equation

$$\sum_{i=1}^{n} \frac{\partial Q(X_i, A_i; \beta)}{\partial \beta} \{Y_i - Q(X_i, A_i; \beta)\} = 0. \tag{2.43}$$

Here, we identify β as θ, and the estimating equation (2.43) involves the estimating function

$$M(z; \beta) = \frac{\partial Q(x, a; \beta)}{\partial \beta} \{Y - Q(x, a; \beta)\}.$$

Assume that the model $Q(x, a; \beta)$ is correctly specified. Then

$$E_\beta \left[\frac{\partial Q(X, A; \beta)}{\partial \beta} \{Y - Q(X, A; \beta)\} \right]$$

$$= E_\beta \left(E_\beta \left[\frac{\partial Q(X, A; \beta)}{\partial \beta} \{Y - Q(X, A; \beta)\} \Big| X, A \right] \right)$$

$$= E_\beta \left[\frac{\partial Q(X, A; \beta)}{\partial \beta} \{E_\beta(Y|X, A) - Q(X, A; \beta)\} \right] = 0,$$

as $E_\beta(Y|X, A) = Q(X, A; \beta)$ for all β, and $M(z; \beta)$ is an unbiased estimating function. Thus, the least squares estimator for β, which is the solution to (2.43), is an M-estimator.

Consequently, $n^{1/2}(\widehat{\beta} - \beta_0)$ converges in distribution to a normal random vector with mean zero and covariance matrix that can be estimated using the sandwich variance estimator $\widehat{\Sigma}$. To deduce this estimator, we must approximate the quantities in (2.40). Differentiation of the estimating function and evaluation at β_0 yields

$$\frac{\partial M(Z; \beta_0)}{\partial \beta^T} = -\frac{\partial Q(X, A; \beta_0)}{\partial \beta} \frac{\partial Q(X, A; \beta_0)}{\partial \beta^T}$$

$$+ \frac{\partial^2 Q(X, A; \beta_0)}{\partial \beta \, \partial \beta^T} \{Y - Q(X, A; \beta_0)\}. \tag{2.44}$$

It is straightforward to show by a conditioning argument like that above that the second term on the right-hand side of (2.44) has expectation zero, so that

$$\left[E\left\{\frac{\partial\, M(Z;\beta_0)}{\partial\beta^T}\right\}\right]^{-1} = \left[-E\left\{\frac{\partial\, Q(X,A;\beta_0)}{\partial\beta}\frac{\partial\, Q(X,A;\beta_0)}{\partial\beta^T}\right\}\right]^{-1},$$

suggesting the estimator

$$\left[-n^{-1}\sum_{i=1}^{n}\left\{\frac{\partial\, Q(X_i,A_i;\widehat{\beta})}{\partial\beta}\frac{\partial\, Q(X_i,A_i;\widehat{\beta})}{\partial\beta^T}\right\}\right]^{-1}. \qquad (2.45)$$

Similarly,

$$E\{M(Z;\beta_0)M^T(Z;\beta_0)\}$$
$$= E\left\{\text{var}(Y|X,A)\frac{\partial\, Q(X,A;\beta_0)}{\partial\beta}\frac{\partial\, Q(X,A;\beta_0)}{\partial\beta^T}\right\}, \qquad (2.46)$$

where

$$\text{var}(Y|X,A) = E[\{Y - Q(X,A;\beta_0)\}^2|X,A].$$

Under the common assumption that $\text{var}(Y|X,A) = \sigma^2$, a constant, which can be estimated in the usual way by the residual mean square $\widehat{\sigma}^2$, (2.45) and (2.46) and substitution in (2.41) lead to

$$\widehat{\Sigma} = \widehat{\sigma}^2\left[-n^{-1}\sum_{i=1}^{n}\left\{\frac{\partial\, Q(X_i,A_i;\widehat{\beta})}{\partial\beta}\frac{\partial\, Q(X_i,A_i;\widehat{\beta})}{\partial\beta^T}\right\}\right]^{-1}. \qquad (2.47)$$

It is straightforward to verify that if $Q(x,a;\beta)$ is a linear model as in (2.26) and (2.27), (2.47) reduces to the familiar expression depending on the associated design matrix. If there is concern that the constant variance assumption is violated, an estimator "robust" to this possibility can be obtained by estimating (2.46) instead by

$$n^{-1}\sum_{i=1}^{n}\left[\{Y_i - Q(X_i,A_i;\widehat{\beta})\}^2\frac{\partial\, Q(X_i,A_i;\widehat{\beta})}{\partial\beta}\frac{\partial\, Q(X_i,A_i;\widehat{\beta})}{\partial\beta^T}\right]. \qquad (2.48)$$

More generally, if $V(x,a)$ is a model for $\text{var}(Y|X = x, A = a)$, and this model and the model $Q(x,a;\beta)$ for $E(Y|X = x, A = a)$ are correctly specified, it can be shown with no other distributional assumptions that the optimal estimator for β solves

$$\sum_{i=1}^{n}\frac{\partial\, Q(X_i,A_i;\beta)}{\partial\beta}V^{-1}(X_i,A_i)\{Y_i - Q(X_i,A_i;\beta)\} = 0. \qquad (2.49)$$

That is, the estimator solving (2.49) has smallest asymptotic variance among all such estimators. Thus, (2.49) implies that the OLS estimator for β is optimal if $\text{var}(Y|X, A)$ is constant. In the case of generalized linear models such as the logistic regression model, the model $V(x, a)$ is a known function of $E(Y|X = x, A = a)$ and thus depends on β. In general, the model $V(x, a)$ might be taken to depend on β and possibly additional parameters that are estimated jointly by solving another estimating equation, so that θ is the collection of β and these additional parameters, and $M(z; \theta)$ is redefined to be (2.49) "stacked" on the additional estimating equation. In these situations, calculations similar to those above can be used to derive the approximate sampling variance. We demonstrate "stacked" estimating equations next in a different context.

We now discuss how the foregoing results can be used to derive the large sample properties of the estimator $\widehat{\delta}_{OR}^*$ in (2.29) for the average causal treatment effect δ^*.

Suppose we have a posited model $Q(x, a; \beta)$, which we assume to be correctly specified, and β is estimated via OLS. The estimator $\widehat{\delta}_{OR}^*$ can be viewed as an M-estimator. Specifically, identify the parameters of interest as $\theta = (\delta^*, \beta^T)^T$. It is straightforward to observe that the estimator $\widehat{\delta}_{OR}^*$ and the OLS estimator $\widehat{\beta}$ solve jointly in θ $(p+1 \times 1)$ the $(p+1 \times 1)$ set of "stacked" estimating equations given by

$$\sum_{i=1}^{n} \{Q(X_i, 1; \beta) - Q(X_i, 0; \beta) - \delta^*\} = 0$$

$$\sum_{i=1}^{n} \frac{\partial Q(X_i, A_i; \beta)}{\partial \beta} \{Y_i - Q(X_i, A_i; \beta)\} = 0, \tag{2.50}$$

so that the estimating function is

$$M(z; \theta) = \begin{pmatrix} Q(x, 1; \beta) - Q(x, 0; \beta) - \delta^* \\ \frac{\partial Q(x, a; \beta)}{\partial \beta} \{y - Q(x, a; \beta)\} \end{pmatrix}. \tag{2.51}$$

The estimating function (2.51) is clearly unbiased.

Letting β_0 and δ_0^* be the true values of β and δ^*, the general M-estimation theory yields

$$n^{1/2} \begin{pmatrix} \widehat{\delta}_{OR}^* - \delta_0^* \\ \widehat{\beta} - \beta_0 \end{pmatrix} \xrightarrow{\mathcal{D}} \mathcal{N}(0, \Sigma),$$

where the $(p+1 \times p+1)$ covariance matrix Σ is given by (2.40) with

$M(z;\theta)$ as in (2.51), and the $(1,1)$ element of $n^{-1}\Sigma$ is then the approximate large sample variance of $\widehat{\delta}^*_{OR}$. Thus, an estimator for the variance of $\widehat{\delta}^*_{OR}$ can be obtained from the $(1,1)$ element of the sandwich variance estimator $\widehat{\Sigma}$.

To derive this estimator, it is straightforward that

$$E_\beta\left[\frac{\partial Q(X,A;\beta)}{\partial\beta}\{Y-Q(X,A;\beta)\}\{Q(X,1;\beta)-Q(X,0;\beta)-\delta^*\}\right]=0,$$

so that $E\{M(z;\theta_0)M^T(z;\theta_0)\}$ is a block diagonal matrix that can be estimated by

$$\begin{pmatrix} A_n & 0 \\ 0 & B_n \end{pmatrix}, \tag{2.52}$$

where

$$A_n = n^{-1}\sum_{i=1}^n\left\{Q(X_i,1;\widehat{\beta})-Q(X_i,0;\widehat{\beta})-\widehat{\delta}^*\right\}^2,$$

$$B_n = n^{-1}\sum_{i=1}^n\left[\{Y_i-Q(X_i,A_i;\widehat{\beta})\}^2\frac{\partial Q(X_i,A_i;\widehat{\beta})}{\partial\beta}\frac{\partial Q(X_i,A_i;\widehat{\beta})}{\partial\beta^T}\right],$$

as in (2.48). It can also be shown that an estimator for

$$\left[E\left\{\frac{\partial M(Z;\theta_0)}{\partial\theta^T}\right\}\right]^{-1}$$

is given by

$$\begin{pmatrix} -1 & C_n^T D_n^{-1} \\ 0 & -D_n^{-1} \end{pmatrix}, \tag{2.53}$$

where

$$C_n = n^{-1}\sum_{i=1}^n\left\{\frac{\partial Q(X_i,1;\widehat{\beta})}{\partial\beta}-\frac{\partial Q(X_i,0;\widehat{\beta})}{\partial\beta}\right\},$$

$$D_n = n^{-1}\sum_{i=1}^n\left\{\frac{\partial Q(X_i,A_i;\widehat{\beta})}{\partial\beta}\frac{\partial Q(X_i,A_i;\widehat{\beta})}{\partial\beta^T}\right\},$$

and (2.53) follows by standard results for inversion of a partitioned matrix. Substituting (2.52) and the inverse of (2.53) in the sandwich variance formula, and isolating the $(1,1)$ element, it can be shown that

$$\widehat{\delta}^*_{OR} \sim N(0, n^{-1}\widehat{\Sigma}_{11}), \qquad \widehat{\Sigma}_{11} = A_n + C_n^T D_n^{-1} B_n D_n^{-1} C_n.$$

If $\text{var}(Y|X,A) = E[\{Y-Q(X,A;\beta_0)\}^2|X,A] = \sigma^2$ as in (2.47), with estimator $\widehat{\sigma}^2$, then this simplifies to $\widehat{\Sigma}_{11} = A_n + \widehat{\sigma}^2 C_n^T D_n^{-1} C_n$.

See Stefanski and Boos (2002) and Boos and Stefanski (2013) for a full introduction to M-estimation.

2.6   Estimation of Causal Effects via the Propensity Score

Another class of estimators for the average causal treatment effect uses the so-called *propensity score.*

2.6.1   The Propensity Score

In the case of two treatment options, so that A is a binary indicator taking values in $\{0,1\}$, the propensity score is defined as

$$\pi(X) = P(A = 1|X);$$

this definition can be generalized to more than two options. This term was introduced by Rosenbaum and Rubin (1983), who coined it to refer to the propensity of receiving one of the treatment options as a function of individual characteristics (covariates).

A fundamental feature of the propensity score that makes it useful for causal inference is given in the following result shown by Rosenbaum and Rubin (1983).

Conditional Independence Given the Propensity Score

If the no unmeasured confounders (strong ignorability) assumption holds, that is, $\{Y^*(1), Y^*(0)\} \perp\!\!\!\perp A|X$, then it is also the case that

$$\{Y^*(1), Y^*(0)\} \perp\!\!\!\perp A|\pi(X). \tag{2.54}$$

Thus, if the no unmeasured confounders assumption holds, then it also holds if we consider only the propensity score. This result is useful because the collection of covariates X that may be required to make the assumption of no unmeasured confounders tenable could be high dimensional, making it challenging to posit an outcome regression model $Q(x, a; \beta)$ for $E(Y|X = x, A = a)$. The propensity score $\pi(X)$ is a one-dimensional function of X and can take on only values between 0 and 1. Thus, if $\pi(X)$ were known, developing models for $E\{Y|\pi(X) = \pi(x), A = a\}$ is likely to be considerably easier.

One way to demonstrate (2.54) is to show that $P\{A = 1|Y^*(1), Y^*(0), \pi(X)\}$ is a function only of $\pi(X)$ and not of $\{Y^*(1), Y^*(0)\}$. By a conditioning argument,

$$P\{A = 1|Y^*(1), Y^*(0), \pi(X)\}$$
$$= E\{I(A = 1)|Y^*(1), Y^*(0), \pi(X)\}$$
$$= E\left[E\{I(A = 1)|Y^*(1), Y^*(0), X\}|Y^*(1), Y^*(0), \pi(X)\right]$$
$$= E\left[P\{A = 1|Y^*(1), Y^*(0), X\}|Y^*(1), Y^*(0), \pi(X)\right]$$

$$= E\left[\underbrace{\pi(X)}|Y^*(1), Y^*(0), \pi(X)\right] \tag{2.55}$$
$$= \pi(X),$$

where $I(B)$ is the indicator function such that $I(B) = 1$ if the event B is true and $= 0$ otherwise, and the equality in (2.55) follows by the no unmeasured confounders assumption.

Under the no unmeasured confounders assumption and SUTVA, using (2.54),

$$E\{Y^*(1)\} = E\left[E\{Y^*(1)|\pi(X)\}\right]$$
$$= E\left[E\{Y^*(1)|\pi(X), A = 1\}\right]$$
$$= E\left[E\{Y|\pi(X), A = 1\}\right],$$

where the outer expectations are with respect to the marginal distribution of $\pi(X)$; and, similarly, $E\{Y^*(0)\} = E\left[E\{Y|\pi(X), A = 0\}\right]$. Thus, the average causal treatment effect can be expressed equivalently as

$$\delta^* = E\left[E\{Y \mid \pi(X), A = 1\} - E\{Y \mid \pi(X), A = 0\}\right]. \tag{2.56}$$

Remark. In a randomized study, the propensity score $\pi(X)$ is known to the investigators and, in general, is in fact independent of X. This is because the treatment options in a clinical trial are typically assigned at random with prespecified, fixed probabilities; with two treatment options, it is often the case that $\pi(x) = 1/2$ for all x. However, in an observational study, the propensity score is not known.

It is thus standard in the analysis of observational studies to posit a model for the propensity score $\pi(x) = P(A = 1|X = x)$. A popular choice is the (parametric) logistic regression model, for example,

$$\text{logit}\{\pi(x; \gamma)\} = \gamma_1 + \gamma_2^T x \quad \text{or} \quad \pi(x; \gamma) = \frac{\exp(\gamma_1 + \gamma_2^T x)}{1 + \exp(\gamma_1 + \gamma_2^T x)}. \tag{2.57}$$

The parameter γ can be estimated based on the data (X_i, A_i), $i = 1, \ldots, n$, by the maximum likelihood estimator $\hat{\gamma}$. In general, for any parametric model $\pi(X; \gamma)$ for the propensity score, the likelihood is

$$\prod_{i=1}^{n}\{\pi(X_i; \gamma)\}^{A_i}\{1 - \pi(X_i; \gamma)\}^{1-A_i},$$

which for the logistic model (2.57) is equal to

$$\prod_{i=1}^{n}\left[\frac{\exp\{(\gamma_1 + \gamma_2^T X_i)A_i\}}{1 + \exp(\gamma_1 + \gamma_2^T X_i)}\right]. \tag{2.58}$$

2.6.2 Propensity Score Stratification

Because of the representation of δ^* in (2.56), Rosenbaum and Rubin (1983, 1984) suggest the following approach to estimation of δ^*. Stratify individuals into S groups based on the values of the estimated propensity scores $\pi(X_i; \widehat{\gamma})$, $i = 1, \dots, n$; that is, choose cutoff values $0 = c_0 < c_1 < \cdots < c_S = 1$ such that individual i belongs to group j if

$$c_{j-1} < \pi(X_i; \widehat{\gamma}) \leq c_j, \ j = 1, \dots, S.$$

The estimator for δ^* is then given by

$$\widehat{\delta}_S^* = \sum_{j=1}^{S} (\overline{Y}_{1j} - \overline{Y}_{0j})\,(n_j/n),$$

where $\overline{Y}_{1j}$ and $\overline{Y}_{0j}$ are the sample average outcomes among individuals in the jth group receiving treatments 1 and 0, respectively; and n_j is the number of individuals (receiving both treatments) in the jth group.

The original suggestion was to take $S = 5$, resulting in stratification of individuals into quintiles, so that $n_j \approx n/5$ for $j = 1, \dots, 5$. Although this is a bit ad hoc, it has been shown to work well in many applications.

Remark. As mentioned previously, an appeal of the propensity score is that it is one dimensional, making it easier in principle to posit outcome regression models for $E\{Y | \pi(X), A\}$ (as in stratification) than it is for $E(Y | X, A)$ when X is high dimensional. Of course, this requires that the analyst posit a model for the propensity score, which likewise involves the challenge of building models with potentially high-dimensional X. In other words, outcome modeling based on the propensity score substitutes one high-dimensional challenge for another.

2.6.3 Inverse Probability Weighting

Another class of estimators for δ^* with a more theoretical justification can be derived formally from semiparametric theory (e.g., Tsiatis, 2006) and is motivated as follows.

If we were able to observe the potential outcomes $\{Y_i^*(1), Y_i^*(0)\}$, $i = 1, \dots, n$, for a sample of individuals from the population, then obvious unbiased estimators for $E\{Y^*(1)\}$ and $E\{Y^*(0)\}$ are

$$n^{-1} \sum_{i=1}^{n} Y_i^*(1) \text{ and } n^{-1} \sum_{i=1}^{n} Y_i^*(0),$$

respectively. However, as formalized in SUTVA, we observe $Y_i^*(1)$ only when $A_i = 1$ and $Y_i^*(0)$ only when $A_i = 0$. Thus, we cannot calculate these estimators because we have what amounts to a "missing data problem" in that we have missing data on $Y^*(1)$ when $A_i = 0$ and missing data on $Y^*(0)$ when $A_i = 1$. This missing data analogy suggests that $E\{Y^*(1)\}$ and $E\{Y^*(0)\}$ can be estimated using so-called inverse probability weighted complete case estimators as originally proposed by Horvitz and Thompson (1952) and developed from a semiparametric perspective in the context of missing data problems in a landmark paper by Robins et al. (1994).

Consider estimation of $E\{Y^*(1)\}$. The propensity score $\pi(X) = P(A = 1|X)$ is the probability that an individual in the population with baseline covariates X is observed to receive treatment option 1. The idea is to construct an estimator in the form of a sample average in which the outcome of an individual having a particular value of X who is observed to receive treatment 1, so with $A = 1$, is weighted by $1/\pi(X)$, so that the individual's outcome represents his own and also those for other individuals sharing that value of X who did not receive treatment 1. For example, if $\pi(X) = 1/3$, then the outcome for such an individual who received treatment 1 is weighted by 3, so that it represents his outcome and those of two other individuals sharing the same X who were likely given treatment 0. The estimator for $E\{Y^*(1)\}$ is thus ideally

$$n^{-1} \sum_{i=1}^{n} \frac{A_i Y_i}{\pi(X_i)}. \tag{2.59}$$

By the same reasoning, an estimator for $E\{Y^*(0)\}$ is

$$n^{-1} \sum_{i=1}^{n} \frac{(1 - A_i) Y_i}{1 - \pi(X_i)}. \tag{2.60}$$

Remark. Clearly, for the estimators (2.59) and (2.60) to be well defined, it is necessary to assume that $0 < \pi(X) < 1$ almost surely. That is, we require

$$P(A = a|X = x) > 0, \quad a = 0, 1 \tag{2.61}$$

for all $x \in \mathcal{X}$ such that $P(X = x) > 0$. This is referred to as the positivity assumption, first mentioned in Section 2.4, and ensures that, for any realized value of X, there are individuals receiving both treatment options.

We can demonstrate formally that (2.59) and (2.60) are unbiased estimators for $E\{Y^*(1)\}$ and $E\{Y^*(0)\}$ as follows. Consider (2.59). Under the positivity assumption, $\pi(X) > 0$ almost surely; and

$$
\begin{aligned}
E\left\{\frac{AY}{\pi(X)}\right\} &= E\left\{\frac{AY^*(1)}{\pi(X)}\right\} \\
&= E\left[E\left\{\frac{AY^*(1)}{\pi(X)}\middle| Y^*(1), X\right\}\right] \\
&= E\left[\frac{E\{A|Y^*(1), X\}Y^*(1)}{\pi(X)}\right] = E\{Y^*(1)\}, \qquad (2.62)
\end{aligned}
$$

where the first equality is due to SUTVA, and the final equality in (2.62) follows because

$$
E\{A|Y^*(1), X\} = E\{A|X\} = P(A = 1|X) = \pi(X)
$$

using the no unmeasured confounders assumption. An analogous argument can be carried out to show that

$$
E\left\{\frac{(1 - A)Y}{1 - \pi(X)}\right\} = E\{Y^*(0)\}.
$$

Consequently, if the propensity score $\pi(x)$ is known for all x and the positivity assumption holds, an unbiased estimator for the average causal treatment effect is

$$
\widehat{\delta}_{IPW}^* = n^{-1}\sum_{i=1}^{n}\left\{\frac{A_i Y_i}{\pi(X_i)} - \frac{(1 - A_i)Y_i}{1 - \pi(X_i)}\right\}. \qquad (2.63)
$$

Of course, in observational studies, the propensity score $\pi(x)$ is ordinarily not known. As noted above, it is customary to posit a model $\pi(x; \gamma)$ such as the logistic regression model (2.57) and to estimate the parameter γ via maximum likelihood. It is natural to substitute the fitted model into (2.63) to obtain the inverse probability weighted estimator

$$
\widehat{\delta}_{IPW}^* = n^{-1}\sum_{i=1}^{n}\left\{\frac{A_i Y_i}{\pi(X_i; \widehat{\gamma})} - \frac{(1 - A_i)Y_i}{1 - \pi(X_i; \widehat{\gamma})}\right\}. \qquad (2.64)
$$

To derive an approximate sampling distribution for $\widehat{\delta}_{IPW}^*$ in (2.64), we recognize that $\widehat{\delta}_{IPW}^*$ and γ can be viewed as M-estimators. With the model (2.57), the maximum likelihood estimator $\widehat{\gamma}$ for γ maximizing (2.58) equivalently solves the estimating (score) equation

$$
\sum_{i=1}^{n}\begin{pmatrix} 1 \\ X_i \end{pmatrix}\left\{A_i - \frac{\exp(\gamma_1 + \gamma_2^T X_i)}{1 + \exp(\gamma_1 + \gamma_2^T X_i)}\right\} = 0.
$$

error

Identifying $\theta = (\delta^*, \gamma^T)^T$, the estimators solve in θ the stacked estimating equations

$$\sum_{i=1}^{n} \left\{ \frac{A_i Y_i}{\pi(X_i; \gamma)} - \frac{(1 - A_i)Y_i}{1 - \pi(X_i; \gamma)} - \delta^* \right\} = 0$$

$$\sum_{i=1}^{n} \begin{pmatrix} 1 \\ X_i \end{pmatrix} \left\{ A_i - \frac{\exp(\gamma_1 + \gamma_2^T X_i)}{1 + \exp(\gamma_1 + \gamma_2^T X_i)} \right\} = 0.$$

(2.65)

The corresponding estimating function can be shown to be unbiased, so that these estimators are M-estimators, and the general theory in Section 2.5 can be used to derive the approximate large sample distribution of $\widehat{\delta}^*_{IPW}$.

Remark. The estimator (2.64) is a competitor to the regression estimator (2.29) and relies on modeling and fitting of the propensity score rather than modeling and fitting of the outcome regression. We thus have identified two classes of estimators for the average causal treatment effect δ^*: those relying on outcome regression modeling and those relying on modeling of the propensity score. Both classes require that the no unmeasured confounders assumption and SUTVA hold.

For the first class, an assumption is made on the conditional distribution of Y given X and A, namely, on the form of $E(Y|X = x, A = a)$. For the regression estimator to be a consistent estimator for δ^*, the posited model $Q(x, a; \beta)$ must be correctly specified. In contrast, for the inverse probability weighted estimator (2.64), no assumption is made on the conditional distribution of Y given X and A; however, an assumption is made instead on the form of $P(A = 1|X = x)$. For the estimator to be consistent for δ^*, the posited model for this probability, $\pi(X; \gamma)$, must be correctly specified; that is, there exists γ_0 such that $\pi(x; \gamma_0) = \pi(x)$, the true propensity score. If not, the motivating argument in (2.62) no longer applies. The underpinnings of both estimators rely on the positivity assumption. In the next section, we discuss estimators that combine both types of modeling and may offer protection against incorrect specification of these models.

We close this section by noting an interesting and possibly counterintuitive feature of inverse probability weighted estimators. Assume that the propensity score model is correctly specified. It can be shown that the estimator (2.64) for δ^*, which substitutes the maximum likelihood estimator $\widehat{\gamma}$ for γ, is more efficient (has smaller asymptotic variance) than the same estimator had the true value of γ been known. That is, it is better from the point of view of precision to estimate the parameter γ, *even if* its true value is known.

We illustrate this general phenomenon in a simple special case. Consider a randomized study with two treatments for which $P(A = 1|X) = 1/2$, so that treatment assignment is independent of baseline covariates X, and the true propensity score is $\pi(x) = 1/2$. Suppose we adopt the (correctly specified) model $\pi(x; \gamma) = \gamma$, so that the true value of γ is $\gamma_0 = 1/2$, and we estimate γ by the obvious estimator

$$\widehat{\gamma} = n^{-1} \sum_{i=1}^{n} A_i,$$

the sample proportion of individuals receiving treatment 1.

Consider the inverse probability weighted estimators for $E\{Y^*(1)\}$ when the propensity score is known and when it is estimated, respectively; namely,

$$n^{-1} \sum_{i=1}^{n} \frac{A_i Y_i}{\pi(X; \gamma_0)} = \sum_{i=1}^{n} \frac{A_i Y_i}{(n/2)} = \widehat{\mu}_1, \tag{2.66}$$

$$n^{-1} \sum_{i=1}^{n} \frac{A_i Y_i}{\pi(X; \widehat{\gamma})} = \frac{n^{-1} \sum_{i=1}^{n} A_i Y_i}{n^{-1} \sum_{i=1}^{n} A_i} = \frac{\sum_{i=1}^{n} A_i Y_i}{\sum_{i=1}^{n} A_i} = \overline{Y}_1. \tag{2.67}$$

The estimator (2.67) based on estimating γ is the usual estimator, the sample average among individuals receiving treatment 1.

As we have shown, in a randomized study, $E\{Y^*(1)\} = E(Y|A = 1) = \mu_1$, say. It is straightforward that

$$E(AY) = E\{AE(Y|A)\} = E(A\mu_1) = \mu_1/2,$$

so that $n^{-1} \sum_{i=1}^{n} A_i Y_i \xrightarrow{p} \mu_1/2$, and $n^{-1} \sum_{i=1}^{n} A_i \xrightarrow{p} 1/2$, and it follows that both (2.66) and (2.67) are consistent estimators for μ_1. From (2.66), algebra yields

$$n^{1/2}(\widehat{\mu}_1 - \mu_1) = 2n^{-1/2} \sum_{i=1}^{n} (A_i Y_i - \mu_1/2). \tag{2.68}$$

Define $\sigma_1^2 = \text{var}(Y|A = 1)$. Now

$$\text{var}(AY) = E\{\text{var}(AY|A)\} + \text{var}\{E(AY|A)\}$$
$$= E(A\sigma_1^2) + \text{var}(A\mu_1) = \sigma_1^2/2 + \mu_1^2/4,$$

so, applying the central limit theorem to the right-hand side of (2.68), after simplification, we have

$$n^{1/2}(\widehat{\mu}_1 - \mu_1) \xrightarrow{D} \mathcal{N}(0, 2\sigma_1^2 + \mu_1^2). \tag{2.69}$$

Similarly, (2.67) can be written as

$$n^{1/2}(\overline{Y}_1 - \mu_1) = \left\{ n^{-1} \sum_{i=1}^{n} A_i \right\}^{-1} n^{-1/2} \sum_{i=1}^{n} A_i(Y_i - \mu_1), \qquad (2.70)$$

and by similar calculations it follows that $E\{A(Y - \mu_1)\} = E[E\{A(Y - \mu_1)|A\}] = 0$ and $\text{var}\{A(Y - \mu_1)\} = E\{A\text{var}(Y - \mu_1)|A)\} + \text{var}[AE(Y - \mu_1)|A)\} = \sigma_1^2/2$. Applying the central limit and Slutsky's theorems to the right-hand side of (2.70) leads to

$$n^{1/2}(\overline{Y}_1 - \mu_1) \xrightarrow{\mathcal{D}} \mathcal{N}(0, 2\sigma_1^2). \qquad (2.71)$$

Comparing (2.69) to (2.71) shows that the usual estimator $\overline{Y}_1$, which uses the estimated propensity score, is relatively more efficient than $\widehat{\mu}_1$, which uses the known propensity score. An entirely similar argument applies for estimation of $E\{Y^*(0)\}$ and thus for estimation of the average causal treatment effect δ^*.

2.7   Doubly Robust Estimation of Causal Effects

As we have noted, the inverse probability weighted estimators in the previous section do not require any assumptions regarding the distribution of Y given X and A, but do require that the assumed model for the propensity score is correctly specified. Under these conditions, the theory of semiparametrics (Tsiatis, 2006) can be used to show that in fact all consistent and asymptotically normal estimators for the average causal treatment effect δ^* are asymptotically equivalent to an estimator of the form

$$\widehat{\delta}^*_{AIPW} = n^{-1} \sum_{i=1}^{n} \left[\frac{A_i Y_i}{\pi(X_i; \widehat{\gamma})} - \frac{(1 - A_i)Y_i}{1 - \pi(X_i; \widehat{\gamma})} - \{A_i - \pi(X_i; \widehat{\gamma})\}h(X_i) \right],$$
$$(2.72)$$

where $h(X_i)$ is any arbitrary function of X_i. The inverse probability weighted estimator (2.64) can be seen to be a special case of (2.72) with $h(X) \equiv 0$. It is straightforward that, under these conditions, with γ_0 the true value of γ,

$$E[\{A - \pi(X; \gamma_0)\}h(X)] = 0$$

for any $h(X)$, so that estimators of the form (2.72) are consistent estimators for the true value of δ^*. The additional term in (2.72) is often said to "augment" the simple inverse probability weighted estimator so as to increase efficiency of estimation of δ^*, and estimators of the form (2.72) are referred to as *augmented inverse probability weighted estimators*.

The theory demonstrates that, among all estimators in the class of estimators (2.72), the efficient estimator, which is the estimator with the smallest asymptotic variance, is obtained by choosing

$$h(X) = \frac{E(Y|X, A = 1)}{\pi(X)} + \frac{E(Y|X, A = 0)}{\{1 - \pi(X)\}}, \qquad (2.73)$$

where $\pi(X)$ is the true propensity score $P(A = 1|X)$. Of course, $E(Y|X, A)$ is not known; if it were, we would use outcome regression modeling to estimate δ^*. However, we can posit a model for $E(Y|X = x, A = a) = Q(x, a; \beta)$ and obtain an estimator $\widehat{\beta}$ as in Section 2.4, which suggests from (2.72) the estimator for δ^* given by

$$\widehat{\delta}^*_{DR} = n^{-1} \sum_{i=1}^{n} \left[\frac{A_i Y_i}{\pi(X_i; \widehat{\gamma})} - \frac{(1 - A_i)Y_i}{1 - \pi(X_i; \widehat{\gamma})} - \frac{\{A_i - \pi(X_i; \widehat{\gamma})\}}{\pi(X_i; \widehat{\gamma})} Q(X_i, 1; \widehat{\beta}) \right.$$
$$\left. - \frac{\{A_i - \pi(X_i; \widehat{\gamma})\}}{1 - \pi(X_i; \widehat{\gamma})} Q(X_i, 0; \widehat{\beta}) \right]. \qquad (2.74)$$

Suppose that $\widehat{\gamma} \xrightarrow{p} \gamma^*$ and $\widehat{\beta} \xrightarrow{p} \beta^*$ as $n \to \infty$ for some values γ^* and β^*. If the propensity score model is correctly specified and $\widehat{\gamma}$ is an M-estimator (maximum likelihood), then $\gamma^* = \gamma_0$, the true value. Otherwise, if $\widehat{\gamma}$ is obtained by fitting an incorrect model with parameters γ, although γ is not a meaningful quantity, $\widehat{\gamma}$ is a function of the data, so it has a limit in probability, denoted by γ^*. Similarly, if the outcome regression model is correctly specified and $\widehat{\beta}$ is an M-estimator, $\widehat{\beta} \xrightarrow{p} \beta_0$, the true value; if the model is not correctly specified, β is a function of the data with limit in probability β^*. In general, then, the estimator $\widehat{\delta}^*_{DR}$ in (2.74) converges in probability to

$$E \left[\frac{AY}{\pi(X; \gamma^*)} - \frac{(1 - A)Y}{1 - \pi(X; \gamma^*)} - \frac{\{A - \pi(X; \gamma^*)\}}{\pi(X; \gamma^*)} Q(X, 1; \beta^*) \right.$$
$$\left. - \frac{\{A - \pi(X; \gamma^*)\}}{1 - \pi(X; \gamma^*)} Q(X, 0; \beta^*) \right]. \qquad (2.75)$$

We now consider the behavior of the limit in probability of (2.75) when either the propensity score model or the outcome regression model (or both) is correctly specified. By SUTVA and algebra,

$$\frac{AY}{\pi(X; \gamma^*)} = \frac{AY^*(1)}{\pi(X; \gamma^*)} = Y^*(1) + \left\{ \frac{A - \pi(X; \gamma^*)}{\pi(X; \gamma^*)} \right\} Y^*(1),$$

$$\frac{(1 - A)Y}{1 - \pi(X; \gamma^*)} = \frac{(1 - A)Y^*(0)}{1 - \pi(X; \gamma^*)} = Y^*(0) - \left\{ \frac{A - \pi(X; \gamma^*)}{1 - \pi(X; \gamma^*)} \right\} Y^*(0).$$

Thus, we can rewrite (2.75) as

$$E\{Y^*(1) - Y^*(0)\}$$
$$+ E\left[\frac{\{A - \pi(X;\gamma^*)\}}{\pi(X;\gamma^*)}\{Y^*(1) - Q(X,1;\beta^*)\}\right] \qquad (2.76)$$
$$+ E\left[\frac{\{A - \pi(X;\gamma^*)\}}{1 - \pi(X;\gamma^*)}\{Y^*(0) - Q(X,0;\beta^*)\}\right]. \qquad (2.77)$$

It follows that $\widehat{\delta}^*_{DR}$ is a consistent estimator for the average causal treatment effect $\delta^* = E\{Y^*(1)\} - E\{Y^*(0)\}$ if the terms in (2.76) and (2.77) are equal to zero.

Note that (2.76) can be written as

$$E\left(E\left[\frac{\{A - \pi(X;\gamma^*)\}}{\pi(X;\gamma^*)}\{Y^*(1) - Q(X,1;\beta^*)\}\middle| X\right]\right)$$
$$= E\left(\frac{E\left[\{A - \pi(X;\gamma^*)\}\middle| X\right]}{\pi(X;\gamma^*)}E[\{Y^*(1) - Q(X,1;\beta^*)\}|X]\right), \quad (2.78)$$

because $Y^*(1) \perp\!\!\!\perp A|X$ by the no unmeasured confounders assumption and using (2.8) with $Z_1 = Y^*(1)$, $Z_2 = A$, and $Z_3 = X$. Similarly, (2.77) becomes

$$E\left(\frac{E\left[\{A - \pi(X;\gamma^*)\}\middle| X\right]}{1 - \pi(X;\gamma^*)}E[\{Y^*(0) - Q(X,0;\beta^*)\}|X]\right). \qquad (2.79)$$

Suppose that the propensity score is correctly specified, while the outcome regression model may or may not be. Then $\gamma^* = \gamma_0$, and $\pi(X;\gamma^*) = \pi(X;\gamma_0) = \pi(X)$, the true propensity score, so that

$$E[\{A - \pi(X;\gamma^*)\}|X] = E[\{A - \pi(X)\}|X] = E(A|X) - \pi(X) = 0,$$

as $E(A|X) = \pi(X)$. Then (2.78) and (2.79) and thus (2.76) and (2.77) are equal to zero. Consequently, if the propensity score model is correctly specified, $\widehat{\delta}^*_{DR}$ is a consistent estimator for δ^* whether or not the outcome regression model is correctly specified.

Conversely, suppose that the outcome regression model is correctly specified, while the propensity score model may or may not be. Then $\beta^* = \beta_0$, so that, by SUTVA and the no unmeasured confounders assumption, $Q(X,a;\beta^*) = Q(X,a;\beta_0) = E(Y|X,A=a) = E\{Y^*(a)|X\}$ for $a = 0,1$, and thus

$$E[\{Y^*(a) - Q(X,a;\beta^*)\}|X] = E[\{Y^*(a) - Q(X,a;\beta_0)\}|X] = 0, \quad a = 0,1.$$

Then, under this condition, (2.78) and (2.79) and thus (2.76) and (2.77) are equal to zero, showing that, if the outcome regression model is correctly specified, $\widehat{\delta}^*_{DR}$ is a consistent estimator for δ^* whether or not the propensity score model is correctly specified.

These developments demonstrate that one need model correctly only one of the propensity score or the outcome regression to render (2.74) a consistent estimator for δ^*. Thus, the estimator (2.74) has built-in "protection" against, or is "robust to," mismodeling in the sense that the analyst has "two tries" to develop a correct model leading to a consistent estimator. This is in contrast to the regression estimator and the inverse probability weighted estimator, which require the outcome regression model or the propensity score model to be correctly specified, respectively, to achieve a consistent estimator for δ^*. As a result, the estimator $\widehat{\delta}^*_{DR}$ in (2.74) is referred to as *doubly robust*.

If both of the propensity score and outcome regression models are correctly specified, then the estimator (2.74) is based on the optimal choice of $h(X)$ given in (2.73). It can be shown in this case that the resulting estimator $\widehat{\delta}^*_{DR}$ achieves the smallest large sample variance among estimators in the class (2.72).

The asymptotic properties of $\widehat{\delta}^*_{DR}$ can be deduced by identifying $\theta = (\delta, \gamma^T, \beta^T)^T$ and viewing the estimators $\widehat{\delta}^*_{DR}$, $\widehat{\gamma}$, and $\widehat{\beta}$ as solving jointly a set of stacked M-estimating equations. For example, if the propensity score is modeled via a logistic regression model as in (2.57) and fitted via maximum likelihood, and the outcome regression model is fitted using OLS, the M-estimating equations are

$$\sum_{i=1}^{n} \left[\frac{A_i Y_i}{\pi(X_i; \gamma)} - \frac{(1 - A_i)Y_i}{1 - \pi(X_i; \gamma)} - \frac{\{A_i - \pi(X_i; \gamma)\}}{\pi(X_i; \gamma)} Q(X_i, 1; \beta) \right.$$
$$\left. - \frac{\{A_i - \pi(X_i; \gamma)\}}{1 - \pi(X_i; \gamma)} Q(X_i, 0; \beta) - \delta^* \right] = 0$$

$$\sum_{i=1}^{n} \begin{pmatrix} 1 \\ X_i \end{pmatrix} \left\{ A_i - \frac{\exp(\gamma_0 + \gamma_1^T X_i)}{1 + \exp(\gamma_0 + \gamma_1^T X_i)} \right\} = 0$$
$$\sum_{i=1}^{n} \frac{\partial Q(X_i, A_i; \beta)}{\partial \beta} \{Y_i - Q(X_i, A_i; \beta)\} = 0.$$

The sandwich variance estimator for the asymptotic variance of $\widehat{\delta}^*_{DR}$ solving these equations can be derived using the general M-estimation theory in Section 2.5.

Remark. We close this section by highlighting the properties of $\widehat{\delta}^*_{IPW}$ and $\widehat{\delta}^*_{DR}$ in the case of a randomized study. Here, the propensity score is known, and thus a correctly specified model for it can be posited. Accordingly, $\widehat{\delta}^*_{IPW}$ constructed with either the known or fitted propensity score is guaranteed to be a consistent estimator for δ^*. Similarly, $\widehat{\delta}^*_{DR}$ is guaranteed to be consistent, and, by the double robustness property, this holds regardless of whether or not the outcome regression model is correctly specified. Moreover, it follows from the semiparametric theory that, in this case, $\widehat{\delta}^*_{DR}$ generally will be a more precise estimator for δ^* than $\widehat{\delta}^*_{IPW}$, even if the outcome regression model is not correctly specified.

2.8   Application

Implementations of the estimators for the average causal treatment effect (2.3) introduced in this chapter are demonstrated on the book's companion website given in the Preface. All codes used to generate simulated data and to implement each method are available on the website.

Chapter 3

Single Decision Treatment Regimes: Fundamentals

3.1 Introduction

The fundamentals of causal inference and potential outcomes in a point exposure study presented in Chapter 2 lay essential groundwork for the statistical framework for the study of single decision dynamic treatment regimes; that is, in the notation of Section 1.4, regimes for which the number of decision points $K = 1$. In this chapter, we present this framework in detail. We show within it how and under what conditions the expected outcome associated with a fixed, specified treatment regime for a single decision point can be estimated from observed data. We then use this framework to characterize formally the notion of an *optimal* single stage dynamic treatment regime. Based on these developments, we motivate and review three main approaches to estimation of an optimal single decision dynamic treatment regime from observed data.

As in most of the literature on this topic, we focus primarily on the situation where the set of possible treatment options $\mathcal{A}_1$ at the single decision point, as defined in Section 1.4, contains two options coded as 0 and 1; that is, $\mathcal{A}_1 = \{0, 1\}$, so that options a_1 in $\mathcal{A}_1$ have possible values 0 or 1. Some of the developments and methods for this case can be extended to $\mathcal{A}_1$ involving a finite number of more than two options, as we indicate in the narrative and demonstrate at the end of the chapter. The methods reviewed involve specification of outcome regression models and related quantities and models for the propensity score. As in Chapter 2, we focus mainly on popular parametric models and defer discussion of nonparametric modeling approaches to the next chapter.

As in Section 1.4, let x_1 be the collection of baseline information available on an individual at this decision point, so that the history available on an individual is $h_1 = x_1$, where $h_1 \in \mathcal{H}_1$. We thus consider dynamic treatment regimes d of the form

$$d = \{d_1(h_1)\},$$

so comprising a single rule $d_1(h_1)$, a function that takes the history h_1 as input and returns either 0 or 1 depending on the value of h_1. If, for a given individual with history h_1, $d_1(h_1) = 0$, then the regime dictates that the individual should receive option 0; if $d_1(h_1) = 1$, the regime dictates that he should receive option 1.

3.2   Treatment Regimes for a Single Decision Point

3.2.1   Class of All Possible Treatment Regimes

As we indicate in Chapter 1, in most situations there is an infinitude of possible rules d_1, and thus regimes d, that can be conceived. With $\mathcal{A}_1 = \{0,1\}$, there are two possible static rules, $d_1(h_1) \equiv 1$ and $d_1(h_1) \equiv 0$ for all $h_1 \in \mathcal{H}_1$, which define two static regimes that dictate that a particular treatment option in $\mathcal{A}_1$ be given regardless of an individual's baseline information. From the discussion in Chapter 2, it should be apparent that comparison of these two static regimes is the focus of interest in a point exposure study; we discuss this further below. These static regimes are of little interest in the context of precision medicine, however, except perhaps for the purpose of comparing the use of a particular treatment option in the entire population to treating the population using a dynamic regime that selects an option in $\mathcal{A}_1$ for an individual based on his or her history h_1.

All other possible rules, and thus dynamic treatment regimes, use the history h_1 in some way. As a simple example, consider Decision 1 in the acute leukemia setting in Section 1.2.1, and suppose that the baseline information includes the variables age (years) and white blood cell count (WBC $\times 10^3/\mu$l). Coding the induction therapy options $\{C_1, C_2\}$ as $\{0,1\}$, the static regimes are "Give C_1," $d_1(h_1) \equiv 0$, and "Give C_2," $d_1(h_1) \equiv 1$, regardless of an individual's age, WBC, or any other component of h_1.

An example of a rule defining a dynamic regime is "If age < 50 and WBC < 10, then give C_2; otherwise, give C_1," which can be written as

$$d_1(h_1) = \text{I}(\text{age} < 50 \text{ and WBC} < 10), \tag{3.1}$$

where again $\text{I}(B)$ is the indicator function such that $\text{I}(B) = 1$ if the event B is true and $= 0$ otherwise. The rule d_1 in (3.1) thus returns a 1 corresponding to induction option C_2 if the event inside the indicator function is true and returns a 0 corresponding to option C_1 if it is not. A different rule and thus different regime would be obtained by taking the threshold value for age to be 51 instead of 50, and likewise for the threshold for WBC. In principle, an infinite number of rules and thus regimes of the form (3.1) can be conceived by traversing all possible combinations of (real-valued) thresholds.

Alternatively, rules and thus regimes that use h_1 differently are possible. For example, consider the rule "if age $+ 8.7 \log(\text{WBC}) - 60 > 0$, give C_2; otherwise give C_1;" that is,

$$d_1(h_1) = \text{I}\{\text{age} + 8.7 \log(\text{WBC}) - 60 > 0\}. \tag{3.2}$$

This is a rule involving a linear combination of functions of elements of h_1. Again, by modifying the coefficients of the linear combination in (3.2), an infinite number of different rules, and thus regimes, is obtained.

Clearly, as this example illustrates, the possibilities for how the information in h_1 is used to form rules and thus regimes to dictate treatment selection at a single decision point can be endless. Only in the simplest cases can all possible rules be enumerated. For instance, if h_1 contains only c binary variables, then there are 2^c possible rules corresponding to each of the 2^c combinations of values that the variables can take on. In most practical settings, h_1 contains continuous and discrete variables and can be high dimensional.

In general, in a specific single decision problem, let $\mathcal{D}$ denote the class of all possible treatment regimes d; that is, defined by all possible functions d_1 of h_1 that return 0 or 1. Except in simple situations, then, $\mathcal{D}$ is an infinite class. Of central interest is deducing an optimal treatment regime in $\mathcal{D}$, where the notion of "optimal" must be defined precisely.

3.2.2 Potential Outcomes Framework

To define the expected outcome for a given regime $d \in \mathcal{D}$ and the concept of an optimal regime in $\mathcal{D}$, we start by defining the potential outcome for any regime $d \in \mathcal{D}$. Consider a randomly chosen individual in the population with baseline information X_1 and thus with history $H_1 = X_1$. As in Chapter 2, we conceive that the individual has potential outcomes $Y^*(0)$ and $Y^*(1)$ that he would achieve if he received treatments 0 and 1, respectively. For any $d \in \mathcal{D}$ characterized by rule d_1, we define the potential outcome that an individual would achieve if assigned treatment according to regime d as

$$Y^*(d) = Y^*(1)\,\mathrm{I}\,\{d_1(H_1) = 1\} + Y^*(0)\,\mathrm{I}\,\{d_1(H_1) = 0\} \qquad (3.3)$$
$$= Y^*(1)d_1(H_1) + Y^*(0)\,\{1 - d_1(H_1)\}.$$

That is, intuitively, the potential outcome $Y^*(d)$ in (3.3) that would be achieved by a randomly chosen individual with history H_1 if the individual were to receive treatment according to d is the outcome the individual would achieve under the treatment option dictated by d for the individual's history H_1. For the static regime d defined by the rule $d_1(h_1) \equiv 1$ for all $h_1 \in \mathcal{H}_1$, note that $Y^*(d) = Y^*(1)$, and similarly $Y^*(d) = Y^*(0)$ for d defined by $d_1(h_1) \equiv 0$.

In the case of $\mathcal{A}_1$ comprising more than two treatment options a_1, so that regimes $d \in \mathcal{D}$ comprise rules $d_1(h_1)$ returning an option $a_1 \in \mathcal{A}_1$ depending on the value of h_1, the definition (3.3) extends straightforwardly. If we let $Y^*(a_1)$ denote the potential outcome that would be achieved by a randomly chosen individual with history H_1 if she were to receive option $a_1 \in \mathcal{A}_1$,

$$Y^*(d) = \sum_{a_1 \in \mathcal{A}_1} Y^*(a_1)\, \mathrm{I}\{d_1(H_1) = a_1\}. \tag{3.4}$$

3.2.3   Value of a Treatment Regime

With the potential outcome associated with a particular fixed regime $d \in \mathcal{D}$ defined as in (3.3) or (3.4), it follows that $E\{Y^*(d)\}$ is the expected outcome if all individuals in the population were to receive treatment according to the rule d_1 characterizing d. In the literature, $E\{Y^*(d)\}$ is often referred to as the *value* of regime $d \in \mathcal{D}$.

If d is one of the two static regimes above, it is immediate that the value of the regime with rule $d_1(h_1) \equiv 1$ is $E\{Y^*(1)\}$ and that for the regime with rule $d_1(h_1) \equiv 0$ is $E\{Y^*(0)\}$. Thus, from Section 2.3, the average causal treatment effect $\delta^* = E\{Y^*(1)\} - E\{Y^*(0)\}$ is the difference in the values corresponding to these two static regimes.

It follows that if, as discussed above, interest focuses on comparing the use of, say, option 1 in the entire population to the use of some fixed dynamic treatment regime $d \in \mathcal{D}$ that selects treatment based on h_1, the difference in values $E\{Y^*(d)\} - E\{Y^*(1)\}$ reflects this comparison and has a causal interpretation. This comparison thus addresses the issue of whether or not it is beneficial on average to use a rule that takes account of individual characteristics to select treatment relative to always administering option 1. In particular, if larger values of the outcome correspond to greater benefit, then interest focuses on whether or not there is sufficient evidence that the true value of this difference is greater than zero.

Remark. In the literature on dynamic treatment regimes, it is common to define the value of a regime $d \in \mathcal{D}$ informally, without explicit reference to potential outcomes. Under this convention, E^d is taken to denote expectation with respect to the probability distribution of the data induced by assigning treatment according to regime $d \in \mathcal{D}$; and, if Y is the outcome variable, the value of regime $d \in \mathcal{D}$ is represented as $E^d(Y)$. Thus, Y is used loosely to refer to both an associated "potential outcome" and the observed outcome. The potential outcome formulation presented in the previous section, in which $Y^*(d)$ is defined precisely as in (3.3) or (3.4), is a formal statement of this notion and allows the assumptions that are required to estimate the value $E\{Y^*(d)\}$ of a fixed $d \in \mathcal{D}$, discussed next, and an optimal regime in $\mathcal{D}$ from observed data, discussed in Sections 3.5.1–3.5.3, to be elucidated explicitly.

We denote the value of a regime $d \in \mathcal{D}$ as

$$\mathcal{V}(d) = E\{Y^*(d)\}.$$

3.3 Estimation of the Value of a Fixed Regime

As for the average causal treatment effect, which we have recognized as being equal to the difference in values for the two static regimes when $\mathcal{A}_1 = \{0, 1\}$, it is thus of interest to estimate the value $\mathcal{V}(d)$ of a given regime $d \in \mathcal{D}$ based on observed data. Such an estimator clearly would be required to compare the value of d to the values of the static regimes and also can be used to compare competing dynamic treatment regimes.

Suppose we have data from a point exposure study, which we now denote by i.i.d.

$$(X_{1i}, A_{1i}, Y_i), \quad i = 1, \dots, n, \tag{3.5}$$

where the subscript "1" emphasizes that the baseline information and treatment received correspond to the single decision point of interest. As in Chapter 2, A_{1i} is the treatment option in $\mathcal{A}_1$ actually received by individual i, and Y_i is the observed outcome for i under that option. Let $H_{1i} = X_{1i}$ be the history for individual i in the sample. As in Section 2.3, the goal is thus to estimate a quantity defined in terms of potential outcomes, $\mathcal{V}(d) = E\{Y^*(d)\}$, based on observed data. Specifically, we wish to deduce the distribution of $Y^*(d)$, which depends on that of $\{X_1, Y^*(1), Y^*(0)\}$, from the distribution of (X_1, A_1, Y).

As we now demonstrate, for $\mathcal{A}_1 = \{0, 1\}$, under SUTVA (2.4), written here as

$$Y_i = Y_i^*(1)A_{1i} + Y_i^*(0)(1 - A_{1i}), \quad i = 1, \dots, n; \tag{3.6}$$

the no unmeasured confounders assumption (2.14),

$$\{Y^*(1), Y^*(0)\} \perp\!\!\!\perp A_1 | H_1, \tag{3.7}$$

which we write in terms of the history $H_1 = X_1$; and the positivity assumption (2.61), now expressed as

$$P(A_1 = a_1 | H_1 = h_1) > 0, \quad a_1 = 0, 1, \tag{3.8}$$

for all $h_1 \in \mathcal{H}_1$ such that $P(H_1 = h_1) > 0$, it is possible to estimate the value $\mathcal{V}(d) = E\{Y^*(d)\}$ of a fixed regime $d \in \mathcal{D}$ from the data (3.5). We discuss two approaches, which are in the spirit of those for estimation of the average causal effect in Sections 2.4 and 2.6.

3.3.1   Outcome Regression Estimator

Consider $\mathcal{A}_1 = \{0, 1\}$. With $d = \{d_1(h_1)\}$, by substitution of (3.3) and manipulations like those in (2.15)–(2.17),

$$E\{Y^*(d)\} = E\left(E\left[Y^*(1)\mathrm{I}\{d_1(H_1) = 1\} + Y^*(0)\mathrm{I}\{d_1(H_1) = 0\} \Big| H_1\right]\right)$$

$$= E\left[E\{Y^*(1)|H_1\}\mathrm{I}\{d_1(H_1) = 1\} + E\{Y^*(0)|H_1\}\mathrm{I}\{d_1(H_1) = 0\}\right]$$

$$\hspace{10cm} (3.9)$$

$$= E\left[E\{Y^*(1)|H_1, A_1 = 1\}\mathrm{I}\{d_1(H_1) = 1\}\right.$$

$$\left. + E\{Y^*(0)|H_1, A_1 = 0\}\mathrm{I}\{d_1(H_1) = 0\}\right] \hspace{2cm} (3.10)$$

$$= E\left[E(Y|H_1, A_1 = 1)\mathrm{I}\{d_1(H_1) = 1\} + E(Y|H_1, A_1 = 0)\mathrm{I}\{d_1(H_1) = 0\}\right]$$

$$\hspace{10cm} (3.11)$$

$$= E\left[E(Y|H_1, A_1 = 1)d_1(H_1) + E(Y|H_1, A_1 = 0)\{1 - d_1(H_1)\}\right],$$

where, analogous to (2.15)–(2.17), the outer expectations are with respect to the marginal distribution of $H_1 = X_1$; (3.10) follows by the no unmeasured confounders assumption (3.7); and (3.11) follows from SUTVA (3.6). As in Section 2.4, the positivity assumption (3.8) ensures that the conditional expectations $E\{Y^*(1)|H_1, A_1 = a_1\}$ and $E(Y|H_1, A_1 = a_1)$, $a_1 = 0, 1$, in (3.10) and (3.11) are well defined.

These developments can be extended to general finite $\mathcal{A}_1$, where $Y^*(d)$ is defined as in (3.4). Under suitable generalizations of SUTVA, the no unmeasured confounders assumption, and the positivity assumption, by analogous calculations,

$$E\{Y^*(d)\} = E\left[\sum_{a_1 \in \mathcal{A}_1} E(Y|H_1, A_1 = a_1)\,\mathrm{I}\{d_1(H_1) = a_1\}\right]. \hspace{1cm} (3.12)$$

The expressions (3.11) and (3.12) show that, under SUTVA and the no unmeasured confounders and positivity assumptions, we can represent the value $\mathcal{V}(d)$ of a given regime $d \in \mathcal{D}$ in terms of the observed data (X_1, A_1, Y). In particular, using notation analogous to that in (2.21), $E\{Y^*(d)\}$ depends on the regression of observed outcome on the history and treatment received,

$$E(Y|H_1 = h_1, A_1 = a_1) = Q_1(h_1, a_1), \hspace{2cm} (3.13)$$

where $Q_1(h_1, a_1)$ is the true function of h_1 and a_1 representing the association between observed outcome and history and treatment received. For $\mathcal{A}_1 = \{0, 1\}$, from (3.11) and using (3.13),

$$E\{Y^*(d)\} = E\left[Q_1(H_1, 1)\mathrm{I}\{d_1(H_1) = 1\} + Q_1(H_1, 0)\mathrm{I}\{d_1(H_1) = 0\}\right],$$

$$\hspace{10cm} (3.14)$$

and similarly for (3.12). If the true function $Q_1(h_1, a_1)$ were known, given the observed data (X_{1i}, A_{1i}, Y_i), $i = 1, \ldots, n$, in (3.5), from (3.14), a natural estimator for the value $\mathcal{V}(d) = E\{Y^*(d)\}$ when $\mathcal{A}_1 = \{0, 1\}$ is then the sample average

$$n^{-1} \sum_{i=1}^{n} \left[Q_1(H_{1i}, 1)I\{d_1(H_{1i}) = 1\} + Q_1(H_{1i}, 0)I\{d_1(H_{1i}) = 0\} \right]; \quad (3.15)$$

similarly, for general $\mathcal{A}_1$, (3.12) is estimated by

$$n^{-1} \sum_{i=1}^{n} \left[\sum_{a_1 \in \mathcal{A}_1} Q_1(H_{1i}, a_1) I\{d_1(H_{1i}) = a_1\} \right]. \quad (3.16)$$

Of course, as in Chapter 2, in practice, the true function $Q_1(h_1, a_1)$ is not known. An obvious approach to using (3.15) or (3.16) to estimate the value of d is thus to posit a model for $Q_1(h_1, a_1)$ and assume that it is correctly specified. We consider a parametric regression model $Q_1(h_1, a_1; \beta_1)$, where now β_1 is a finite-dimensional vector of parameters characterizing the model, and this model can be linear or nonlinear in β_1 as in the examples in Section 2.4. For example, if Y is a continuous outcome and $\mathcal{A}_1 = \{0, 1\}$,

$$Q_1(h_1, a_1; \beta_1) = \beta_{11} + \beta_{12}^T h_1 + \beta_{13} a_1 + \beta_{14}^T h_1 a_1, \quad \beta_1 = (\beta_{11}, \beta_{12}^T, \beta_{13}, \beta_{14}^T)^T,$$

analogous to (2.25); similarly, for binary outcome Y, a logistic regression model analogous to (2.27) can be posited. More complex linear models replacing h_1 by a vector $\tilde{h}_1$ of known features constructed from h_1, including polynomial and other nonlinear basis functions and interaction terms, can also be specified.

Given a suitable estimator $\widehat{\beta}_1$ based on the observed data, for example, derived via M-estimation techniques as in Section 2.5, the regression estimator for the value $\mathcal{V}(d) = E\{Y^*(d)\}$ of a fixed regime $d \in \mathcal{D}$ is obtained by substitution of the model $Q_1(h_1, a_1; \beta_1)$ in the sample average (3.15) or (3.16), evaluated at $\widehat{\beta}_1$; for the former, the estimator is thus

$$\widehat{\mathcal{V}}_Q(d) \quad (3.17)$$

$$= n^{-1} \sum_{i=1}^{n} \left[Q_1(H_{1i}, 1; \widehat{\beta}_1)I\{d_1(H_{1i}) = 1\} + Q_1(H_{1i}, 0; \widehat{\beta}_1)I\{d_1(H_{1i}) = 0\} \right],$$

and similarly for general $\mathcal{A}_1$. As long as the model $Q_1(h_1, a_1; \beta_1)$ is correctly specified, so that there exists true value $\beta_{1,0}$ such that $Q_1(h_1, a_1; \beta_{1,0}) = Q_1(h_1, a_1)$; $\widehat{\beta}_1$ is a consistent estimator for $\beta_{1,0}$; and SUTVA and the no unmeasured confounders and positivity assumptions hold, $\widehat{\mathcal{V}}_Q(d)$ in (3.17) is a consistent estimator for the true value $\mathcal{V}(d)$.

Under these conditions, an approximate large sample distribution for $\widehat{V}_Q(d)$ can be obtained by viewing $\widehat{V}_Q(d)$ and $\widehat{\beta}_1$ as solving a set of stacked M-estimating equations and appealing to the general M-estimation theory in Section 2.5.

3.3.2 *Inverse Probability Weighted Estimator*

An alternative approach to estimation of $\mathcal{V}(d)$ is motivated by considerations analogous to those for estimation of the average causal effect in Section 2.6.3; see, for example, Zhang et al. (2012b). We restrict our discussion to the case of two treatment options, $\mathcal{A}_1 = \{0, 1\}$; extension to general $\mathcal{A}_1$ is possible but is more involved; see Section 3.5.5. We continue to assume that SUTVA (3.6), the no unmeasured confounders assumption (3.7), and the positivity assumption (3.8) hold.

If, for fixed regime $d \in \mathcal{D}$ characterized by rule d_1, we were able to observe the potential outcomes $Y_i^*(d)$, $i = 1, \ldots, n$, for each individual in a sample from the population, then the obvious estimator for the value $\mathcal{V}(d) = E\{Y^*(d)\}$ is

$$n^{-1} \sum_{i=1}^{n} Y_i^*(d).$$

Of course, we cannot observe $Y_i^*(d)$ for all individuals i. From (3.3),

$$Y_i^*(d) = Y_i^*(1)\mathrm{I}\{d_1(H_{1i}) = 1\} + Y_i^*(0)\mathrm{I}\{d_1(H_{1i}) = 0\},$$

and, by SUTVA (3.6),

$$Y_i = Y_i^*(1)A_{1i} + Y_i^*(0)(1 - A_{1i}).$$

It is straightforward to observe that if $A_{1i} = d_1(H_{1i})$, so that the treatment option actually received by i coincides with that dictated by regime d, then $Y_i = Y_i^*(d)$, so that we do in fact observe $Y_i^*(d)$ for such an individual. For example, if $d_1(H_{1i}) = 1$ and individual i received treatment option 1, $A_{1i} = 1$, then $Y_i^*(d) = Y_i^*(1)$ and $Y_i = Y_i^*(1)$, and similarly for option 0. Otherwise, if $A_i \neq d_1(H_{1i})$, then clearly $Y_i \neq Y_i^*(d)$. For such individuals, although we do observe an outcome, it does not reflect the outcome that the individual would have had under regime d; that is, $Y_i^*(d)$ is "missing."

As in Section 2.6.3, this missing data analogy implies that the same considerations used to deduce the inverse probability weighted estimators for $E\{Y^*(1)\}$ and $E\{Y^*(0)\}$ in (2.59) and (2.60) can be invoked here. Let

$$\mathcal{C}_d = \mathrm{I}\{A_1 = d_1(H_1)\} = A_1\mathrm{I}\{d_1(H_1) = 1\} + (1 - A_1)\mathrm{I}\{d_1(H_1) = 0\}$$

$$\tag{3.18}$$

be the indicator of whether or not the treatment option actually received coincides with the option dictated by d for an individual with history H_1; for brevity, we suppress dependence of $\mathcal{C}_d$ on A_1 and H_1. Thus, if $\mathcal{C}_d = 1$, $Y^*(d)$ is observed; otherwise, it is missing. Then

$$\pi_{d,1}(H_1) = P(\mathcal{C}_d = 1|H_1) \tag{3.19}$$

is the propensity for receiving treatment consistent with regime d given an individual's history. This suggests constructing an estimator for $\mathcal{V}(d) = E\{Y^*(d)\}$ in the form of a sample average, where the observed outcome of an individual with a particular value of H_1 who received treatment coinciding with that dictated by d, so with $Y = Y^*(d)$, is weighted by $1/\pi_{d,1}(H_1)$ so as to represent the individual's own outcome and those of other individuals with the same H_1 who did not. That is,

$$\widehat{\mathcal{V}}_{IPW}(d) = n^{-1} \sum_{i=1}^{n} \frac{\mathcal{C}_{d,i} Y_i}{\pi_{d,1}(H_{1i})}. \tag{3.20}$$

From (3.18) and (3.19), it is straightforward to deduce that

$$\pi_{d,1}(H_1) = E\left[A_1 I\{d_1(H_1) = 1\} + (1 - A_1)I\{d_1(H_1) = 0\}|H_1\right]$$
$$= \pi_1(H_1)I\{d_1(H_1) = 1\} + \{1 - \pi_1(H_1)\}I\{d_1(H_1) = 0\} \tag{3.21}$$
$$= \pi_1(H_1)^{d_1(H_1)}\{1 - \pi_1(H_1)\}^{1-d_1(H_1)},$$

where $\pi_1(H_1) = P(A_1 = 1|H_1)$ is the propensity score defined in Section 2.6 written in terms of the history H_1. Note that, for the estimator (3.20) to be well defined, it must be that $\pi_{d,1}(H_1) > 0$ for all $d \in \mathcal{D}$; this holds under the positivity assumption (3.8), which implies that $0 < \pi_1(H_1) < 1$ almost surely.

That (3.20) is an unbiased estimator for the value $\mathcal{V}(d) = E\{Y^*(d)\}$ follows by an argument similar to that in Section 2.6.3. Specifically, using SUTVA and the definition of $Y^*(d)$,

$$E\left\{\frac{\mathcal{C}_d Y}{\pi_{d,1}(H_1)}\right\} = E\left\{\frac{\mathcal{C}_d Y^*(d)}{\pi_{d,1}(H_1)}\right\} = E\left[E\left\{\frac{\mathcal{C}_d Y^*(d)}{\pi_{d,1}(H_1)}\bigg| Y^*(1), Y^*(0), H_1\right\}\right]$$
$$= E\left[\frac{E\{\mathcal{C}_d|Y^*(1), Y^*(0), H_1\}Y^*(d)}{\pi_1(H_1)I\{d_1(H_1) = 1\} + \{1 - \pi_1(H_1)\}I\{d_1(H_1) = 0\}}\right]$$
$$= E\{Y^*(d)\} \tag{3.22}$$

almost surely using (3.21), where the last equality follows because

$$E\{\mathcal{C}_d|Y^*(1), Y^*(0), H_1\}$$
$$= E\left[A_1 I\{d_1(H_1) = 1\} + (1 - A_1)I\{d_1(H_1) = 0\} \bigg| Y^*(1), Y^*(0), H_1\right]$$

$$= E(A_1|H_1)\mathrm{I}\{d_1(H_1) = 1\} + E(1 - A_1|H_1)\mathrm{I}\{d_1(H_1) = 0\}$$
$$= \pi_1(H_1)\mathrm{I}\{d_1(H_1) = 1\} + \{1 - \pi_1(H_1)\}\mathrm{I}\{d_1(H_1) = 0\}$$

almost surely by the no unmeasured confounders assumption.

If the observed data (X_{1i}, A_{1i}, Y_i), $i = 1, \ldots, n$, in (3.5) are from a randomized study, then the propensity score $\pi_1(h_1)$ is known and often independent of the history h_1, in which case the "propensity of consistency with d" $\pi_{d,1}(h_1)$ is also known. In this case, the estimator $\widehat{\mathcal{V}}_{IPW}(d)$ in (3.20) can be used to estimate the value as is; as discussed at the end of Section 2.6.3, it might be advantageous to substitute a fitted version of $\pi_1(h_1)$.

If the data are from an observational study, as in Section 2.6.3, $\pi_{d,1}(h_1)$ is not known in general because $\pi_1(h_1)$ is not known. Accordingly, a model $\pi_1(h_1; \gamma_1)$ for the propensity score $P(A_1 = 1|H_1 = h_1)$ must be posited, such as the logistic regression model

$$\pi_1(h_1; \gamma_1) = \frac{\exp(\gamma_{11} + \gamma_{12}^T h_1)}{1 + \exp(\gamma_{11} + \gamma_{12}^T h_1)}, \quad \gamma_1 = (\gamma_{11}, \gamma_{12}^T)^T, \tag{3.23}$$

as in (2.57), which induces a model $\pi_{d,1}(h_1; \gamma_1)$. If $\widehat{\gamma}_1$ is the maximum likelihood estimator for γ_1, then substitution of the fitted model in (3.20) yields the inverse probability weighted estimator

$$\widehat{\mathcal{V}}_{IPW}(d) = n^{-1} \sum_{i=1}^{n} \frac{\mathcal{C}_{d,i} Y_i}{\pi_{d,1}(H_{1i}; \widehat{\gamma}_1)}. \tag{3.24}$$

From (3.24) and the above argument, if the propensity score model $\pi_1(h_1; \gamma_1)$ is correctly specified, so that there exists $\gamma_{1,0}$ such that $\pi_1(h_1; \gamma_{1,0}) = \pi_1(h_1)$, then the induced model $\pi_{d,1}(h_1; \gamma_1)$ is correctly specified, and $\widehat{\mathcal{V}}_{IPW}(d)$ is a consistent estimator for the true value $\mathcal{V}(d)$.

An alternative to (3.24) that can enjoy considerably smaller sampling variation in practice is a weighted average of the observed Y_i, namely,

$$\widehat{\mathcal{V}}_{IPW*}(d) = \left\{ \sum_{i=1}^{n} \frac{\mathcal{C}_{d,i}}{\pi_{d,1}(H_{1i}; \widehat{\gamma}_1)} \right\}^{-1} \sum_{i=1}^{n} \frac{\mathcal{C}_{d,i} Y_i}{\pi_{d,1}(H_{1i}; \widehat{\gamma}_1)}. \tag{3.25}$$

It can be shown by the same manipulations as in (3.22) that, when the propensity model is correctly specified and $\gamma_{1,0}$ substituted for $\widehat{\gamma}_1$, n^{-1} times the sum in the first inverse term on the right-hand side of (3.25) has expectation equal to one. Thus, (3.25) is also a consistent estimator for $\mathcal{V}(d)$ and has been advocated as preferable to (3.24) in practice.

As for the regression estimator, viewing the estimators (3.24) or (3.25) and the maximum likelihood estimator $\widehat{\gamma}_1$ as M-estimators solving a stacked set of estimating equations analogous to (2.65), the theory in

Section 2.5 can be used to derive the approximate large sample distribution of $\widehat{\mathcal{V}}_{IPW}(d)$ or $\widehat{\mathcal{V}}_{IPW*}(d)$.

Remark. When $\mathcal{C}_d = 1$, so that $A_1 = d_1(H_1)$ almost surely, it is straightforward to observe that $\widehat{\mathcal{V}}_{IPW}(d)$ and $\widehat{\mathcal{V}}_{IPW*}(d)$ are unchanged if $\pi_{d,1}(H_{1i}; \widehat{\gamma}_1)$ is replaced for each i by

$$\pi_1(H_{1i}; \widehat{\gamma}_1)\mathrm{I}(A_{1i} = 1) + \{1 - \pi_1(H_{1i}; \widehat{\gamma}_1)\}\mathrm{I}(A_{1i} = 0)$$
$$= \pi_1(H_{1i}; \widehat{\gamma}_1)A_{1i} + \{1 - \pi_1(H_{1i}; \widehat{\gamma}_1)\}(1 - A_{1i}) \qquad (3.26)$$
$$= \pi_1(H_{1i}; \widehat{\gamma}_1)^{A_{1i}}\{1 - \pi_1(H_{1i}; \widehat{\gamma}_1)\}^{(1-A_{1i})}.$$

Accordingly, some literature accounts define (3.24) with (3.26) as the denominator of the ith summand. As above, the motivation for $\widehat{\mathcal{V}}_{IPW}(d)$ implies the form of the denominator in (3.24).

Remark. The tradeoff between the regression estimator (3.17) and the inverse probability weighted estimators (3.24) and (3.25) is analogous to that discussed for estimation of the average causal effect at the end of Section 2.6.3. The first requires correct modeling of the outcome regression relationship, while the latter requires correct modeling of the propensity score. Moreover, the counterintuitive result discussed at the end of Section 2.6 that it is preferable to estimate the parameter in the propensity score model even if it is known (provided that the model is correct) persists in this setting.

If the data are from a randomized study, so that the true form of $\pi_1(h_1)$ is known, the inverse probability weighted estimator using $\pi_1(h_1)$ directly or a fitted version of it has the advantage that it is guaranteed to be consistent, whereas consistency of the regression estimator is still predicated on a correct outcome regression model.

3.3.3 Augmented Inverse Probability Weighted Estimator

In the same spirit as for estimation of the average causal effect, the requirement of correct modeling of the outcome regression relationship for the regression estimator (3.17) or of the propensity score for the inverse probability weighted estimator (3.24) to achieve consistent estimation of the value motivates consideration of the broader class of augmented inverse probability weighted estimators for the value $\mathcal{V}(d)$ similar to that discussed in Section 2.7.

As in that section, the inverse probability weighted estimator (3.24) requires that the propensity score model is correctly specified, but does not require that an assumption be made on the distribution of Y given H_1 and A_1. Under these conditions, appealing to the theory of semiparametrics (Robins et al., 1994; Tsiatis, 2006), similar to the developments in Section 2.7, all consistent and asymptotically normal estimators for the value $\mathcal{V}(d)$ are asymptotically equivalent to an estimator of the form

$$\widehat{\mathcal{V}}_{AIPW}(d) = n^{-1} \sum_{i=1}^{n} \left[\frac{\mathcal{C}_{d,i} Y_i}{\pi_{d,1}(H_{1i}; \widehat{\gamma}_1)} - \frac{\mathcal{C}_{d,i} - \pi_{d,1}(H_{1i}; \widehat{\gamma}_1)}{\pi_{d,1}(H_{1i}; \widehat{\gamma}_1)} L_1(H_{1i}) \right],$$

(3.27)

where now $L_1(H_1)$ is an arbitrary function of H_1; and the second, "augmentation term" in (3.27) has conditional expectation given H_{1i} equal to zero when evaluated at the true value $\gamma_{1,0}$.

It follows from the theory that the optimal choice of $L_1(H_1)$ leading to the efficient estimator in the class (3.27) with smallest asymptotic variance is

$$L_1(H_1) = E\{Y^*(d) | H_1\}$$
$$= Q_1(H_1, 1) \mathrm{I}\{d_1(H_1) = 1\} + Q_1(H_1, 0) \mathrm{I}\{d_1(H_1) = 0\}, \quad (3.28)$$

where the second equality follows from (3.11) and (3.14) under SUTVA and the no unmeasured confounders and positivity assumptions. This suggests positing a model for $E(Y|H_1 = h_1, A_1 = a_1) = Q_1(h_1, a_1)$, $Q_1(h_1, a_1; \beta_1)$, say; and representing (3.28) as

$$\mathcal{Q}_{d,1}(H_1; \beta_1) = Q_1(H_1, 1; \beta_1) \mathrm{I}\{d_1(H_1) = 1\} + Q_1(H_1, 0; \beta_1) \mathrm{I}\{d_1(H_1) = 0\}.$$

(3.29)

If $\widehat{\beta}_1$ is a suitable estimator for β_1, substituting in (3.27) then leads to the estimator

$$\widehat{\mathcal{V}}_{AIPW}(d) = n^{-1} \sum_{i=1}^{n} \left[\frac{\mathcal{C}_{d,i} Y_i}{\pi_{d,1}(H_{1i}; \widehat{\gamma}_1)} - \frac{\mathcal{C}_{d,i} - \pi_{d,1}(H_{1i}; \widehat{\gamma}_1)}{\pi_{d,1}(H_{1i}; \widehat{\gamma}_1)} \mathcal{Q}_{d,1}(H_{1i}; \widehat{\beta}_1) \right].$$

(3.30)

Note that the second "augmentation term" in the summand of (3.30) depends on the data from all n individuals in the data set and thus can be interpreted as attempting to improve precision by "capturing back" some of the information from those for whom $\mathcal{C}_d = 0$ and thus did not receive treatment consistent with regime d.

Remark. From the previous section, $\widehat{\mathcal{V}}_{AIPW}(d)$ is unchanged by replacing $\pi_{d,1}(H_{1i}; \widehat{\gamma}_1)$ in the leading "inverse weighted" term of (3.30) by (3.26). Writing the quotient in the augmentation term of (3.30) as $\{\mathcal{C}_{d,i}/\pi_{d,1}(H_{1i}; \widehat{\gamma}_1) - 1\}$, it is straightforward to observe that $\widehat{\mathcal{V}}_{AIPW}(d)$ is unaltered if this same substitution is made in this term.

By an argument similar to that in Section 2.7, the augmented inverse probability weighted estimator $\widehat{\mathcal{V}}_{AIPW}(d)$ in (3.30) can be shown to be doubly robust. That is, it is a consistent estimator for the true value $\mathcal{V}(d)$

if either the propensity score model $\pi_1(h_1; \gamma_1)$ or the outcome regression model $Q_1(h_1, a_1; \beta_1)$ is correctly specified, so offers protection against mismodeling. If the data are from a randomized study, so that the form of $\pi_1(h_1; \gamma_1)$ is known, as in the remark at the end of Section 3.3.2, the double robustness property thus ensures that $\widehat{\mathcal{V}}_{AIPW}(d)$ is consistent, regardless of whether or not the outcome regression model is correct.

If both models are correctly specified, then the estimator uses the optimal choice of $L_1(H_1)$ given in (3.28), and it can be shown that it achieves the smallest large sample variance among estimators of the form (3.27) and is referred to as a locally efficient estimator. In particular, the estimator $\widehat{\mathcal{V}}_{AIPW}(d)$ in (3.30) is relatively more efficient than the simple inverse weighted estimator $\widehat{\mathcal{V}}_{IPW}(d)$ in (3.24), which is based on taking $L(H_1) \equiv 0$. In fact, as with any simple inverse weighted estimator, $\widehat{\mathcal{V}}_{IPW}(d)$ can be unstable in practice if the value of $\pi_{d,1}(H_{1i}; \widehat{\gamma}_1)$ is very small for some individuals in the sample. Interestingly, the additional augmentation term in $\widehat{\mathcal{V}}_{AIPW}(d)$ often serves to mitigate this instability.

As for the other estimators in this section, (3.30) can be cast as an M-estimator that solves jointly the maximum likelihood estimating equations for $\widehat{\gamma}_1$ and appropriate estimating equations for obtaining $\widehat{\beta}_1$. Viewing these equations as a set of stacked M-estimating equations, the theory in Section 2.5 can be used to derive the approximate large sample distribution of $\widehat{\mathcal{V}}_{AIPW}(d)$.

Remark. Recall that the regression estimator (3.17) requires that the outcome regression relationship $Q_1(h_1, a_1)$ be modeled correctly to yield a consistent estimator for the value. If this model is indeed correctly specified, the resulting estimator $\widehat{\mathcal{V}}_Q(d)$, which is outside the class of estimators (3.27), is more efficient than (3.30) in general, even if both the outcome regression and propensity score models are correctly specified. However, the gain in efficiency over (3.30) is often negligible in this case, making the doubly robust, augmented inverse probability weighted estimator, which offers protection against possible mismodeling, an attractive alternative.

3.4 Characterization of an Optimal Regime

As we have noted, the class of all possible treatment regimes $\mathcal{D}$ is typically infinite. Although evaluation of specific, fixed regimes in $\mathcal{D}$ is of some interest, as described in the last section, a further objective is to identify an optimal treatment regime within $\mathcal{D}$. As a first step toward estimation of an optimal regime from data, armed with the potential outcome framework in Section 3.2.2, we consider a precise characterization of an optimal regime.

As noted in Section 3.2.3, the conventional comparison of treatment options, which in this context are static regimes, is based on contrasting the expected outcomes that would be achieved if all individuals in the population were to receive each option; that is, on contrasting the associated values. Likewise, comparison of these static regimes to competing dynamic regimes is also based on the values. If the outcome is defined so that larger values correspond to greater benefit, which we assume henceforth, then regimes with larger associated values, so leading to greater benefit on average if used to select treatment in the population, are preferred. Thus, intuitively, if we consider all regimes $d \in \mathcal{D}$, it is natural to define an optimal regime in $\mathcal{D}$ as one that leads to the maximum value among all $d \in \mathcal{D}$.

Formally, then, an optimal regime d^{opt}, say, is one that maximizes the value among all $d \in \mathcal{D}$, namely,

$$d^{opt} = \arg\max_{d \in \mathcal{D}} E\{Y^*(d)\} = \arg\max_{d \in \mathcal{D}} \mathcal{V}(d)$$

or, equivalently,

$$E\{Y^*(d^{opt})\} \geq E\{Y^*(d)\} \text{ for all } d \in \mathcal{D}. \tag{3.31}$$

Remark. In principle, it is possible that there is more than one regime d^{opt} satisfying (3.31), so that there is more than one regime achieving the maximum value; we discuss this further below. Accordingly, to be precise, we usually refer to "an" rather than "the" optimal regime. In the literature, it is commonplace to downplay this technicality and to refer to "the" optimal regime.

It is straightforward to derive the form of an optimal treatment regime $d^{opt} = \{d_1^{opt}(h_1)\}$. We first give an intuitive demonstration and then a formal argument, focusing on $\mathcal{A}_1 = \{0, 1\}$.

Consider any regime $d \in \mathcal{D}$ with rule $d_1(h_1)$, and recall the definition of $Y^*(d)$ in (3.3), namely,

$$Y^*(d) = Y^*(1)\mathrm{I}\{d_1(H_1) = 1\} + Y^*(0)\,\mathrm{I}\{d_1(H_1) = 0\}.$$

Using this definition, we can write the value $\mathcal{V}(d) = E\{Y^*(d)\}$ of d as

$$E\{Y^*(d)\} = E\left[E\{Y^*(d)|H_1\}\right] \tag{3.32}$$
$$= E\left[E\{Y^*(1)|H_1\}\mathrm{I}\{d_1(H_1) = 1\} + E\{Y^*(0)|H_1\}\mathrm{I}\{d_1(H_1) = 0\}\right].$$

Inspection of the right-hand side of (3.32) shows that the expression inside the outer expectation (which is with respect to the distribution of H_1), evaluated at any h_1, will be as large as possible if the rule $d_1(h_1)$

is such that $d_1(h_1) = 1$ when $E\{Y^*(1)|H_1 = h_1\} > E\{Y^*(0)|H_1 = h_1\}$ and $d_1(h_1) = 0$ when $E\{Y^*(1)|H_1 = h_1\} < E\{Y^*(0)|H_1 = h_1\}$; that is, if $d_1(h_1)$ chooses the treatment option $a_1 \in \mathcal{A}_1$ that maximizes $E\{Y^*(a_1)|H_1 = h_1\}$ for all h_1. If $d_1(h_1)$ satisfies this requirement, then it is clear that the expectation of the inside expression in (3.32) with respect to the distribution of H_1 will be as large as possible, and thus $E\{Y^*(d)\}$ will be as large as possible.

These developments suggest that an optimal regime d^{opt} is characterized formally by the rule

$$d_1^{opt}(h_1) = \arg\max_{a_1 \in \mathcal{A}_1} E\{Y^*(a_1)|H_1 = h_1\} \tag{3.33}$$

for all h_1. The rule $d_1^{opt}(h_1)$ in (3.33) chooses the treatment option in $\mathcal{A}_1$ having the maximum expected outcome conditional on the history (baseline information). This result makes intuitive sense: the best decision on treatment for a patient whose realized history is h_1 is to choose the option that maximizes the expected value of the outcome that would be achieved for such a patient and thus is expected to provide the patient with the most benefit given her history is h_1.

In the above, we did not consider the situation where

$$E\{Y^*(1)|H_1 = h_1\} = E\{Y^*(0)|H_1 = h_1\}$$

for some h_1. If there is a value of h_1 such that this is true, then a rule of the form (3.33) that chooses treatment option 1 for this h_1 and a rule that instead chooses option 0 define different regimes that both achieve the maximum value, underscoring the point above that there may be more than one optimal regime. If a unique representation is desired, one can designate one of the options to be the default option when both options are equally beneficial for a given h_1. Here, we take option 0 to be the default for definiteness; because in many contexts 0 codes a a control or standard of care option and 1 an experimental option, this represents a conservative choice. Under this choice, (3.33) can be written equivalently for all h_1 as

$$d_1^{opt}(h_1) = \mathrm{I}\left[E\{Y^*(1)|H_1 = h_1\} > E\{Y^*(0)|H_1 = h_1\}\right]. \tag{3.34}$$

For completeness, we now present the formal result and proof.

Characterization of an Optimal Single Decision Treatment Regime

The regime d^{opt} with rule d_1^{opt} given in (3.33),

$$d_1^{opt}(h_1) = \arg\max_{a_1 \in \mathcal{A}_1} E\{Y^*(a_1)|H_1 = h_1\} \quad \text{for all } h_1,$$

satisfies (3.31) and is thus an optimal treatment regime.

Proof. Choose any arbitrary $d \in \mathcal{D}$, where $d = \{d_1(h_1)\}$. Because $E\{Y^*(d)\} = E\left[E\{Y^*(d)|H_1\}\right]$ and $E\{Y^*(d^{opt})\} = E\left[E\{Y^*(d^{opt})|H_1\}\right]$, the result follows if we can show that

$$E\{Y^*(d^{opt})|H_1 = h_1\} \geq E\{Y^*(d)|H_1 = h_1\} \quad \text{for all } h_1.$$

Because d^{opt} is defined by (3.33), it follows that

$$E\{Y^*(d^{opt})|H_1 = h_1\} = \max_{a_1 \in \mathcal{A}_1} E\{Y^*(a_1)|H_1 = h_1\} = V_1(h_1) \quad (3.35)$$

for any h_1. Thus, using (3.35), the definition of $Y^*(d)$ in (3.3), and the fact that $I\{d_1(h_1) = 1\} + I\{d_1(h_1) = 0\} = 1$,

$$E\{Y^*(d^{opt})|H_1 = h_1\} = \max_{a_1 \in \mathcal{A}_1} E\{Y^*(a_1)|H_1 = h_1\}$$

$$= \max_{a_1 \in \mathcal{A}_1} E\{Y^*(a_1)|H_1 = h_1\}\left[I\{d_1(h_1) = 1\} + I\{d_1(h_1) = 0\}\right]$$

$$\geq E\{Y^*(1)|H_1 = h_1\}I\{d_1(h_1) = 1\} + E\{Y^*(0)|H_1 = h_1\}I\{d_1(h_1) = 0\}$$

$$= E\left[Y^*(1)I\{d_1(h_1) = 1\} + Y^*(0)I\{d_1(h_1) = 0\}\Big| H_1 = h_1\right]$$

$$= E\{Y^*(d)|H_1 = h_1\},$$

demonstrating the result.   □

In (3.35), we define $V_1(h_1)$ to be the expected outcome that is achieved using the option selected by the rule $d_1^{opt}(h_1)$ for given h_1. In the multiple decision setting presented in Chapters 5 and 7, $V_1(h_1)$ and analogous quantities are referred to as *value functions*. From (3.33),

$$E\{V_1(H_1)\} = E\left[E\{Y^*(d^{opt})|H_1\}\right] = E\{Y^*(d^{opt})\} = \mathcal{V}(d^{opt}). \quad (3.36)$$

In Chapters 5 and 7, the role of value functions in characterizing an optimal, multiple decision regime is demonstrated in detail.

Remark. It is important to distinguish between the optimal treatment option for a randomly chosen patient and an optimal decision as to which option to administer given the patient's history H_1. The optimal option is arg $\max_{a_1 \in \mathcal{A}_1} Y^*(a_1)$; that is, the option corresponding to the largest (potential) outcome that can be achieved by the patient. In practice, the values of the potential outcomes are not known at the time of the treatment decision, so it is not possible to identify the optimal option. All that is known is the patient's history, H_1. By the construction above, $d_1^{opt}(H_1)$ yields the treatment option that corresponds to the largest expected outcome given knowledge of this history. It is straightforward using the definition of $Y^*(d)$ in (3.3) to see that

$$Y^*(d) \leq \max\{Y^*(1), Y^*(0)\} \quad \text{for all } d \in \mathcal{D},$$

so that $Y^*(d^{opt}) \leq \max\{Y^*(1), Y^*(0)\}$ almost surely. Thus, an optimal regime may not necessarily select the "best" treatment for a given individual. Rather, an optimal regime dictates the "best" decision that can be made using the information available on the individual at the time of the decision.

Remark. Our presentation has been in the context of $\mathcal{A}_1 = \{0, 1\}$. Intuitively, for general, finite $\mathcal{A}_1$, given the definition of $Y^*(d)$ in (3.4) in this case, it is possible to demonstrate that the definition of an optimal regime in (3.33) applies to general $\mathcal{A}_1$.

The foregoing developments characterize an optimal dynamic treatment regime in terms of potential outcomes. To estimate an optimal treatment regime in practice, as for estimation of the value of a fixed regime in Section 3.3, it must be possible to identify an optimal regime from observed data (X_{1i}, A_{1i}, Y_i), $i = 1, \ldots, n$. This is immediate under SUTVA (3.6) and the no unmeasured confounders (3.7) and positivity (3.8) assumptions. Specifically, under these conditions, we have shown in (3.9)–(3.11) that

$$E\{Y^*(a_1)|H_1\} = E\{Y^*(a_1)|H_1, A_1 = a_1\} = E(Y|H_1, A_1 = a_1) \quad (3.37)$$

for $a_1 = 0, 1$, which in fact holds for any $a_1 \in \mathcal{A}_1$ for general, finite $\mathcal{A}_1$.

Applying (3.37) to the expression for $d_1^{opt}(h_1)$ in (3.33) yields the equivalent representation

$$d_1^{opt}(h_1) = \underset{a_1 \in \mathcal{A}_1}{\arg\max}\, E(Y|H_1 = h_1, A_1 = a_1) \quad (3.38)$$

in terms of the observed data. Thus, defining as in (3.13)

$$E(Y|H_1 = h_1, A_1 = a_1) = Q_1(h_1, a_1),$$

we can write (3.38) as

$$d_1^{opt}(h_1) = \underset{a_1 \in \mathcal{A}_1}{\arg\max}\, Q_1(h_1, a_1). \quad (3.39)$$

In the case of $\mathcal{A}_1 = \{0, 1\}$, and taking option 0 to be the default when $E(Y|H_1 = h_1, A_1 = 1) = E(Y|H_1 = h_1, A_1 = 0)$, (3.34) can be expressed in terms of the observed data as

$$d_1^{opt}(h_1) = I\{Q_1(h_1, 1) > Q_1(h_1, 0)\}. \quad (3.40)$$

From (3.35) and (3.36), the maximum value achieved by d^{opt} can be written in terms of the observed data as

$$\mathcal{V}(d^{opt}) = E\{V_1(H_1)\} = E\left\{\max_{a_1 \in \mathcal{A}_1} Q_1(H_1, a_1)\right\}, \quad (3.41)$$

where again the outer expectation is with respect to the distribution of H_1.

3.5 Estimation of an Optimal Regime

3.5.1 Regression-based Estimation

The representations of an optimal regime in (3.39) and (3.40) in terms of the true function $Q_1(h_1, a_1)$ suggest immediately estimating d^{opt} from observed data (X_{1i}, A_{1i}, Y_i), $i = 1, \ldots, n$, for which SUTVA and the no unmeasured confounders and positivity assumptions are thought to hold by positing a parametric regression model $Q_1(h_1, a_1; \beta_1)$ as in Section 3.3.1, assuming this model is correctly specified, and substituting the fitted model in these expressions. For example, if Y is continuous and $\mathcal{A}_1 = \{0, 1\}$, a linear model

$$Q_1(h_1, a_1; \beta_1) = \beta_{11} + \beta_{12}^T h_1 + \beta_{13} a_1 + \beta_{14}^T h_1 a_1 \qquad (3.42)$$

might be adopted, where the estimator $\widehat{\beta}_1$ for $\beta_1 = (\beta_{11}, \beta_{12}^T, \beta_{13}, \beta_{14}^T)^T$ is obtained by a suitable M-estimation technique. A logistic model might be posited for binary outcome Y, where the associated β_1 is estimated by an M-estimator (maximum likelihood).

In general, assuming that the posited model is correct, where β_1 is estimated by $\widehat{\beta}_1$, the estimator $\widehat{d}_Q^{opt}$ for d^{opt} is characterized by the estimated rule

$$\widehat{d}_{Q,1}^{opt}(h_1) = \arg\max_{a_1 \in \mathcal{A}_1} Q_1(h_1, a_1; \widehat{\beta}_1), \qquad (3.43)$$

which is equivalent to

$$\widehat{d}_{Q,1}^{opt}(h_1) = \mathrm{I}\{Q_1(h_1, 1; \widehat{\beta}_1) > Q_1(h_1, 0; \widehat{\beta}_1)\} \qquad (3.44)$$

when $\mathcal{A}_1 = \{0, 1\}$ and option 0 is the default. That is, the regression-based estimator for d^{opt} is

$$\widehat{d}_Q^{opt} = \{\widehat{d}_{Q,1}^{opt}(h_1)\}, \qquad (3.45)$$

where $\widehat{d}_{Q,1}^{opt}(h_1)$ is as in (3.43). From (3.41), $\mathcal{V}(d^{opt})$ can be estimated by the sample average

$$\widehat{\mathcal{V}}_Q(d^{opt}) = n^{-1} \sum_{i=1}^n \max_{a_1 \in \mathcal{A}_1} Q_1(H_{1i}, a_1; \widehat{\beta}_1). \qquad (3.46)$$

In the case of the linear model (3.42) and $\mathcal{A}_1 = \{0, 1\}$ with option 0 the default, for example, it is straightforward that (3.44) becomes

$$\widehat{d}_{Q,1}^{opt}(h_1) = \mathrm{I}(\widehat{\beta}_{13} + \widehat{\beta}_{14}^T h_1 > 0),$$

and

$$\max_{a_1 \in \mathcal{A}_1} Q_1(H_1, a_1; \widehat{\beta}_1) = \widehat{\beta}_{11} + \widehat{\beta}_{12}^T H_1 + (\widehat{\beta}_{13} + \widehat{\beta}_{14}^T H_1) \mathrm{I}(\widehat{\beta}_{13} + \widehat{\beta}_{14}^T H_1 > 0),$$

so that, from (3.46),

$$\widehat{\mathcal{V}}_Q(d^{opt})$$

$$= n^{-1} \sum_{i=1}^{n} \left\{ \widehat{\beta}_{11} + \widehat{\beta}_{12}^T H_{1i} + (\widehat{\beta}_{13} + \widehat{\beta}_{14}^T H_{1i}) \mathrm{I}(\widehat{\beta}_{13} + \widehat{\beta}_{14}^T H_{1i} > 0) \right\}.$$

Remark. This approach to estimation of an optimal regime and its associated value based on a posited regression model for $Q_1(h_1, a_1) = E(Y|H_1 = h_1, A_1 = a_1)$ is a special case in the single decision setting of the method known as *Q-learning* for estimation of an optimal multiple decision regime and its value, discussed in detail in Chapters 5 and 7.

As for a fixed regime, it is of interest to establish the large sample properties of the estimator $\widehat{\mathcal{V}}_Q(d^{opt})$ for the value associated with d^{opt}. As in Section 3.3, it is natural to view $\widehat{\mathcal{V}}_Q(d^{opt})$ and $\widehat{\beta}_1$ as solving a set of stacked M-estimating equations and to appeal to the usual M-estimation theory in Section 2.5. For example, if β_1 is estimated by OLS, then $\widehat{\mathcal{V}}_Q(d^{opt})$ and $\widehat{\beta}_1$ solve jointly

$$\sum_{i=1}^{n} \left\{ \max_{a_1 \in \mathcal{A}_1} Q_1(H_{1i}, a_1; \beta_1) - \mathcal{V}(d^{opt}) \right\} = 0 \tag{3.47}$$

$$\sum_{i=1}^{n} \frac{\partial Q_1(H_{1i}, A_i; \beta_1)}{\partial \beta_1} \{Y_i - Q_1(H_{1i}, A_i; \beta_1)\} = 0. \tag{3.48}$$

However, because of the involvement of the max operator in (3.47), this may not be straightforward. In the standard M-estimation argument to derive asymptotic normality in Section 2.5, differentiability of the estimating function with respect to its parameters, $\mathcal{V}(d^{opt})$ and β_1 here, is assumed implicitly to justify the Taylor series expansion (2.33). The max operator is not differentiable everywhere, which leads to some difficulty. We illustrate in a simple special case.

Example: Nonregularity of $\widehat{\mathcal{V}}_Q(d^{opt})$

Suppose that H_1 is one dimensional, $\mathcal{A}_1 = \{0, 1\}$ with option 0 the default, and

$$Q_1(h_1, a_1; \beta_1) = \beta_{11} + \beta_{12}h_1 + \beta_{13}a_1 \tag{3.49}$$

is a correctly specified model for the true $Q_1(h_1, a_1)$, with true value $\beta_{1,0} = (\beta_{11,0}, \beta_{12,0}, \beta_{13,0})^T$ of β_1. It follows that

$$\max_{a_1 \in \mathcal{A}_1} Q_1(h_1, a_1; \beta_1) = \beta_{11} + \beta_{12}h_1 + \beta_{13}\mathrm{I}(\beta_{13} > 0). \tag{3.50}$$

Note that (3.50) is not differentiable in β_{13} when $\beta_{13} = 0$, which corresponds to the null hypothesis of no treatment difference; this will be important momentarily. Because the model (3.49) is correctly specified, from (3.50), the true value of d^{opt} is

$$\mathcal{V}(d^{opt}) = E\left\{\max_{a_1 \in \mathcal{A}_1} Q_1(H_1, a_1; \beta_{1,0})\right\}$$

$$= \beta_{11,0} + \beta_{12,0} E(H_1) + \beta_{13,0} I(\beta_{13,0} > 0),$$

and the estimator $\widehat{\mathcal{V}}_Q(d^{opt})$ solving (3.47) is

$$\widehat{\mathcal{V}}_Q(d^{opt}) = n^{-1} \sum_{i=1}^{n} \left\{\widehat{\beta}_{11} + \widehat{\beta}_{12} H_{1i} + \widehat{\beta}_{13} I(\widehat{\beta}_{13} > 0)\right\}$$

$$= \widehat{\beta}_{11} + \widehat{\beta}_{12}\overline{H}_1 + \widehat{\beta}_{13} I(\widehat{\beta}_{13} > 0), \quad \overline{H}_1 = n^{-1} \sum_{i=1}^{n} H_{1i},$$

where $\widehat{\beta}_1$ solves (3.48). Consequently,

$$n^{1/2}\left\{\widehat{\mathcal{V}}_Q(d^{opt}) - \mathcal{V}(d^{opt})\right\}$$

$$= n^{1/2}(\widehat{\beta}_{11} - \beta_{11,0}) + n^{1/2}(\widehat{\beta}_{12} - \beta_{12,0})E(H_1) \qquad (3.51)$$

$$+ n^{1/2}(\widehat{\beta}_{12} - \beta_{12,0})\{\overline{H}_1 - E(H_1)\} \qquad (3.52)$$

$$+ n^{1/2}\{\widehat{\beta}_{13} I(\widehat{\beta}_{13} > 0) - \beta_{13,0} I(\beta_{13,0} > 0)\}; \qquad (3.53)$$

and by the usual M-estimation theory,

$$n^{1/2}\begin{pmatrix} \widehat{\beta}_{11} - \beta_{11,0} \\ \widehat{\beta}_{12} - \beta_{12,0} \\ \widehat{\beta}_{13} - \beta_{13,0} \end{pmatrix} \xrightarrow{\mathcal{D}} \begin{pmatrix} Z_1 \\ Z_2 \\ Z_3 \end{pmatrix} \sim \mathcal{N}(0, \Sigma), \qquad (3.54)$$

where Z_1, Z_2, and Z_3 are random variables with joint normal distribution with mean zero and covariance matrix Σ. Regardless of the value of $\beta_{12,0}$, because $\overline{H}_1 - E(H_1) \xrightarrow{P} 0$, the term in (3.52) converges in probability to zero, and the terms in (3.51) converge in distribution to Z_1 and $Z_2 E(H_1)$, respectively.

Consider (3.53). The function $g(u) = u\,I(u > 0)$ is continuous for all u but, as noted above, is not differentiable at $u = 0$. If $\beta_{13,0} \neq 0$, then $g(u)$ is differentiable in an open interval containing $\beta_{13,0}$, so that a standard Taylor series (delta method) argument can be applied to (3.53) to conclude that this term converges in distribution to $g'(\beta_{13,0})Z_3$, where $g'(\beta_{13,0}) = \{dg(u)/du\}|_{u=\beta_{13,0}} = 0$ if $\beta_{13,0} < 0$ and $= 1$ if $\beta_{13,0} > 0$; i.e., $g'(\beta_{13,0}) = I(\beta_{13,0} > 0)$. Thus, because $n^{1/2}(\widehat{\beta}_{11} - \beta_{11,0})$, $n^{1/2}(\widehat{\beta}_{12} - $

$\beta_{12,0}$), and (3.53) converge jointly in distribution to $\{Z_1, Z_2, Z_3 \mathrm{I}(\beta_{13,0} > 0)\}^T$, by the continuous mapping theorem (e.g., van der Vaart, 2000, Theorem 2.3) and Slutsky's theorem,

$$n^{1/2} \left\{ \widehat{\mathcal{V}}_Q(d^{opt}) - \mathcal{V}(d^{opt}) \right\} \xrightarrow{\mathcal{D}} Z_1 + Z_2 E(H_1) + Z_3 \mathrm{I}(\beta_{13,0} > 0), \quad (3.55)$$

so that the large sample distribution of the left-hand side is the same as the distribution of the linear combination of jointly normal random variables on the right-hand side. Thus, when the true $\beta_{13,0} \neq 0$, the estimator for the value, $\widehat{\mathcal{V}}(d^{opt})$, is asymptotically normal with large sample distribution following from (3.55).

Now suppose that $\beta_{13,0} = 0$. Then (3.53) becomes

$$n^{1/2} \widehat{\beta}_{13} \mathrm{I}(\widehat{\beta}_{13} > 0),$$

and, from (3.54), $n^{1/2} \widehat{\beta}_{13} \xrightarrow{\mathcal{D}} Z_3$. Because $\mathrm{I}(\widehat{\beta}_{13} > 0) = \mathrm{I}(n^{1/2} \widehat{\beta}_{13} > 0)$, applying the continuous mapping and Slutsky's theorems, it follows that

$$n^{1/2} \left\{ \widehat{\mathcal{V}}_Q(d^{opt}) - \mathcal{V}(d^{opt}) \right\} \xrightarrow{\mathcal{D}} Z_1 + Z_2 E(H_1) + Z_3 \mathrm{I}(Z_3 > 0).$$

Thus, when the true coefficient of treatment in (3.49) $\beta_{13,0} = 0$, at which $\max_{a_1 \in \mathcal{A}_1} Q_1(h_1, a_1; \beta_1)$ in (3.50) is not differentiable, the large sample distribution of the left-hand side is the same as the distribution $Z_1 + Z_2 E(H_1) + Z_3 \mathrm{I}(Z_3 > 0)$, which, even though Z_1, Z_2, and Z_3 are jointly normal, is not normal. Under these conditions, then, the estimator $\widehat{\mathcal{V}}(d^{opt})$ does not follow conventional asymptotic theory.

These developments demonstrate that $\widehat{\mathcal{V}}_Q(d^{opt})$ is an example of a *nonregular* estimator. Although the estimator follows standard asymptotic theory when $\beta_{13,0} \neq 0$, the usual large sample normal approximation to its sampling distribution is not valid when $\beta_{13,0} = 0$. In (3.49) $\beta_{13,0} = 0$ corresponds to the situation where there is no difference in expected outcome between the two treatment options 0 and 1 for any h_1, which cannot be ruled out in practice. Thus, technically, it is not possible to disregard the behavior of the estimator at $\beta_{13,0} = 0$ and appeal to the standard theory, which complicates derivation of measures of uncertainty for estimators for the value of an optimal regime. Even if $\beta_{13,0} \neq 0$, so that the standard normal asymptotic theory does hold, if $\beta_{13,0}$ is close to zero, in finite samples the normal approximation can be poor, resulting in unreliable inference in practice.

Although we showed this problem in a simple special case, it is a general phenomenon resulting from the inherent nonsmoothness of (3.47) due to the max operator. Indeed, because an optimal dynamic treatment regime is characterized by the max operation, large sample properties of estimators for an optimal regime and its associated value by any other method, including those discussed in the next two sections, are subject to similar difficulties. This is a well-known challenge for inference for optimal dynamic treatment regimes. In Chapter 10, we discuss statistical inference in nonsmooth problems and approaches that have been advocated for circumventing this complication to derive valid inference.

3.5.2 Estimation via A-learning

In this and the next section, we restrict attention to $\mathcal{A}_1 = \{0, 1\}$ and for definiteness continue to take treatment option 0 to be the default. Under these conditions, from (3.40), an optimal regime involves a rule satisfying

$$d_1^{opt}(h_1) = I\{Q_1(h_1, 1) > Q_1(h_1, 0)\} = I\{Q_1(h_1, 1) - Q_1(h_1, 0) > 0\}.$$

The equivalent form of the rule on the far right-hand side shows that it depends on the *contrast function*

$$C_1(h_1) = Q_1(h_1, 1) - Q_1(h_1, 0), \tag{3.56}$$

so that the rule characterizing an optimal regime can be written as

$$d_1^{opt}(h_1) = I\{C_1(h_1) > 0\}. \tag{3.57}$$

The basic premise of the class of techniques for estimation of an optimal regime referred to as *advantage learning* or *A-learning* (Blatt et al., 2004) is that full knowledge of the function $Q_1(h_1, a_1)$ is not required to characterize and estimate an optimal regime. Rather, it suffices to consider only the contrast function (3.56). Because a_1 is a binary indicator, any arbitrary function $Q_1(h_1, a_1)$ can be written as

$$Q_1(h_1, a_1) = \nu_1(h_1) + a_1 C_1(h_1), \tag{3.58}$$

where $\nu_1(h_1) = Q_1(h_1, 0)$. From (3.58), $Q_1(h_1, a_1)$ is maximized by taking $a_1 = I\{C_1(h_1) > 0\}$, as required, so does not depend on $\nu_1(h_1)$; and the maximum itself is given by

$$V_1(h_1) = \nu_1(h_1) + C_1(h_1)I\{C_1(h_1) > 0\}. \tag{3.59}$$

Robins (2004) refers to $Q_1(h_1, a_1) - Q_1(h_1, 0) = a_1 C_1(h_1)$ as the *optimal blip to zero function*, which compares the expected difference in outcome between using the option coded as 0, viewed as a reference or control treatment, and using a_1 among patients with history h_1.

Motivated by these observations, A-learning methods are based on positing a model $C_1(h_1; \psi_1)$ for the contrast function, and thus the optimal blip to zero function, depending on a finite-dimensional parameter

ψ_1, and leaving $\nu_1(h_1)$ unspecified. This is equivalent to specifying a model for $Q_1(h_1, a_1)$ of the form

$$\nu_1(h_1) + a_1 C_1(h_1; \psi_1), \tag{3.60}$$

where $\nu_1(h_1)$ is an arbitrary function of h_1. Because only the contrast function component of (3.60) must be correctly specified to yield a valid estimator for d^{opt}, this approach is expected to enjoy some robustness relative to the regression-based method in the previous section (Q-learning), which requires correct specification of an entire model $Q_1(h_1, a_1; \beta_1)$.

As long as there is some value of ψ_1 for which $C_1(h_1; \psi_1) = 0$, the model (3.60) preserves the *causal null hypothesis* of no treatment effect; that is, there is no difference in expected outcome in the population between options 0 and 1. Specifically, when $C_1(h_1; \psi_1) = 0$, (3.60) implies that $Q_1(h_1, 1) = Q_1(h_1, 0) = \nu_1(h_1)$, where $\nu_1(h_1)$ is arbitrary, and thus $E\{Q_1(H_1, 1) - Q_1(H_1, 0)\} = 0$, so that the model includes the causal null hypothesis as a possibility. A model $C_1(h_1; \psi_1)$ with this property is the simplest example of a *structural nested mean model*; these models were originally proposed by Robins (1986) and in this context are a framework for estimating the average causal effect of a treatment option relative to a reference or control coded as 0.

Under this formulation of the problem, the goal is to estimate ψ_1 in $C_1(h_1; \psi_1)$ based on observed data (X_{1i}, A_{1i}, Y_i), $i = 1, \ldots, n$, for which SUTVA and the no unmeasured confounders and positivity assumptions hold. The fitted model for the contrast function can then be substituted in (3.57) to yield an estimator for an optimal regime.

We present a particular A-learning method for estimation of ψ_1 in a model $C_1(h_1; \psi_1)$ for the contrast function developed by Robins (2004) and referred to as *g-estimation*. As in Sections 3.3.2 and 3.3.3, let $\pi_1(h_1) = P(A_1 = 1 | H_1 = h_1)$ be the propensity score. Using the theory of semiparametrics (Robins et al., 1994; Tsiatis, 2006), assuming that the propensity score is known or correctly specified, Robins (2004) showed that all consistent and asymptotically normal estimators for ψ_1 solve an estimating equation of the form

$$\sum_{i=1}^{n} \lambda_1(H_{1i}) \{A_{1i} - \pi_1(H_{1i})\} \{Y_i - A_{1i} C_1(H_{1i}; \psi_1) + \theta_1(H_{1i})\} = 0 \tag{3.61}$$

for arbitrary function $\lambda_1(h_1)$ that is the same dimension as ψ_1 and arbitrary real-valued function $\theta_1(h_1)$.

It is straightforward to see that (3.61) is an M-estimating equation by observing that the estimating function in (3.61) is unbiased. Using the notation in Section 2.5 to denote expectation with respect to the distribution of the data evaluated at ψ_1,

$$
\begin{aligned}
E_{\psi_1}&[\lambda_1(H_1)\{A_1 - \pi_1(H_1)\}\{Y - A_1 C_1(H_1; \psi_1) + \theta_1(H_1)\}]\\
&= E_{\psi_1}[\lambda_1(H_1)\{A_1 - \pi_1(H_1)\}\\
&\qquad\qquad \times \{E_{\psi_1}(Y|H_1, A_1) - A_1 C_1(H_1; \psi_1) + \theta_1(H_1)\}]\\
&= E_{\psi_1}[\lambda_1(H_1)\{A_1 - \pi_1(H_1)\}\{\nu_1(H_1) + \theta_1(H_1)\}]\\
&= E_{\psi_1}\Big(E_{\psi_1}[\lambda_1(H_1)\{A_1 - \pi_1(H_1)\}\{\nu_1(H_1) + \theta_1(H_1)\}|H_1]\Big)\\
&= E_{\psi_1}[\lambda_1(H_1)\{E(A_1|H_1) - \pi_1(H_1)\}\{\nu_1(H_1) + \theta_1(H_1)\}]\\
&= 0, \qquad\qquad\qquad\qquad\qquad\qquad\qquad\qquad\qquad\qquad (3.62)
\end{aligned}
$$

where the first equality follows by an iterated conditional expectation given (H_1, A_1), the second follows by substituting the expression for $Q_1(H_1, A_1)$ in (3.60) for $E(Y|H_1, A_1)$, and (3.62) follows using the definition of the propensity score.

The specific functions $\lambda_1(h_1)$ and $\theta(h_1)$ that lead to the estimator for ψ_1 with smallest asymptotic variance among those solving an estimating equation of the form (3.61) follow from Robins (2004). The optimal choices in this sense are $\theta_1(h_1) = -\nu_1(h_1)$ and

$$
\lambda_1(h_1) = \frac{\partial C_1(h_1; \psi_1)}{\partial \psi_1}\Big[\{1 - \pi_1(h_1)\}v(h_1, 1) + \pi_1(h_1)v(h_1, 0)\Big]^{-1},
$$

where $v(h_1, a_1) = \mathrm{var}(Y|H_1 = h_1, A_1 = a_1)$, and $\pi_1(h_1)$ is the true propensity score. When $\mathrm{var}(Y|H_1, A_1)$ does not depend on H_1 or A_1 and is thus constant, the latter reduces to $\lambda_1(h_1) = \partial C_1(h_1; \psi_1)/\partial \psi_1$. In the following, we take $\mathrm{var}(Y|H_1, A_1)$ to be constant.

Of course, $\nu_1(h_1)$ is taken to be arbitrary in (3.60), which is the basis for the appeal of this approach. However, for the purpose of obtaining a consistent, asymptotically normal estimator for ψ_1, it is possible to proceed as follows. Posit a model for the true $\nu_1(h_1)$, $\nu_1(h_1; \phi_1)$, say, in terms of a finite-dimensional parameter ϕ_1, and estimate ϕ_1 jointly with ψ_1 in the model for the contrast function, $C_1(h_1; \psi_1)$, by solving the set of stacked estimating equations

$$
\sum_{i=1}^{n} \frac{\partial C_1(H_{1i}; \psi_1)}{\partial \psi_1} \{A_{1i} - \pi_1(H_{1i})\}
$$
$$
\times \{Y_i - A_{1i}C_1(H_{1i}; \psi_1) - \nu_1(H_{1i}; \phi_1)\} = 0 \qquad (3.63)
$$
$$
\sum_{i=1}^{n} \frac{\partial \nu_1(H_{1i}; \phi_1)}{\partial \phi_1} \{Y_i - A_{1i}C_1(H_{1i}; \psi_1) - \nu_1(H_{1i}; \phi_1)\} = 0. \qquad (3.64)
$$

As we now demonstrate, if the model for the contrast function is correctly specified, so that the true contrast function is $C_1(h_1; \psi_{1,0})$ for some $\psi_{1,0}$;

and the propensity score is known or correctly specified, even if the model $\nu_1(h_1; \phi_1)$ is not, the estimator $\widehat{\psi}_1$ solving these equations jointly with the estimator $\widehat{\phi}_1$ is a consistent, asymptotically normal estimator for the true value $\psi_{1,0}$ of ψ_1.

Suppose that the model $\nu_1(h_1; \phi_1)$ is misspecified. We show that $(\widehat{\psi}_1^T, \widehat{\phi}_1^T)^T$ solving the estimating equations converges in probability to $(\psi_{1,0}^T, \phi_1^{*T})^T$, where ϕ_1^* is the solution to

$$E\left[\frac{\partial \nu_1(H_1; \phi_1^*)}{\partial \phi_1}\{\nu_1(H_1) - \nu(H_1; \phi_1^*)\}\right] = 0. \tag{3.65}$$

From the theory of M-estimation, under regularity conditions, this follows if the estimating function corresponding to these estimating equations has mean zero when evaluated at $(\psi_{1,0}^T, \phi_1^{*T})$; that is, if

$$E\left[\frac{\partial C_1(H_1; \psi_{1,0})}{\partial \psi_1}\{A_1 - \pi_1(H_1)\}\right.$$
$$\left. \times \{Y - A_1 C_1(H_1; \psi_{1,0}) - \nu_1(H_1; \phi_1^*)\}\right] = 0 \tag{3.66}$$

$$E\left[\frac{\partial \nu_1(H_1; \phi_1^*)}{\partial \phi_1}\{Y - A_1 C_1(H_1; \psi_{1,0}) - \nu_1(H_1; \phi_1^*)\}\right] = 0. \tag{3.67}$$

Using iterated conditional expectations as above, conditioning on (H_1, A_1), the left-hand sides of (3.66) and (3.67) are equal to

$$E\left[\frac{\partial C_1(H_1; \psi_{1,0})}{\partial \psi_1}\{A_1 - \pi_1(H_1)\}\{\nu_1(H_1) - \nu_1(H_1; \phi_1^*)\}\right] \tag{3.68}$$

and

$$E\left[\frac{\partial \nu_1(H_1; \phi_1^*)}{\partial \phi_1}\{\nu_1(H_1) - \nu_1(H_1; \phi_1^*)\}\right], \tag{3.69}$$

respectively. The expectation in (3.69) is immediately seen to be equal to zero by the definition of ϕ_1^* in (3.65). Likewise, using an iterated conditional expectation given H_1, (3.68) is equal to

$$\left[\frac{\partial C_1(H_1; \psi_{1,0})}{\partial \psi_1}\{E(A_1|H_1) - \pi_1(H_1)\}\{\nu_1(H_1) - \nu_1(H_1; \phi_1^*)\}\right] = 0,$$

where we use the fact that the propensity score is correctly specified.

Thus, we conclude that $\widehat{\psi}_1$ solving the g-estimation equations (3.63)–(3.64) is a consistent and asymptotically normal estimator for the true value $\psi_{1,0}$ characterizing the true contrast function, regardless of whether or not the model $\nu_1(H_1; \phi_1)$ is misspecified. Note that if $\nu_1(h_1; \phi_1)$ is in fact also correctly specified, so that the true function $\nu_1(h_1) = \nu_1(h_1; \phi_{1,0})$ for some $\phi_{1,0}$, then $\phi_1^* = \phi_{1,0}$, and $\widehat{\phi}_1$ is a consistent and asymptotically normal estimator for $\phi_{1,0}$.

The foregoing discussion takes the propensity score $\pi_1(h_1)$ to be known and correctly specified. Although this may be the case in a randomized study, if the data are from an observational study, as in Sections 3.3.2 and 3.3.3, it is necessary to posit and fit a model $\pi_1(h_1; \gamma_1)$; for example, a logistic regression model as in (3.23), which could be fitted by maximum likelihood. In this case, assuming (3.23), the estimator for ψ_1 is found by solving jointly in $(\psi_1^T, \phi_1^T, \gamma_1^T)^T$ the stacked estimating equations

$$\sum_{i=1}^{n} \frac{\partial C_1(H_{1i}; \psi_1)}{\partial \psi_1} \{A_{1i} - \pi_1(H_{1i}; \gamma_1)\}$$

$$\times \{Y_i - A_{1i}C_1(H_{1i}; \psi_1) - \nu_1(H_{1i}; \phi_1)\} = 0$$

$$\sum_{i=1}^{n} \frac{\partial \nu_1(H_{1i}; \phi_1)}{\partial \phi_1} \{Y_i - A_{1i}C_1(H_{1i}; \psi_1) - \nu_1(H_{1i}; \phi_1)\} = 0 \quad (3.70)$$

$$\sum_{i=1}^{n} \begin{pmatrix} 1 \\ H_{1i} \end{pmatrix} \left\{ A_{1i} - \frac{\exp(\gamma_{11} + \gamma_{12}^T H_{1i})}{1 + \exp(\gamma_{11} + \gamma_{12}^T H_{1i})} \right\} = 0.$$

If the propensity score model is correctly specified, then the argument above can be extended to conclude that, if the model for the contrast function is correctly specified, $\widehat{\psi}_1$ solving these estimating equations jointly in $(\psi_1^T, \phi_1^T, \gamma_1^T)^T$ is a consistent and asymptotically normal estimator for $\psi_{1,0}$ even if the model $\nu_1(H_1; \phi_1)$ is misspecified. In fact, it is possible to show by similar manipulations that if, instead, the model $\nu_1(H_1; \phi_1)$ is correctly specified but the propensity score model $\pi_1(H_1; \gamma_1)$ is not, $\widehat{\psi}_1$ is a consistent and asymptotically normal estimator for $\psi_{1,0}$. In this sense, the estimator $\widehat{\psi}_1$ can be viewed as doubly robust: only one of the models $\nu_1(H_1; \phi_1)$ or $\pi_1(H_1; \gamma_1)$ need be correctly specified for $\widehat{\psi}_1$ to be a consistent and asymptotically normal estimator for $\psi_{1,0}$ characterizing the true contrast function.

Given $\widehat{\psi}_1$, from (3.57), the rule d_1^{opt} characterizing an optimal treatment regime can be estimated as

$$\widehat{d}_{A,1}^{opt}(h_1) = I\{C_1(h_1; \widehat{\psi}_1) > 0\}. \quad (3.71)$$

The estimator for d^{opt} is then given by

$$\widehat{d}_A^{opt} = \{\widehat{d}_{A,1}^{opt}(h_1)\},$$

where $\widehat{d}_{A,1}^{opt}(h_1)$ is as in (3.71).

Alternative estimating equations based on a different formulation are also possible. Murphy (2003) proposes an A-learning approach based on the so-called *advantage* or *regret function*

$$C_1(H_1) \left[I\{C_1(H_1) > 0\} - A_1 \right] \quad (3.72)$$

rather than the blip function. For an individual with history H_1 who receives treatment A_1, the advantage is the increase in expected outcome the individual would achieve if instead she received the optimal treatment option. That is, if $C_1(H_1) = Q_1(H_1, 1) - Q_1(H_1, 0) > 0$, then option 1 is the optimal decision for such an individual. If $A_1 = 1$, then the individual incurs no advantage, whereas if $A_1 = 0$, the advantage is $C_1(H_1)$. Conversely, if $Q_1(H_1, 1) - Q_1(H_1, 0) \leq 0$, option 0 is the optimal decision, and the individual would incur no advantage if $A_1 = 0$, while if $A_1 = 1$, the advantage would be $-C_1(H_1)$. This leads to (3.72), representing the "advantage" in expected outcome if the optimal option were given relative to that actually received, or, equivalently, the "regret" incurred by not using the optimal option. Note that (3.72) depends on the contrast function. Murphy (2003) and Blatt et al. (2004) develop A-learning methods based on direct modeling of the advantage function rather than the contrast function. These methods and the relationship between them and the g-estimation approach presented here, based on direct modeling of the contrast function, including the relationship between advantage and blip functions, are discussed and compared by Robins (2004) and Moodie et al. (2007).

Remark. As discussed by Chakraborty et al. (2010) and Schulte et al. (2014), in certain special cases, the regression-based (Q-learning) estimator for an optimal regime and the estimator obtained via the A-learning method presented above are identical. This holds if the propensity score $\pi_1(h_1) = P(A_1 = 1 | H_1 = h_1)$ does not depend on h_1, as in a randomized study; and the regression model $Q_1(h_1, a_1; \beta_1)$ and the model for $Q_1(h_1, a_1)$ implied by the models $C_1(h_1; \psi_1)$ and $\nu_1(h_1; \phi_1)$ are linear in functions of h_1 and are compatible in the sense that $Q_1(h_1, a_1; \beta_1)$ and

$$\nu_1(h_1; \phi_1) + a_1 C_1(h_1; \psi_1)$$

are of the same functional form. For example, this is the case when $Q_1(h_1, a_1; \beta_1) = \beta_{11} + \beta_{12}^T h_1 + \beta_{13} a_1 + \beta_{14}^T h_1 a_1$ as in (3.42) and

$$\nu_1(h_1; \phi_1) = \phi_{11} + \phi_{12}^T h_1, \qquad C_1(h_1; \psi_1) = \psi_{11} + \psi_{12}^T h_1. \qquad (3.73)$$

Under these conditions, with $\pi(h_1) = \gamma_1$, a constant; $\text{var}(Y|H_1, A_1)$ not depending on H_1 or A_1; and thus $\lambda_1(h_1) = \partial C_1(h_1; \psi_1)/\partial \psi_1$, the A-learning estimating equations (3.63)–(3.64) become

$$\sum_{i=1}^n \frac{\partial C_1(H_{1i}; \psi_1)}{\partial \psi_1}(A_{1i} - \gamma_1)\{Y_i - A_{1i}C_1(H_{1i}; \psi_1) - \nu_1(H_{1i}; \phi_1)\} = 0$$

$$(3.74)$$

$$\sum_{i=1}^n \frac{\partial \nu_1(H_{1i}; \phi_1)}{\partial \phi_1}\{Y_i - A_{1i}C_1(H_{1i}; \psi_1) - \nu_1(H_{1i}; \phi_1)\} = 0.$$

Writing $\beta_1 = (\phi_1^T, \psi_1^T)^T$ and

$$Q_1(h_1, a_1; \beta_1) = \nu_1(h_1; \phi_1) + a_1 C_1(h_1; \psi_1),$$

the OLS estimating equation for β_1 assuming that $\text{var}(Y|H_1, A_1)$ is constant is, from (3.48),

$$\sum_{i=1}^{n} \frac{\partial Q_1(H_{1i}, A_i; \beta_1)}{\partial \beta_1} \{Y_i - A_{1i} C_1(H_{1i}; \psi_1) - \nu_1(H_{1i}; \phi_1)\} = 0,$$

where

$$\frac{\partial Q_1(H_{1i}, A_i; \beta_1)}{\partial \beta_1} = \begin{pmatrix} A_{1i} \dfrac{\partial C_1(H_{1i}; \psi_1)}{\partial \psi_1} \\ \dfrac{\partial \nu_1(H_{1i}; \phi_1)}{\partial \phi_1} \end{pmatrix}.$$

Then, as long as terms of the form in $C_1(h_1; \psi_1)$ are contained in $\nu_1(h_1; \phi_1)$, as in (3.73),

$$\sum_{i=1}^{n} \frac{\partial C_1(H_{1i}; \psi_1)}{\partial \psi_1} \{Y_i - A_{1i} C_1(H_{1i}; \psi_1) - \nu_1(H_{1i}; \phi_1)\} = 0.$$

Substituting this in (3.74) shows that the estimating equations for $\beta_1 = (\phi_1^T, \psi_1^T)^T$ are identical. It follows that the resulting estimators for d^{opt} are also identical.

We conclude this section by discussing estimation of the value $\mathcal{V}(d^{opt})$ following estimation of d^{opt} via A-learning methods. Recall from (3.41) that

$$\mathcal{V}(d^{opt}) = E\{V_1(H_1)\} = E\left\{ \max_{a_1 \in \mathcal{A}_1} Q(H_1, a_1) \right\}.$$

Because the premise of A-learning is that only a model for the contrast or the advantage function need be specified, we cannot appeal to this definition directly. However, as we now demonstrate, the value function $V_1(H_1)$ can be expressed in terms of the advantage function, which leads to an estimator for $\mathcal{V}(d^{opt})$.

Note that

$$E\left(Y + C_1(H_1)[I\{C_1(H_1) > 0\} - A_1] \,\Big|\, H_1\right)$$
$$= E\left\{ E\left(Y + C_1(H_1)[I\{C_1(H_1) > 0\} - A_1] \,\Big|\, H_1, A_1\right) \,\Big|\, H_1 \right\}$$
$$= E\left(E(Y|H_1, A_1) + C_1(H_1)[I\{C_1(H_1) > 0\} - A_1] \,\Big|\, H_1 \right)$$
$$= E\left(Q_1(H_1, 0) + A_1 C_1(H_1) + C_1(H_1)[I\{C_1(H_1) > 0\} - A_1] \,\Big|\, H_1 \right)$$

$$= E[Q_1(H_1,0) + C_1(H_1)I\{C_1(H_1) > 0\}|H_1]$$
$$= Q_1(H_1,0) + C_1(H_1)I\{C_1(H_1) > 0\} = V_1(H_1)$$

almost surely by (3.59). Then an obvious estimator for $\mathcal{V}(d^{opt})$ is

$$\widehat{\mathcal{V}}_A(d^{opt}) = n^{-1} \sum_{i=1}^{n} \left(Y_i + C_1(H_{1i}; \widehat{\psi}_1) \left[I\{C_1(H_{1i}; \widehat{\psi}_1) > 0\} - A_{1i} \right] \right),$$
$$(3.75)$$

where $\widehat{\psi}_1$ is obtained via an A-learning method.

As in the previous section, although in principle (3.75) can be reexpressed in the form of an estimating equation and "stacked" with the estimating equations for A-learning, appealing to the usual M-estimation theory to derive large sample properties of $\widehat{\mathcal{V}}_A(d^{opt})$ in (3.75) is subject to the same considerations discussed at the end of Section 3.5.1. In particular, the advantage function, on which (3.75) depends, with a model for the contrast function depending on ψ_1 substituted, is not differentiable for all values of ψ_1. Thus, $\widehat{\mathcal{V}}_A(d^{opt})$ in (3.75) is a nonregular estimator.

3.5.3 Value Search Estimation

We continue to take $\mathcal{A}_1 = \{0, 1\}$, with treatment option 0 the default. The methods for estimation of an optimal dynamic treatment regime in the previous two sections are based on posited models for either the entire regression relationship $Q_1(h_1, a_1) = E(Y|H_1 = h_1, A_1 = a_1)$ or for the contrast function $C_1(h_1) = Q_1(h_1, 1) - Q_1(h_1, 0)$. Thus, in both approaches, the form of the posited model dictates the form of the rules d_1^{opt} under consideration.

For example, suppose that $h_1 = x_1 = (x_{11}, x_{12})^T$, where x_{11} and x_{12} are scalar baseline covariates, and we posit

$$Q_1(h_1, a_1; \beta_1) = \beta_{11} + \beta_{12}x_{11} + \beta_{13}x_{12} + a_1(\beta_{14} + \beta_{15}x_{11} + \beta_{16}x_{12}). \quad (3.76)$$

It follows that the rule d_1^{opt} implied by this model is of the form

$$d_1^{opt}(h_1) = I(\beta_{14} + \beta_{15}x_{11} + \beta_{16}x_{12} > 0). \quad (3.77)$$

Similarly, if we were to posit the contrast function model

$$C_1(h_1; \psi_1) = \psi_{11} + \psi_{12}x_{11} + \psi_{13}x_{12}, \quad (3.78)$$

the implied rule is of the form

$$d_1^{opt}(h_1) = I(\psi_{11} + \psi_{12}x_{11} + \psi_{13}x_{12} > 0). \quad (3.79)$$

Both (3.77) and (3.79) are in the form of a hyperplane in two-dimensional space determined by the values of $(\beta_{14}, \beta_{15}, \beta_{16})^T$ or $(\psi_{11}, \psi_{12}, \psi_{13})^T$, respectively, so that the treatment option assigned depends on which side of the hyperplane an individual's covariates (x_{11}, x_{12}) lie.

This demonstrates that a posited model for the regression relationship or contrast function induces a *class* of regimes, $\mathcal{D}_\eta$, indexed by a parameter η, say, in which the search for an optimal regime is implicitly restricted. In the above example, $\mathcal{D}_\eta$ is the class of all regimes characterized by rules of the form

$$d_1(h_1; \eta_1) = \mathrm{I}(\eta_{11} + \eta_{12}x_{11} + \eta_{13}x_{12} > 0), \quad \eta_1 = (\eta_{11}, \eta_{12}, \eta_{13})^T \in \mathbb{R}^3,$$
$$(3.80)$$

which are indexed by values of η_1. Here, the subscript "1" emphasizes that η_1 corresponds to rules for the single decision point under consideration. In our discussion of multiple decision problems involving K rules later in the book, η is the collection of K parameters corresponding to the K rules. Consistent with this convention, here, with $K = 1$ decision, η comprises the single parameter η_1; that is, $\eta = \eta_1$.

Because the chosen model restricts consideration to the induced class $\mathcal{D}_\eta$, of concern are the consequences of positing a model that is incorrectly specified. For definiteness, continue to let $h_1 = (x_{11}, x_{12})^T$, and suppose that the true outcome regression relationship is

$$E(Y|H_1 = h_1, A_1 = a_1)$$
$$= \exp\{1 + x_{11} + 2x_{12} + 3x_{11}x_{12} + a_1(1 - 2x_{11} + x_{12})\}. \quad (3.81)$$

It is straightforward to deduce that the true rule d_1^{opt} characterizing an optimal regime $d^{opt} \in \mathcal{D}$ is

$$d_1^{opt}(h_1) = \mathrm{I}(1 - 2x_{11} + x_{12} > 0), \tag{3.82}$$

so that a true optimal regime in the class of all regimes $\mathcal{D}$ is contained in the class $\mathcal{D}_\eta$ comprising regimes with rules of the form (3.80). Suppose that we posit a linear model of the form (3.76). This model is incorrectly specified, as there is no value of β_1 such that the model coincides with the true relationship (3.81). Even though the model is misspecified, it implies rules of the form (3.77); thus, it induces the class $\mathcal{D}_\eta$ containing a true optimal regime characterized by the rule (3.82). However, if we were to fit the model (3.76) using, e.g., OLS, to obtain the estimator $\widehat{\beta}_1$, the estimated optimal regime characterized by the estimated rule

$$\widehat{d}_{Q,1}^{opt}(h_1) = \mathrm{I}\{\widehat{\beta}_{14} + \widehat{\beta}_{15}x_{11} + \widehat{\beta}_{16}x_{12} > 0\}$$

may be a poor estimator for d_1^{opt} in (3.82). This is because $\widehat{\beta}_1$ is unlikely to reflect the true values of the coefficients in the exponential function characterizing the true regression relationship (3.81) and thus those in the true rule (3.82). Similar considerations apply when the contrast function is modeled as in (3.78).

Indeed, if we posit an incorrect model for $Q_1(h_1, a_1)$ or $C_1(h_1)$ that does not imply rules of the form (3.80), the class of regimes induced by the model does not contain $d^{opt} \in \mathcal{D}$ characterized by the true rule (3.82). In this case, it is clear that the estimated optimal regime based on the misspecified model is possibly quite far from a true optimal regime in $\mathcal{D}$.

This discussion suggests a different perspective on deducing an optimal regime. Because estimation of an optimal regime in $\mathcal{D}$ using the methods in the previous two sections is predicated on correct specification of models for the outcome regression relationship or contrast function, identifying an optimal regime d^{opt} within the class $\mathcal{D}$ of all possible regimes is challenging. A more realistic and practically relevant objective is to restrict attention directly to a class of regimes $\mathcal{D}_\eta \subset \mathcal{D}$, indexed by a parameter η, whether or not $\mathcal{D}_\eta$ contains d^{opt}, and to focus on estimation of an optimal regime within the restricted class $\mathcal{D}_\eta$.

As above, the class $\mathcal{D}_\eta$ can be motivated by a posited model. Alternatively, $\mathcal{D}_\eta$ can be based on scientific and practical considerations related to implementation of an optimal regime, such as cost, feasibility, or interpretability. For instance, regimes that involve thresholds for the values of components of h_1 may be more straightforward to implement in practice and more interpretable by clinicians and patients than regimes based on hyperplanes and thus on linear combinations of functions of patient covariates. For example, with $h_1 = (x_{11}, x_{12})^T$ as above, $\mathcal{D}_\eta$ might be taken to comprise regimes characterized by rules of the form

$$d_1(h_1; \eta_1) = \mathrm{I}(x_{11} < \eta_{11}, x_{12} < \eta_{12}), \qquad \eta_1 = (\eta_{11}, \eta_{12})^T \in \mathbb{R}^2, \quad (3.83)$$

so involving rectangular regions in the covariate space defined by the thresholds η_{11} and η_{12}; here, the form of $d_1(h_1; \eta_1)$ presupposes that option 1 is favored for smaller values of x_{11} and x_{12}. Alternatively, for one-dimensional $h_1 = x_1$, the class $\mathcal{D}_\eta$ of regimes defined by rules

$$d_1(h_1; \eta_1) = \mathrm{I}(h_1 \geq \eta_{11})\eta_{12} + \mathrm{I}(h_1 < \eta_{11})(1 - \eta_{12})$$

for $\eta_{11} \in \mathbb{R}$ and $\eta_{12} \in \{0, 1\}$ allows either treatment option to be selected if h_1 exceeds or falls below a real-valued threshold. Likewise, if h_1 is high dimensional and contains components that are not collected routinely in practice and the goal is to develop an optimal regime for use in a resource limited setting, it is natural to restrict attention to a class $\mathcal{D}_\eta$ with elements characterized by rules that depend in a simple way on only a key subset of the components of h_1.

In general, if we deliberately restrict attention to a class of regimes $\mathcal{D}_\eta$, with elements $d_\eta = \{d_1(h_1; \eta_1)\}$, where the form of the rules

$d_1(h_1; \eta_1)$ is chosen based on the above considerations, then it is of interest to estimate an *optimal restricted regime* d_η^{opt} in $\mathcal{D}_\eta$, where d_η^{opt} is characterized by the rule

$$d_1(h_1; \eta_1^{opt}), \quad \eta_1^{opt} = \arg\max_{\eta_1} \mathcal{V}(d_\eta), \qquad (3.84)$$

so that

$$d_\eta^{opt} = \{d_1(h_1; \eta_1^{opt})\}.$$

That is, an optimal restricted regime in $\mathcal{D}_\eta$ is one that achieves the maximum value among all regimes in $\mathcal{D}_\eta$, which is attained when $\eta_1 = \eta_1^{opt}$. Thus, estimating an optimal regime in $\mathcal{D}_\eta$ is equivalent to estimating η_1^{opt} defined in (3.84).

If the class $\mathcal{D}_\eta$ is induced by a posited outcome regression or contrast function model, it is natural to consider estimation of η_1^{opt} by fitting the model assuming it is correct and substituting the resulting estimator $\widehat{\eta}_1$ in $d_1(h_1; \eta_1)$. However, if the posited model is misspecified, the estimator $\widehat{\eta}_1$ may be far from the value η_1^{opt} that satisfies (3.84).

This suggests an alternative approach based on the definition of η_1^{opt} in (3.84). Given an estimator for the value of a fixed regime d, $\widehat{\mathcal{V}}(d)$, say, the idea is to estimate $\mathcal{V}(d_\eta)$ by $\widehat{\mathcal{V}}(d_\eta)$ for any fixed $\eta = \eta_1$, treat $\widehat{\mathcal{V}}(d_\eta)$ as a function of η_1, and then maximize $\widehat{\mathcal{V}}(d_\eta)$ in η_1; that is, estimate η_1^{opt} by

$$\widehat{\eta}_1^{opt} = \arg\max_{\eta_1} \widehat{\mathcal{V}}(d_\eta). \qquad (3.85)$$

The estimator for the rule $d_1(h_1; \eta_1^{opt})$ characterizing an optimal regime in $\mathcal{D}_\eta$ is then

$$d_1(h_1; \widehat{\eta}_1^{opt}), \qquad (3.86)$$

and the estimator $\widehat{d}_\eta^{opt}$ for an optimal regime d_η^{opt} in $\mathcal{D}_\eta$ defined by (3.85) and (3.86) is

$$\widehat{d}_\eta^{opt} = \{d_1(h_1, \widehat{\eta}_1^{opt})\}.$$

We refer to $\widehat{d}_\eta^{opt}$ as a *value search estimator*, as this approach involves searching over the parameter space of $\eta = \eta_1$ for $\widehat{\eta}_1^{opt}$ maximizing an estimator of the value $\widehat{\mathcal{V}}(d_\eta)$. This estimator has also been referred to as a *direct* or *policy search* estimator; the latter term arises from analogous work in computer science, where a dynamic treatment regime is referred to as a policy in the literature on reinforcement learning. We discuss this connection further in Chapters 5 and 7.

As proposed by Zhang et al. (2012b), it is natural to base this on the inverse probability weighted and augmented inverse probability weighted estimators for the value of a fixed regime d, $\widehat{\mathcal{V}}_{IPW}(d)$ and $\widehat{\mathcal{V}}_{AIPW}(d)$, respectively, introduced in Sections 3.3.2 and 3.3.3. Specifically, consider a regime $d_\eta \in \mathcal{D}_\eta$ for fixed $\eta = \eta_1$ characterized by rule $d_1(h_1; \eta_1)$. Analogous to (3.18), (3.19), and (3.21), let

$$\mathcal{C}_{d_\eta} = I\{A_1 = d_1(H_1; \eta_1)\}, \tag{3.87}$$

which depends on η_1; and let

$$\pi_{d_\eta,1}(H_1; \eta_1, \gamma_1) \tag{3.88}$$
$$= \pi_1(H_1; \gamma_1)I\{d_1(H_1; \eta_1) = 1\} + \{1 - \pi_1(H_1; \gamma_1)\}I\{d_1(H_1; \eta_1) = 0\}$$

be a model for $P(\mathcal{C}_{d_\eta} = 1 | H_1)$, which is induced by a model $\pi_1(h_1; \gamma_1)$ for the propensity score. Thus, for this fixed $\eta = \eta_1$, $\mathcal{C}_{d_\eta}$ in (3.87) is the indicator of whether or not the treatment option actually received by an individual with history H_1 coincides with the option dictated by regime d_η, and (3.88) is the propensity for receiving treatment consistent with d_η given an individual's history.

With these definitions, from (3.24), a simple inverse probability weighted estimator for $\mathcal{V}(d_\eta)$ for fixed $\eta = \eta_1$ is

$$\widehat{\mathcal{V}}_{IPW}(d_\eta) = n^{-1} \sum_{i=1}^{n} \frac{\mathcal{C}_{d_\eta,i} Y_i}{\pi_{d_\eta,1}(H_{1i}; \eta_1, \widehat{\gamma}_1)}, \tag{3.89}$$

where $\widehat{\gamma}_1$ is an estimator for γ_1 as before. As in Section 3.3.2, under SUTVA and the no unmeasured confounders and positivity assumptions and with the propensity score model $\pi_1(h_1; \gamma_1)$ correctly specified, (3.89) is a consistent estimator for the true value $\mathcal{V}(d_\eta)$ of d_η for fixed η. As for (3.24), if the data are from a randomized study, the form of $\pi_1(h_1; \gamma_1)$ is known, guaranteeing that the estimator $\widehat{\mathcal{V}}_{IPW}(d_\eta)$ is consistent for the true $\mathcal{V}(d_\eta)$ in this case.

Similarly, following the developments in Section 3.3.3, from (3.30), the augmented inverse probability weighted estimator corresponding to the efficient estimator for $\mathcal{V}(d_\eta)$ for fixed $\eta = \eta_1$ is

$$\widehat{\mathcal{V}}_{AIPW}(d_\eta) = n^{-1} \sum_{i=1}^{n} \left[\frac{\mathcal{C}_{d_\eta,i} Y_i}{\pi_{d_\eta,1}(H_{1i}; \eta_1, \widehat{\gamma}_1)} \right. \tag{3.90}$$
$$\left. - \frac{\mathcal{C}_{d_\eta,i} - \pi_{d_\eta,1}(H_{1i}; \eta_1, \widehat{\gamma}_1)}{\pi_{d_\eta,1}(H_{1i}; \eta_1, \widehat{\gamma}_1)} \mathcal{Q}_{d_\eta,1}(H_{1i}; \eta_1, \widehat{\beta}_1) \right],$$

where

$$\mathcal{Q}_{d_\eta,1}(H_1; \eta_1, \beta_1) = Q_1(H_1, 1; \beta_1)I\{d_1(H_1; \eta_1) = 1\} \tag{3.91}$$
$$+ Q_1(H_1, 0; \beta_1)I\{d_1(H_1; \eta_1) = 0\},$$

$Q_1(h_1, a_1; \beta_1)$ is a model for $Q_1(h_1, a_1) = E(Y | H_1 = h_1, A_1 = a_1)$ as

before, and $\widehat{\beta}_1$ is a suitable estimator for β_1. Under SUTVA and the no
unmeasured confounders and positivity assumptions and for fixed η, as
in Section 3.3.3, (3.90) is a consistent estimator for the true value $\mathcal{V}(d_\eta)$
if either the propensity score model $\pi_1(h_1; \gamma_1)$ or the outcome regression
model $Q_1(h_1, a_1; \beta_1)$ is correctly specified, so is doubly robust. If both
models are correctly specified, then the estimator $\widehat{\mathcal{V}}_{AIPW}(d_\eta)$ for fixed
$\eta = \eta_1$ has smallest asymptotic variance among augmented estimators
of the form (3.27), as in the discussion following (3.30). As for (3.30), if
the data are from a randomized study, so that the form of $\pi_1(h_1; \gamma_1)$ is
known, double robustness ensures that $\widehat{\mathcal{V}}_{AIPW}(d_\eta)$ is consistent for the
true value $\mathcal{V}(d_\eta)$, regardless of whether or not the outcome regression
model is correct.

Zhang et al. (2012b) advocate maximizing $\widehat{\mathcal{V}}_{IPW}(d_\eta)$ or $\widehat{\mathcal{V}}_{AIPW}(d_\eta)$
in $\eta = \eta_1$ to obtain $\widehat{\eta}_{1,IPW}^{opt}$ or $\widehat{\eta}_{1,AIPW}^{opt}$, respectively, and then estimating
the rule characterizing an optimal regime by substitution in $d_1(h_1; \eta_1)$
as in (3.86), leading to the competing estimators

$$\widehat{d}_{\eta,IPW}^{opt} = \{d_1(h_1, \widehat{\eta}_{1,IPW}^{opt})\} \quad \text{and} \quad \widehat{d}_{\eta,AIPW}^{opt} = \{d_1(h_1, \widehat{\eta}_{1,AIPW}^{opt})\}$$

for an optimal regime $d_\eta^{opt} \in \mathcal{D}_\eta$ as above. The associated value achieved
by d_η^{opt}, $\mathcal{V}(d_\eta^{opt})$, can be estimated in the obvious way by substituting $\widehat{\eta}_{1,IPW}^{opt}$ or $\widehat{\eta}_{1,AIPW}^{opt}$ for η_1 in (3.89) or (3.90) to yield estimators
$\widehat{\mathcal{V}}_{IPW}(d_\eta^{opt})$ and $\widehat{\mathcal{V}}_{AIPW}(d_\eta^{opt})$.

Intuition suggests that the estimator $\widehat{d}_{\eta,AIPW}^{opt}$ based on maximiz-
ing $\widehat{\mathcal{V}}_{AIPW}(d_\eta)$ should be of higher quality than $\widehat{d}_{\eta,IPW}^{opt}$ maximizing
$\widehat{\mathcal{V}}_{IPW}(d_\eta)$ in some sense, given that $\widehat{\mathcal{V}}_{AIPW}(d_\eta)$ is a more efficient and
stable estimator for the true value. This is borne out in simulation stud-
ies reported by Zhang et al. (2012b), which demonstrate that using the
estimated regime $\widehat{d}_{\eta,AIPW}^{opt}$ to assign treatment in the simulated population results in higher average outcome, approaching the true value
$\mathcal{V}(d_\eta^{opt})$ achieved by d_η^{opt}, than that achieved using $\widehat{d}_{\eta,IPW}^{opt}$.

Similarly, $\widehat{\mathcal{V}}_{AIPW}(d_\eta^{opt})$ is expected to be a more efficient estimator
for $\mathcal{V}(d_\eta^{opt})$ than $\widehat{\mathcal{V}}_{IPW}(d_\eta^{opt})$. The simulations performed by Zhang et al.
(2012b) also support this contention. Moreover, these authors present
evidence that $\widehat{\mathcal{V}}_{AIPW}(d_\eta^{opt})$ exhibits double robustness as predicted by
the theory when one of the propensity or outcome regression models is
misspecified. In their simulation studies, this estimator yields a Monte
Carlo average that is almost identical to the true value $\mathcal{V}(d_\eta^{opt})$ of d_η^{opt},
while that based on $\widehat{\mathcal{V}}_{IPW}(d_\eta^{opt})$ overestimates the true value, even when
the propensity score model is correctly specified. This is likely a conse-
quence of the instability of simple inverse weighting, as discussed earlier.

It is possible to generalize the foregoing developments to the case where $\mathcal{A}_1$ comprises a finite, arbitrary number of treatment options. We defer discussion of this formulation and of inverse probability weighted and augmented inverse probability weighted estimators analogous to (3.89) and (3.90) to Section 3.5.5.

In contrast to regression-based (Q-learning) estimation of the value and that based on A-learning in Sections 3.5.1 and 3.5.2, estimation of the value by $\widehat{\mathcal{V}}_{IPW}(d_\eta^{opt})$ and $\widehat{\mathcal{V}}_{AIPW}(d_\eta^{opt})$ cannot be cast as the solving a set of stacked M-estimating equations, as these estimators are obtained by maximizing the objective functions (3.89) or (3.90) in η_1 and substituting the result, which cannot be expressed in this way. This precludes a direct demonstration of nonstandard asymptotic behavior of $\widehat{\mathcal{V}}_{IPW}(d_\eta^{opt})$ and $\widehat{\mathcal{V}}_{AIPW}(d_\eta^{opt})$ like that at the end of Section 3.5.1 for the regression-based estimator. However, that these estimators do not follow conventional asymptotic theory can be appreciated by examining the true value $\mathcal{V}(d_\eta^{opt})$, as can be seen in the following simple example.

Example: Nonregularity of $\widehat{\mathcal{V}}_{IPW}(d_\eta^{opt})$ and $\widehat{\mathcal{V}}_{AIPW}(d_\eta^{opt})$

Suppose that H_1 is one dimensional and satisfies $H_1 \sim \mathcal{N}(0,1)$ and that we take the restricted class $\mathcal{D}_\eta$ to comprise regimes d_η characterized by rules of the form

$$d_1(h_1; \eta) = I(h_1 > \eta_1), \quad \eta_1 \in \mathbb{R}. \qquad (3.92)$$

Thus, regimes in $\mathcal{D}_\eta$ select treatment option 0 or 1 depending on the value of h_1 relative to a real-valued threshold η_1, where it is assumed a priori that option 1 is favored for larger values of h_1. Suppose further that Y is a continuous outcome and that the true outcome regression relationship is

$$Q_1(h_1, a_1) = E(Y|H_1 = h_1, A_1 = a_1)$$
$$= \beta_{11,0} + \beta_{12,0}h_1 + \beta_{13,0}a_1 + \beta_{14,0}h_1a_1,$$

where $(\beta_{11,0}, \beta_{12,0}, \beta_{13,0}, \beta_{14,0})^T$ are the true values of the coefficients in $Q_1(h_1, a_1)$, and $\beta_{14,0} \geq 0$. Thus, an optimal regime in $\mathcal{D}_\eta$ is characterized by the threshold η_1^{opt} maximizing the value $\mathcal{V}(d_\eta)$ in η_1, where d_η is a fixed regime in $\mathcal{D}_\eta$ characterized by a rule of the form (3.92). It follows from (3.11) that

$$\mathcal{V}(d_\eta) = E\Big[\{\beta_{11,0} + \beta_{12,0}H_1 + \beta_{13,0} + \beta_{14,0}H_1\}I(H_1 > \eta_1)$$
$$+ \{\beta_{11,0} + \beta_{12,0}H_1\}\{1 - I(H_1 > \eta_1)\}\Big]$$
$$= \beta_{11,0} + \beta_{12,0}E(H_1) + \beta_{13,0}E\{I(H_1 > \eta_1)\} + \beta_{14,0}E\{H_1I(H_1 > \eta_1)\}$$
$$= \beta_{11,0} + \beta_{13,0}\{1 - \Phi(\eta_1)\} + \beta_{14,0}\varphi(\eta_1), \qquad (3.93)$$

where $\Phi(\cdot)$ and $\varphi(\cdot)$ are the cumulative distribution function and density of the standard normal distribution, respectively. From (3.93), $\mathcal{V}(d_\eta)$ is a smooth function in η_1, and it is straightforward that

$$\frac{\partial \mathcal{V}(d_\eta)}{\partial \eta_1} = -(\beta_{13,0} + \beta_{14,0}\eta_1)\varphi(\eta_1) \tag{3.94}$$

$$\frac{\partial^2 \mathcal{V}(d_\eta)}{\partial \eta_1^2} = (\beta_{14,0}\eta_1^2 + \beta_{13,0}\eta_1 - \beta_{14,0})\varphi(\eta_1). \tag{3.95}$$

Consider the behavior of $\mathcal{V}(d_\eta)$ in (3.93). First suppose that $\beta_{14,0} = 0$, so that (3.93) reduces to

$$\mathcal{V}(d_\eta) = \beta_{11,0} + \beta_{13,0}\{1 - \Phi(\eta_1)\}.$$

If $\beta_{13,0} > 0$, it is immediate that there is no unique maximum of $\mathcal{V}(d_\eta)$ in $-\infty < \eta_1 < \infty$, as $\Phi(\eta_1) \to 0$ as $\eta_1 \to -\infty$, so that $\mathcal{V}(d_\eta)$ approaches its largest possible value as $\eta_1 \to -\infty$. In this case, an optimal regime dictates that all individuals in the population should receive treatment option 1, regardless of their h_1. Analogously, if $\beta_{13,0} < 0$, there is also no unique maximum, as $\Phi(\eta_1) \to 1$ as $\eta_1 \to \infty$, and an optimal regime dictates that all individuals in the population should receive option 0. If $\beta_{13,0} = 0$, then $\mathcal{V}(d_\eta)$ is constant for all values of η_1, and again there is no unique maximum, and selection of a treatment option is ambiguous. Thus, when $\beta_{14,0} = 0$, $\mathcal{V}(d_\eta)$ does not have a unique maximum in η_1, so that η_1^{opt} and thus an optimal regime $d_\eta^{opt} \in \mathcal{D}_\eta$ and corresponding $\mathcal{V}(d_\eta^{opt})$ are not well defined. It follows that standard asymptotic theory, which requires these quantities to be well defined, cannot be applied to yield approximations to the large sample behavior of $\widehat{\mathcal{V}}_{IPW}(d_\eta^{opt})$ and $\widehat{\mathcal{V}}_{AIPW}(d_\eta^{opt})$.

Suppose instead that $\beta_{14,0} > 0$. Setting (3.94) equal to zero yields $\eta_1 = -\beta_{13,0}/\beta_{14,0}$. It is immediate that this value of η_1 corresponds to a unique maximum of $\mathcal{V}(d_\eta)$, as it can be verified that (3.95) evaluated at this value of η_1 is less than zero. Thus, η_1^{opt} and an optimal regime $d_\eta^{opt} \in \mathcal{D}_\eta$ and $\mathcal{V}(d_\eta^{opt})$ are well defined. Under these conditions, namely, that $\mathcal{V}(d_\eta)$ is a smooth function in η_1 with a unique maximum, Zhang et al. (2012b) sketch a heuristic argument demonstrating that standard asymptotic results can be applied to deduce an approximate normal sampling distribution for either estimator $\widehat{\mathcal{V}}_{IPW}(d_\eta^{opt})$ or $\widehat{\mathcal{V}}_{AIPW}(d_\eta^{opt})$ whose variance can be estimated using the sandwich technique.

Summarizing these developments, for $\mathcal{D}_\eta$ comprising regimes characterized by rules as in (3.92), as long as $\beta_{14,0} > 0$, $\widehat{\mathcal{V}}_{IPW}(d_\eta^{opt})$ and $\widehat{\mathcal{V}}_{AIPW}(d_\eta^{opt})$ have standard asymptotic theory, but this is not the case if $\beta_{14,0} = 0$. Because $\beta_{14,0} = 0$ (and $\beta_{13,0} \neq 0$) corresponds to the situation that all individuals in the population should receive option 0 or

1 depending on the sign of $\beta_{13,0}$, regardless of their realized h_1, which cannot be dismissed as a possibility in practice, technically, it is not possible to derive a conventional large sample approximate (normal) sampling distribution for $\widehat{\mathcal{V}}_{IPW}(d_\eta^{opt})$ or $\widehat{\mathcal{V}}_{AIPW}(d_\eta^{opt})$ that is relevant for all $\beta_{14,0} \geq 0$. Thus, these estimators are nonregular. Luedtke and van der Laan (2016a) discuss this phenomenon in more generality and propose approaches to deriving valid asymptotic approximations for such nonregular estimators.

Zhang et al. (2012b) present simulation studies over a range of scenarios where the true distribution of the data does not correspond to a situation analogous to $\beta_{14,0} = 0$ in the above example. Their results suggest that appealing to standard asymptotic theory under these conditions leads to reliable estimators of uncertainty (standard errors and confidence intervals) for the estimators $\widehat{\mathcal{V}}_{IPW}(d_\eta^{opt})$ and $\widehat{\mathcal{V}}_{AIPW}(d_\eta^{opt})$, and particularly the latter. However, it is important to recognize that standard theory can fail. Indeed, even if the true distribution is only "close to" involving such difficulty, as would be the case in the example if $\beta_{14,0} > 0$ but is close to zero, the approximation based on standard theory can be poor.

As noted at the end of Section 3.5.1, in Chapter 10, we present a detailed account of statistical inference on the value of an optimal dynamic treatment regime and on the parameters characterizing an optimal regime.

3.5.4 Implementation and Practical Performance

The three main approaches reviewed in Sections 3.5.1–3.5.3 offer researchers a range of alternatives for estimation of an optimal dynamic treatment regime in a single decision problem based on data from a point exposure study. Key considerations for practice are ease of implementation and relative performance, which we now discuss.

Implementation

The regression-based (Q-learning) estimators for an optimal regime and its value discussed in Section 3.5.1 are straightforward to implement, as they require fitting only of a posited outcome regression model, which ordinarily can be carried out using established methods and software. Likewise, the A-learning methods discussed in Section 3.5.2 involve solution of the stacked M-estimating equations (3.70). The final equation for the parameter in the propensity score model can be solved using standard methods for binary regression, and the estimator for γ_1 substituted in the first equation. The first and second equations in (3.70) then often can be solved using regression software.

Implementation of value search methods is a bit more challenging, as these methods involve maximization of $\widehat{\mathcal{V}}_{IPW}(d_\eta)$ or $\widehat{\mathcal{V}}_{AIPW}(d_\eta)$, which are nonsmooth functions of η_1. Accordingly, conventional optimization techniques (e.g., Newton-Raphson) cannot be used to maximize these quantities in η_1, and alternative nonsmooth optimization methods are required. Zhang et al. (2012b) describe use of a genetic algorithm as discussed by Goldberg (1989), as implemented in the R package rgenoud (Mebane and Sekhon, 2011). When the dimension of η_1 is not large, Zhang et al. (2012b) also discuss maximization by way of a direct grid search; that is, by evaluation of $\widehat{\mathcal{V}}_{IPW}(d_\eta)$ and $\widehat{\mathcal{V}}_{AIPW}(d_\eta)$ over all combinations of values of the components of η_1 defined by a grid of possible values in each dimension. Both approaches work well in their examples. As η_1 is likely to be low dimensional in situations where the restricted class of regimes is chosen deliberately for interpretability or ease of implementation, either method is feasible for practical use. However, when η_1 is high dimensional, maximization is subject to the usual curse of dimensionality, so that the computational burden can be substantial and practical performance unstable.

Practical Performance

Of obvious interest is how these methods compare under different conditions. An important measure of performance of an estimator for an optimal regime is the extent to which the value of the estimator approaches the true maximum achievable value of a true optimal regime. That is, it is natural to compare the average outcome achieved if an estimated regime $\widehat{d}^{opt}$ is used to select treatment for the entire patient population, $\mathcal{V}(\widehat{d}^{opt})$, say, to the true $\mathcal{V}(d^{opt})$. It is important to distinguish $\mathcal{V}(\widehat{d}^{opt})$ from $\widehat{\mathcal{V}}(d^{opt})$. The latter is an estimator for the true maximum achievable value $\mathcal{V}(d^{opt})$ based on $\widehat{d}^{opt}$, so that it is entirely possible that its numerical value for any given data set could be greater or less than the true $\mathcal{V}(d^{opt})$. In contrast, $\mathcal{V}(\widehat{d}^{opt})$ can be thought of as $E\{Y^*(d)\}$ viewed as a function of d evaluated at $\widehat{d}^{opt}$ for a given data set, which by the definition of d^{opt} must be such that $\mathcal{V}(\widehat{d}^{opt}) \leq \mathcal{V}(d^{opt})$.

It is ordinarily not possible to derive an analytical expression for $\mathcal{V}(\widehat{d}^{opt})$ that can be evaluated numerically for a given data set, but an empirical version can be deduced and has been employed in simulation studies reported in the literature. In particular, in a simulation study, the value of an estimated regime, $\mathcal{V}(\widehat{d}^{opt})$, for a single simulated data set can be approximated by generating a large number (e.g., 10^6) individuals from the generative data scenario, selecting treatment for each using the estimated regime, and calculating the average outcome across these simulated individuals. These average outcomes are then averaged across all simulated data sets and this overall average compared to the value of a true optimal regime $\mathcal{V}(d^{opt})$. In many cases, derivation of $\mathcal{V}(d^{opt})$ is itself analytically intractable and is also calculated by averaging outcomes under d^{opt} across a large number of simulated individuals. Zhang et al. (2012b) and Schulte et al. (2014) describe these calculations.

These authors present results from extensive simulation studies using this measure of performance to compare competing estimators for optimal treatment regimes, where it is assumed that larger outcomes are more beneficial and where SUTVA and the no unmeasured confounders and positivity assumptions hold. Zhang et al. (2012b) report on several studies of the relative performance of regression-based (Q-learning) and value search methods in finite samples across a range of generative data scenarios. In their simulations, in moderate sample sizes, if the posited outcome regression model $Q_1(h_1, a_1; \beta_1)$ is correctly specified, the regression-based estimator $\widehat{d}_Q^{opt}$ in (3.45) can achieve a value $\mathcal{V}(\widehat{d}_Q^{opt})$ virtually the same as the true $\mathcal{V}(d^{opt})$, and the Monte Carlo average of the estimated values $\widehat{\mathcal{V}}_Q(d^{opt})$ is usually very close to $\mathcal{V}(d^{opt})$, reflecting the consistency of the estimator $\widehat{\mathcal{V}}_Q(d^{opt})$. Likewise, when the class $\mathcal{D}_\eta$ contains the true d^{opt}, the value search estimator $\widehat{d}_{\eta,AIPW}^{opt}$ achieves comparable performance to $\widehat{d}_Q^{opt}$ when the model $Q_1(h_1, a_1; \beta_1)$ is correctly specified, regardless of whether or not the propensity score model is correct, in that $\mathcal{V}(\widehat{d}_{\eta,AIPW}^{opt})$ is very close to $\mathcal{V}(d^{opt})$; and $\widehat{\mathcal{V}}_{AIPW}(d_\eta^{opt})$ consistently estimates $\mathcal{V}(d^{opt})$, as the double robustness property suggests. In fact, with $d^{opt} \in \mathcal{D}_\eta$, $\widehat{d}_{\eta,AIPW}^{opt}$ shows only mild degradation of performance even if the model $Q_1(h_1, a_1; \beta_1)$ is also misspecified.

In contrast, and not surprisingly, $\mathcal{V}(\widehat{d}_Q^{opt})$ can be considerably smaller than $\mathcal{V}(d^{opt})$ if the outcome regression model is misspecified. The extent of this poor performance of $\widehat{d}_Q^{opt}$ under a misspecified model is dependent on the generative data scenario and the assumed model $Q_1(h_1, a_1; \beta_1)$. As discussed in Section 3.5.3, scenarios can be constructed for which the misspecified model includes or excludes d^{opt}. For example, if $h_1 = (x_{11}, x_{12})^T$ and the simulated data are generated from the true regression relationship (3.81),

$$Q_1(h_1, a_1) = \exp\{1 + x_{11} + 2x_{12} + 3x_{11}x_{12} + a_1(1 - 2x_{11} + x_{12})\},$$

so that $d_1^{opt}(h_1) = \mathrm{I}(1 - 2x_{11} + x_{12} > 0)$ as in (3.82), the misspecified model

$$Q_1(h_1, a_1; \beta_1) = \beta_{11} + \beta_{12}x_{11} + \beta_{13}x_{12} + a_1(\beta_{14} + \beta_{15}x_{11} + \beta_{16}x_{12})$$

as in (3.76) induces rules of the form $\mathrm{I}(\beta_{14} + \beta_{15}x_{11} + \beta_{16}x_{12} > 0)$, which includes $d_1^{opt}(h_1)$. If instead the true relationship is

$$Q_1(h_1,a_1) = \exp\left[2 - 0.2x_{11} + 0.2x_{12}\right.$$
$$\left. + a_1\{2\text{sign}(x_{12} - x_{11}^2 + 1)/(2 + |x_{12} - x_{11}^2 + 1|)\}\right],$$

so that $d^{opt}(h_1) = \text{I}(1 - x_{11}^2 + x_{12} > 0)$, the rules induced by this misspecified model do not include $d_1^{opt}(h_1)$.

Zhang et al. (2012b) present simulations under both types of scenario. When the misspecified model includes d^{opt} and $d^{opt} \in \mathcal{D}_\eta$, the value achieved by $\widehat{d}_Q^{opt}$ is considerably less than that achieved by $\widehat{d}_{\eta,AIPW}^{opt}$ with misspecified $Q_1(h_1,a_1;\beta_1)$. This is not surprising, as $\widehat{d}_{\eta,AIPW}^{opt}$ enjoys the double robustness property, whereas $\widehat{d}_Q^{opt}$ depends directly on the assumed outcome regression model. When the misspecified model does not include d^{opt} and $d^{opt} \notin \mathcal{D}_\eta$, as might be expected, both $\widehat{d}_Q^{opt}$ and $\widehat{d}_{\eta,AIPW}^{opt}$ yield values that fail to achieve the true optimal $\mathcal{V}(d^{opt})$. However, $\mathcal{V}(\widehat{d}_{\eta,AIPW}^{opt})$ is much closer to $\mathcal{V}(d^{opt})$ than is $\mathcal{V}(\widehat{d}_Q^{opt})$, even if the propensity score model is incorrect, and the value achieved by $\widehat{d}_{\eta,AIPW}^{opt}$ is very close to $\mathcal{V}(d_\eta^{opt})$, whether or not the propensity score model is also misspecified.

Zhang et al. (2012b) do not recommend the use of $\widehat{d}_{\eta,IPW}^{opt}$, citing its unstable behavior when there are small values of $\pi_{d_\eta,1}(H_{1i};\eta_1,\widehat{\gamma}_1)$ for some i, which leads to overestimation of the true value $\mathcal{V}(d^{opt})$. Taylor et al. (2015) argue that the findings of Zhang et al. (2012b) regarding the performance of $\widehat{d}_Q^{opt}$ with a misspecified model may be more pessimistic than need be, suggesting that a careful data analyst employing regression diagnostics would recognize a poorly fitting model $Q_1(h_1,a_1;\beta_1)$ and thus be able to develop a model that captures the salient features of the true outcome regression relationship. See Section 4.5 for discussion.

The foregoing conclusions with misspecified model $Q_1(h_1,a_1;\beta_1)$ are difficult to generalize, as they are highly scenario dependent, particularly when the model does not include d^{opt}. Accordingly, Schulte et al. (2014) present a suite of simulation studies comparing Q- and A-learning methods in which they restrict attention to generative data scenarios where the contrast function model $C_1(h_1;\psi_1)$ is correctly specified, so that d^{opt} is included in all models, and focus on the impact of increasing amounts of misspecification of other model components. Namely, they consider scenarios where the true $Q_1(h_1,a_1)$ is written as

$$Q_1(h_1,a_1) = \nu_1(h_1) + a_1 C_1(h_1)$$

as in (3.58), and the true propensity score is $\pi_1(h_1)$. For Q-learning, they consider outcome regression models of the form

$$Q_1(h_1,a_1;\beta_1) = \nu_1(h_1;\phi_1) + a_1 C_1(h_1;\psi_1), \quad \beta_1 = (\phi_1^T, \psi_1^T)^T,$$

where there exists $\psi_{1,0}$ such that $C_1(h_1; \psi_{1,0}) = C_1(h_1)$, and where $\nu_1(h_1; \phi_1)$ may or may not be correctly specified. For A-learning, they use the same correct model $C_1(h_1; \psi_1)$ and consider models $\nu_1(h_1; \phi_1)$ and $\pi(h_1; \gamma_1)$, where one or both of these may be misspecified.

When all models are correctly specified, so that $Q_1(h_1, a_1; \beta_1)$ is correctly specified for Q-learning, Q-learning performs slightly better than A-learning in their simulations; that is, $\mathcal{V}(\widehat{d}_Q^{opt})$ is somewhat closer to $\mathcal{V}(d^{opt})$ than $\mathcal{V}(\widehat{d}_A^{opt})$. When the propensity score model is misspecified but $\nu_1(h_1; \phi_1)$ is correct, so that $Q_1(h_1, a_1; \beta_1)$ continues to be correctly specified, not unexpectedly, $\mathcal{V}(\widehat{d}_Q^{opt})$ is closer to the true $\mathcal{V}(d^{opt})$ than $\mathcal{V}(\widehat{d}_A^{opt})$ over a range of increasing levels of misspecification. Conversely, when $\nu_1(h_1; \phi_1)$ is misspecified, so that $Q_1(h_1, a_1; \beta_1)$ is incorrect, but the propensity score is correct, A-learning dominates Q-learning as the extent of misspecification increases. When both models are misspecified, both estimators suffer degradation of performance. Schulte et al. (2014) offer extensive discussion of the roles of the respective model components in the trade-off between Q- and A-learning.

In all of these studies of performance, an interesting finding is that, although the quality of estimation of the parameters β_1, ψ_1, or η_1 defining the induced or assumed class of regimes can be poor under misspecified models, this does not necessarily translate into poor performance of the resulting estimated regime $\widehat{d}^{opt}$. Specifically, $\mathcal{V}(\widehat{d}^{opt})$ can nonetheless be reasonably close to $\mathcal{V}(d^{opt})$.

Overall, these and other studies of relative performance of these methods do not offer definitive evidence that any one method is uniformly preferable for use in practice. All are dependent in complicated ways on the underlying distribution of the data and the quality of model specification by the data analyst. A reasonable approach in applications is to implement more than one of them under modeling assumptions that yield the same form of decision rules characterizing optimal regimes; that is, where the form of the rules induced by models $Q_1(h_1, a_1; \beta_1)$ or $C_1(h_1; \psi_1)$ for Q- or A-learning and those dictated by the choice of $\mathcal{D}_\eta$ for value search estimation coincide. The extent to which the results are in qualitative agreement together with subject matter knowledge will provide the analyst with informal insight, including on whether or not the true d^{opt} is contained in the induced class of regimes.

3.5.5 More than Two Treatment Options

As noted at the outset, we have focused in this chapter mainly on the case of two treatment options coded as 0 and 1, $\mathcal{A}_1 = \{0, 1\}$. This focus is consistent with much of the literature on the single decision problem. Moreover, presentation of the fundamental ideas and results is simplified in this setting, allowing the reader to concentrate on the conceptual underpinnings without the distraction of more complex notation and arguments.

Of course, as we have indicated throughout, the definitions of the potential outcome $Y^*(d)$ associated with a fixed regime $d \in \mathcal{D}$ in (3.4) and thus its value $\mathcal{V}(d) = E\{Y^*(d)\}$ in (3.12) extend straightforwardly to general $\mathcal{A}_1$, as do SUTVA (3.6), the no unmeasured confounders assumption (3.7), and the positivity assumption (3.8) in the obvious way. Likewise, as in Section 3.4, the characterization of an optimal regime $d^{opt} \in \mathcal{D}$ given in (3.33) can be demonstrated for general $\mathcal{A}_1$ by an argument that is somewhat messier but not conceptually more difficult than the one given in that section.

As noted in Sections 3.3.1 and Section 3.5.1, estimation of the value of a fixed regime $d \in \mathcal{D}$ and of an optimal regime $d^{opt} \in \mathcal{D}$ via outcome regression-based methods is straightforward for general $\mathcal{A}_1$. However, the presentations in Sections 3.3.2 and 3.3.3 of estimation of the value of a fixed $d \in \mathcal{D}$ and of value search estimation of an optimal regime in a restricted class $\mathcal{D}_\eta$ in Section 3.5.3 based on inverse probability weighting and of estimation of an optimal regime $d^{opt} \in \mathcal{D}$ via A-learning in Section 3.5.2 are deliberately restricted to the case $\mathcal{A}_1 = \{0, 1\}$ to allow accessible introductions to the rationales underlying these methods. We now discuss how these approaches extend to general $\mathcal{A}_1$ involving $m_1 \geq 2$ treatment options.

Inverse Probability Weighted Estimators and Value Search Estimation

First consider estimation of the value of a fixed regime based on inverse and augmented inverse probability weighted estimators, where the m_1 treatment options in $\mathcal{A}_1$ are coded as $1, \ldots, m_1$; i.e., $\mathcal{A}_1 = \{1, \ldots, m_1\}$. For brevity, we present the estimators in the context of estimation of $d_\eta \in \mathcal{D}_\eta$ for fixed $\eta = \eta_1$ and restricted class $\mathcal{D}_\eta$, but the development of course is relevant to estimation of $\mathcal{V}(d)$ for a fixed $d \in \mathcal{D}$ with the obvious modifications.

Let

$$\omega_1(h_1, a_1) = P(A_1 = a_1 | H_1 = h_1), \qquad (3.96)$$

where, of necessity,

$$\omega_1(h_1, m_1) = 1 - \sum_{a_1=1}^{m_1-1} \omega_1(h_1, a_1).$$

In the rest of this book, we often refer to the probabilities (3.96) as "propensities," representing the propensity for receiving treatment a_1

given observed history. As before,

$$Q_1(h_1, a_1) = E(Y|H_1 = h_1, A_1 = a_1)$$

for all h_1 and $a_1 \in \mathcal{A}_1$. Similar to modeling of the propensity score as in this and the previous chapter, a multinomial (polytomous) logistic regression model can be posited for the propensities $\omega_1(h_1, a_1)$ in (3.96); for example, generalizing (3.23),

$$\omega_1(h_1, a_1; \gamma_1) = \frac{\exp(\widetilde{h}_1^T \gamma_{1,a_1})}{1 + \sum_{j=1}^{m_1-1} \exp(\widetilde{h}_1^T \gamma_{1j})}, \quad a_1 = 1, \ldots, m_1 - 1,$$

$$\omega_1(h_1, m_1; \gamma_1) = \frac{1}{1 + \sum_{j=1}^{m_1-1} \exp(\widetilde{h}_1^T \gamma_{1j})}, \quad (3.97)$$

where, $\widetilde{h}_1 = (1, h_1^T)^T$ or some other vector of features of h_1, and $\gamma_1 = (\gamma_{11}^T, \ldots, \gamma_{1,m_1-1}^T)^T$. The model can be fitted via maximum likelihood. Likewise, as in Sections 3.3.3 and 3.5.3, a model $Q_1(h_1, a_1; \beta_1)$ for $Q_1(h_1, a_1)$ can be posited and fitted using suitable techniques.

Analogous to (3.87), (3.88), and (3.91) in the case $m_1 = 2$, define

$$\mathcal{C}_{d_\eta} = \mathrm{I}\{A_1 = d_1(H_1; \eta_1)\};$$

$$\pi_{d_\eta,1}(H_1; \eta_1, \gamma_1) = \sum_{a_1=1}^{m_1} \mathrm{I}\{d_1(H_1; \eta_1) = a_1\} \omega_1(H_1, a_1; \gamma_1),$$

a model for $P(\mathcal{C}_{d_\eta} = 1|H_1)$ induced by the model for $\omega_1(H_1, a_1)$; and

$$\mathcal{Q}_{d_\eta,1}(H_1; \eta_1, \beta_1) = \sum_{a_1=1}^{m_1} \mathrm{I}\{d_1(H_1; \eta_1) = a_1\} Q_1(H_1, a_1; \beta_1). \quad (3.98)$$

Then, with $\widehat{\gamma}_1$ and $\widehat{\beta}_1$ suitable estimators for γ_1 and β_1, parallel to the developments in Sections 3.3.3 and 3.5.3, the augmented inverse probability weighted estimator corresponding to the efficient estimator for $\mathcal{V}(d_\eta)$ for fixed $\eta = \eta_1$ is

$$\widehat{\mathcal{V}}_{AIPW}(d_\eta) = n^{-1} \sum_{i=1}^{n} \left[\frac{\mathcal{C}_{d_\eta,i} Y_i}{\pi_{d_\eta,1}(H_{1i}; \eta_1, \widehat{\gamma}_1)} \right. \quad (3.99)$$

$$\left. - \frac{\mathcal{C}_{d_\eta,i} - \pi_{d_\eta,1}(H_{1i}; \eta_1, \widehat{\gamma}_1)}{\pi_{d_\eta,1}(H_{1i}; \eta_1, \widehat{\gamma}_1)} \mathcal{Q}_{d_\eta,1}(H_{1i}; \eta_1, \widehat{\beta}_1) \right].$$

The simple inverse weighted estimator $\widehat{\mathcal{V}}_{IPW}(d_\eta)$ analogous to (3.89) is obtained by taking $Q_1(h_1, a_1; \beta_1) \equiv 0$ in (3.99).

As in the case of $m_1 = 2$ treatment options, for fixed d_η, under generalizations of SUTVA and the no unmeasured confounders and positivity assumptions, $\widehat{\mathcal{V}}_{AIPW}(d_\eta)$ in (3.99) is doubly robust in that it is a consistent estimator for $\mathcal{V}(d_\eta)$ if either of the models $\omega_1(h_1, a_1; \gamma_1)$ or $Q_1(h_1, a_1; \beta_1)$ is correctly specified, and $\widehat{\mathcal{V}}_{AIPW}(d_\eta)$ is guaranteed to be consistent if the data are from a randomized study, in which case $\omega_1(h_1, a_1)$ is known. Moreover, if both models are correctly specified, $\widehat{\mathcal{V}}_{AIPW}(d_\eta)$ has smallest asymptotic variance among all estimators for $\mathcal{V}(d_\eta)$ in the class of augmented inverse probability weighted estimators analogous to (3.27) for general $\mathcal{A}_1$.

Value search estimation of an optimal restricted regime d_η^{opt} in $\mathcal{D}_\eta$ defined as in (3.84) is then immediate via maximization of $\widehat{\mathcal{V}}_{AIPW}(d_\eta)$ in (3.99) or the simpler estimator $\widehat{\mathcal{V}}_{IPW}(d_\eta)$ in $\eta = \eta_1$, analogous to the approach for $m_1 = 2$ in Section 3.5.3. As in that section, the resulting estimator $\widehat{d}_{\eta, AIPW}^{opt}$ obtained by maximizing $\widehat{\mathcal{V}}_{AIPW}(d_\eta)$ should be preferred to $\widehat{d}_{\eta, IPW}^{opt}$ maximizing $\widehat{\mathcal{V}}_{IPW}(d_\eta)$, and $\widehat{\mathcal{V}}_{AIPW}(d_\eta)$ should relatively more efficient than $\widehat{\mathcal{V}}_{IPW}(d_\eta)$ as an estimator for $\mathcal{V}(d_\eta^{opt})$.

A-learning

We now sketch briefly how the A-learning technique for estimation of an optimal regime $d^{opt} \in \mathcal{D}$ in Section 3.5.2 extends to general $\mathcal{A}_1$. Consistent with the notion of an optimal blip to zero function in the case $m_1 = 2$, code the m_1 options so that $\mathcal{A}_1 = \{0, 1, \ldots, m_1 - 1\}$, where the option coded as 0 is a reference or control treatment. From (3.39), an optimal rule is thus of the form

$$d_1^{opt}(h_1) = \underset{j \in \{0, 1, \ldots, m_1 - 1\}}{\arg\max} \; Q_1(h_1, j).$$

Analogous to (3.56), defining the contrast functions

$$C_{1j}(h_1) = Q_1(h_1, j) - Q_1(h_1, 0), \quad j = 0, 1, \ldots, m_1 - 1, \qquad (3.100)$$

where obviously $C_{10}(h_1) \equiv 0$, we can express an optimal rule equivalently as

$$d_1^{opt}(h_1) = \underset{j \in \{0, 1, \ldots, m_1 - 1\}}{\arg\max} \; C_{1j}(h_1). \qquad (3.101)$$

As in the case of two options in Section 3.5.2, (3.101) demonstrates that it is sufficient to consider the contrast functions (3.100) to characterize and estimate an optimal regime.

As in (3.58), because a_1 takes on a finite number of values, any arbitrary function $Q_1(h_1, a_1)$ can be written as

$$Q_1(h_1, a_1) = \nu_1(h_1) + \sum_{j=1}^{m_1-1} C_{1j}(h_1) I(a_1 = j), \qquad (3.102)$$

where $\nu(h_1) = Q_1(h_1, 0)$. From (3.102), $Q_1(h_1, a_1)$ is maximized in a_1 by taking

$$a_1 = \underset{j \in \{0,1,\dots,m_1-1\}}{\arg\max} C_{1j}(h_1),$$

so does not depend on $\nu(h_1)$, and the maximum itself is given by, analogous to (3.59),

$$V_1(h_1) = \nu_1(h_1) + \underset{j \in \{0,1,\dots,m_1-1\}}{\max} C_{1j}(h_1). \qquad (3.103)$$

As in Section 3.5.2, these considerations suggest positing models for the contrast functions (3.100). In the most general case, models of the form

$$C_{1j}(h_1; \psi_1)$$

depending on a common finite-dimensional parameter ψ_1 can be specified. For example, for a continuous outcome, one could posit models of the form

$$C_{1j}(h_1; \psi_1) = \psi_{11,j} + \psi_{12}^T h_1, \quad \psi_1 = (\psi_{11,1}, \dots, \psi_{11,m_1-1}, \psi_{12}^T)^T,$$

so that all models share the component ψ_{12}. Analogous to (3.61), ψ_1 can be estimated via g-estimation , which in its most general form involves solving an estimating equation

$$\sum_{i=1}^{n} \left(\left[\sum_{j=1}^{m_1-1} \lambda_{1j}(H_{1i}) \left\{ I(A_{1i} = j) - \omega_1(H_{1i}, j) \right\} \right] \right. \qquad (3.104)$$

$$\left. \times \left\{ Y_i - \sum_{j=1}^{m_1-1} I(A_{1i} = j) C_{1j}(H_{1i}; \psi_1) + \theta_1(H_{1i}) \right\} \right) = 0$$

for arbitrary vector-valued functions $\lambda_{1j}(h_1)$, $j = 1, \dots, m_1 - 1$, of the same dimension as ψ_1 and arbitrary real-valued function $\theta_1(h_1)$, where, from (3.96),

$$\omega_1(h_1, j) = P(A_1 = j | H_1 = h_1).$$

Alternatively, one can posit contrast function models

$$C_{1j}(h_1; \psi_{1j}), \quad j = 1, \dots, m_1 - 1,$$

say, where ψ_{1j}, $j = 1, \dots, m_1 - 1$, are finite-dimensional parameters, so that ψ_1 comprises the distinct elements of $(\psi_{11}^T, \dots, \psi_{1,m_1-1}^T)^T$; e.g., for a continuous outcome, one might specify

$$C_{1j}(h_1; \psi_{1j}) = \psi_{11,j} + \psi_{12,j}^T h_1, \quad \psi_{1j} = (\psi_{11,j}, \psi_{12,j}^T)^T.$$

If the parameters ψ_{1j}, $j = 1, \ldots, m_1 - 1$ are nonoverlapping, so are variationally independent, solving (3.104) reduces to solving separately the equations

$$
\sum_{i=1}^{n} \left[\lambda_{1j}(H_{1i}) \left\{ I(A_{1i} = j) - \omega_1(H_{1i}, j) \right\} \right.
$$
(3.105)

$$
\left. \times \left\{ Y_i - \sum_{j=1}^{m_1-1} I(A_{1i} = j) C_{1j}(H_{1i}; \psi_{1j}) + \theta_1(H_{1i}) \right\} \right] = 0
$$

for $j = 1, \ldots, m_1 - 1$, where now $\lambda_{1j}(h_1)$ are arbitrary vector-valued functions of the same dimension as ψ_{1j}, $j = 1, \ldots, m_1 - 1$. As in Section 3.5.2, it can be shown that these estimating equations are unbiased; the argument is left as an exercise for the interested reader.

On the basis of efficiency, as in Section 3.5.2, $\theta_1(h_1) = -\nu_1(h_1)$ is the optimal choice; and, if $\text{var}(Y|H_1, A_1)$ does not depend on H_1 or A_1, the optimal choices for $\lambda_{1j}(h_1)$ are

$$
\frac{\partial C_{1j}(h_1; \psi_1)}{\partial \psi_1} \quad \text{and} \quad \frac{\partial C_{1j}(h_1; \psi_{1j})}{\partial \psi_{1j}}
$$

in (3.104) and (3.105), respectively. A model $\nu_1(h_1; \phi_1)$ for the true $\nu_1(h_1)$ can be specified; and, given a model $\omega_1(h_1, a_1; \gamma_1)$, stacked estimating equations analogous to those in that section can be solved to yield the A-learning estimator for d^{opt}. Namely, in the case of (3.105), for example, from (3.101),

$$
\widehat{d}_{A,1}^{opt}(h_1) = \underset{j \in \{0,1,\ldots,m_1-1\}}{\arg\max} \; C_{1j}(h_1; \widehat{\psi}_{1j}).
$$

By an argument similar to that at the end of Section 3.5.2, it is straightforward to demonstrate that

$$
E \left\{ Y + \underset{j \in \{0,1,\ldots,m_1-1\}}{\max} C_{1j}(H_1) - \sum_{j=1}^{m_1-1} C_{1j}(H_1) I(A_1 = j) \,\middle|\, H_1 \right\} = V_1(H_1)
$$

almost surely using (3.103). This suggests the estimator for $\mathcal{V}(d^{opt})$ given by, in the case of models $C_{1j}(h_1; \psi_{1j})$, $j = 1, \ldots, m_1 - 1$ involving distinct parameters estimated via (3.105),

$$
\widehat{\mathcal{V}}_A(d^{opt}) = n^{-1} \sum_{i=1}^{n} \left\{ Y_i + \underset{j \in \{0,1,\ldots,m_1-1\}}{\max} C_{1j}(H_{1i}; \widehat{\psi}_{1j}) \right.
$$

$$
\left. - \sum_{j=1}^{m_1-1} C_{1j}(H_1; \widehat{\psi}_{1j}) I(A_{1i} = j) \right\}.
$$

See Robins (2004) and Moodie et al. (2007) for further discussion of this and related methods.

3.6   Application

Implementations of several of the estimators for an optimal single decision treatment regime introduced in this chapter are demonstrated on the book's companion website given in the Preface. All codes used to generate simulated data and to implement each method are available on the website.

Chapter 4

Single Decision Treatment Regimes: Additional Methods

4.1 Introduction

In Chapter 3, we discuss fundamental approaches to estimation of an optimal single decision treatment regime and its associated value. In their standard forms, the outcome regression and A-learning estimators for an optimal regime $d^{opt} \in \mathcal{D}$ and the value search estimators for d_η^{opt} in a restricted class $\mathcal{D}_\eta$ found by maximizing simple and augmented inverse probability weighted value estimators are based on low-dimensional parametric models for the outcome regression, contrast function, and/or propensity score. For the outcome regression and A-learning estimators, the class of regimes effectively is restricted by the choice of outcome regression and contrast function model, respectively. Likewise, value search estimators are predicated on the explicitly specified restricted class $\mathcal{D}_\eta$, and the dimension of $\eta = \eta_1$ in its elements $d_\eta = \{d_1(h_1; \eta_1)\}$ must be relatively low to render feasible in practice optimization of $\widehat{\mathcal{V}}_{IPW}(d_\eta)$ and $\widehat{\mathcal{V}}_{AIPW}(d_\eta)$ in η_1. Thus, all of these methods limit the search for an optimal regime to a restricted class that is specified either indirectly through posited models or directly and whose elements typically are characterized by a parameter of low dimension.

In this chapter, we discuss additional approaches to estimation of an optimal regime within particular restricted classes and consider two of these in some detail. The first class of methods follows from recognizing that estimation of an optimal treatment regime can be viewed as a weighted classification problem. This allows the extensive work on classification methods and machine learning in the statistical and computer science literature to be exploited to define a restricted class of regimes and to estimate an optimal regime within the restricted class. Here, the rules characterizing regimes can be likened to classifiers and thus, as in this literature, can be potentially complex, involving high-dimensional parameterizations and thus highly flexible functions of the available information. The methods can be implemented using algorithms and software that have been developed specifically for this purpose.

In another type of method, the restricted class is instead deliberately chosen to comprise regimes characterized by decision rules that are easy to understand, interpret, and present to clinicians and patients. In Section 4.4, we discuss the particular case where rules are taken to be in the form of a *decision list*. A decision list comprises a set of "if-then" clauses, each of which assigns a treatment option on the basis of individual information.

In Section 4.5, we review further proposals in the recent literature.

The developments in this chapter rely heavily on those in Sections 3.3.2, 3.3.3, and 3.5.3; accordingly, the reader may wish to review these sections before proceeding. As in Chapter 3, we adopt the potential outcomes framework in Section 3.2.2 and take the available data to be i.i.d.

$$(X_{1i}, A_{1i}, Y_i), \; i = 1, \ldots, n,$$

where A_1 takes values in a set of treatment options $\mathcal{A}_1$, and $H_1 = X_1$. Throughout this chapter, we take SUTVA (3.6) and the no unmeasured confounders (3.7) and positivity (3.8) assumptions to hold.

4.2   Optimal Regimes from a Classification Perspective

4.2.1   Generic Classification Problem

We first review the generic classification problem. For the purpose of this description, let Z denote the "label" or "class," where we restrict attention to binary Z taking on values in $\{0, 1\}$; and let X be a vector of "features" or covariates, taking values in $\mathcal{X}$, the "feature space." Let $\mathcal{D}$ be a family of classifiers, where $d \in \mathcal{D}$ is a classifier such that $d : \mathcal{X} \to \{0, 1\}$. For example, with $X = (X_1, X_2)^T$, where X_1 and X_2 are scalar variables, classifiers in $\mathcal{D}$ may be in the form of hyperplanes, as in

$$d(X) = \mathrm{I}(\eta_{11} + \eta_{12} X_1 + \eta_{13} X_2 > 0), \tag{4.1}$$

or rectangular regions, e.g.,

$$d(X) = \mathrm{I}(X_1 < \eta_{11}) + \mathrm{I}(X_1 \geq \eta_{11}, X_2 < \eta_{12}). \tag{4.2}$$

In the generic classification problem, a training data set (X_i, Z_i), $i = 1, \ldots, n$, is available, and the goal is to find (estimate) the classifier $d \in \mathcal{D}$ that minimizes the classification error

$$\sum_{i=1}^{n} \{Z_i - d(X_i)\}^2 = \sum_{i=1}^{n} \mathrm{I}\{Z_i \neq d(X_i)\}$$

or the weighted classification error

$$\sum_{i=1}^{n} w_i \{Z_i - d(X_i)\}^2 = \sum_{i=1}^{n} w_i \, \mathrm{I}\{Z_i \neq d(X_i)\}, \tag{4.3}$$

where w_i, $i = 1, \ldots, n$, are fixed, known, nonnegative weights. This problem is a form of supervised learning, one approach within the broad area of machine learning.

Numerous techniques for solving the classification problem or approximations to it have been proposed, along with accompanying algorithms and software. For example, when the approach of *linear support vector machines* (Cortes and Vapnik, 1995) is used, the family $\mathcal{D}$ comprises classifiers in the form of hyperplanes as in (4.1). The general support vector machines approach leads to classifiers involving boundaries distinguishing the classes that can be nonlinear. With *classification and regression trees* (CART) (Breiman et al., 1984), the search is restricted to the class $\mathcal{D}$ with elements defining rectangular regions as in (4.2). A full discussion of these and other approaches to the classification problem is beyond our scope here.

4.2.2 Classification Analogy

Consider the setting of two treatment options, so that $\mathcal{A}_1 = \{0, 1\}$. Following Zhang et al. (2012a), we now describe how estimation of an optimal treatment regime d_η^{opt} within a restricted class $\mathcal{D}_\eta$, as discussed in Section 3.5.3, can be viewed as a weighted classification problem as in (4.3), which allows us to take advantage of the above developments. As in Section 3.5.3, for any fixed regime $d_\eta = \{d_1(h_1; \eta_1)\}$ in $\mathcal{D}_\eta$, indexed by $\eta = \eta_1$, define

$$\mathcal{C}_{d_\eta} = \mathrm{I}\{A_1 = d_1(H_1; \eta_1)\}$$
$$= A_1 \mathrm{I}\{d_1(H_1; \eta_1) = 1\} + (1 - A_1)\mathrm{I}\{d_1(H_1; \eta_1) = 0\},$$

the indicator of whether or not the treatment option received coincides with that recommended by d_η; let

$$\pi_{d_\eta, 1}(H_1; \eta_1, \gamma_1)$$
$$= \pi_1(H_1; \gamma_1)\mathrm{I}\{d_1(H_1; \eta_1) = 1\} + \{1 - \pi_1(H_1; \gamma_1)\}\mathrm{I}\{d_1(H_1; \eta_1) = 0\}$$

be a model for $P(\mathcal{C}_{d_\eta} = 1|H_1)$, where $\pi_1(h_1; \gamma_1)$ is a model for the propensity score $\pi_1(h_1) = P(A_1 = 1|H_1 = h_1)$; and let

$$\mathcal{Q}_{d_\eta, 1}(H_1; \eta_1, \beta_1) \tag{4.4}$$
$$= Q_1(H_1, 1; \beta_1)\mathrm{I}\{d_1(H_1; \eta_1) = 1\} + Q_1(H_1, 0; \beta_1)\mathrm{I}\{d_1(H_1; \eta_1) = 0\},$$

where $Q_1(h_1, a_1; \beta_1)$ is a model for the outcome regression $Q_1(h_1, a_1) = E(Y|H_1 = h_1, A_1 = a_1)$.

Consider the augmented inverse probability weighted estimator for the value $\mathcal{V}(d_\eta)$ given in (3.90); namely,

$$\widehat{\mathcal{V}}_{AIPW}(d_\eta) = n^{-1} \sum_{i=1}^{n} \left[\frac{\mathcal{C}_{d_\eta,i} Y_i}{\pi_{d_\eta,1}(H_{1i}; \eta_1, \widehat{\gamma}_1)} \right. \tag{4.5}$$

$$\left. - \frac{\mathcal{C}_{d_\eta,i} - \pi_{d_\eta,1}(H_{1i}; \eta_1, \widehat{\gamma}_1)}{\pi_{d_\eta,1}(H_{1i}; \eta_1, \widehat{\gamma}_1)} \mathcal{Q}_{d_\eta,1}(H_{1i}; \eta_1, \widehat{\beta}_1) \right],$$

where $\widehat{\beta}_1$ and $\widehat{\gamma}_1$ are suitable estimators for β_1 and γ_1 yielding fitted models $Q_1(h_1, a_1; \widehat{\beta}_1)$ and $\pi_1(h_1; \widehat{\gamma}_1)$, respectively. As discussed in Section 3.5.3, a value search estimator for $d_\eta^{opt} = \{d_1(h_1; \eta_1^{opt})\}$, where $\eta_1^{opt} = \arg\max_{\eta_1} \mathcal{V}(d_\eta)$, is $\widehat{d}_{\eta,AIPW}^{opt} = \{d_1(h_1; \widehat{\eta}_{1,AIPW}^{opt})\}$, and $\widehat{\eta}_{1,AIPW}^{opt}$ maximizes $\widehat{\mathcal{V}}_{AIPW}(d_\eta)$ in η_1.

Using the above definitions,

$$\frac{\mathcal{C}_{d_\eta} Y}{\pi_{d_\eta,1}(H_1; \eta_1, \gamma_1)} \tag{4.6}$$

$$= \frac{[A_1 I\{d_1(H_1; \eta_1) = 1\} + (1 - A_1) I\{d_1(H_1; \eta_1) = 0\}] Y}{\pi_1(H_1; \gamma_1) I\{d_1(H_1; \eta_1) = 1\} + \{1 - \pi_1(H_1; \gamma_1)\} I\{d_1(H_1; \eta_1) = 0\}}$$

$$= \frac{A_1 Y}{\pi_1(H_1; \gamma_1)} I\{d_1(H_1; \eta_1) = 1\} + \frac{(1 - A_1) Y}{\{1 - \pi_1(H_1; \gamma_1)\}} I\{d_1(H_1; \eta_1) = 0\},$$

where the last equality follows by considering the cases $d_1(H_1; \eta_1) = 1$ and $d_1(H_1; \eta_1) = 0$ in turn. Likewise, by similar manipulations,

$$\frac{\mathcal{C}_{d_\eta} - \pi_{d_\eta,1}(H_1; \eta_1, \gamma_1)}{\pi_{d_\eta,1}(H_1; \eta_1, \gamma_1)} \mathcal{Q}_{d_\eta,1}(H_1; \eta_1, \beta_1) \tag{4.7}$$

$$= \frac{\{A_1 - \pi_1(H_1; \gamma_1)\}}{\pi_1(H_1; \gamma_1)} Q_1(H_1, 1; \beta_1) I\{d_1(H_1; \eta_1) = 1\}$$

$$- \frac{\{A_1 - \pi_1(H_1; \gamma_1)\}}{1 - \pi_1(H_1; \gamma_1)} Q_1(H_1, 0; \beta_1) I\{d_1(H_1; \eta_1) = 0\}.$$

Define

$$\psi_1(H_1, A_1, Y) = \frac{A_1 Y}{\pi_1(H_1)} - \frac{\{A_1 - \pi_1(H_1)\}}{\pi_1(H_1)} Q_1(H_1, 1), \tag{4.8}$$

$$\psi_0(H_1, A_1, Y) = \frac{(1 - A_1) Y}{1 - \pi_1(H_1)} + \frac{\{A_1 - \pi_1(H_1)\}}{1 - \pi_1(H_1)} Q_1(H_1, 0). \tag{4.9}$$

Then, from the above, it follows that $\widehat{\mathcal{V}}_{AIPW}(d_\eta)$ in (4.5) can be expressed equivalently as

$$\widehat{\mathcal{V}}_{AIPW}(d_\eta) = n^{-1} \sum_{i=1}^{n} \Big[\widehat{\psi}_1(H_{1i}, A_{1i}, Y_i) \mathrm{I}\{d_1(H_{1i}; \eta_1) = 1\}$$
$$+ \widehat{\psi}_0(H_{1i}, A_{1i}, Y_i) \mathrm{I}\{d_1(H_{1i}; \eta_1) = 0\} \Big], \quad (4.10)$$

where $\widehat{\psi}_1(H_{1i}, A_{1i}, Y_i)$ and $\widehat{\psi}_0(H_{1i}, A_{1i}, Y_i)$ are (4.8) and (4.9) evaluated at (H_{1i}, A_{1i}, Y_i) with $Q_1(H_1, 1; \widehat{\beta}_1)$, $Q_1(H_1, 0; \widehat{\beta}_1)$, and $\pi_1(H_1; \widehat{\gamma}_1)$ substituted for $Q_1(H_1, 1)$, $Q_1(H_1, 0)$, and $\pi_1(H_1)$.

The equivalent expression for $\widehat{\mathcal{V}}_{AIPW}(d_\eta)$ in (4.10) can in fact be deduced directly. Under SUTVA and the no unmeasured confounders and positivity assumptions and using arguments similar to those in (2.62) and Section 2.7,

$$E\{\psi_1(H_1, A_1, Y)|H_1\} = E\{Y^*(1)|H_1\} = Q_1(H_1, 1),$$
$$E\{\psi_0(H_1, A_1, Y)|H_1\} = E\{Y^*(0)|H_1\} = Q_1(H_1, 0) \quad (4.11)$$

almost surely. From Section 3.3.1,

$$\mathcal{V}(d_\eta) = E\{Y^*(d_\eta)\}$$
$$= E[E\{Y^*(1)|H_1\}\mathrm{I}\{d_1(H_1; \eta_1) = 1\} + E\{Y^*(0)|H_1\}\mathrm{I}\{d_1(H_1; \eta_1) = 0\}]$$
$$= E\left[Q_1(H_1, 1)\mathrm{I}\{d_1(H_1; \eta_1) = 1\} + Q_1(H_1, 0)\mathrm{I}\{d_1(H_1; \eta_1) = 0\}\right], \quad (4.12)$$

so that

$$\mathcal{V}(d_\eta) = E[E\{\psi_1(H_1, A_1, Y)|H_1\}\mathrm{I}\{d_1(H_1; \eta_1) = 1\}$$
$$+ E\{\psi_0(H_1, A_1, Y)|H_1\}\mathrm{I}\{d_1(H_1; \eta_1) = 0\}]$$

$$= E[\psi_1(H_1, A_1, Y)\mathrm{I}\{d_1(H_1; \eta_1) = 1\}$$
$$+ \psi_0(H_1, A_1, Y)\mathrm{I}\{d_1(H_1; \eta_1) = 0\}]. \quad (4.13)$$

Thus, (4.10) follows as an estimator for $\mathcal{V}(d_\eta)$ directly from (4.13).

The equivalent expression (4.10) for $\widehat{\mathcal{V}}_{AIPW}(d_\eta)$ leads to the weighted classification problem interpretation as follows. Noting that

$$\mathrm{I}\{d_1(H_1; \eta_1) = 1\} = d_1(H_1; \eta_1), \quad \mathrm{I}\{d_1(H_1; \eta_1) = 0\} = 1 - d_1(H_1; \eta_1),$$

by straightforward algebra, (4.10) can be rewritten as

$$\widehat{\mathcal{V}}_{AIPW}(d_\eta) = n^{-1} \sum_{i=1}^{n} \Big[d_1(H_{1i}; \eta_1) \big\{ \widehat{\psi}_1(H_{1i}, A_{1i}, Y_i) - \widehat{\psi}_0(H_{1i}, A_{1i}, Y_i) \big\}$$
$$+ \widehat{\psi}_0(H_{1i}, A_{1i}, Y_i) \Big]. \quad (4.14)$$

Recall the definition of the contrast function

$$C_1(h_1) = Q_1(h_1, 1) - Q_1(h_1, 0)$$

in (3.56). From (4.11), it follows that

$$E\{\psi_1(H_1, A_1, Y) - \psi_0(H_1, A_1, Y)|H_1\} = C_1(H_1) \tag{4.15}$$

almost surely. Thus, we can view

$$\widehat{C}_1(H_{1i}, A_{1i}, Y_i) = \widehat{\psi}_1(H_{1i}, A_{1i}, Y_i) - \widehat{\psi}_0(H_{1i}, A_{1i}, Y_i) \tag{4.16}$$

in the first term in the summand on the right-hand side of (4.14) as a predictor of the contrast function $C_1(H_{1i})$ for individual i.

As above, the value search estimator $\widehat{d}^{opt}_{\eta, AIPW}$ is found by maximizing (4.5), and thus (4.14), in η_1. Because the second term on the right-hand side of (4.14) does not depend on η_1, substituting (4.16) in (4.14), it follows that maximizing (4.5) in η_1 is equivalent to maximizing

$$n^{-1} \sum_{i=1}^{n} d_1(H_{1i}; \eta_1)\widehat{C}_1(H_{1i}, A_{1i}, Y_i). \tag{4.17}$$

A further manipulation is possible. Because for any a, $a = \mathrm{I}(a > 0)|a| - \mathrm{I}(a \leq 0)|a|$, and using shorthand

$$d_{\eta_1, 1i} = d_1(H_{1i}; \eta_1), \quad \widehat{C}_{1i} = \widehat{C}_1(H_{1i}, A_{1i}, Y_i),$$

a summand in (4.17) can be reexpressed as

$$
\begin{aligned}
d_{\eta_1, 1i}\widehat{C}_{1i} &= d_{\eta_1, 1i}\mathrm{I}(\widehat{C}_{1i} > 0)|\widehat{C}_{1i}| - d_{\eta_1, 1i}\mathrm{I}(\widehat{C}_{1i} \leq 0)|\widehat{C}_{1i}| \\
&= \mathrm{I}(\widehat{C}_{1i} > 0)|\widehat{C}_{1i}| - |\widehat{C}_{1i}|\{(1 - d_{\eta_1, 1i})\mathrm{I}(\widehat{C}_{1i} > 0) + d_{\eta_1, 1i}\mathrm{I}(\widehat{C}_{1i} \leq 0)\} \\
&= \mathrm{I}(\widehat{C}_{1i} > 0)|\widehat{C}_{1i}| - |\widehat{C}_{1i}|\{\mathrm{I}(\widehat{C}_{1i} > 0) - d_{\eta_1, 1i}\}^2, \tag{4.18}
\end{aligned}
$$

where the last equality in (4.18) follows because $d_1(H_1; \eta_1)$ takes on only the values $\{0, 1\}$. Substituting the result in (4.18) into (4.17) and recognizing that the first term in (4.18) does not depend on η_1, it follows that maximizing (4.17) and thus $\widehat{\mathcal{V}}_{AIPW}(d_\eta)$ in (4.5) in η_1 is equivalent to minimizing in η_1

$$
n^{-1} \sum_{i=1}^{n} |\widehat{C}_1(H_{1i}, A_{1i}, Y_i)| \left[\mathrm{I}\{\widehat{C}_1(H_{1i}, A_{1i}, Y_i) > 0\} - d_1(H_{1i}; \eta_1) \right]^2
$$

$$
= n^{-1} \sum_{i=1}^{n} |\widehat{C}_1(H_{1i}, A_{1i}, Y_i)| \mathrm{I}\left[\mathrm{I}\{\widehat{C}_1(H_{1i}, A_{1i}, Y_i) > 0\} \neq d_1(H_{1i}; \eta_1) \right].
$$

$$\tag{4.19}$$

Comparison of (4.19) to the weighted classification error in (4.3) shows that $|\widehat{C}_1(H_{1i}, A_{1i}, Y_i)|$ can be identified as the "weight" w_i, $\text{I}\{\widehat{C}_1(H_{1i}, A_{1i}, Y_i) > 0\}$ as the "label" Z_i, and the rule $d_1(h_1; \eta_1)$ as the "classifier" d; and the restricted class $\mathcal{D}_\eta$ can be identified with the family of classifiers, where classifiers in the family are the rules characterizing regimes in $\mathcal{D}_\eta$. The formulation (4.19) has an intuitive interpretation. Recall from (3.57) that $d^{opt} \in \mathcal{D}$, the class of all possible regimes, is characterized by the rule satisfying

$$d_1^{opt}(h_1) = \text{I}\{C_1(h_1) > 0\}$$

when we assume as in Sections 3.4 and 3.5 that treatment option 0 is the default when both treatment options are equally beneficial. Thus, the quantity in brackets in a summand of (4.19) compares a predictor of the option selected by a global optimal rule to that selected by a rule characterizing a regime in $\mathcal{D}_\eta$ for the ith individual. The "weight" $|\widehat{C}_1(H_{1i}, A_{1i}, Y_i)|$ attaches greater importance to the contributions of individuals for whom the absolute difference in expected outcomes achieved using the two treatment options, measured by the predicted contrast function, is large.

The above developments are equally relevant if we consider estimation of $\mathcal{V}(d_\eta)$ by maximizing instead the 'inverse probability weighted estimator given in (3.89); namely,

$$\widehat{\mathcal{V}}_{IPW}(d_\eta) = n^{-1} \sum_{i=1}^{n} \frac{\mathcal{C}_{d_\eta,i} Y_i}{\pi_{d_\eta,1}(H_{1i}; \eta_1, \widehat{\gamma}_1)}, \qquad (4.20)$$

which is a special case of $\widehat{\mathcal{V}}_{AIPW}(d_\eta)$ in (4.5) found by taking $Q_1(h_1, a_1) \equiv 0$. Here, from (4.6) and redefining

$$\psi_1(H_1, A_1, Y) = \frac{A_1 Y}{\pi_1(H_1)}, \quad \psi_0(H_1, A_1, Y) = \frac{(1 - A_1) Y}{1 - \pi_1(H_1)}, \qquad (4.21)$$

(4.20) can be rewritten analogous to (4.14) as

$$\widehat{\mathcal{V}}_{IPW}(d_\eta) = n^{-1} \sum_{i=1}^{n} \Big[d_1(H_{1i}; \eta_1) \big\{ \widehat{\psi}_1(H_{1i}, A_{1i}, Y_i) - \widehat{\psi}_0(H_{1i}, A_{1i}, Y_i) \big\}$$
$$+ \widehat{\psi}_0(H_{1i}, A_{1i}, Y_i) \Big],$$

where now $\widehat{\psi}_1(H_{1i}, A_{1i}, Y_i)$ and $\widehat{\psi}_0(H_{1i}, A_{1i}, Y_i)$ are as in (4.21) evaluated at $(H_{1i}, A_{1i}, Y_i,)$ with the fitted model $\pi_1(H_1; \widehat{\gamma}_1)$ substituted. Then, recognizing that (4.11) holds with $\psi_1(H_1, A_1, Y)$ and $\psi_0(H_1, A_1, Y)$ defined as in (4.21), so that

$$E\{\psi_1(H_1, A_1, Y) - \psi_0(H_1, A_1, Y) | H_1\} = C_1(H_1)$$

analogous to (4.15), the same manipulations leading to (4.19) can be carried out to demonstrate that maximizing $\widehat{V}_{IPW}(d_\eta)$ in (4.20) in η_1 is equivalent to minimizing in η_1

$$n^{-1} \sum_{i=1}^{n} |\widehat{C}_1(H_{1i}, A_{1i}, Y_i)| \Big[I\{\widehat{C}_1(H_{1i}, A_{1i}, Y_i) > 0\} - d_1(H_{1i}; \eta_1) \Big]^2$$

$$= n^{-1} \sum_{i=1}^{n} |\widehat{C}_1(H_{1i}, A_{1i}, Y_i)| I \Big[I\{\widehat{C}_1(H_{1i}, A_{1i}, Y_i) > 0\} \neq d_1(H_{1i}; \eta_1) \Big],$$

$$(4.22)$$

where now

$$\widehat{C}_1(H_{1i}, A_{1i}, Y_i) = \widehat{\psi}_1(H_{1i}, A_{1i}, Y_i) - \widehat{\psi}_0(H_{1i}, A_{1i}, Y_i)$$

$$= \frac{A_{1i} Y_i}{\pi_1(H_{1i}; \widehat{\gamma}_1)} - \frac{(1 - A_{1i}) Y_i}{1 - \pi_1(H_{1i}; \widehat{\gamma}_1)}. \qquad (4.23)$$

We refer to this formulation in the discussion of the method known as outcome weighted learning in the next section.

Summarizing, the foregoing arguments demonstrate that value search estimation of an optimal restricted regime d_η^{opt} by maximizing the estimators $\widehat{V}_{IPW}(d_\eta)$ or $\widehat{V}_{AIPW}(d_\eta)$ can be likened to solving a weighted classification problem. Given this equivalence, estimation of d_η^{opt} can be accomplished using off-the-shelf software and algorithms for deducing a classifier from a training data set by minimizing the weighted classification error (4.3), with "weights" $|\widehat{C}_1(H_{1i}, A_{1i}, Y_i)|$, "labels" $I\{\widehat{C}_1(H_{1i}, A_{1i}, Y_i) > 0\}$, and $d_1(h_1; \eta_1)$ playing the role of the classifier. The choice of classification approach dictates the restricted class of regimes $\mathcal{D}_\eta$. For example, this can be carried out using the R package rpart (Therneau et al., 2015), which implements the CART approach and thus restricts the class of regimes to be those characterized by rules in the form of rectangular regions. Alternatively, one can appeal to one of the many packages available in R or other platforms to implement versions of the support vector machine approach; see, for example, Karatzoglou et al. (2006).

It is important to recognize that the challenges of implementation of value search estimation as presented in Section 3.5.3 are not circumvented by appealing to this analogy to a classification problem. As discussed in Section 3.5.4 in the context of the original forms of $\widehat{V}_{IPW}(d_\eta)$ and $\widehat{V}_{AIPW}(d_\eta)$, the objective functions (4.19) and (4.22) to be minimized are nonsmooth in η_1. In fact, this representation provides further insight into this difficulty. A little thought reveals that a rule $d_1(h_1; \eta_1)$ can be written as

$$d_1(h_1; \eta_1) = I\{f_1(h_1; \eta_1) > 0\} \qquad (4.24)$$

for some function $f_1(h_1; \eta_1)$; for example, with $H_1 = X_1 = (X_{11}, X_{12})^T$, for rules involving hyperplanes as in (3.80),

$$f_1(h_1; \eta_1) = \eta_{11} + \eta_{12} x_{11} + \eta_{13} x_{12}. \tag{4.25}$$

Writing again $\widehat{C}_{1i} = \widehat{C}_1(H_{1i}, A_{1i}, Y_i)$ for brevity, where $\widehat{C}_1(H_{1i}, A_{1i}, Y_i)$ is defined as in either (4.16) or (4.23), it is straightforward to observe that

$$I\{I(\widehat{C}_{1i} > 0) \neq d_1(H_{1i}; \eta_1)\} = I\left[\{2I(\widehat{C}_{1i} > 0) - 1\} f_1(H_{1i}; \eta_1) \leq 0\right].$$

Thus, letting

$$\ell_{0\text{-}1}(x) = I(x \leq 0) \tag{4.26}$$

be the so-called 0-1 loss function, the objective functions (4.19) and (4.22) corresponding to $\widehat{\mathcal{V}}_{AIPW}(d_\eta)$ and $\widehat{\mathcal{V}}_{IPW}(d_\eta)$, respectively, can be reexpressed as

$$n^{-1} \sum_{i=1}^n |\widehat{C}_1(H_{1i}, A_{1i}, Y_i)| \, \ell_{0\text{-}1}\left(\left[2I\{\widehat{C}_1(H_{1i}, A_{1i}, Y_i) > 0\} - 1\right] f_1(H_{1i}; \eta_1)\right).$$

$$\tag{4.27}$$

The loss function (4.26) is nonconvex. Optimization of objective functions such as (4.27) involving nonconvex loss functions is notoriously challenging, and standard optimization techniques cannot be used. Thus, (4.27) shows that the difficulty of implementation of value search estimation is a consequence of this issue.

Approaches to optimization of nonsmooth, nonconvex objective functions have been well studied in the literature on classification and incorporated in software like that mentioned above. Thus, viewing value search estimation as a weighted classification problem allows these developments and implementations to be exploited for the purpose of estimating an optimal treatment regime. In the next section, we discuss this further in the context of a special case of the foregoing formulation.

4.3 Outcome Weighted Learning

Zhao et al. (2012) propose an approach to estimation of an optimal treatment regime within a restricted class that they refer to as *outcome weighted learning* (OWL). As we now show, the motivation for OWL follows as a special case of the developments in the previous section, starting from the simple inverse weighted estimator $\widehat{\mathcal{V}}_{IPW}(d_\eta)$ in (4.20). We continue to focus on the setting where $\mathcal{A}_1 = \{0, 1\}$.

Consider again estimation of an optimal restricted regime d_η^{opt} in a restricted class $\mathcal{D}_\eta$ by maximizing in $\eta = \eta_1$ the simple inverse probability weighted estimator $\widehat{\mathcal{V}}_{IPW}(d_\eta)$ given in (4.20). As shown in the previous section, this is equivalent to minimizing (4.22), with $\widehat{C}_1(H_{1i}, A_{1i}, Y_i)$ as defined in (4.23). Using the definitions of $\mathcal{C}_{d_\eta,i}$ and $\pi_{d_\eta,1}(H_{1i}; \eta_1, \widehat{\gamma}_1)$, by straightforward algebra,

$$\widehat{C}_1(H_{1i}, A_{1i}, Y_i) = \frac{Y_i\{A_{1i} - \pi_1(H_{1i}; \widehat{\gamma}_1)\}}{\pi_1(H_{1i}; \widehat{\gamma}_1)\{1 - \pi_1(H_{1i}; \widehat{\gamma}_1)\}}. \tag{4.28}$$

Zhao et al. (2012) impose the condition that Y is bounded and $Y \geq 0$, with larger values preferred. Under the positivity assumption (3.8), $0 < \pi(H_1) < 1$ almost surely, we expect that $0 < \pi_1(H_1; \widehat{\gamma}_1) < 1$ and the denominator of (4.28) to be positive. Thus, with $Y \geq 0$, it is clear that

$$\mathrm{I}\{\widehat{C}_1(H_{1i}, A_{1i}, Y_i) > 0\} = \mathrm{I}(A_{1i} = 1) = A_{1i}. \tag{4.29}$$

Moreover, under these conditions,

$$|\widehat{C}_1(H_{1i}, A_{1i}, Y_i)| = \frac{Y_i|A_{1i} - \pi_1(H_{1i}; \widehat{\gamma}_1)|}{\pi_1(H_{1i}; \widehat{\gamma}_1)\{1 - \pi_1(H_{1i}; \widehat{\gamma}_1)\}}$$

$$= \begin{cases} \dfrac{Y_i}{\pi_1(H_{1i}; \widehat{\gamma}_1)} & \text{if } A_{1i} = 1, \\[2mm] \dfrac{Y_i}{1 - \pi_1(H_{1i}; \widehat{\gamma}_1)} & \text{if } A_{1i} = 0, \end{cases}$$

which can be written concisely as

$$|\widehat{C}_1(H_{1i}, A_{1i}, Y_i)| = \frac{Y_i}{A_{1i}\pi_1(H_{1i}; \widehat{\gamma}_1) + (1 - A_{1i})\{1 - \pi_1(H_{1i}; \widehat{\gamma}_1)\}}. \tag{4.30}$$

Substituting (4.29) and (4.30) in (4.22) then yields that maximizing $\widehat{\mathcal{V}}_{IPW}(d_\eta)$ in η_1 under these conditions is equivalent to minimizing the weighted classification error

$$n^{-1} \sum_{i=1}^{n} \frac{Y_i}{A_{1i}\pi_1(H_{1i}; \widehat{\gamma}_1) + (1 - A_{1i})\{1 - \pi_1(H_{1i}; \widehat{\gamma}_1)\}} \left\{A_{1i} - d_1(H_{1i}; \eta_1)\right\}^2$$

$$= n^{-1} \sum_{i=1}^{n} \left[\frac{Y_i}{A_{1i}\pi_1(H_{1i}; \widehat{\gamma}_1) + (1 - A_{1i})\{1 - \pi_1(H_{1i}; \widehat{\gamma}_1)\}} \right.$$

$$\left. \times \mathrm{I}\{A_{1i} \neq d_1(H_{1i}; \eta_1)\} \right]. \tag{4.31}$$

In (4.31), the treatment indicator A_{1i} plays the role of the "label," and the "weight" is given in (4.30).

Outcome Weighted Learning

In their original formulation, Zhao et al. (2012) restrict attention to the setting of a randomized clinical trial, where the propensity score $\pi_1(H_1) = P(A_1 = 1|H_1) = P(A_1 = 1) = \pi_1$, say, a known constant. In addition, they code the treatment options as $\{-1, 1\}$, as is common in the classification literature in computer science. Under these conditions, the weighted classification error (4.31) becomes, in our notation,

$$n^{-1} \sum_{i=1}^{n} \frac{Y_i}{A_{1i}\pi_1 + (1 - A_{1i})/2} I\{A_{1i} \neq d_1(H_{1i}; \eta_1)\}, \qquad (4.32)$$

where the true π_1 can be replaced by an estimator (the sample proportion receiving treatment option 1).

With the treatment options coded as 1 and -1, so reexpressing $\mathcal{A}_1 = \{1, -1\}$, any rule $d_1(h_1; \eta_1)$ takes on values 1 or -1 and, similar to the representation of $d_1(h_1; \eta_1)$ in (4.24) at the end of the last section, can be expressed as

$$d_1(h_1; \eta_1) = \text{sign}\{f_1(h_1; \eta_1)\}, \qquad (4.33)$$

where $f_1(h_1; \eta_1)$ is some function of h_1, referred to by Zhao et al. (2012) as a decision function. With this definition, the weighted classification error (4.32) can be reexpressed as in Equation (2.1) of Zhao et al. (2012) as

$$n^{-1} \sum_{i=1}^{n} \frac{Y_i}{A_{1i}\pi_1 + (1 - A_{1i})/2} I[A_{1i} \neq \text{sign}\{f_1(H_{1i}; \eta_1)\}]. \qquad (4.34)$$

Thus, ideally, if as in the previous section one chooses a particular family of classifiers, so restricting attention to decision functions $f_1(h_1; \eta_1)$ of the specific form dictated by this choice and thus to regimes characterized by rules of the form $d_1(h_1; \eta_1) = \text{sign}\{f_1(h_1; \eta_1)\}$, one minimizes (4.34) in η_1 to estimate the optimal decision function, and thus optimal regime, within the induced restricted class.

As in the previous section, (4.34) is nonsmooth and involves the nonconvex 0-1 loss function (4.26), as

$$I[A_{1i} \neq \text{sign}\{f_1(H_{1i}; \eta_1)\}] = I\{A_{1i} f_1(H_{1i}; \eta_1) \leq 0\}$$
$$= \ell_{0\text{-}1}\{A_{1i} f_1(H_{1i}; \eta_1)\},$$

which makes minimization in η_1 challenging. To address this difficulty, Zhao et al. (2012) invoke a standard tactic used in the classification literature wherein the nonconvex 0-1 loss function is replaced by a convex "surrogate," yielding a so-called convex relaxation of (4.34). They propose adopting the popular convex surrogate used in the context of the support vector machine approach, the so-called "hinge loss" function

$$\ell_{hinge}(x) = (1 - x)_+, \quad x_+ = \max(0, x). \tag{4.35}$$

Thus, rather than minimizing (4.34), Zhao et al. (2012) replace $\ell_{0-1}(\cdot)$ by $\ell_{hinge}(\cdot)$ and advocate minimizing in η_1

$$n^{-1} \sum_{i=1}^{n} \frac{Y_i}{A_{1i}\pi_1 + (1 - A_{1i})/2} \{1 - A_{1i}f_1(H_{1i}; \eta_1)\}_+ + \lambda_n \|f_1\|^2, \tag{4.36}$$

where $\| \cdot \|$ is a suitable norm for f_1; λ_n is a scalar tuning parameter possibly depending on n; and the second term in (4.36) thus penalizes the complexity of the estimated decision function to avoid overfitting, which is a challenge with high-dimensional information h_1.

Zhao et al. (2012) refer to minimization of (4.36) as OWL. Letting $\widehat{\eta}_{1,OWL}^{opt}$ be the minimizer of (4.36), the estimated optimal restricted regime arising from OWL is then

$$\widehat{d}_{\eta,OWL}^{opt} = \{d_1(h_1; \widehat{\eta}_{1,OWL}^{opt})\} = [\text{sign}\{f_1(h_1; \widehat{\eta}_{1,OWL}^{opt})\}].$$

Zhao et al. (2012) advocate a class of decision functions, and thus regimes, that allows great flexibility to accommodate high-dimensional h_1 and the likely complex relationships between elements of h_1 and treatment options. In particular, they appeal to developments from the literature on penalized regression methods for estimation of complex functions and represent decision functions as residing within a reproducing kernel Hilbert space, thus inducing a rich and flexible corresponding restricted class $\mathcal{D}_\eta$. This includes decision functions of the form in (4.25) as a special case but also allows complicated decision functions with very high-dimensional η_1. We refer the reader to Sections 2.3–2.4 of Zhao et al. (2012) for details and discussion of this formulation and implementation.

It is important to recognize that minimization of (4.36) is a different optimization problem from that involving minimization of (4.34), so that the value of η_1 minimizing (4.36) is not necessarily the same as that minimizing the original objective function corresponding to maximization of a consistent estimator for $\mathcal{V}(d_\eta)$. Accordingly, the resulting estimator $\widehat{d}_{\eta,OWL}^{opt}$ and that obtained by maximizing (4.34) are not necessarily equivalent. Zhao et al. (2012) present theoretical arguments justifying the use of the hinge loss as a surrogate for 0-1 loss and large sample results regarding the choice of λ_n and the extent to which $\widehat{d}_{\eta,OWL}^{opt}$ resembles a true optimal regime; see Sections 3.2–3.5 of Zhao et al. (2012).

Remark. The strategy of Zhao et al. (2012) is equally applicable in the more general case of the objective functions (4.19) and (4.22) corresponding to $\widehat{\mathcal{V}}_{AIPW}(d_\eta)$ and $\widehat{\mathcal{V}}_{IPW}(d_\eta)$. These objective functions can be reexpressed as in (4.27), in terms of a decision function $f_1(h_1; \eta_1)$ as in (4.24). One then can replace the 0-1 loss function in (4.27) by the hinge loss (4.35) and invoke a highly flexible representation of the decision function as proposed by Zhao et al. (2012), and, analogous to (4.36), minimize a penalized version of the resulting objective function in η_1. As above, the estimator for an optimal regime obtained by this approach applied to $\widehat{\mathcal{V}}_{AIPW}(d_\eta)$ and $\widehat{\mathcal{V}}_{IPW}(d_\eta)$ is not necessarily equivalent to that maximizing $\widehat{\mathcal{V}}_{AIPW}(d_\eta)$ and $\widehat{\mathcal{V}}_{IPW}(d_\eta)$, respectively. However, as demonstrated by Zhao et al. (2012) in the case of (4.34), the resulting estimator can approach the performance of a true optimal regime.

Residual Weighted Learning

An obvious limitation of OWL is the requirement that $Y \geq 0$. An additional drawback is that an estimated optimal restricted regime is not robust to a simple shift in the outcome. To address these issues and also to allow the propensity $\pi_1(h_1)$ to depend on h_1, Zhou et al. (2017) propose a modification of OWL that they refer to as *residual weighted learning* (RWL). We present the approach in the case $\mathcal{A}_1 = \{0, 1\}$.

Briefly, assuming that the propensity $\pi_1(h_1)$ is known, which can be relaxed to assuming that the model $\pi_1(h_1; \gamma_1)$ is correctly specified, with true value $\gamma_{1,0}$ of γ_1, in the context of (4.31), Zhou et al. (2017) note that the decision rule minimizing the expectation of a summand of (4.31) with $\widehat{\gamma}_1$ replaced by $\gamma_{1,0}$ is unchanged if Y is replaced by a $Y - g_1(H_1)$ for any function $g_1(h_1)$ not depending on η_1 as in

$$\frac{Y - g_1(H_1)}{A_1 \pi_1(H_1; \gamma_{1,0}) + (1 - A_1)\{1 - \pi_1(H_1; \gamma_{1,0})\}} \mathrm{I}\{A_1 \neq d_1(H_1; \eta_1)\}.$$
(4.37)

Zhou et al. (2017) note that an intuitively reasonable choice for $g_1(H_1)$ is that minimizing the variance of (4.37), given by

$$Q_1(H_1, 1)\mathrm{I}\{d_1(H_1; \eta_1) \neq 1\} + Q_1(H_1, 0)\mathrm{I}\{d_1(H_1; \eta_1) \neq 0\},$$

which does depend on η_1. They thus suggest the compromise choice

$$g_1^*(H_1) = \frac{Q_1(H_1, 1) + Q_0(H_1, 0)}{2}$$

$$= E\left(\left.\frac{Y}{2[A_1\pi_1(H_1; \gamma_{1,0}) + (1 - A_1)\{1 - \pi_1(H_1; \gamma_{1,0})\}]}\right| H_1\right).$$
(4.38)

Thus, instead of minimizing (4.31) in η_1, they propose minimizing in η_1

the weighted classification error

$$n^{-1} \sum_{i=1}^{n} \left[\frac{Y_i - \widehat{g}_1^*(H_{1i}; \widehat{\beta}_1)}{A_{1i}\pi_1(H_{1i}; \widehat{\gamma}_1) + (1 - A_{1i})\{1 - \pi_1(H_{1i}; \widehat{\gamma}_1)\}} \right.$$

$$\left. \times \; \mathrm{I}\{A_{1i} \neq d_1(H_{1i}; \eta_1)\} \right], \tag{4.39}$$

where $\widehat{g}_1^*(h_1; \widehat{\beta}_1)$ is obtained by positing a linear model directly for the expectation in (4.38) and fitting it using a version of weighted least squares (WLS). Zhou et al. (2017) refer to estimation of an optimal restricted regime in $\mathcal{D}_\eta$ via minimization of (4.39) in η_1 as RWL. As for OWL, writing $d_1(H_1; \eta_1)$ in terms of a decision function as above, implementation is accomplished by replacing the nonconvex 0-1 loss function by a smooth surrogate loss function that, although still nonconvex, has computational advantages. See Zhou et al. (2017) for further details.

The RWL approach involves incorporation of a regression model for (4.38) into an inverse probability weighted estimator. It is thus natural to contemplate the connection between RWL and value search estimation via maximization of the doubly robust augmented inverse probability weighted estimator (4.5) for $\mathcal{V}(d_\eta)$ or, equivalently, minimization of (4.19), which involves a model for $Q_1(h_1, a_1)$, and, from Section 3.3.3, for fixed $d_1(h_1; \eta_1)$ has smallest asymptotic variance among estimators of the form (3.27). It can be shown via straightforward algebra that minimizing in η_1 (4.39) with $\widehat{g}_1^*(H_1; \widehat{\beta}_1)$ replaced by an arbitrary function $L_1(H_1)$ that does not depend on $d_1(H_1; \eta_1)$ is equivalent to maximizing the augmented estimator (3.27) based on the same function $L_1(H_1)$ in the augmentation term. However, minimizing in η_1 (4.39) with $\widehat{g}_1^*(H_1; \widehat{\beta}_1)$ the fitted regression model for (4.38) as proposed by Zhou et al. (2017) does not coincide with maximizing (4.5), which involves taking $L_1(H_1)$ equal to the fitted $\mathcal{Q}_{d_\eta,1}(H_1; \eta_1, \widehat{\beta}_1)$ in (4.4) and does depend on $d_1(H_1; \eta_1)$. Accordingly, intuition suggests that, as in Section 3.5.3, the estimator for d_η^{opt} obtained by maximizing $\widehat{\mathcal{V}}_{AIPW}(d_\eta)$ should be of higher quality than the RWL estimator in the sense described in that section. See Liu et al. (2018) for further proposals to improve on OWL based on augmented inverse probability weighted estimation of the value.

4.4   Interpretable Treatment Regimes via Decision Lists

When the classification approach outlined in the previous two sections is implemented using very flexible machine learning techniques, as in OWL, this can lead to an induced class of regimes with complex, highly parameterized decision rules. Although such regimes can synthesize high-dimensional patient information and, owing to the flexibility with which the rules are represented, achieve performance close to that of an optimal regime in $\mathcal{D}$, they are difficult to understand and thus may regarded with skepticism as a "black box" by clinicians and patients. Moreover, scientific insights on the interplay between patient characteristics and treatment options that can inform future research may be challenging to deduce from such complicated decision rules.

Motivated by these considerations, Zhang et al. (2015) take a perspective on specification of a restricted class of regimes that emphasizes parsimony and interpretability. These authors argue that there is strong practical appeal to regimes whose rules can be understood and interpreted easily by clinicians and patients, to whom they can be presented through accessible short text descriptions or flowchart diagrams. Likewise, such interpretable decision rules can generate new scientific insights and hypotheses.

In this spirit, Zhang et al. (2015) focus on the class of regimes where the decision rule characterizing a given regime is in the form of a *decision list* (Rivest, 1987; Letham et al., 2015), developed in computer science to represent interpretable classifiers. A decision list is a sequence of if-then clauses, where, in the present context, the "if" component is a condition involving patient information that, if true, leads to recommendation of a treatment option in the set of available options $\mathcal{A}_1$. As will be clear shortly, this formulation lends itself naturally to the situation where $\mathcal{A}_1$ contains a finite but arbitrary number of treatment options.

For definiteness, consider the setting of acute leukemia in Sections 1.2.1 and 3.2.1 and the first decision point involving selection of induction chemotherapy, where the available patient information h_1 includes the variables age and WBC. Recall the very simple example of a decision rule given in (3.1), where there are two chemotherapeutic options $\{C_1, C_2\}$ coded as $\{0, 1\}$, namely,

$$d_1(h_1) = I(\text{age} < 50 \text{ and WBC} < 10).$$

It should be clear that this rule can be expressed as the decision list

If age < 50 and WBC < 10 then C_2;

else C_1.

As a slightly richer example, suppose instead that there are three chemotherapeutic options, $\mathcal{A}_1 = \{C_1, C_2, C_3\}$, which may be different agents and/or different doses of the same agent. A decision rule in the

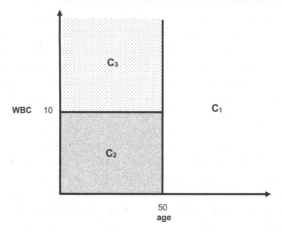

Figure 4.1 *Graphical depiction of the decision rule characterized by the decision list in (4.40).*

form of a decision list is

$$\text{If age} < 50 \text{ and WBC} < 10 \text{ then } C_2;$$

$$\text{else if age} \geq 50 \text{ then } C_1; \tag{4.40}$$

$$\text{else } C_3.$$

This rule is depicted graphically in Figure 4.1. Implementation of a rule in the form of a decision list involves checking the condition in each if-then clause and continuing to the next clause until a condition is true or the final clause is reached. Thus, to follow (4.40), age and WBC are first ascertained and checked against the condition in the first clause. If the condition {age < 50 and WBC < 10} is true, C_2 is recommended (shaded region of the figure). If this condition is not true, then it must be that at least one of age ≥ 50 or WBC ≥ 10 holds. If it is true that age ≥ 50, then the condition in the second clause holds, and C_1 is assigned (unshaded region). Otherwise, it must be that, while age < 50, WBC ≥ 10, and C_3 is recommended (dotted region).

The foregoing examples are chosen deliberately to be simple, involving only two patient variables, to illustrate the basic premise of a decision list. However, there is no restriction on the dimension of the patient information involved in the conditions of each clause or in the length of the decision list. Suppose in the second example that the patient information also includes Eastern Cooperative Oncology Group (ECOG) Performance Status ECOG, a measure on an ordinal scale describing a cancer patient's level of daily living functioning; and platelet count PLAT (platelets/ml). A more complex rule in the form of a decision list is

> If age < 50 and ECOG < 2 then C_2;
>
> else if WBC ≥ 20 then C_1;
>
> else if PLAT > 300 then C_1;
>
> else C_3.

$$(4.41)$$

In the implementation of rule (4.41), a patient whose age < 50 and ECOG < 2 would receive C_2, regardless of his WBC and PLAT status. For a patient for whom age ≥ 50 or ECOG ≥ 2 (so for whom the condition in the first clause is not satisfied), if WBC ≥ 20, C_1 is recommended. By the third clause in (4.41), a patient for whom the first two conditions are not satisfied, so with age ≥ 50 or ECOG ≥ 2 and WBC < 20, if PLAT > 300, would also receive C_1. A patient not satisfying any of the previous conditions, so for whom age ≥ 50 or ECOG ≥ 2, WBC < 20, and PLAT ≤ 300, would receive C_3. As with the rule in (4.40), the if-then clauses partition the four-dimensional space defined by these variables into regions where the three treatment options are recommended. See Zhang et al. (2015) for further examples of rules in the form of a decision list.

We now describe the general formulation for the single decision case as presented by Zhang et al. (2015). For $\mathcal{A}_1$ involving $m_1 \geq 2$ treatment options and baseline history h_1, a rule in the form of a decision list of length L_1 is characterized generically as

> If c_{11} then a_{11};
>
> else if c_{12} then a_{12};
>
> $\vdots$
>
> else if c_{1L_1} then a_{1L_1};
>
> else a_{10},

$$(4.42)$$

which can be summarized as $\{(c_{11}, a_{11}), \ldots, (c_{1L_1}, a_{1L_1}), a_{10}\}$. Here, $c_{11}, \ldots, c_{1L_1}$ are logical conditions as in the examples above that are true or false for each h_1; and $a_{1\ell}$, $\ell = 0, 1, \ldots, L_1$, are the recommended treatment options, which are elements of $\mathcal{A}_1$. Thus, for example, in (4.41), $L_1 = 3$, $c_{11} = \{$ age < 50 and ECOG $< 2\}$, and $a_{11} = C_2$. As demonstrated in (4.41), options can be repeated in different clauses. The case $L_1 = 0$ corresponds to the static rule that recommends option a_{10} regardless of the value of h_1.

Zhang et al. (2015) provide a formal expression for a rule in the form of a decision list as follows, focusing on the situation where all components of h_1 are (approximately) viewed as real-valued. Let

$$\mathcal{T}_1(c_{1\ell}) = \{h_1 : c_{1\ell} \text{ is true }\}, \quad \ell = 1, \ldots, L_1,$$

and define the sets $\mathcal{R}_{11} = \mathcal{T}_1(c_{11})$,

$$\mathcal{R}_{1\ell} = \{\cap_{j<\ell} \mathcal{T}_1(c_{1j})^c\} \bigcap \mathcal{T}_1(c_{1\ell}), \quad \ell = 2, \ldots, L_1,$$

$$\mathcal{R}_{10} = \bigcap_{j=1}^{L_1} \mathcal{T}_1(c_{1j})^c,$$

where $\mathcal{T}^c$ is the complement of the set $\mathcal{T}$.

Each of the sets $\mathcal{R}_{1\ell}$, $\ell = 0, \ldots, L_1$, is simply a mathematical representation of the conditions that must be satisfied for a patient to receive the treatment recommended by the ℓth clause. For example, in (4.41), if h_1 contains age, ECOG, WBC, and PLAT as well as other variables, $\mathcal{R}_{11} = \mathcal{T}_1(c_{11})$ is the set of h_1 values for which age < 50 and ECOG < 2 is satisfied, $\mathcal{T}_1(c_{12})$ is the set of h_1 for which WBC ≥ 20, and $\mathcal{T}_1(c_{13})$ is the set of h_1 with PLAT > 300. Then, by definition, $\mathcal{R}_{12}$ is the set of h_1 for which age ≥ 50 or ECOG ≥ 2 (i.e., $\mathcal{T}_1(c_{11})^c$) and WBC ≥ 20 ($\mathcal{T}_1(c_{12})$), which is the set of h_1 values for which the rule recommends that patients receive C_1. Similarly, $\mathcal{R}_{13}$ is the set of h_1 for which age ≥ 50 or ECOG ≥ 2 ($\mathcal{T}_1(c_{11})^c$), WBC < 20, ($\mathcal{T}_1(c_{12})^c$), and PLAT > 300 ($\mathcal{T}_1(c_{13})$); that is, the set of h_1 for which the rule also recommends C_1. Finally, $\mathcal{R}_{10}$ is the set of h_1 for which none of the previous conditions are satisfied; that is, for which age ≥ 50 or ECOG ≥ 2 ($\mathcal{T}_1(c_{11})^c$), WBC < 20, ($\mathcal{T}_1(c_{12})^c$), and PLAT ≤ 300 ($\mathcal{T}_1(c_{13})^c$), and C_3 is recommended.

With these definitions, it is straightforward to observe that a given value h_1 can be an element of at most one of the sets $\mathcal{R}_{1\ell}$, $\ell = 0, 1, \ldots, L_1$. Thus, a decision rule in the form of a decision list defining a regime can be written formally as

$$d_1(h_1) = \sum_{\ell=0}^{L_1} a_{1\ell} \, I(h_1 \in \mathcal{R}_{1\ell}). \tag{4.43}$$

From (4.43) and the definitions of the sets $\mathcal{R}_{1\ell}$, $\ell = 0, \ldots, L_1$, a specific such rule is characterized by a set of L_1 logical conditions and corresponding treatment options in $\mathcal{A}_1$; that is, by $\{(c_{11}, a_{11}), \ldots, (c_{1L_1}, a_{1L_1}), a_{10}\}$.

As noted by Zhang et al. (2015), the conditions $c_{1\ell}$, $\ell = 1, \ldots, L_1$, in principle can involve h_1 in arbitrarily complex ways. To achieve the goal of parsimony and interpretability, the authors restrict attention to $c_{1\ell}$ that involve at most two components of h_1 in statements involving thresholds. That is, if h_1 has p_1 components, letting $j_1 < j_2 \in \{1, \ldots, p_1\}$ be the indices of two arbitrary components of h_1, the sets $\mathcal{T}_1(c_{1\ell})$ are restricted to be of any of the forms

$$\begin{aligned}
&\{h_1 : h_{1j_1} \leq \tau_{11}\} &&\{h_1 : h_{1j_1} \leq \tau_{11} \text{ or } h_{1j_2} \leq \tau_{12}\} \\
&\{h_1 : h_{1j_1} \leq \tau_{11} \text{ and } h_{1j_2} \leq \tau_{12}\} &&\{h_1 : h_{1j_1} \leq \tau_{11} \text{ or } h_{1j_2} > \tau_{12}\} \\
&\{h_1 : h_{1j_1} \leq \tau_{11} \text{ and } h_{1j_2} > \tau_{12}\} &&\{h_1 : h_{1j_1} > \tau_{11} \text{ or } h_{1j_2} \leq \tau_{12}\} \\
&\{h_1 : h_{1j_1} > \tau_{11} \text{ and } h_{1j_2} \leq \tau_{12}\} &&\{h_1 : h_{1j_1} > \tau_{11} \text{ or } h_{1j_2} > \tau_{12}\} \\
&\{h_1 : h_{1j_1} > \tau_{11} \text{ and } h_{1j_2} > \tau_{12}\} &&\{h_1 : h_{1j_1} > \tau_{11}\},
\end{aligned}$$

$$(4.44)$$

where τ_{11} and τ_{12} are scalar threshold values. Zhang et al. (2015) argue that clauses that involve conditions of the forms in (4.44) and thus the resulting decision rules are more easily interpretable and explained than clauses that involve, for example, linear combinations of elements of h_1.

Up until now, we have viewed the rules in a restricted class of regimes as being indexed by a vector-valued parameter η_1, but there is no conceptual reason that rules cannot be indexed by a more complex construct. Accordingly, define η_1 to be a collection $\{(c_{11}, \mathsf{a}_{11}), \ldots, (c_{1L_1}, \mathsf{a}_{1L_1}), \mathsf{a}_{10}\}$ comprising L_1 logical conditions, each of which is of the form of those in one of the sets $\mathcal{T}_1(c_{1\ell})$ in (4.44), involving possibly different thresholds τ_{11} and, if needed, τ_{12}; and a set of corresponding treatment options in $\mathcal{A}_1$, $\mathsf{a}_{11}, \ldots, \mathsf{a}_{1L_1}, \mathsf{a}_{10}$. With this definition of η_1, a rule (4.43) can be written as $d_1(h_1; \eta_1)$, and the restricted class $\mathcal{D}_\eta$ consists of all possible regimes d_η with rules characterized by η_1 of this form.

In addition to parsimony and interpretability, an appealing feature of decision rules of this form, with at most two variables involved in any condition, is that they allow patient characteristics to be ascertained in sequence. That is, in (4.41), age and ECOG must be available for any patient, but WBC need only be measured on patients who do not satisfy the first condition c_{11} and PLAT only on patients who do not satisfy the first and second conditions c_{11} and c_{12}. This "short circuiting" of the need to ascertain all patient characteristics up front at the time of the treatment decision can be important in settings where some patient variables can be expensive or burdensome to collect.

This feature can be exploited by recognizing that a decision list need not be unique. Formally, for a decision list described by $\eta_1 = \{(c_{11}, \mathsf{a}_{11}), \ldots, (c_{1L_1}, \mathsf{a}_{1L_1}), \mathsf{a}_{10}\}$ and corresponding decision rule $d_1(h_1; \eta_1)$, there may exist another decision list described by $\eta_1' = \{(c_{11}', \mathsf{a}_{11}'), \ldots, c_{1L_1'}', \mathsf{a}_{1L_1'}'), \mathsf{a}_{10}'\}$ with corresponding rule $d_1(h_1; \eta_1')$, say, such that $d_1(h_1; \eta_1) = d_1(h_1; \eta_1')$ for all h_1 but $L_1 \neq L_1'$ or $L_1 = L_1'$ but $c_{1j} \neq c_{1j}'$ or $\mathsf{a}_{1j} \neq \mathsf{a}_{1j}'$ for some $j = 1, \ldots, L_1$. That is, for decision rules in the form of a decision list, it is possible to represent the same rule using several alternative decision lists. To appreciate this, consider the decision list in (4.40). Inspection of the graphical depiction of this list in Figure 4.1 shows that it has the following alternative representation, with the same L_1 ($= 2$) but with different definitions of a_{11} and a_{12} and different clauses c_{1j}, yielding the same recommended treatment options as (4.40) for all h_1:

If age $\geq$ 50 then C$_1$;

else if WBC $<$ 10 then C$_2$;   (4.45)

else C$_3$.

Thus, (4.40) and (4.45) are two different representations, or versions, of the rule that recommends treatment based on age and WBC as depicted in Figure 4.1.

In general, then, equivalent versions of the rule characterizing a regime $d_\eta \in \mathcal{D}_\eta$ corresponding to alternative representations of the defining decision list are possible. Of course, it follows that the value $\mathcal{V}(d_\eta)$ of d_η is the same regardless of which version of the rule is considered. Here, for any $d_\eta \in \mathcal{D}_\eta$, as in (3.4), with $Y^*(a_1)$ the potential outcome if a randomly chosen patient with history H_1 were to receive option $a_1 \in \mathcal{A}_1$, the potential outcome under d_η is given by

$$Y^*(d_\eta) = \sum_{a_1 \in \mathcal{A}_1} Y^*(a_1)\, \mathrm{I}\{d_1(H_1; \eta_1) = a_1\},$$

and

$$\mathcal{V}(d_\eta) = E\{Y^*(d_\eta)\}. \qquad (4.46)$$

This suggests that, if we wish to estimate an optimal restricted regime $d_\eta^{opt} \in \mathcal{D}_\eta$ characterized by a rule

$$d_1(h_1; \eta_1^{opt}), \quad \eta_1^{opt} = \arg\max_{\eta_1} \mathcal{V}(d_\eta)$$

as in (3.84) achieving the maximum value $\mathcal{V}(d_\eta^{opt})$, if there are equivalent versions of an optimal rule corresponding to alternative representations of the defining decision list, we should seek to estimate the one that is the least costly and/or burdensome to implement in the patient population. For example, if a particular component of h_1 is expensive to ascertain, a representation of the defining decision list in which this characteristic does not appear in any of the clauses until well down the list will be less costly than one in which it appears in the first clause.

Zhang et al. (2015) propose an approach to estimation of an optimal restricted regime $d_\eta^{opt} \in \mathcal{D}_\eta$ focused on this objective. Specifically, as in Sections 3.5.3 and 3.5.5, they advocate value search estimation of an optimal regime d_η^{opt} by maximizing in η_1 an augmented inverse probability weighted estimator for the value $\mathcal{V}(d_\eta)$ for fixed d_η in (4.46) subject to the requirement that, among all versions of an optimal regime corresponding to different representations of the defining decision list achieving the maximum value $\mathcal{V}(d_\eta^{opt})$, that minimizing some measure of the expected "cost" of implementation is targeted.

We first describe the estimator for $\mathcal{V}(d_\eta)$ and then discuss how the minimal expected cost requirement can be formalized. As in Section 3.5.5, code the m_1 treatment options in $\mathcal{A}_1$ as $1, \ldots, m_1$, so that $\mathcal{A}_1 = \{1, \ldots, m_1\}$; and, as in (3.96), let

$$\omega_1(h_1, a_1) = P(A_1 = a_1 | H_1 = h_1), \quad \omega_1(h_1, m_1) = 1 - \sum_{a_1=1}^{m_1-1} \omega_1(h_1, a_1).$$

As in (3.97), posit a multinomial (polytomous) logistic regression model $\omega_1(h_1, a_1; \gamma_1)$ for $\omega(h_1, a_1)$; and, with

$$Q_1(h_1, a_1) = E(Y | H_1 = h_1, A_1 = a_1)$$

for all h_1 and $a_1 \in \mathcal{A}_1$, posit and fit a model $Q_1(h_1, a_1; \beta_1)$ by suitable techniques. As in Section 3.5.5, defining

$$\mathcal{C}_{d_\eta} = \mathrm{I}\{A_1 = d_1(H_1; \eta_1)\}; \tag{4.47}$$

$$\pi_{d_\eta,1}(H_1; \eta_1, \gamma_1) = \sum_{a_1=1}^{m_1} \mathrm{I}\{d_1(H_1; \eta_1) = a_1\} \omega_1(H_1, a_1; \gamma_1), \tag{4.48}$$

a model for $P(\mathcal{C}_{d_\eta} = 1 | H_1)$ induced by the model for $\omega_1(H_1, a_1)$; and

$$\mathcal{Q}_{d_\eta,1}(H_1; \eta_1, \beta_1) = \sum_{a_1=1}^{m_1} \mathrm{I}\{d_1(H_1; \eta_1) = a_1\} Q_1(H_1, a_1; \beta_1), \tag{4.49}$$

with $\widehat{\gamma}_1$ and $\widehat{\beta}_1$ suitable estimators for γ_1 and β_1, the augmented inverse probability weighted estimator corresponding to the efficient estimator for $\mathcal{V}(d_\eta)$ for fixed $\eta = \eta_1$ is given in (3.99); namely

$$\widehat{\mathcal{V}}_{AIPW}(d_\eta) = n^{-1} \sum_{i=1}^{n} \left[\frac{\mathcal{C}_{d_\eta,i} Y_i}{\pi_{d_\eta,1}(H_{1i}; \eta_1, \widehat{\gamma}_1)} \right. \tag{4.50}$$
$$\left. - \frac{\mathcal{C}_{d_\eta,i} - \pi_{d_\eta,1}(H_{1i}; \eta_1, \widehat{\gamma}_1)}{\pi_{d_\eta,1}(H_{1i}; \eta_1, \widehat{\gamma}_1)} \mathcal{Q}_{d_\eta,1}(H_{1i}; \eta_1, \widehat{\beta}_1) \right].$$

Noting that (4.47) can be written equivalently as

$$\mathcal{C}_{d_\eta} = \sum_{a_1=1}^{m_1} \mathrm{I}\{d_1(H_1; \eta_1) = a_1\} \mathrm{I}(A_1 = a_1),$$

by substitution of this expression and (4.48) and (4.49) in (4.50) and manipulations generalizing those in (4.6) and (4.7), it can be shown that (4.50) can be written equivalently as

$$\widehat{\mathcal{V}}_{AIPW}(d_\eta)$$

$$= n^{-1} \sum_{i=1}^{n} \sum_{a_1=1}^{m_1} \left(\left[\frac{\mathrm{I}(A_{1i} = a_1)}{\omega_1(H_{1i}, a_1; \widehat{\gamma}_1)} \left\{ Y_i - Q_1(H_{1i}, a_1; \widehat{\beta}_1) \right\} \right. \right. \tag{4.51}$$

$$\left. \left. + Q_1(H_{1i}, a_1; \widehat{\beta}_1) \right] \mathrm{I}\{d_1(H_{1i}; \eta_1) = a_1\} \right),$$

which is the expression for the estimator for $\mathcal{V}(d_\eta)$ given in Equation (2) of Zhang et al. (2015).

We now formalize the notion of the expected cost of a decision list. For any regime $d_\eta \in \mathcal{D}_\eta$ characterized by rule $d_1(h_1; \eta_1)$ for $\eta_1 = \{(c_{11}, \mathsf{a}_{11}), \ldots, (c_{1L_1}, \mathsf{a}_{1L_1}), \mathsf{a}_{10}\}$, let $\mathcal{N}_{1\ell}$ be the cost of measuring the components of h_1 necessary to check conditions $c_{11}, \ldots, c_{1\ell}$. Ideally, the costs $\mathcal{N}_{1\ell}$, $\ell = 1, \ldots, L_1$, can be specified according to subject matter considerations, reflecting monetary costs, risk, burden, and so on. For simplicity in demonstrating the principle, Zhang et al. (2015) take $\mathcal{N}_{1\ell}$ to be equal to the number of components of h_1 that must be available to check conditions $c_{11}, \ldots, c_{1\ell}$, the rationale being that the fewer comparisons to thresholds made, the better. In this case, the expected cost of implementing regime d_η with rule

$$d_1(h_1; \eta_1) = \sum_{\ell=0}^{L_1} \mathsf{a}_{1\ell} \, \mathrm{I}(h_1 \in \mathcal{R}_{1\ell})$$

as in (4.43) in the population of patients is given by

$$N_1(d_\eta) = \sum_{\ell=1}^{L_1} \mathcal{N}_{1\ell} P(H_1 \in \mathcal{R}_{1\ell}) + \mathcal{N}_{1L_1} P(H_1 \in \mathcal{R}_{10}). \tag{4.52}$$

Note that (4.52) is smaller than the cost of measuring all components of h_1 involved in the full set of conditions $c_{11}, \ldots, c_{1L_1}$, given by

$$\mathcal{N}_{1L_1} = \mathcal{N}_{1L_1} \sum_{\ell=0}^{L_1} P(H_1 \in \mathcal{R}_{1\ell}),$$

using the fact that, clearly, $\sum_{\ell=0}^{L_1} P(H_1 \in \mathcal{R}_{1\ell}) = 1$.

As an example, consider the decision rule depicted in Figure 4.1. For the decision list in (4.45), $L_1 = 2$, $\mathcal{N}_{11} = 1$, $\mathcal{N}_{12} = 2$, and the expected cost of implementing the regime characterized by the rule represented in this form is

$$N_1(d_\eta) = \mathcal{N}_{11} P(\mathsf{age} \geq 50) + \mathcal{N}_{12} P(\mathsf{age} < 50, \mathsf{WBC} < 10)$$
$$+ \mathcal{N}_{12} P(\mathsf{age} < 50, \mathsf{WBC} \geq 10)$$

$$= \mathcal{N}_{11}P(\text{age} \geq 50) + \mathcal{N}_{12}P(\text{age} < 50)$$
$$= P(\text{age} \geq 50) + 2P(\text{age} < 50).$$

In contrast, the alternative list in (4.40) has $\mathcal{N}_{11} = 2$ and $\mathcal{N}_{12} = 2$, and the expected cost of implementing the regime characterized by its corresponding rule is

$$\mathcal{N}_{12} = 2 = 2\{P(\text{age} \geq 50) + P(\text{age} < 50)\}$$
$$> P(\text{age} \geq 50) + 2P(\text{age} < 50)$$

as long as $P(\text{age} \geq 50) > 0$. Thus, the version of the regime with rule as in Figure 4.1 characterized by the decision list (4.45) involves lower expected cost than the version in (4.40).

The approach to estimation of an optimal regime in $\mathcal{D}_\eta$, the class of all possible regimes d_η with rules $d_1(h_1; \eta_1)$ in the form of decision lists with clauses that involve conditions as in (4.44) proposed by Zhang et al. (2015) is then as follows. Among all $d_\eta \in \mathcal{D}_\eta$ achieving the maximum value $\mathcal{V}(d_\eta^{opt})$, estimate the one whose corresponding rule can be represented by a decision list that minimizes expected cost. Formally, letting

$$\mathcal{L}(v) = \{d_\eta \in \mathcal{D}_\eta : \mathcal{V}(d_\eta) = v\},$$

the set of all regimes $d_\eta \in \mathcal{D}_\eta$ achieving value v, the goal is to estimate d_η^{opt} in the set

$$\underset{d_\eta \in \mathcal{L}\{\mathcal{V}(d_\eta^{opt})\}}{\arg\min} \; N_1(d_\eta)$$

of regimes achieving the maximum value with minimal expected cost.

To achieve this objective, Zhang et al. (2015) replace $\mathcal{V}(d_\eta)$ by the augmented inverse probability weighted estimator $\widehat{\mathcal{V}}_{AIPW}(d_\eta)$ in (4.50) and estimate the expected cost of a regime d_η by $\widehat{N}_1(d_\eta)$ found by replacing the probabilities $P(H_1 \in \mathcal{R}_{1\ell})$ in the definition of $N_1(d_\eta)$ in (4.52) by sample proportions. Specifically, define

$$\widehat{\mathcal{L}}(v) = \{d_\eta \in \mathcal{D}_\eta : \widehat{\mathcal{V}}_{AIPW}(d_\eta) = v\}.$$

Then if $\widehat{d}_\eta^{opt}$ is an estimator for an optimal regime, so maximizes $\widehat{\mathcal{V}}_{AIPW}(d_\eta)$ in η_1, the proposed estimator $\widehat{d}_{\eta,DL}^{opt}$ is constructed so as to belong to the set

$$\underset{d_\eta \in \widehat{\mathcal{L}}\{\widehat{\mathcal{V}}_{AIPW}(\widehat{d}_\eta^{opt})\}}{\arg\min} \; \widehat{N}_1(d_\eta). \tag{4.53}$$

Zhang et al. (2015) propose a computational algorithm for finding $\widehat{d}_{\eta,DL}^{opt}$, where a maximum list length of $L_{1,max}$ is imposed. The algorithm involves two steps: find a $\widehat{\eta}^{opt}$ and thus $\widehat{d}_{\eta}^{opt}$ maximizing $\widehat{\mathcal{V}}_{AIPW}(d_{\eta})$, and then find an element of the set (4.53). Owing to the tree structure of a decision list, it is a greedy algorithm in the spirit of CART (Breiman et al., 1984) and is rather involved. The approach is described in detail in Zhang et al. (2015) and the associated supplementary material. Zhang et al. (2018) describe an alternative algorithm.

4.5   Additional Approaches

The approaches discussed in the preceding sections are only a small subset of those proposed in an extensive, evolving literature on estimation of optimal treatment regimes for single decision problems, including methods specifically focused on a single decision and others that include single decision problems as a special case. The coverage of fundamentals in Chapter 3 and the detailed account of the estimators derived from the classification perspective in Sections 4.2 and 4.3 and based on the concept of decision lists in Section 4.4 provide a foundation for further study of this literature. We review briefly here selected additional approaches, recognizing that an exhaustive survey of this area is not possible.

In Section 3.5.1, we discuss estimation of an optimal regime based directly on modeling of the outcome regression $Q_1(h_1, a_1) = E(Y|H_1 = h_1, A_1 = a_1)$; that is, the method referred to as Q-learning. As noted in Section 4.1, this is conventionally implemented using a fully parametric model for $Q_1(h_1, a_1)$ of typically low dimension. Accordingly, recognizing that the true relationship is likely considerably more complex than can be represented by such a model, it is natural to be concerned that the resulting estimator may be far from a true optimal regime. Several authors have proposed using this approach with various forms of nonparametric regression models for $Q_1(h_1, a_1)$, including Qian and Murphy (2011), Zhao et al. (2011), and Moodie et al. (2014), such as generalized additive models, support vector regression (Vapnik et al., 1997), and random forests (Breiman, 2001). Here, the resulting estimated decision rule will likely be quite complicated and difficult to interpret, as it is based directly on the fitted nonparametric representation of $Q_1(h_1, a_1)$. Shi et al. (2016) and Song et al. (2017) propose methods for estimation of an optimal single decision regime based on the assumption of a so-called semiparametric single index model, which is in the spirit of the idea underlying A-learning, involving a parametric representation of the contrast function with the main effects of h_1 left unspecified.

Other authors consider parametric modeling but focus on techniques for correct model specification and identification of treatment-covariate interactions; work along these lines includes Gunter et al. (2007, 2011b,c), Biernot and Moodie (2010), Gunter et al. (2011a), Lu et al. (2013), and Tian et al. (2014).

Based on (4.12), namely,

$$\mathcal{V}(d_\eta) = E\left[Q_1(H_1,1)\mathrm{I}\{d_1(H_1;\eta_1) = 1\} + Q_1(H_1,0)\mathrm{I}\{d_1(H_1;\eta_1) = 0\}\right],$$

Taylor et al. (2015) propose estimating an optimal regime in a specified restricted class $\mathcal{D}_\eta$ with elements $d_\eta = \{d_1(h_1;\eta_1)\}$ by maximizing

$$\widehat{\mathcal{V}}(d_\eta) \tag{4.54}$$

$$= n^{-1}\sum_{i=1}^{n}\left[\widehat{Q}_1(H_1,1)\mathrm{I}\{d_1(H_1;\eta_1) = 1\} + \widehat{Q}_1(H_1,0)\mathrm{I}\{d_1(H_1;\eta_1) = 0\}\right],$$

in η_1, where $\widehat{Q}_1(h_1,a_1)$ is a nonparametric estimator for $Q_1(h_1,a_1)$ obtained using random forests; any flexible nonparametric regression estimator could of course be substituted. Here, in contrast to the outcome regression (Q-learning) techniques in the previous paragraph, for which the form of the estimated optimal regime is determined directly by the representation of $Q_1(h_1,a_1)$, the class of regimes of interest is predefined, and flexible modeling of $Q_1(h_1,a_1)$ is meant only to ensure faithful representation of the value $\mathcal{V}(d_\eta)$. Indeed, this is a value search approach in that an estimator for the value is maximized in η_1. However, in contrast to the value search methods based on inverse probability weighted or augmented inverse probability weighted estimators for the value, which are guaranteed to be consistent estimators for the true value if the data are from a randomized study, $\widehat{\mathcal{V}}(d_\eta)$ above need not be a consistent estimator for the true value of d_η unless the model for $Q_1(h_1,a_1)$ is correctly specified. Similarly, the methods in the previous paragraph are predicated on such correct specification. The hope is that, by using a flexible nonparametric model for $Q_1(h_1,a_1)$ that is thus "nearly correct," this concern is mitigated.

Note that a variation of the conventional value search approach based on the augmented inverse probability weighted estimator given in (3.90) and (4.5) would be to replace the fitted fully parametric model for $Q_1(h_1,a_1)$ in the "augmentation term" by a flexible nonparametric estimator. As pointed out in the rejoinder to Taylor et al. (2015), the resulting estimator for the value is locally efficient.

Rubin and van der Laan (2012) present a classification analogy formulation similar to that in Section 4.2.2. Other authors propose additional methods inspired by the classification perspective (Kang et al., 2014; Xu et al., 2015). The implementation of the methods in Section 4.2 by Zhang et al. (2012a) using CART and the methods proposed by Laber and Zhao (2015) and Zhu et al. (2017) are tree-based approaches that yield estimated optimal regimes similar in spirit to those in Section 4.4. Mi et al. (2019) propose a version of OWL using a representation of the decision rule based on an ensemble of deep neural networks. Related methods in the context of subgroup identification include Su et al. (2009), Foster et al. (2011) and Lipkovich et al. (2011).

Some work proposes departures from the framework considered here. For example, Fan et al. (2017) propose a method for estimation of an optimal regime using a different criterion for optimality based on concordance of outcomes from individuals assigned the same treatment option. Additional approaches predicated on alternative optimality criteria are discussed in Section 7.4.8. Chen et al. (2016) develop a version of OWL for the case of an infinite set of treatment options along a continuous range of safe doses.

The fundamental classification problem is binary, involving two classes or labels; accordingly, the classification perspective on estimation of optimal treatment regimes taken in Section 4.2 is focused on the case of exactly two treatment options. Tao and Wang (2017) and Lou et al. (2018) propose approaches in the case of three or more treatment options; the latter can be viewed as an extension of OWL. Huang et al. (2019) propose a general framework for this problem in the single decision case.

Additional references proposing methods for multiple decision problems, which of course include the single decision setting as a special case, are given in Section 7.4.8.

4.6   Application

Implementations of several of the estimators for an optimal single decision treatment regime introduced in this chapter are demonstrated on the book's companion website given in the Preface. All codes used to generate simulated data and to implement each method are available on the website.

Chapter 5

Multiple Decision Treatment Regimes: Overview

5.1 Introduction

In this and the next two chapters, we present a comprehensive review of dynamic treatment regimes in the setting where there are $K > 1$ decision points at which treatment selection will take place. As in the single decision case covered in Chapters 3 and 4, a statistical framework is required in which the value of a multiple decision regime, which is the expected outcome if all individuals in the population were to receive treatment at each of the K decision points according to the regime, and the notion of an optimal multiple decision regime can be formalized. Analogous to the single decision case, this framework involves suitably defined potential outcomes and concepts of causal inference.

This fundamental causal inference framework for sequential treatment and decision making was conceived and set forth in a landmark paper by James Robins (Robins, 1986) and in numerous subsequent works (e.g., Robins, 1987, 1989, 1997, 2004). Robins was the first to present a cohesive formulation of causal inference in the context of time-dependent treatments; a historical perspective on the contributions of Robins is given in Richardson and Rotnitzky (2014).

Owing to the time-dependent nature of sequential decision making, this framework, definition of the value of a fixed regime and characterization of an optimal regime within it, and conditions under which the value of a fixed regime and an optimal regime and its value can be estimated from data are considerably more complex than in the single decision setting. Likewise, the methodology is substantially more involved.

In this chapter, to set the stage for the precise, detailed account of the statistical formulation, conditions, and methodology given in Chapters 6 and 7, we present an overview of the K-decision problem in which many of the technical details underlying the developments are downplayed. This narrative introduces the concepts and results in a less formal way and thus provides a high level preview of the more rigorous presentation in the following two chapters. This is not to imply that this chapter is not challenging in its own right, however. This chapter can stand alone for readers interested mainly in the "big picture" without the distraction of detailed proofs and arguments. The methods discussed in this chapter involve specification of various models. As in Chapters 2 and 3, we focus mainly on the use of parametric models; considerations for modeling and more flexible approaches are discussed in Section 5.7.4.

Because the developments in these chapters are generalizations of those for the single decision case, the reader may wish to review Chapters 2–4 before proceeding.

5.2   Multiple Decision Treatment Regimes

We begin by restating the basic definition of a regime involving K decision rules introduced in Section 1.4. As noted there, we take the number of decision points $K \geq 1$ at which treatment decisions must be made to be known and finite. The decision points may correspond to milestones in the disease or disorder process where a treatment decision is required, to the occurrence of events that necessitate a treatment decision, or to planned clinic visits at which a patient is evaluated and decisions on treatment are to be made.

For example, in the setting of acute leukemia in Section 1.2.1, with $K = 2$, Decision 1, at which induction chemotherapy is selected, is made at the milestone of diagnosis; Decision 2, at which maintenance or salvage therapy is chosen based on response status of the patient, corresponds to the milestone of evaluation of response to initial induction therapy. As in Section 1.2.3, an HIV-infected patient may return to the clinic at monthly intervals following initiation of antiretroviral therapy for assessment of his virologic and immunologic status, evaluation of which may lead the clinician to continue, modify, withdraw, or restart treatment. For a cardiovascular disease patient who has undergone percutaneous coronary intervention and implantation of a stent, a decision to place her on one of several possible anti-platelet regimens is made. If she experiences a subsequent myocardial infarction, a second decision must be made on how to adjust her treatment following this event.

From a statistical perspective, in the case of planned clinic visits as in the HIV infection example, the decision points can be regarded as taking place at fixed times (measured from baseline). In contrast, in the leukemia setting, times to achievement of response (or not) may be different for different individuals, so that initiation of maintenance or salvage therapy at Decision 2 does not occur at the same fixed time from baseline for all. In this case, the time of this decision point is better regarded as random. When there are K decision points that all individuals would experience, the distinction between the situations where the timing of the K decisions is the same or different for different individuals, so between fixed versus random times, is not important; what matters is that there are K decisions for all individuals, and both cases are handled by the same formulation. In this and Chapters 6 and 7 on multiple decision regimes, as in most of the literature, we assume that any individual following a K-decision regime would reach all K decisions, and the development is based on this K-decision formulation.

In the cardiovascular disease example, the decision on anti-platelet regimen may take place at a fixed time following implantation of the stent for any patient, but not all patients will experience a subsequent myocardial infarction, so that the second decision point is never reached for such patients. Patients who do experience a subsequent myocardial infarction will do so at different times as well. This situation is an example of the more complex setting in which there is a maximum of K possible decision points that can be reached at different (random) times for different individuals, but it is possible that different individuals will not reach all of them. One key setting in which this is relevant is when the outcome is a time to an event that can occur at any time post-baseline, such as overall or progression-free survival time, which is often of interest in chronic disease. If the event occurs before an individual has experienced all K decisions, the number of decision points he does reach is itself random. We defer discussion of this setting to Chapter 8, where we present an appropriate statistical framework that accommodates these features in the context of a time-to-event outcome.

Henceforth, then, we assume that all individuals will experience all K decisions. For $k = 1, \ldots, K$, let $\mathcal{A}_k$ be the set of treatment options available at Decision k, where a_k denotes an option in $\mathcal{A}_k$. Assume that the number of options in $\mathcal{A}_k$, $k = 1, \ldots, K$, is finite, as is typically the case in most disease or disorder contexts. As noted in Section 1.4, $\mathcal{A}_k$ could also be an infinite set, as when the treatment options are doses within a continuous range. We focus on a finite number of options in this book; continuous does are discussed in Section 9.2.3.

It is also possible that some options in $\mathcal{A}_k$ are infeasible for some individuals. As discussed in Section 1.4, this is the case at Decision 2 in the acute leukemia example, where $\mathcal{A}_k$ comprises four options: the two maintenance therapies, which are appropriate only for patients who respond to the induction therapy selected at Decision 1, and the two salvage options, which would be given only to patients who did not respond. In much of the literature on dynamic treatment regimes, this restriction is typically not highlighted, so it is tacitly assumed in the notation and discussion that all options $a_k \in \mathcal{A}_k$ are feasible for all individuals. In this chapter, we similarly downplay this feature, as it requires additional notation and technical considerations that can distract from the main ideas. In Section 6.2.2, we present a careful definition of sets of feasible treatment options, and the formal account of multiple decision regimes in Chapters 6 and 7 incorporates this notion throughout.

Following Section 1.4, we now define the information available at each decision point that potentially could be implicated in selection of a treatment option and thus in a decision rule for this purpose. As in that section and the discussion of single decision regimes in Chapters 2 and 3, we can define this information and thus a treatment regime comprising a set of such rules without reference to observed data, as rules for selecting treatment using information available on a patient can be conceived based on subject matter expertise, practical considerations, and so on. Of course, that observed data on this information can be used to make inference on treatment regimes is the premise of this book.

Let x_1 be information available on an individual at Decision 1, which as is customary we refer to as baseline. Likewise, let x_k, $k = 2,\ldots,K$, be the additional information that may become available on an individual between Decisions $k-1$ and k, so after initiation of the treatment option selected at Decision $k-1$ up to and immediately preceding Decision k. The initial information x_1 can include demographics, medical history variables, genetic and genomic characteristics, baseline physiological and clinical measures, and environmental and lifestyle factors. Subsequent x_k can include updated physiological and clinical measures, timing of adverse events related to prior treatments, concomitant conditions, response status to prior treatments, adherence to previous treatments, and so on. In general, let $\mathcal{X}_k$ denote the support of x_k, $k = 1,\ldots,K$.

At Decision 1, the accrued information, or history, available on an individual is x_1, which we denote by $h_1 = x_1$. Let $a_1 \in \mathcal{A}_1$ be the treatment option administered at Decision 1. At Decision 2, the accrued information or history available includes all of the baseline information, the treatment option administered at Decision 1, and the additional information arising between Decisions 1 and 2; that is, $h_2 = (x_1, a_1, x_2)$. In general, at the kth decision point, the accrued information/history is

$$h_1 = x_1,$$
$$h_k = (x_1, a_1, \ldots, x_{k-1}, a_{k-1}, x_k), \quad k = 2,\ldots,K. \qquad (5.1)$$

Let $\mathcal{H}_k$ denote support of h_k, $k = 1,\ldots,K$.

An alternative representation of (5.1) is also useful. Define

$$\overline{x}_k = (x_1,\ldots,x_k), \quad \overline{a}_k = (a_1,\ldots,a_k), \quad k = 1,\ldots,K, \qquad (5.2)$$

$$\overline{\mathcal{A}}_k = \mathcal{A}_1 \times \cdots \times \mathcal{A}_k, \quad k = 1,\ldots,K,$$

as in Section 1.4, and similarly

$$\overline{\mathcal{X}}_k = \mathcal{X}_1 \times \cdots \times \mathcal{X}_k, \quad k = 1,\ldots,K,$$

so that $\overline{x}_k$ takes values in $\overline{\mathcal{X}}_k$, and $\overline{a}_k$ takes values in $\overline{\mathcal{A}}_k$. It follows that $\mathcal{H}_1 = \mathcal{X}_1$, $h_k = (\overline{x}_k, \overline{a}_{k-1})$, and

$$\mathcal{H}_k = \overline{\mathcal{X}}_k \times \overline{\mathcal{A}}_{k-1}, \quad k = 2,\ldots,K.$$

It is commonplace in the literature to write for brevity $\bar{a} = \bar{a}_K$, $\bar{x} = \bar{x}_K$, and similarly for other quantities; we adopt this convention here.

A *decision rule* at Decision k is a function $d_k(h_k)$ that maps an individual's history to a treatment option in $\mathcal{A}_k$; that is,

$$d_k : \mathcal{H}_k \to \mathcal{A}_k \quad k = 1, \ldots, K.$$

Thus, the rule $d_k(h_k)$ takes as input the accrued information or history available on an individual at Decision k and returns a treatment option from among those in $\mathcal{A}_k$. A *dynamic treatment regime* is then a collection of decision rules, one rule corresponding to each of the K decision points, written as

$$d = \{d_1(h_1), \ldots, d_K(h_K)\}.$$

We sometimes use the streamlined representation $d = (d_1, \ldots, d_K)$.

Of course, a decision rule $d_k(h_k)$ need only depend on a subset of the elements of h_k. As discussed in Section 1.4, a static rule is one that does not use any of the information in h_k to assign treatment; that is, a static rule selects the same treatment option in $\mathcal{A}_k$ regardless of the value of h_k. A static regime is thus one in which each of its rules $d_k(h_k)$, $k = 1, \ldots, K$, is static. Static regimes are of little interest in precision medicine, and, indeed, may be unethical or nonsensical in situations where some treatment options are not appropriate for individuals with certain histories, as in the case of maintenance therapy for a leukemia patient who did not respond to initial induction therapy.

As in the single decision case, an infinitude of possible rules at each decision point, and thus an infinitude of possible regimes, can be conceived. Accordingly, for given K, we now let $\mathcal{D}$ denote the (infinite) class of all possible K-decision regimes. Of obvious importance is characterizing the performance of any given regime $d \in \mathcal{D}$ and identifying an optimal regime $d^{opt} \in \mathcal{D}$. Given a specific outcome of interest, as in the single decision setting, the performance of a regime $d \in \mathcal{D}$ is reflected by the expected outcome that would be achieved were all individuals in the population to be assigned treatment at each of the K decision points according to its K rules; that is, the *value* of d. If larger outcomes are preferred, which we continue to assume, an optimal regime $d^{opt} \in \mathcal{D}$ is then one that maximizes the value among all $d \in \mathcal{D}$.

We require an appropriate statistical framework in which the value of a K-decision regime can be defined precisely. In the next section, we present a potential outcomes formulation for the K-decision problem within which a formal definition of the value can be made, which makes explicit the greater complexity of the multiple decision setting relative to the single decision case.

Example: Two-Decision Regime for Acute Leukemia

For definiteness, we present a simple example of a regime in the case $K = 2$ in the acute leukemia setting in Section 1.2.1. As in Section 3.2.1, at Decision 1, $\mathcal{A}_1 = \{C_1, C_2\}$, and suppose again that the baseline history h_1 includes age (years) and baseline white blood cell count (WBC$_1$ $\times 10^3/\mu l$). Then, defining the set

$$\mathcal{C} = \{\text{age} < 50, \text{WBC}_1 < 10\},$$

equivalent to (3.1), an example of a rule at Decision 1 is

$$d_1(h_1) = C_2\, I(\mathcal{C}) + C_1\, I(\mathcal{C}^c). \tag{5.3}$$

At Decision 2, $\mathcal{A}_2 = \{M_1, M_2, S_1, S_2\}$. Suppose that the intervening information x_2 between Decisions 1 and 2, and thus the history h_2, includes white blood cell count at Decision 2, WBC$_2$; ECOG Performance Status, ECOG, defined in Section 4.4; EVENT, an indicator of a grade 3 or higher adverse hematologic event resulting from induction therapy; and RESP, an indicator of response to induction therapy. Define the sets

$$\mathcal{M} = \{\text{WBC}_1 < 11.2, \text{WBC}_2 < 10.5, \text{EVENT} = 0, \text{ECOG} \leq 2\},$$

$$\mathcal{S} = \{\text{age} > 60, \text{WBC}_2 < 11.0, \text{ECOG} \geq 2\}.$$

Then an example of a Decision 2 rule is

$$\begin{aligned} d_2(h_2) = I(\text{RESP} = 1)\{M_1\, I(\mathcal{M}) + M_2\, I(\mathcal{M}^c)\} \\ + I(\text{RESP} = 0)\{S_1\, I(\mathcal{S}) + S_2\, I(\mathcal{S}^c)\}. \end{aligned} \tag{5.4}$$

In the Decision 2 rule (5.4), an individual responding to the induction therapy selected at Decision 1 receives one of the two maintenance options depending on whether or not his values of WBC$_1$, WBC$_2$, EVENT, and ECOG satisfy the conditions in the set $\mathcal{M}$; likewise, an individual who does not respond receives one of the two salvage options according to whether or not his age, WBC$_2$, and ECOG values satisfy the conditions in $\mathcal{S}$. Together, the rules (5.3) and (5.4) define a regime $d = (d_1, d_2)$.

Of course, alternative rules that involve, for example, linear combinations or other functions of the components of h_1 and h_2 are also possible.

We close this section by discussing a key feature of regimes $d \in \mathcal{D}$. Analogous to the "overbar" notation used in (5.2), it is convenient to refer to the subset of the first k rules in a K-decision regime d as

$$\bar{d}_k = (d_1, \ldots, d_k), \quad k = 1, \ldots, K, \quad d = \bar{d}_K = (d_1, \ldots, d_K). \tag{5.5}$$

This notation facilitates the following.

By considering each Decision $1, \ldots, K$ in turn, one can see that, if the K rules in $d = (d_1, \ldots, d_K) \in \mathcal{D}$ are followed by an individual, the treatment options selected at each decision point depend only on the evolving realizations $x_1, \ldots, x_K$ of the intervening information. Specifically, if an individual presents with baseline information $h_1 = x_1$, the option selected at Decision 1 is $d_1(h_1) = d_1(x_1)$. At Decision 2, with rule $d_2(h_2) = d_2(\overline{x}_2, a_1)$, the option selected depends on that selected at Decision 1 through the argument a_1. Thus, the option selected at Decision 2 for an individual following $\underline{d}$ is

$$d_2\{\overline{x}_2, d_1(x_1)\},$$

where the option $d_1(x_1)$ selected at Decision 1 is substituted for a_1. At Decision 3, with rule $d_3(h_3) = d_3(\overline{x}_3, \overline{a}_2) = d_3(\overline{x}_3, a_1, a_2)$, the option selected is

$$d_3[\overline{x}_3, d_1(x_1), d_2\{\overline{x}_2, d_1(x_1)\}].$$

Clearly, this construction continues through all K decisions.

To represent this formulation concisely, define recursively

$$\begin{aligned}
\overline{d}_2(\overline{x}_2) &= [d_1(x_1), d_2\{\overline{x}_2, d_1(x_1)\}] \\
\overline{d}_3(\overline{x}_3) &= [d_1(x_1), d_2\{\overline{x}_2, d_1(x_1)\}, d_3\{\overline{x}_3, \overline{d}_2(\overline{x}_2)\}] \\
&\ \ \vdots \qquad\qquad\qquad\qquad\qquad\qquad\qquad\qquad (5.6) \\
\overline{d}_K(\overline{x}_K) &= [d_1(x_1), d_2\{\overline{x}_2, d_1(x_1)\}, \ldots, d_K\{\overline{x}_K, \overline{d}_{K-1}(\overline{x}_{K-1})\}],
\end{aligned}$$

so that $\overline{d}_k(\overline{x}_k)$, $k = 2, \ldots, K$, comprises the treatment options selected through Decision k for an individual following $\underline{d}$. For brevity, and consistent with notation elsewhere, write $\overline{d}(\overline{x}) = \overline{d}_K(\overline{x}_K)$ This recursive representation is important in showing that it is possible to estimate the value of a fixed regime $d \in \mathcal{D}$ from observed data, presented in Section 5.4, and in methods for estimation of $\mathcal{V}(d)$ for fixed $d \in \mathcal{D}$, discussed in Section 5.5.

This development demonstrates that defining treatment regimes in terms of rules $d_k(h_k) = d_k(\overline{x}_k, \overline{a}_{k-1})$ for $k = 2, \ldots, K$ is redundant from the point of view of an individual following its K rules. If an individual follows regime d through Decision k, then the treatment options selected at Decisions $1, \ldots, k$ are determined recursively through only the baseline and intervening information up to that point. That is, a_1 is determined by x_1, and then a_2 is determined by $(\overline{x}_2, a_1) = (x_1, a_1, x_2)$, but because a_1 is a function of x_1, a_2 is determined by $\overline{x}_2 = (x_1, x_2)$, and so on. The definition of rule d_k as a function of the history $h_k = (\overline{x}_k, \overline{a}_{k-1})$, so as mapping values in $\mathcal{H}_k$ to $\mathcal{A}_k$, $k = 2, \ldots, K$, is, however, important in the characterization of an optimal regime and in formulation of methods for estimation of an optimal regime; see Sections 5.6 and 5.7.

Example: Simple Two-Decision Regime

We illustrate the foregoing points with a simple example with $K = 2$ and two treatment options coded as 0 and 1 at each decision point; i.e., $\mathcal{A}_1 = \{0, 1\}$, $\mathcal{A}_2 = \{0, 1\}$. Take both the baseline information x_1 and intervening information x_2 between Decisions 1 and 2 to be binary variables, so that $\mathcal{X}_1 = \{0, 1\}$ and $\mathcal{X}_2 = \{0, 1\}$, say. Consider a regime $d = (d_1, d_2) \in \mathcal{D}$, where, by definition, $d_1(h_1) = d_1(x_1)$ maps values in $\mathcal{H}_1 = \mathcal{X}_1$ to $\mathcal{A}_1$ and $d_2(h_2) = d_2(\overline{x}_2, a_1)$ maps values in $\mathcal{H}_2 = \overline{\mathcal{X}}_2 \times \mathcal{A}_1$ to $\mathcal{A}_2$. Thus, for each of the two possible values of $h_1 = x_1$, d_1 must return a value in $\mathcal{A}_1$; suppose that d_1 is such that

$$d_1(x_1 = 0) = 0$$
$$d_1(x_1 = 1) = 1,$$

where we note the arguments of the rules explicitly here and below for emphasis. Similarly, for each of the eight possible values of $h_2 = (x_1, x_2, a_1)$, d_2 must return a value in $\mathcal{A}_2$; suppose that d_2 is such that

$$d_2(x_1 = 0, x_2 = 0, a_1 = 0) = 0$$
$$d_2(x_1 = 0, x_2 = 0, a_1 = 1) = 1* \qquad (5.7)$$
$$d_2(x_1 = 0, x_2 = 1, a_1 = 0) = 1$$
$$d_2(x_1 = 0, x_2 = 1, a_1 = 1) = 1*$$
$$d_2(x_1 = 1, x_2 = 0, a_1 = 0) = 0*$$
$$d_2(x_1 = 1, x_2 = 0, a_1 = 1) = 1$$
$$d_2(x_1 = 1, x_2 = 1, a_1 = 0) = 0*$$
$$d_2(x_1 = 1, x_2 = 1, a_1 = 1) = 0.$$

Although this definition indeed is such that d_2 returns an option in $\mathcal{A}_2$ for all values of h_2, the configurations indicated by an asterisk are superfluous in the following sense. If an individual were to follow regime d, treatment at Decision 1 is determined by x_1, so that a configuration for which the value of a_1 is not equal to $d_1(x_1)$ could not occur. For example, consider (5.7); because $x_1 = 0$, Decision 1 treatment is determined as $d_1(x_1) = 0$, so that $a_1 = 1$ is not possible.

5.3   Statistical Framework

5.3.1   *Potential Outcomes for K Decisions*

We now sketch the salient features of the potential outcomes framework for K decisions. A precise account is given in Section 6.2.

As in the single decision case, assume that there is an outcome of interest that is determined following all K decisions, which either can be ascertained only after Decision K or can be defined using the baseline and intervening information, where larger outcomes are preferred. For example, as in Section 1.2.3, consider a regime for treatment of HIV infection, where, as above, individuals following its rules report to the clinic at K planned visits for evaluation and decisions on administration of antiretroviral therapy. Treatment benefit might be measured by viral load, the amount of HIV genetic material in a blood sample (viral RNA copies/ml), reflecting virologic status, ascertained at a final visit subsequent to the Kth decision point one year after initiation of therapy. Because smaller viral load is more desirable, consistent with the convention that larger outcomes are better, we could take outcome to be negative viral load. Alternatively, suppose that an individual's CD4 T cell count (cells/mm^3), where lower counts indicate poorer immunologic status so that larger counts are preferred, is ascertained at visits $k = 2, \ldots, K$, prior to administration of the treatment option selected at Decision k. Then CD4 count is part of the intervening information between Decisions $k-1$ and k, $k = 2, \ldots, K$. Suppose that CD4 count is measured again at a final visit subsequent to Decision K (at visit $K+1$, say). The final outcome might then be the total number of CD4 measures among those taken at visits $2, \ldots, K, K+1$ that were above 200 cells/mm^3. Here, the outcome is based on intervening information on CD4 count collected between Decisions $k-1$ and k, $k = 2, \ldots, K$, and following the final, Kth visit. This flexibility in defining the outcome is implicit in the following development.

Consider a randomly chosen individual in the population of interest. At Decision 1, she presents with baseline information given by the random variable X_1, and suppose that she receives treatment option $a_1 \in \mathcal{A}_1$. It is not difficult to appreciate that, from this point forward, the evolution of her disease or disorder process will be influenced by a_1. For instance, physiological and clinical measures ascertained after Decision 1 as well as events that occur after Decision 1 reflect the effects of a_1; moreover, these measures and events might be different from those she would have experienced under a different option $a_1' \in \mathcal{A}_1$, say. In general, then, the information that would accrue on this individual between Decisions 1 and 2 clearly depends on the treatment option she received at Decision 1. To formalize this, we can conceive of a random variable $X_2^*(a_1)$, say, representing the potential intervening information between Decisions 1 and 2 that would arise if a randomly chosen individual were to receive option $a_1 \in \mathcal{A}_1$ at Decision 1.

Now suppose that an individual receives option $a_1 \in \mathcal{A}_1$ at Decision 1 and $a_2 \in \mathcal{A}_2$ at Decision 2. Analogous to Decision 1, we expect her disease or disorder process subsequent to Decision 2 to be influenced by both a_1 and a_2. In particular, measures ascertained and events occurring between Decisions 2 and 3 will reflect the effects of a_1 followed by a_2; that is, the sequence $\bar{a}_2$. Accordingly, we can conceive of the potential intervening information between Decisions 2 and 3 if a randomly chosen individual were to receive a_1 at Decision 1 and a_2 at Decision 2, represented by the random variable $X_3^*(\bar{a}_2)$.

Continuing, following administration of the sequence $\bar{a}_{k-1}$ at Decisions 1 to $k - 1$, the potential intervening information that would arise between Decisions $k - 1$ and k is represented by the random variable $X_k^*(\bar{a}_{k-1})$, $k = 2, \ldots, K$. If options $a_1, \ldots, a_K$ were given at all K decisions, it of course follows that the outcome that would be achieved would reflect the effects of all K treatment options. Accordingly, let

$$Y^*(\bar{a}_K) = Y^*(\bar{a})$$

denote the outcome that would be achieved if a randomly chosen individual were to receive treatment sequence $\bar{a} = \bar{a}_K$ across all K decision points.

Summarizing, the potential information arising between decision points over the course of the K decisions and the potential outcome arising if an individual were to receive the options $\bar{a} = (a_1, \ldots, a_K)$ are

$$\{X_1, X_2^*(a_1), X_3^*(\bar{a}_2), \ldots, X_K^*(\bar{a}_{K-1}), Y^*(\bar{a})\}. \qquad (5.8)$$

The random variables $X_k^*(\bar{a}_{k-1})$, $k = 2, \ldots, K$, and $Y^*(\bar{a})$ are referred to as potential outcomes, where the former are intermediate to the final outcome of interest after Decision K. Note that, strictly speaking, as a pretreatment variable, X_1 it is not a "potential outcome" in the sense of these other random variables; however, we include X_1 in (5.8) for convenience later and refer to (5.8) as "potential outcomes."

Implicit in these developments is the assumption that the potential intervening information arising between Decisions $k - 1$ and k depends only on the treatment options received through Decision $k - 1$ and is not influenced by options administered in the future.

Clearly, there is a set of potential outcomes for every $\bar{a} \in \overline{\mathcal{A}}$. Accordingly, define the set of all possible potential outcomes as

$$W^* = \Big\{ X_2^*(a_1), X_3^*(\bar{a}_2), \ldots, X_K^*(\bar{a}_{K-1}), Y^*(\bar{a}),$$
$$\text{for } a_1 \in \mathcal{A}_1, \bar{a}_2 \in \overline{\mathcal{A}}_2, \ldots, \bar{a}_{K-1} \in \overline{\mathcal{A}}_{K-1}, \bar{a} \in \overline{\mathcal{A}} \Big\}. \qquad (5.9)$$

In some accounts in the literature, the baseline information X_1 is included in W^*, although it is not "potential" as noted above.

Now consider a regime $d \in \mathcal{D}$. Informally, we can conceive of potential outcomes if a randomly chosen individual from the population were to receive treatment options at Decisions 1 to K by following the rules in d. If an individual with baseline information X_1 were to be assigned treatment according to regime d, at Decision 1, the treatment received is determined by rule d_1. As above, the resulting intervening information that would arise between Decisions 1 and 2 would depend on the option selected by d_1. We thus write $X_2^*(d_1)$ to denote the potential information that would arise if a randomly chosen individual were to receive treatment according to the rules in d. Implicitly, it is assumed as above that this potential intervening information is affected only by the option received at Decision 1 and thus only by the result of rule d_1 and is not influenced by the results of applying subsequent rules. Similarly, define $X_k^*(\bar{d}_{k-1})$ as the potential information that would arise between Decisions $k-1$ and k if the first $k-1$ rules in d were used to determine treatment at Decisions 1 through $k-1$ for $k = 2, \ldots, K$, and let

$$Y^*(d) = Y^*(\bar{d}_K)$$

be the potential outcome that would be achieved if an individual were to receive treatment according to the K rules in d.

Intuitively, then, we write the potential outcomes that would be achieved under regime $d \in \mathcal{D}$ as

$$\{X_1, X_2^*(d_1), X_3^*(\bar{d}_2), \ldots, X_K^*(\bar{d}_{K-1}), Y^*(d)\}, \qquad (5.10)$$

where we again include X_1 for convenience later.

As in (3.3) and (3.4) in Section 3.2.2 for the single decision case, a formal definition of the potential outcomes in (5.10) is in terms of the set of all potential outcomes W^* in (5.9). In Section 6.2.3, we present a precise such statement, which demonstrates that the definition of each quantity in (5.10) depends on that of the previous elements. For our purposes here, it suffices to appreciate that each $d \in \mathcal{D}$ has a corresponding set of potential outcomes (5.10) and in particular a potential outcome of interest $Y^*(d)$ resulting from following the rules in d.

As in Section 3.2.3, we thus define the value of regime $d \in \mathcal{D}$ as

$$\mathcal{V}(d) = E\{Y^*(d)\}, \qquad (5.11)$$

where $Y^*(d)$ is defined as above. Here, the value $\mathcal{V}(d)$ in (5.11) is the expected outcome that would be achieved if all K rules in d were followed to select treatment.

Likewise, as in Section 3.4, an optimal regime $d^{opt} \in \mathcal{D}$ is one that maximizes the value (5.11) among all $d \in \mathcal{D}$. That is, analogous to (3.31),

$$E\{Y^*(d^{opt})\} \geq E\{Y^*(d)\} \text{ for all } d \in \mathcal{D}, \qquad (5.12)$$

or, equivalently,

$$d^{opt} = \arg\max_{d \in \mathcal{D}} E\{Y^*(d)\} = \arg\max_{d \in \mathcal{D}} \mathcal{V}(d).$$

In contrast to that for the single decision case in Section 3.4, the derivation of the form of an optimal regime

$$d^{opt} = \{d_1^{opt}(h_1), \ldots, d_K^{opt}(h_K)\}$$

satisfying (5.12) is considerably more involved. We defer discussion to Section 5.6.

5.3.2   Data

The foregoing developments suggest that, ideally, estimation of the value of a fixed regime $d \in \mathcal{D}$ and of an optimal regime in $\mathcal{D}$ and its value require data from a longitudinal study in which baseline and intervening information across all K decisions is collected from all participants, along with the treatments actually received at each decision point and the final outcome of interest. In particular, the desired data for a randomly chosen participant can be summarized in time order as

$$(X_1, A_1, X_2, A_2, \ldots, X_K, A_K, Y). \tag{5.13}$$

In (5.13), X_1 is the baseline information available at Decision 1, taking values in $\mathcal{X}_1$. The random variables A_k, $k = 1, \ldots, K$, taking values in $\mathcal{A}_k$, $k = 1, \ldots, K$, respectively, are the treatment options actually received, and X_k, $k = 2, \ldots, K$, taking values in $\mathcal{X}_k$, $k = 2, \ldots, K$, are the collections of information actually arising in the intervening periods between Decisions $k - 1$ and k. The observed outcome is Y. As noted in Section 5.3.1, Y is determined following all K decisions and is either ascertained entirely after Decision K or is defined as a function of the intervening information $X_2, \ldots, X_K$ and additional information collected subsequent to Decision K.

As in Section 5.2, define for $k = 1, \ldots, K$

$$\overline{X}_k = (X_1, \ldots, X_k), \qquad \overline{A}_k = (A_1, \ldots, A_k),$$
$$\overline{X} = \overline{X}_K = (X_1, \ldots, X_K), \quad \overline{A} = \overline{A}_K = (A_1, \ldots, A_K), \tag{5.14}$$

so that the observed data (5.13) on a randomly chosen individual can be written succinctly as

$$(\overline{X}_K, \overline{A}_K, Y) = (\overline{X}, \overline{A}, Y).$$

Analogous to (5.1), denote the observed history at each decision point as

$$H_1 = X_1, \tag{5.15}$$
$$H_k = (X_1, A_1, \ldots, X_{k-1}, A_{k-1}, X_k) = (\overline{X}_k, \overline{A}_{k-1}), \quad k = 2, \ldots, K,$$

where H_k takes values in $\mathcal{H}_k$, $k = 1, \ldots, K$. Here and in Chapters 6 and 7, we use both types of notation (5.14) and (5.15) interchangeably. The "overbar" notation proves convenient when it is necessary to refer to specific components of the history, as will be evident shortly.

A natural source of data of the form (5.13) is a longitudinal observational study, such as a prospective cohort study or a retrospective study using an existing database. Of course, such "real-world" observational data are subject to the usual concerns over confounding reviewed in Section 2.3.3 in the case of a point exposure study, where a single treatment decision is the focus. In that setting, individuals who received certain treatment options may have different (baseline) characteristics from those who received other options and thus be prognostically different. Moreover, characteristics associated with both potential outcome and treatment selection may or may not be recorded in the data. Indeed, this issue is considerably more complicated with K decisions. At each decision, individuals who receive different treatment options may have different histories and be prognostically different. In fact, an individual's history at Decision k, characteristics of which may have been used by clinicians to select treatment at k, is influenced by previous treatment decisions, and the individual's subsequent evolving characteristics will be both affected by the option received at k and be used to select treatment options at Decision $k + 1$ and beyond. As in the single decision setting, characteristics associated with both treatment selection and future characteristics and ultimate prognosis may or may not be captured in the data.

The possibility for such time-dependent confounding poses a significant challenge for using observational data to compare options at each decision point and more generally for making inferences on full K-decision treatment regimes with a causal interpretation. Clearly, a generalization of the no unmeasured confounders assumption (3.7) that applies to each of the K decision points is required and involves the potential outcomes (5.9) and observed data in a complicated way. Moreover, it is apparent that generalizations of SUTVA (3.6) and the positivity assumption (3.8) are needed. We introduce such assumptions in the next section. Intuitively, as noted above, a generalization of the no unmeasured confounders assumption requires that the history H_k of accrued information at each of the $k = 1, \ldots, K$ decision points recorded in the data for each individual include all characteristics that were actually used to make treatment decisions and that are related to prognosis. It may be optimistic to expect that such a condition would hold for data not collected for the purpose of making inference on sequential treatment decisions and thus on treatment regimes.

As discussed in Section 2.3.2 and subsequently for the single decision case, data from a well-conducted randomized study are not subject to confounding and facilitate evaluation of causal effects of treatment options. Intuition thus suggests that a study in which participants are randomized to the available treatment options at each of the K decisions of interest similarly would yield data that are not subject to time-dependent confounding and accordingly would support inference on multistage treatment regimes with a causal interpretation. As noted in Section 1.4, the *sequential multiple assignment randomized trial* (SMART) design has been advocated specifically for this purpose.

In a SMART, participants are randomly assigned to the feasible treatment options at each decision point. As an example, Figure 5.1 shows the design of a SMART that could be implemented to evaluate the treatment options for the $K = 2$ treatment decisions discussed in Section 1.2.1 in the setting of acute leukemia and thus would yield data that are not subject to confounding and could be used to study treatment regimes. A participant in this trial is first randomized to one of the two induction chemotherapy options; after ascertainment of response status, a participant responding to induction therapy is randomized to one of the maintenance therapies, and a participant who does not respond is randomly assigned to one of the salvage options. In a SMART, baseline information X_1 and extensive additional information X_2 accruing in the period between initiation of induction therapy (Decision 1) and ascertainment of response status (Decision 2) would be collected deliberately to inform the formulation of fixed regimes and estimation of an optimal regime, where X_2 includes response status.

SMARTs are discussed in detail in Chapter 9. For our purposes in this chapter, as argued in the next section, they represent a "gold standard" data source for the study of multistage treatment regimes.

In summary, the observed data arising from either a longitudinal observational study or SMART involving n participants are

$$(X_{1i}, A_{1i}, \ldots, X_{Ki}, A_{Ki}, Y_i), \quad i = 1, \ldots, n, \qquad (5.16)$$

written in streamlined form as

$$(\overline{X}_i, \overline{A}_i, Y_i), \quad i = 1, \ldots, n,$$

which, as for a point exposure study, are assumed to be i.i.d. In a longitudinal observational study, the treatment options actually received, $A_{1i}, \ldots, A_{Ki}$, are chosen at the discretion of clinicians and patients; in a SMART, participants are randomly assigned to the options in $\mathcal{A}_1, \ldots, \mathcal{A}_K$, respectively.

We close this section by raising a key point. Separate studies, be they observational or randomized, may have been conducted comparing the treatment options at each decision point. For definiteness, consider the acute leukemia setting, for which $K = 2$. Suppose that a clinical

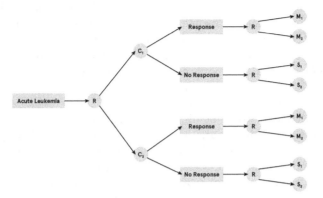

Figure 5.1 *Schematic depiction the design of a SMART for studying the treatment options at the two key decision points in the setting of acute leukemia discussed in Section 1.2.1. At Decision 1, trial participants are randomized to the two induction chemotherapy options* C_1 *and* C_2. *At Decision 2, subjects for whom a response is induced are randomized to the two maintenance options* M_1 *and* M_2, *and subjects for whom no response is induced are randomized to the two salvage options* S_1 *and* S_2. *The symbol* ® *denotes randomization.*

trial comparing the Decision 1 induction options in $\mathcal{A}_1$ on the basis of response has been conducted. Suppose further that data from a clinical trial comparing Decision 2 maintenance options in subjects who responded to any induction therapy on the basis of a survival outcome are also available, as are data from yet another trial comparing Decision 2 salvage options among nonresponders for this outcome. In each study, characteristics of each individual at the time of treatment assignment are also recorded. As these are entirely separate studies, the participants involved in each are distinct and moreover may be from different patient populations. It is natural to ask if these separate data sources can be combined to study treatment regimes and in particular to estimate an optimal treatment regime.

It is tempting to hope that one could use the methods in Chapters 3 and 4 for a single decision to estimate an optimal decision rule for selecting an induction option based on the data from the first trial, and, in separate analyses, use these methods to estimate optimal decision rules selecting a maintenance option for responders and a salvage option for nonresponders using the data from second and third studies, respectively. One could then "piece together" these estimated optimal decision rules to comprise an estimated optimal regime. Unfortunately, one challenge that makes this approach suspect, even if the participants in all studies were drawn from the same patient population, is the possibility for "delayed effects" of the treatments. For example, suppose that one of the Decision 1 induction chemotherapies yields a lower response rate than the other but has enhanced long-term effects that result in a larger expected survival time for responders when it is followed by a certain maintenance option. Without data from subjects for whom the entire sequence of receipt of Decision 1 induction therapy, ascertainment of response status, receipt of Decision 2 treatment, and subsequent survival time is available, it would be difficult for this feature to be deduced and accounted for in estimation of an optimal regime. In fact, it is common for new clinical trials to build on results of previous studies, so if the first trial showed sufficient evidence of a larger response rate for C_2, say, subsequent studies of maintenance and salvage options might be carried out in subjects who had received C_2 previously, so that delayed effects of C_1 could never be revealed.

This complication supports the contention that data of the form (5.16), for which all n subjects are observed over all K decisions, are required for inference on multistage treatment regimes. In this chapter and in Chapters 6 and 7, we assume that such data are available from a longitudinal observational study or a SMART. (This requirement is relaxed somewhat for a possibly censored time-to-event outcome in Chapter 8.)

5.3.3 Identifiability Assumptions

We have introduced a potential outcomes framework in which the value of a fixed regime $d \in \mathcal{D}$ as well as an optimal regime $d^{opt} \in \mathcal{D}$ and its value can be defined formally, and we have characterized the data to be used to estimate these and other quantities. As in the single decision setting, the key challenge is thus to deduce the distribution of the potential outcomes, in terms of which these quantities of interest are defined, from the distribution of these observed data.

Specifically, recall from Section 3.3 that, in the single decision case with $\mathcal{A}_1 = \{0, 1\}$, the potential outcomes are $\{Y^*(1), Y^*(0)\}$, in terms of which the potential outcome under $d \in \mathcal{D}$, $Y^*(d)$, is defined in (3.3). Thus, the goal is to identify the distribution of $Y^*(d)$, or more generally the joint distribution of $\{X_1, Y^*(d)\}$, which depends on that of $\{X_1, Y^*(1), Y^*(0)\}$, in terms of the distribution of the observed data (X_1, A_1, Y). We demonstrated in Sections 3.3–3.5 that this distribution can be identified based on the observed data under SUTVA (3.6) and the no unmeasured confounders (3.7) and positivity (3.8) assumptions. In particular, we showed that it is possible to identify the functional $E\{Y^*(d)\}$ of the distribution of $\{X_1, Y^*(d)\}$ from the observed data under these assumptions, which makes possible estimation of the value $\mathcal{V}(d) = E\{Y^*(d)\}$ and an optimal regime d^{opt}. Although we presented arguments in the particular case where $\mathcal{A}_1$ comprises two treatment options, these extend straightforwardly to general $\mathcal{A}_1$.

In the multiple decision setting, by extension, the analogous question is whether or not it is possible to identify the distribution of the potential outcomes

$$\{X_1, X_2^*(d_1), X_3^*(\overline{d}_2), \ldots, X_K^*(\overline{d}_{K-1}), Y^*(d)\}$$

in (5.10) associated with a fixed regime $d \in \mathcal{D}$, which depends on that of $\{X_1, W^*\}$, from the distribution of the observed data

$$(X_1, A_1, X_2, A_2, \ldots, X_K, A_K, Y)$$

in (5.13). As above, if this is possible, we can then identify any functional of the distribution of these potential outcomes, such as the value $\mathcal{V}(d) = E\{Y^*(d)\}$, from the distribution of the observed data.

We now state and discuss assumptions under which this is possible, which are generalizations of SUTVA and the no unmeasured confounders and positivity assumptions in the single decision case.

SUTVA (Consistency Assumption)

This assumption states that the observed intervening information between decision points and the observed outcome are those that potentially would be achieved under the treatments actually received; that is

$$X_k = X_k^*(\overline{A}_{k-1}) = \sum_{\overline{a}_{k-1} \in \overline{\mathcal{A}}_{k-1}} X_k^*(\overline{a}_{k-1}) \mathrm{I}(\overline{A}_{k-1} = \overline{a}_{k-1}), \quad k = 2, \ldots, K,$$

$$(5.17)$$

$$Y = Y^*(\overline{A}) = \sum_{\overline{a} \in \overline{\mathcal{A}}} Y^*(\overline{a}) \mathrm{I}(\overline{A} = \overline{a}).$$

As discussed for the single decision case in Section 2.3, SUTVA (5.17), also referred to as the *consistency assumption*, states that a treatment option is consistent regardless of how it was administered, and potential intervening information and outcomes for any one individual in the population are unaffected by the treatment assignments or potential information and outcomes of other individuals.

Sequential Randomization Assumption

The sequential randomization assumption (SRA), first discussed by Robins (1986), is a generalization of the no unmeasured confounders assumption to the multiple decision case. Because the multiple decision

setting is considerably more complex, different versions of this assumption are possible, some of which are stronger than others. The strongest
version, which suffices for our purposes, states that

$$W^* \perp\!\!\!\perp A_k | \overline{X}_k, \overline{A}_{k-1}, \quad k = 1, \ldots, K, \quad \text{where } A_0 \text{ is null}, \qquad (5.18)$$

which can be written equivalently in terms of the history variables H_k
as

$$W^* \perp\!\!\!\perp A_k | H_k, \quad k = 1, \ldots, K. \qquad (5.19)$$

Remark. In (5.18) and in the rest of this book, when discussing condition-
ing on $H_k = (\overline{X}_k, \overline{A}_{k-1})$ and realizations $h_k = (\overline{x}_k, \overline{a}_{k-1})$, to streamline
the presentation, we often do not distinguish the case $k = 1$, and thus
in such situations it is understood that A_0 and a_0 are null.

The SRA (5.18) and (5.19) states that, conditional on the past history of treatment assignment and accruing information at Decision k,
treatment selection at k is made independently of all potential information and outcomes, past, present, and future, and thus certainly of
future prognosis as reflected by future potential information and outcome. That is, treatment selection at Decision k depends only on an
individual's observed history H_k, $k = 1, \ldots, K$, and not additionally on
potential outcomes. A weaker version of the SRA requires that treatment selection at Decision k is made independently of only all future
potential information and outcomes given past history.

Remark. In a SMART, treatment options are randomized at each decision point. As will be made precise in Section 6.2.2, the feasible treatment options at Decision k among those in $\mathcal{A}_k$ for a participant are often
determined by his history. For example, in the acute leukemia SMART
in Figure 5.1, the feasible options at Decision 2 to which a subject can
be randomized are determined by response status, which is ascertained
in the intervening period between Decisions 1 and 2 and so is contained
in X_2. Thus, in a SMART, given a participant's history at Decision k,
because of randomization, assignment to one of the feasible options at k
is independent of all potential outcomes. That is, the strong SRA (5.18)
holds by design in a SMART.

As noted above and discussed in Section 5.4, the strong SRA (5.18),
SUTVA (5.17), and the positivity assumption given next allow the distribution of potential outcomes to be expressed in terms of that of the
observed data. This is also possible under weaker versions of the SRA
at the price of more complex arguments (Robins, 1986, 1987).

In clinical practice, it is almost certainly true that treatment decisions made by clinicians and patients are based on a patient's history and not on potential outcomes that are not observed. As discussed for the single decision setting in Section 2.3, the difficulty in observational studies is that accrued information that was used in the decisions may not be captured in the observed data. Thus, implicit in the SRA is that all information used to make each treatment decision for $k = 1, \ldots, K$ is contained in the observed, available histories $H_1, \ldots, H_K$, respectively.

Of course, it is clear that the SRA (5.18) cannot be verified from the observed data, as at any decision point it is impossible to determine from the data that are available if there are additional measures associated with both treatment selection and past, present, and future prognosis that are not recorded. As in the single decision case, whether or not the SRA is plausible for data from an observational study must be determined based on domain science expertise.

Remark. Justification of the no unmeasured confounders assumption for an observational point exposure study, so with a single decision point only, is often tenuous. It follows that, for $K > 1$ decision points, when working with observational data that were not collected for the purpose of studying sequential treatment decisions and treatment regimes, it may be even more difficult to have confidence that the SRA holds. That the strong SRA (5.18) holds automatically for a SMART makes the data from such a study a "gold standard" for this objective.

Positivity Assumption

We defer a precise statement of the positivity assumption to Section 6.2.4, where we present a formal definition in terms of sets of feasible treatment options at each decision point based on an individual's history. For our purposes in this chapter, we express the positivity assumption informally as follows.

Intuitively, whether or not it is possible to deduce the distribution of the potential outcomes $\{X_1, X_2^*(d_1), X_3^*(\bar{d}_2), \ldots, X_K^*(\bar{d}_{K-1}), Y^*(d)\}$ in (5.10) for any fixed $d \in \mathcal{D}$ from the observed data is predicated on the feasible treatment options at each decision point k for each possible history being represented in the data. That is, for each k and each possible realized history $h_k = (\bar{x}_k, \bar{a}_{k-1})$, there must be some individuals who actually received each of the feasible options for this history that a regime could select. If this is not the case, then it is not possible to study regimes that select from among the feasible options for any possible history.

The positivity assumption is

$$P(A_k = a_k|H_k = h_k) = P(A_k = a_k|\overline{X}_k = \overline{x}_k, \overline{A}_{k-1} = \overline{a}_{k-1}) > 0,$$
$$k = 1, \ldots, K, \tag{5.20}$$

for all options a_k that are feasible for history h_k and for all possible histories; that is, histories h_k satisfying

$$P(H_k = h_k) = P(\overline{X}_k = \overline{x}_k, \overline{A}_{k-1} = \overline{a}_{k-1}) > 0, \quad k = 1, \ldots, K. \tag{5.21}$$

Remark. As noted in Chapters 1 and 2, to circumvent measure theoretic subtleties, we present the positivity assumption (5.20) treating all random variables as discrete. Thus, for example, (5.21) can be viewed as the joint density $p_{\overline{X}_k, \overline{A}_{k-1}}(\overline{x}_k, \overline{a}_{k-1})$ when some elements of $\overline{X}_k$ are not discrete. We make heavy use of this convention in the sequel.

5.4   The g-Computation Algorithm

We are now in a position to state the main identifiability result.

It can be shown that, under SUTVA (5.17), the SRA (5.18), and the positivity assumption (5.20), the distribution of

$$\{X_1, X_2^*(d_1), X_3^*(\overline{d}_2), \ldots, X_K^*(\overline{d}_{K-1}), Y^*(d)\}$$

in (5.10) for any $d \in \mathcal{D}$ can be identified from the distribution of the observed data

$$(X_1, A_1, X_2, A_2, \ldots, X_K, A_K, Y).$$

As discussed previously, if this holds, it is possible to identify functionals of interest involving the potential outcomes, such as the value $\mathcal{V}(d) = E\{Y^*(d)\}$, from the observed data. We present this result, which is due to Robins (1986), without proof; the detailed argument is given in Section 6.3.

We first state what is usually referred to as the *g-computation algorithm*, also known as the *g-formula* (Robins, 1986), which is in the context of sequences of treatment options $\overline{a}$. As noted in the remark at the end of Chapter 1 and above, for simplicity, we treat all random variables as discrete. Denote the joint density of the observed data evaluated at realization $(x_1, a_1, \ldots, x_K, a_K, y) = (\overline{x}_K, \overline{a}_K, y) = (\overline{x}, \overline{a}, y)$ as

$$p_{X_1, A_1, \ldots, X_K, A_K, Y}(x_1, a_1, \ldots, x_K, a_K, y) \tag{5.22}$$
$$= P(X_1 = x_1, A_1 = a_1, \ldots, X_K = x_K, A_K = a_K, Y = y).$$

As long as (5.22) is positive, it is straightforward to factorize (5.22) as, in obvious notation,

$$p_{Y|\overline{X},\overline{A}}(y|\overline{x},\overline{a})\times p_{A_K|\overline{X}_K,\overline{A}_{K-1}}(a_K|\overline{x}_K,\overline{a}_{K-1})$$

$$\times p_{X_K|\overline{X}_{K-1},\overline{A}_{K-1}}(x_K|\overline{x}_{K-1},\overline{a}_{K-1})\times p_{A_{K-1}|\overline{X}_{K-1},\overline{A}_{K-2}}(a_{K-1}|\overline{x}_{K-1},\overline{a}_{K-2})$$

$$\vdots \tag{5.23}$$

$$\times p_{X_2|X_1,A_1}(x_2|x_1,a_1)\times p_{A_1|X_1}(a_1|x_1)$$

$$\times p_{X_1}(x_1).$$

In its basic form, the g-computation algorithm states that the joint density of the potential outcomes corresponding to any $\overline{a}_K = \overline{a} \in \overline{\mathcal{A}}$,

$$\{X_1, X_2^*(a_1), X_3^*(\overline{a}_2), \ldots, X_K^*(\overline{a}_{K-1}), Y^*(\overline{a})\},$$

can be written in terms of that of the observed data given in (5.23) as

$$p_{X_1,X_2^*(a_1),X_3^*(\overline{a}_2),\ldots,X_K^*(\overline{a}_{K-1}),Y^*(\overline{a})}(x_1,x_2,\ldots,x_K,y)$$
$$= p_{Y|\overline{X},\overline{A}}(y|\overline{x},\overline{a})$$
$$\times p_{X_K|\overline{X}_{K-1},\overline{A}_{K-1}}(x_K|\overline{x}_{K-1},\overline{a}_{K-1})$$
$$\vdots \tag{5.24}$$
$$\times p_{X_2|X_1,A_1}(x_2|x_1,a_1)$$
$$\times p_{X_1}(x_1).$$

Note that the representation (5.24) depends only on the components on the left-hand side of the factorization (5.23) of the joint density of the observed data, which correspond to the conditional densities of intervening information given past history. The conditional densities of treatment received given past history on the right-hand side are not involved in (5.24). Thus, (5.24) effectively treats $a_1, \ldots, a_K$ as fixed.

We show (5.24) in the case $K = 2$; readers uninterested in the details can skip this demonstration without loss of continuity.

Demonstration of the g-Computation Algorithm (5.24) for $K = 2$

Proof. Here, the set of all possible potential outcomes in (5.9) is

$$W^* = \left\{X_2^*(a_1), Y^*(\overline{a}) \text{ for } a_1 \in \mathcal{A}_1, \overline{a}_2 \in \overline{\mathcal{A}}_2\right\},$$

and the observed data are (X_1, A_1, X_2, A_2, Y). Consider a realization $(x_1, a_1, x_2, a_2, y) = (\overline{x}_2, \overline{a}_2, y) = (\overline{x}, \overline{a}, y)$ such that

$$p_{X_1,X_2^*(a_1),Y^*(\overline{a})}(x_1,x_2,y) = P\{X_1 = x_1, X_2^*(a_1) = x_2, Y^*(\overline{a}) = y\} > 0. \tag{5.25}$$

For $K = 2$, the g-computation algorithm (5.24) states that

$$p_{X_1, X_2^*(a_1), Y^*(\bar{a})}(x_1, x_2, y)$$
$$= p_{Y|\overline{X}, \overline{A}}(y|\overline{x}, \bar{a})\, p_{X_2|X_1, A_1}(x_2|x_1, a_1)\, p_{X_1}(x_1). \qquad (5.26)$$

We now demonstrate that the first and middle terms on the right-hand side of (5.26) can be reexpressed such that the right-hand side is equal to the joint density of $\{X_1, X_2^*(a_1), Y^*(\bar{a})\}$.

The middle term on the right-hand side of (5.26) is

$$p_{X_2|X_1, A_1}(x_2|x_1, a_1) = P(X_2 = x_2|X_1 = x_1, A_1 = a_1).$$

By (5.25) and the positivity assumption (5.20),

$$P(X_1 = x_1, A_1 = a_1) = P(A_1 = a_1 \mid X_1 = x_1)\, P(X_1 = x_1) > 0. \quad (5.27)$$

Thus, the middle term is well defined, and we have that

$$p_{X_2|X_1, A_1}(x_2|x_1, a_1) = P(X_2 = x_2|X_1 = x_1, A_1 = a_1)$$
$$= P\{X_2^*(a_1) = x_2|X_1 = x_1, A_1 = a_1\} \qquad (5.28)$$
$$= P\{X_2^*(a_1) = x_2|X_1 = x_1\} = p_{X_2^*(a_1)|X_1}(x_2|x_1), \qquad (5.29)$$

where (5.28) follows by SUTVA (5.17), and (5.29) follows by the SRA (5.18). Likewise, the first term on the right-hand side of (5.26) is

$$p_{Y|\overline{X}, \overline{A}}(y|\overline{x}, \bar{a}) = P(Y = y|\overline{X} = \overline{x}, \overline{A} = \bar{a}). \qquad (5.30)$$

Note that

$$P(\overline{X} = \overline{x}, \overline{A} = \bar{a}) = P(A_2 = a_2 \mid \overline{X} = \overline{x}, A_1 = a_1)$$
$$\times P(X_2 = x_2 \mid X_1 = x_1, A_1 = a_1)\, P(X_1 = x_1, A_1 = a_1)$$
$$= P(A_2 = a_2 \mid \overline{X} = \overline{x}, A_1 = a_1)$$
$$\times P(X_2^*(a_1) = x_2 \mid X_1 = x_1)\, P(X_1 = x_1, A_1 = a_1) > 0,$$

which follows by the positivity assumption (5.20), (5.25), (5.27), and (5.29), so that (5.30) is well defined. Thus, we have

$$p_{Y|\overline{X}, \overline{A}}(y|\overline{x}, \bar{a}) = P(Y = y \mid \overline{X} = \overline{x}, \overline{A} = \bar{a})$$
$$= P\{Y^*(\bar{a}) = y \mid \overline{X} = \overline{x}, A_1 = a_1, A_2 = a_2\} \qquad (5.31)$$
$$= P\{Y^*(\bar{a}) = y \mid X_1 = x_1, X_2 = x_2, A_1 = a_1\} \qquad (5.32)$$
$$= P\{Y^*(\bar{a}) = y \mid X_1 = x_1, X_2^*(a_1) = x_2, A_1 = a_1\} \qquad (5.33)$$
$$= \frac{P\{Y^*(\bar{a}) = y, X_2^*(a_1) = x_2|X_1 = x_1, A_1 = a_1\}}{P\{X_2^*(a_1) = x_2|X_1 = x_1, A_1 = a_1\}}$$

$$= \frac{P\{Y^*(\overline{a}) = y, X_2^*(a_1) = x_2 | X_1 = x_1\}}{P\{X_2^*(a_1) = x_2 | X_1 = x_1\}} \tag{5.34}$$

$$= P\{Y^*(\overline{a}) = y \mid X_1 = x_1, X_2^*(a_1) = x_2\}$$

$$= p_{Y^*(\overline{a})|X_1, X_2^*(a_1)}(y|x_1, x_2), \tag{5.35}$$

where (5.31) follows by SUTVA (5.17); (5.32) follows by the SRA (5.18), $W^* \perp\!\!\!\perp A_2 | \overline{X}_2, A_1$; (5.33) follows by SUTVA; and (5.34) follows by the SRA, $W^* \perp\!\!\!\perp A_1 | X_1$.

Substituting (5.29) and (5.35) in (5.26) yields

$$p_{Y|\overline{X},\overline{A}}(y|\overline{x},\overline{a}) \, p_{X_2|X_1,A_1}(x_2|x_1,a_1) \, p_{X_1}(x_1)$$

$$= p_{Y^*(\overline{a})|X_1,X_2^*(a_1)}(y|x_1,x_2) \, p_{X_2^*(a_1)|X_1}(x_2|x_1) \, p_{X_1}(x_1),$$

$$= p_{X_1, X_2^*(a_1), Y^*(\overline{a})}(x_1, x_2, y),$$

demonstrating the validity of the g-computation algorithm. In Section 6.2.4, we present results that can be used to demonstrate the g-computation algorithm for general K. □

The representation of the density of the potential outcomes $\{X_1, X_2^*(a_1), X_3^*(\overline{a}_2), \ldots, X_K^*(\overline{a}_{K-1}), Y^*(\overline{a})\}$ for any $\overline{a} \in \overline{\mathcal{A}}$ in terms of that of the observed data as in (5.24) can be used to obtain an expression for $E\{Y^*(\overline{a})\}$, analogous to the developments in Section 2.4 for a single decision point. Write (5.24) compactly as

$$p_{X_1, X_2^*(a_1), X_3^*(\overline{a}_2), \ldots, X_K^*(\overline{a}_{K-1}), Y^*(\overline{a})}(x_1, x_2, \ldots, x_K, y)$$

$$= p_{Y|\overline{X},\overline{A}}(y|\overline{x},\overline{a})$$

$$\times \left\{ \prod_{k=2}^{K} p_{X_k|\overline{X}_{k-1},\overline{A}_{k-1}}(x_k|\overline{x}_{k-1},\overline{a}_{k-1}) \right\} p_{X_1}(x_1). \tag{5.36}$$

The marginal density of $Y^*(\overline{a})$ can be obtained by integration of the right-hand side of (5.36); that is,

$$p_{Y^*(\overline{a})}(y) = \int_{\overline{\mathcal{X}}} \left[\; p_{Y|\overline{X},\overline{A}}(y|\overline{x},\overline{a}) \right. \tag{5.37}$$

$$\left. \times \left\{ \prod_{k=2}^{K} p_{X_k|\overline{X}_{k-1},\overline{A}_{k-1}}(x_k|\overline{x}_{k-1},\overline{a}_{k-1}) \right\} \times p_{X_1}(x_1) \right] d\nu_K(x_K) \cdots d\nu_1(x_1),$$

where, analogous to (2.18), $d\nu_K(x_K) \cdots d\nu_1(x_1)$ is the dominating measure. It follows that $E\{Y^*(\overline{a})\}$ can be obtained from (5.37); in the case where all random variables are discrete, so that integration is with respect to the counting measure and yields a summation over all $\overline{x}$ in $\overline{\mathcal{X}}$, it is straightforward that

$$
E\{Y^*(\overline{a})\} = \sum_{\overline{x} \in \overline{\mathcal{X}}} \Bigg[\quad E(Y|\overline{X} = \overline{x}, \overline{A} = \overline{a}) \tag{5.38}
$$

$$
\times \left\{ \prod_{k=2}^{K} P(X_k = x_k|\overline{X}_{k-1} = \overline{x}_{k-1}, \overline{A}_{k-1} = \overline{a}_{k-1}) \right\} P(X_1 = x_1) \Bigg].
$$

Because expectations of potential outcomes are central to causal inference, (5.38) itself is sometimes referred to as the g-computation algorithm or g-formula.

We now present the version of the g-computation algorithm corresponding to a fixed regime $d \in \mathcal{D}$, which builds on this development. As in the discussion at the end of Section 5.2, this relies on the fact that, if d is followed by an individual, then the treatment options selected at each decision point depend only on the intervening information, so that the treatments received through Decision k for an individual presenting with baseline information $h_1 = x_1$, $k = 2, \ldots, K$, can be represented by the recursion in (5.6); namely

$$
\overline{d}_k(\overline{x}_k) = [d_1(x_1), d_2\{\overline{x}_2, d_1(x_1)\}, \ldots, d_k\{\overline{x}_k, \overline{d}_{k-1}(\overline{x}_{k-1})\}].
$$

The g-computation algorithm states that, for any $d \in \mathcal{D}$, under SUTVA (5.17), the SRA (5.18), and the positivity assumption (5.20), analogous to (5.24), the joint density of the potential outcomes $\{X_1, X_2^*(d_1), X_3^*(\overline{d}_2), \ldots, X_K^*(\overline{d}_{K-1}), Y^*(d)\}$ can be obtained as

$$
p_{X_1, X_2^*(d_1), X_3^*(\overline{d}_2), \ldots, X_K^*(\overline{d}_{K-1}), Y^*(d)}(x_1, \ldots, x_K, y) \tag{5.39}
$$

$$
= p_{Y|\overline{X},\overline{A}}\{y|\overline{x}, \overline{d}(\overline{x})\}
$$

$$
\times p_{X_K|\overline{X}_{K-1}, \overline{A}_{K-1}}\{x_K|\overline{x}_{K-1}, \overline{d}_{K-1}(\overline{x}_{K-1})\}
$$

$$
\vdots \tag{5.40}
$$

$$
\times p_{X_2|X_1, A_1}\{x_2|x_1, d_1(x_1)\}
$$

$$
\times p_{X_1}(x_1),
$$

for any realization $(x_1, x_2, \ldots, x_K, y)$ for which (5.39) is positive. As in (5.36), this joint density can be expressed compactly as

$$
p_{X_1, X_2^*(d_1), X_3^*(\overline{d}_2), \ldots, X_K^*(\overline{d}_{K-1}), Y^*(d)}(x_1, \ldots, x_K, y)
$$

$$
= p_{Y|\overline{X},\overline{A}}\{y|\overline{x}, \overline{d}_K(\overline{x})\} \tag{5.41}
$$

$$
\times \left[\prod_{k=2}^{K} p_{X_k|\overline{X}_{k-1}, \overline{A}_{k-1}}\{x_k|\overline{x}_{k-1}, \overline{d}_{k-1}(\overline{x}_{k-1})\} \right] p_{X_1}(x_1).
$$

In Section 6.3, we present a proof of (5.40).

The representations in (5.40) and (5.41) of the density of $\{X_1, X_2^*(d_1), X_3^*(\bar{d}_2), \ldots, X_K^*(\bar{d}_{K-1}), Y^*(d)\}$ for any $d \in \mathcal{D}$ demonstrate that it can be identified from the observed data. Accordingly, as in (5.37), the marginal density of $Y^*(d)$ can be obtained as

$$p_{Y^*(d)}(y) = \int_{\overline{\mathcal{X}}} \left(\quad p_{Y|\overline{X},\overline{A}}\{y|\overline{x}, \overline{d}(\overline{x})\} \right. \tag{5.42}$$
$$\times \left[\prod_{k=2}^{K} p_{X_k|\overline{X}_{k-1},\overline{A}_{k-1}}\{x_k|\overline{x}_{k-1}, \overline{d}_{k-1}(\overline{x}_{k-1})\} \right] p_{X_1}(x_1) \Bigg)$$
$$\times d\nu_K(x_K) \cdots d\nu_1(x_1),$$

where, as in (5.37), $d\nu_K(x_K) \cdots d\nu_1(x_1)$ is the dominating measure. It follows that

$$E\{Y^*(d)\} = \int_{\overline{\mathcal{X}}} \left(\quad E\{Y|\overline{X} = \overline{x}, \overline{A} = \overline{d}(\overline{x})\} \right. \tag{5.43}$$
$$\times \left[\prod_{k=2}^{K} p_{X_k|\overline{X}_{k-1},\overline{A}_{k-1}}\{x_k|\overline{x}_{k-1}, \overline{d}_{k-1}(\overline{x}_{k-1})\} \right] p_{X_1}(x_1) \Bigg)$$
$$\times d\nu_K(x_K) \cdots d\nu_1(x_1),$$

which, in the case where all random variables are discrete, can be written as

$$E\{Y^*(d)\} = \sum_{\overline{x} \in \overline{\mathcal{X}}} \left(\quad E\{Y|\overline{X} = \overline{x}, \overline{A} = \overline{d}(\overline{x})\} \right. \tag{5.44}$$
$$\times \left[\prod_{k=2}^{K} P\{\overline{X}_k = \overline{x}_k|\overline{X}_{k-1} = \overline{x}_{k-1}, \overline{A}_{k-1} = \overline{d}_{k-1}(\overline{x}_{k-1})\} \right] P(X_1 = x_1) \Bigg).$$

The foregoing results demonstrate that, as long as the analyst is willing to adopt SUTVA, the SRA, and the positivity assumption, inference on a fixed regime $d \in \mathcal{D}$ from observed data, and in particular estimation of the value $\mathcal{V}(d) = E\{Y^*(d)\}$ of d, is possible. The expressions (5.42) and (5.43) suggest an approach to estimation of $\mathcal{V}(d)$, discussed next, that involves developing models for either the density $p_{Y|\overline{X},\overline{A}}(y|\overline{x}, \overline{a})$ or

$$Q_K(h_K, a_K) = Q_K(\overline{x}_K, \overline{a}_K) = Q_K(\overline{x}, \overline{a}) = E(Y|\overline{X} = \overline{x}, \overline{A} = \overline{a}), \tag{5.45}$$

and the densities

$$p_{X_1}(x_1), \quad p_{X_k|\overline{X}_{k-1},\overline{A}_{k-1}}(x_k|\overline{x}_{k-1}, \overline{a}_{k-1}), \quad k = 2, \ldots, K.$$

5.5   Estimation of the Value of a Fixed Regime

5.5.1   Estimation via g-Computation

The developments in the last section demonstrate that, in principle, estimation of the marginal density $p_{Y^*(d)}(y)$ of $Y^*(d)$ and of the value $E\{Y^*(d)\}$ for a fixed $d \in \mathcal{D}$ can be accomplished by positing models for each of the components on the right-hand sides of (5.42) and (5.43), respectively; fitting these models by appropriate methods; and substituting the fitted models into (5.42) and (5.43). In particular, for (5.42), we might posit parametric models, in obvious notation,

$$p_{Y|\overline{X},\overline{A}}(y|\overline{x},\overline{a};\zeta_{K+1}),$$

$$p_{X_k|\overline{X}_{k-1},\overline{A}_{k-1}}(x_k|\overline{x}_{k-1},\overline{a}_{k-1};\zeta_k), \quad k = 2,\ldots,K, \qquad (5.46)$$

$$p_{X_1}(x_1;\zeta_1),$$

depending on a parameter $\zeta = (\zeta_1^T,\ldots,\zeta_{K+1}^T)^T$. We discuss specification of such models below.

Given the observed data in (5.16),

$$(X_{1i}, A_{1i},\ldots,X_{Ki}, A_{Ki}, Y_i) = (\overline{X}_i, \overline{A}_i, Y_i), \quad i = 1,\ldots,n,$$

ζ can be estimated by maximizing the partial likelihood

$$\prod_{i=1}^n \left\{ p_{Y|\overline{X},\overline{A}}(Y_i|\overline{X}_i, \overline{A}_i; \zeta_{K+1}) \right.$$

$$\left. \prod_{k=2}^K p_{X_k|\overline{X}_{k-1},\overline{A}_{k-1}}(X_{ki}|\overline{X}_{k-1,i}, \overline{A}_{k-1,i}; \zeta_k)\, p_{X_1}(X_{1i};\zeta_1) \right\} \qquad (5.47)$$

in ζ to obtain the estimator $\widehat{\zeta} = (\widehat{\zeta}_1^T,\ldots,\widehat{\zeta}_{K+1}^T)^T$. Usually, the models for these densities would be such that the ζ_k, $k = 1,\ldots,K+1$, are distinct and nonoverlapping; that is, the ζ_k are variationally independent. In this case, the estimators $\widehat{\zeta}_k$ can be obtained by maximizing each component in (5.47) separately in ζ_k; (5.47) accommodates the situation where the ζ_k share components across k.

A major obstacle to this approach is that (5.42) and (5.43) involve integration over the sample space $\overline{\mathcal{X}} = \mathcal{X}_1 \times \cdots \times \mathcal{X}_K$ of all realizations $\overline{x} = (x_1,\ldots,x_K)$ of intervening information. When all of $x_1,\ldots,x_K$ are discrete and of low dimension, and the $\mathcal{X}_k$ are finite, so that the integrals are sums as in (5.44) over manageable sets of values, direct evaluation of (5.42) and (5.43) might be feasible in practice. However, in the much more realistic situation where $x_1,\ldots,x_K$ are possibly high dimensional, with discrete and continuous components, the required integration is likely to be computationally insurmountable, and estimation of $p_{Y^*(d)}(y)$ and $E\{Y^*(d)\}$ by direct evaluation is not possible.

To address this difficulty, Robins (1986) suggested approximating the distribution of $Y^*(d)$ for $d \in \mathcal{D}$ by positing and fitting models as in (5.46) and then using Monte Carlo integration. Specifically, for $r = 1, \ldots, M$, simulate a realization from the distribution of $Y^*(d)$ as follows:

1. Generate random x_{1r} from $p_{X_1}(x_1; \widehat{\zeta}_1)$.

2. Generate random x_{2r} from $p_{X_2|X_1,A_1}\{x_2|x_{1r}, d_1(x_{1r}); \widehat{\zeta}_2\}$.

3. Continue in this fashion, generating random x_{kr} from

$$p_{X_k|\overline{X}_{k-1},\overline{A}_{k-1}}\{x_k|\overline{x}_{k-1,r}, \overline{d}_{k-1}(\overline{x}_{k-1,r}); \widehat{\zeta}_k\}, \quad k = 3, \ldots, K.$$

4. Generate random y_r from $p_{Y|\overline{X},\overline{A}}\{y|\overline{x}_r, \overline{d}_K(\overline{x}_r); \widehat{\zeta}_{K+1}\}$.

Here, $\overline{x}_r = (x_{1r}, \ldots, x_{Kr})$. The values $y_1, \ldots, y_M$ so obtained are a random sample from the estimated distribution of $Y^*(d)$ represented in terms of the observed data by the fitted models in (5.46).

Given this random sample, the value $\mathcal{V}(d) = E\{Y^*(d)\}$ for a fixed regime $d \in \mathcal{D}$ can then be estimated by

$$\widehat{\mathcal{V}}_{GC}(d) = M^{-1} \sum_{r=1}^{M} y_r. \tag{5.48}$$

Likewise, any other functional of the distribution of $Y^*(d)$ can be estimated by the analogous sample quantity. This general approach has been referred to as estimation by the g-computation algorithm.

Although estimation via this approach is possible in principle, there are significant challenges to its practical implementation. Development of the models (5.46) can be a daunting task in practice, particularly when K is large and/or the collections of intervening information $x_1, \ldots, x_K$ are complex and high dimensional. With univariate outcome Y as we have assumed throughout, specification of a model

$$p_{Y|\overline{X},\overline{A}}(y|\overline{x}, \overline{a}; \zeta_{K+1}) \tag{5.49}$$

may be feasible; e.g., if Y is continuous, one might take (5.49) to be a normal density with mean and possibly variance depending on $(\overline{x}, \overline{a})$. However, developing models

$$p_{X_k|\overline{X}_{k-1},\overline{A}_{k-1}}(x_k|\overline{x}_{k-1}, \overline{a}_{k-1}; \zeta_k), \quad k = 2, \ldots, K, \tag{5.50}$$

$$p_{X_1}(x_1; \zeta_1), \tag{5.51}$$

when X_k, $k = 1, \ldots, K$, are multivariate, even if not high dimensional, involves several difficulties. Suppose that X_k comprises both continuous components X_{k1} and discrete components X_{k2}. One might factorize (5.50) as either

$$p_{X_{k1}|X_{k2},\overline{X}_{k-1},\overline{A}_{k-1}}(x_{k1}|x_{k2},\overline{x}_{k-1},\overline{a}_{k-1};\zeta_{k1})$$
$$\times\, p_{X_{k2}|\overline{X}_{k-1},\overline{A}_{k-1}}(x_{k2}|\overline{x}_{k-1},\overline{a}_{k-1};\zeta_{k2}) \qquad (5.52)$$

or

$$p_{X_{k2}|X_{k1},\overline{X}_{k-1},\overline{A}_{k-1}}(x_{k2}|x_{k1},\overline{x}_{k-1},\overline{a}_{k-1};\zeta_{k2})$$
$$\times\, p_{X_{k1}|\overline{X}_{k-1},\overline{A}_{k-1}}(x_{k1}|\overline{x}_{k-1},\overline{a}_{k-1};\zeta_{k1}) \qquad (5.53)$$

and similarly for (5.51), and specify models for each conditional density. For example, one might represent the first term in (5.52) as a multivariate normal density with mean and covariance matrix depending on the conditioning set. If the components of X_{k2} are all binary, the second term in (5.52) can be factorized further into univariate components, ordered in some sensible or arbitrary fashion, each of which is modeled by a Bernoulli density with success probability depending on the relevant conditioning set. One can develop models for the terms in the alternative factorization (5.53) similarly. Clearly, then, there is no unique representation of the densities (5.50) and (5.51), so that estimation of any functional of the distribution of $Y^*(d)$, and in particular $\mathcal{V}(d)$, is entirely predicated on the chosen representation. Moreover, once a particular representation is adopted, there are myriad modeling choices for how each component of the representation depends on the variables in the conditioning set. The extent to which the results are sensitive to the modeling strategy is likely problem specific.

Even if such models are developed, simulation of random deviates from the required distributions in each step itself can be demanding when $x_1,\ldots,x_K$ are high dimensional and comprise discrete and continuous components. Moreover, derivation of approximate standard errors for $\widehat{\mathcal{V}}_{GC}(d)$ in (5.48) is not straightforward. Use of a parametric bootstrap, where the posited models are taken as true, has been suggested to obtain approximate measures of uncertainty. This is of necessity computationally intensive, as derivation of each bootstrap sample embeds M simulations.

Because of these considerations, estimation of the value $\mathcal{V}(d)$ for a fixed $d \in \mathcal{D}$ using the g-computation algorithm is not commonplace in practice. The g-formula is most useful as a demonstration that it is possible in principle to identify and estimate $\mathcal{V}(d)$ from observed data under SUTVA, the SRA, and the positivity assumption. In the next section, we discuss an approach to estimation of $\mathcal{V}(d)$ that may be somewhat more straightforward to implement but involves other drawbacks; further methods are presented in Chapter 6.

Remark. If interest focuses on estimation of an optimal regime $d^{opt} \in \mathcal{D}$ satisfying (5.12), it is clear that estimating d^{opt} by maximizing $\widehat{\mathcal{V}}_{GC}(d)$ in (5.48) in d is a formidable computational challenge. Assuming that the required models can be developed and fitted, estimation of $\mathcal{V}(d) = E\{Y^*(d)\}$ for each fixed $d \in \mathcal{D}$ requires carrying out a Monte Carlo simulation. Thus, optimization of $\widehat{\mathcal{V}}_{GC}(d)$ requires evaluation of $\widehat{\mathcal{V}}_{GC}(d)$ by simulation for each of numerous $d \in \mathcal{D}$. We defer further discussion of estimation of an optimal regime $d^{opt} \in \mathcal{D}$ to later in this chapter.

5.5.2 Inverse Probability Weighted Estimator

Because of the form of the g-formula, estimation based on the g-computation algorithm does not require specification of models for the densities of treatment received given past history, namely,

$$p_{A_1|X_1}(a_1|x_1) = p_{A_1|H_1}(a_1|h_1), \tag{5.54}$$
$$p_{A_k|\overline{X}_k,\overline{A}_{k-1}}(a_k|\overline{x}_k,\overline{a}_{k-1}) = p_{A_k|H_k}(a_k|h_k), \quad k = 2,\ldots,K.$$

Under SUTVA, the SRA, and the positivity assumption, an alternative demonstration that $p_{Y^*(d)}(y)$ and $E\{Y^*(d)\}$ can be represented in terms of the observed data is possible, which suggests another approach to estimation of the value $\mathcal{V}(d)$ for given $d \in \mathcal{D}$ using inverse probability weighting based on models for the densities in (5.54). We sketch this result here for $E\{Y^*(d)\}$; a rigorous proof is deferred to Section 6.4.3.

Using the notation defined in (5.6), the event $\{\overline{A} = \overline{d}(\overline{X})\}$; that is,

$$[A_1 = d_1(X_1), A_2 = d_2\{\overline{X}_2, d_1(X_1)\}, \ldots, A_K = d_K\{\overline{X}_K, \overline{d}_{K-1}(\overline{X}_{K-1})\}],$$

corresponds to the situation where the treatment options actually received by a randomly chosen individual are consistent with those selected by the rules in d at all K decision points. Thus, analogous to the development for a single decision in Section 3.3.2, let

$$\mathcal{C}_d = \mathrm{I}\{\overline{A} = \overline{d}(\overline{X})\} \qquad \text{compatibility indicator} \tag{5.55}$$

be the indicator of whether or not the treatment options received by an individual coincide with those selected by d for all K decisions. Let

$$\pi_{d,1}(X_1) = p_{A_1|X_1}\{d_1(X_1)|X_1\}, \tag{5.56}$$
$$\pi_{d,k}(\overline{X}_k) = p_{A_k|\overline{X}_k,\overline{A}_{k-1}}[d_k\{\overline{X}_k, \overline{d}_{k-1}(\overline{X}_{k-1})\}|\overline{X}_k, \overline{d}_{k-1}(\overline{X}_{k-1})],$$
$$k = 2,\ldots,K;$$

that is, $\pi_{d,1}(X_1)$ and $\pi_{d,k}(\overline{X}_k)$, $k = 2, \ldots, K$, are the densities of A_1 given X_1 and A_k given $\overline{X}_k$ and $\overline{A}_{k-1}$ evaluated at $d_1(X_1)$ and $d_k\{\overline{X}_k, \overline{d}_{k-1}(\overline{X}_{k-1})\}$, respectively.

Then it is shown rigorously in Section 6.4.3 that

end of followup ✗

$$\widehat{\mathcal{V}}_{IPW}(d)$$

$$= n^{-1} \sum_{i=1}^{n} \frac{I\{\overline{A}_i = \overline{d}(\overline{X}_i)\}Y_i}{\prod_{k=1}^{K} p_{A_k|\overline{X}_k,\overline{A}_{k-1}}[d_k\{\overline{X}_{ki}, \overline{d}_{k-1}(\overline{X}_{k-1,i})\}|\overline{X}_{ki}, \overline{d}_{k-1}(\overline{X}_{k-1,i})]}$$

$$= n^{-1} \sum_{i=1}^{n} \frac{\mathcal{C}_{d,i} Y_i}{\left\{\prod_{k=2}^{K} \pi_{d,k}(\overline{X}_{ki})\right\} \pi_{d,1}(X_{1i})} \tag{5.57}$$

is an unbiased estimator for $\mathcal{V}(d) = E\{Y^*(d)\}$.

Sketch of Proof of (5.57)

Proof. The following informal demonstration relies on a conditioning argument analogous to that in (3.22) for $K = 1$. Define

$$\overline{X}_k^*(\overline{d}_{k-1}) = \{X_1, X_2^*(d_1), X_3^*(\overline{d}_2), \ldots, X_k^*(\overline{d}_{k-1})\}, \quad k = 2, \ldots, K.$$

Then   *compatibility indicator*

$$E\left[\frac{\mathcal{C}_d Y}{\left\{\prod_{k=2}^{K} \pi_{d,k}(\overline{X}_k)\right\} \pi_{d,1}(X_1)}\right]$$

$$= E\left(\frac{\mathcal{C}_d Y^*(d)}{\left[\prod_{k=2}^{K} \pi_{d,k}\{\overline{X}_k^*(\overline{d}_{k-1})\}\right] \pi_{d,1}(X_1)}\right)$$

$$= E\left\{E\left(\frac{I\{\overline{A} = \overline{d}(\overline{X})\}Y^*(d)}{\left[\prod_{k=2}^{K} \pi_{d,k}\{\overline{X}_k^*(\overline{d}_{k-1})\}\right] \pi_{d,1}(X_1)}\bigg| X_1, W^*\right)\right\},$$

$$= E\left(\frac{P\{\overline{A} = \overline{d}(\overline{X})|X_1, W^*\}Y^*(d)}{\left[\prod_{k=2}^{K} \pi_{d,k}\{\overline{X}_k^*(\overline{d}_{k-1})\}\right] \pi_{d,1}(X_1)}\right), \tag{5.58}$$

where the first equality holds because $Y = Y^*(d)$ and $\overline{X}_k = \overline{X}_k^*(\overline{d}_{k-1})$, $k = 2, \ldots, K$, when $\mathcal{C}_d = 1$ by SUTVA; and (5.58) follows because $Y^*(d)$ and the denominator are functions of $\{X_1, W^*\}$. It is shown in Section 6.4.3 that, under SUTVA, the SRA, and the positivity assumption,

$$P\{\overline{A} = \overline{d}(\overline{X})|X_1, W^*\} > 0$$

almost surely and that the denominator in (5.58),

$$\left[\prod_{k=2}^{K} \pi_{d,k}\{\overline{X}_k^*(\overline{d}_{k-1})\}\right] \pi_{d,1}(X_1) = P\{\overline{A} = \overline{d}(\overline{X})|X_1, W^*\}$$

almost surely, so that

$$E\left[\frac{\mathcal{C}_d Y}{\left\{\prod_{k=2}^{K} \pi_{d,k}(\overline{X}_k)\right\} \pi_{d,1}(X_1)}\right] = E\{Y^*(d)\}. \tag{5.59}$$

The result (5.59) thus demonstrates that the value $\mathcal{V}(d) = E\{Y^*(d)\}$ can be identified in terms of the observed data. □

As in the single decision case, the estimator (5.57) can be motivated via a missing data analogy. As is evident in the argument above, when $\mathcal{C}_d = 1$, $Y^*(d)$ is observed; otherwise, it is missing. Under SUTVA, the SRA, and the positivity assumption, the denominator

$$\left\{\prod_{k=2}^{K} \pi_{d,k}(\overline{X}_k)\right\} \pi_{d,1}(X_1) \qquad \text{probability of remaining uncensored}$$

can be interpreted as the propensity for receiving treatment consistent with regime d through all K decisions, given the observed history. Thus, the inverse probability weighting is in the spirit discussed in Section 3.3.2; however, the formulation is considerably more complex and is presented formally in Section 6.4.3.

Analogous to the single decision case, if the observed data are from a SMART,

$$p_{A_1|X_1}(a_1|x_1) = p_{A_1|H_1}(a_1|h_1) = P(A_1 = a_1|H_1 = h_1),$$
$$p_{A_k|\overline{X}_k, \overline{A}_{k-1}}(a_k|\overline{x}_k, \overline{a}_{k-1}) = p_{A_k|H_k}(a_k|h_k) = P(A_k = a_k|H_k = h_k),$$
$$k = 2, \ldots, K,$$

in (5.54) are known, so that $\pi_{d,1}(X_1)$ and $\pi_{d,k}(\overline{X}_k)$, $k = 2, \ldots, K$, can be calculated for each individual, and the estimator (5.57) can be used as is. If the data are from an observational study, the analyst must posit models for each density.

Two Options at Each Decision Point

We illustrate in the case where there are two treatment options at each decision point, coded as 0 and 1; that is, $\mathcal{A}_k = \{0, 1\}$, $k = 1, \ldots, K$, as in the development for a single decision in Section 3.3.2. Of course, the actual options coded as 0 and 1 at each decision point need not be the same across $k = 1, \ldots, K$. Define the propensities to receive the option coded as 1 at each decision as a function of history as

$$\pi_k(h_k) = P(A_k = 1 | H_k = h_k), \quad k = 1, \ldots, K, \qquad (5.60)$$

where we can write (5.60) equivalently as

$$\pi_1(h_1) = \pi_1(x_1) = P(A_1 = 1 | X_1 = x_1),$$
$$\pi_k(h_k) = \pi_k(\overline{x}_k, \overline{a}_{k-1}) = P(A_k = 1 | \overline{X}_k = \overline{x}_k, \overline{A}_{k-1} = \overline{a}_{k-1}),$$
$$k = 2, \ldots, K.$$

Then it is straightforward that

$$p_{A_1|X_1}(a_1|x_1) = p_{A_1|H_1}(a_1|h_1) = \pi_1(h_1)^{a_1}\{1 - \pi_1(h_1)\}^{1-a_1}$$
$$p_{A_k|\overline{X}_k,\overline{A}_{k-1}}(a_k|\overline{x}_k, \overline{a}_{k-1}) = p_{A_k|H_k}(a_k|h_k) = \pi_k(h_k)^{a_k}\{1 - \pi_k(h_k)\}^{1-a_k}$$
$$k = 2, \ldots, K;$$

that is, each of these densities is that of a Bernoulli distribution. It follows from (5.56) that

$$\pi_{d,1}(X_1) = \pi_1(X_1)^{d_1(X_1)}\{1 - \pi_1(X_1)\}^{1-d_1(X_1)}$$
$$\pi_{d,k}(\overline{X}_k) = \pi_k\{\overline{X}_k, \overline{d}_{k-1}(\overline{X}_{k-1})\}^{d_k\{\overline{X}_k,\overline{d}_{k-1}(\overline{X}_{k-1})\}} \qquad (5.61)$$
$$\times [1 - \pi_k\{\overline{X}_k, \overline{d}_{k-1}(\overline{X}_{k-1})\}]^{1-d_k\{\overline{X}_k,\overline{d}_{k-1}(\overline{X}_{k-1})\}},$$
$$k = 2, \ldots, K.$$

We can posit parametric propensity models for the $\pi_k(h_k)$

$$\pi_k(h_k; \gamma_k), \quad k = 1, \ldots, K,$$

in terms of parameters $\gamma = (\gamma_1^T, \ldots, \gamma_K^T)^T$; e.g., logistic regression models

$$\pi_k(h_k; \gamma_k) = \frac{\exp(\gamma_{k1} + \gamma_{k2}^T \widetilde{h}_k)}{1 + \exp(\gamma_{k1} + \gamma_{k2}^T \widetilde{h}_k)}, \quad \gamma_k = (\gamma_{k1}, \gamma_{k2}^T)^T, \quad k = 1, \ldots, K,$$

with $\widetilde{h}_k$ functions of elements of h_k, which can be fitted by maximizing

$$\prod_{i=1}^{n} \left\{ \prod_{k=1}^{K} \{\pi_k(H_{ki}; \gamma_k)\}^{A_{ki}} \{1 - \pi_k(H_{ki}; \gamma_k)\}^{1-A_{ki}} \right\} \qquad (5.62)$$

to obtain estimators $\widehat{\gamma}_k$, $k = 1, \ldots, K$. Ordinarily, the γ_k are distinct, and maximization can be carried out for each k separately, but (5.62) accommodates the situation where the γ_k share components as in (5.47).

The posited models can be substituted directly in (5.61) to obtain

$$\pi_{d,1}(X_1; \gamma_1) = \pi_1(X_1; \gamma_1)^{d_1(X_1)} \{1 - \pi_1(X_1; \gamma_1)\}^{1-d_1(X_1)} \tag{5.63}$$

$$\pi_{d,k}(\overline{X}_k; \gamma_k) = \pi_k\{\overline{X}_k, \overline{d}_{k-1}(\overline{X}_{k-1}); \gamma_k\}^{d_k\{\overline{X}_k, \overline{d}_{k-1}(\overline{X}_{k-1})\}}$$
$$\times [1 - \pi_k\{\overline{X}_k, \overline{d}_{k-1}(\overline{X}_{k-1}); \gamma_k\}]^{1-d_k\{\overline{X}_k, \overline{d}_{k-1}(\overline{X}_{k-1})\}},$$
$$k = 2, \ldots, K;$$

and the estimator for the value is then

$$\widehat{\mathcal{V}}_{IPW}(d) = n^{-1} \sum_{i=1}^{n} \frac{\mathcal{C}_{d,i} Y_i}{\left\{\prod_{k=2}^{K} \pi_{d,k}(\overline{X}_{ki}; \widehat{\gamma}_k)\right\} \pi_{d,1}(X_{1i}; \widehat{\gamma}_1)}. \tag{5.64}$$

Inspection of (5.64) and the definitions of $\pi_{d,k}(\overline{X}_k; \gamma_k)$ in (5.63) show that, when $K = 1$, (5.64) reduces to the inverse probability weighted estimator (3.24). Moreover, the argument leading to the identifiability result (5.59) demonstrates that, if the propensity models $\pi_k(h_k; \gamma_k)$ are correctly specified, so that there exists $\gamma_{k,0}$ such that $\pi_k(h_k; \gamma_{k,0}) = \pi_k(h_k)$, then the induced models $\pi_{d,k}(\overline{X}_k; \gamma_k)$ are also correctly specified for $k = 1, \ldots, K$. It follows that $\widehat{\mathcal{V}}_{IPW}(d)$ is a consistent estimator for the true value $\mathcal{V}(d)$. If the observed data are from a SMART, for which the propensities are known, then $\widehat{\mathcal{V}}_{IPW}(d)$ is guaranteed to be consistent if the known or fitted $\pi_k(h_k)$ are substituted in (5.64).

More than Two Options at Each Decision Point

When the sets $\mathcal{A}_k$, $k = 1, \ldots, K$, comprise finite but arbitrary numbers of options m_k at each decision point, coded as $1, \ldots, m_k$, so that $\mathcal{A}_k = \{1, \ldots, m_k\}$, a similar formulation is possible analogous to that in Section 3.5.5 in the single decision case. The densities in (5.54) are now multinomial as in (3.96), depending on the propensities

$$\omega_k(h_k, a_k) = P(A_k = a_k | H_k = h_k), \quad k = 1, \ldots, K; \tag{5.65}$$

or, equivalently,

$$\omega_k(\overline{x}_k, \overline{a}_{k-1}, a_k) = P(A_k = a_k | \overline{X}_k = \overline{x}_k, \overline{A}_{k-1} = \overline{a}_{k-1}),$$

$$\omega_k(h_k, m_k) = 1 - \sum_{a_k=1}^{m_k-1} \omega_k(h_k, a_k). \tag{5.66}$$

Then from (5.56),

$$\pi_{d,1}(X_1) = \prod_{a_1=1}^{m_1} \omega_1(X_1, a_1)^{I\{d_1(X_1)=a_1\}} = \sum_{a_1=1}^{m_1} I\{d_1(X_1) = a_1\} \omega_1(X_1, a_1)$$

$$\pi_{d,k}(\overline{X}_k) = \prod_{a_k=1}^{m_k} \omega_k\{\overline{X}_k, \overline{d}_{k-1}(\overline{X}_{k-1}), a_k\}^{\mathrm{I}[d_k\{\overline{X}_k, \overline{d}_{k-1}(\overline{X}_{k-1})\}=a_k]},$$

$$= \sum_{a_k=1}^{m_k} \mathrm{I}[d_k\{\overline{X}_k, \overline{d}_{k-1}(\overline{X}_{k-1})\} = a_k]\omega_k\{\overline{X}_k, \overline{d}_{k-1}(\overline{X}_{k-1}), a_k\},$$

$$k = 2, \ldots, K.$$

Polytomous logistic regression models $\omega_k(h_k, a_k; \gamma_k)$ can be posited for each k and estimators $\widehat{\gamma}_k$ obtained as discussed in Section 3.5.5 and substituted in these expressions to yield $\pi_{d,1}(X_1; \widehat{\gamma}_1)$ and $\pi_{d,k}(\overline{X}_k; \widehat{\gamma}_k)$, $k = 2, \ldots, K$, in the denominator of (5.64).

A large sample approximation to the sampling distribution of $\widehat{\mathcal{V}}_{IPW}(d)$ can be derived by viewing $\widehat{\mathcal{V}}_{IPW}(d)$ and $\widehat{\gamma} = (\widehat{\gamma}_1^T, \ldots, \widehat{\gamma}_K^T)^T$ maximizing (5.62) or the analogous objective function for polytomous logistic regression, so solving the K estimating equations obtained by differentiation of the objective function, as M-estimators and appealing to the standard theory in Section 2.5.

Remark. Although the inverse probability weighted estimator $\widehat{\mathcal{V}}_{IPW}(d)$ in (5.64) is consistent and has routine large sample theory as an M-estimator, it has considerable drawbacks. Except for estimation of γ, the estimator makes use of data only from individuals i for whom $\mathcal{C}_{d,i} = 1$; that is, for whom $\overline{A}_i = \overline{d}(\overline{X}_i)$. As the number of decision points K and the number of treatment options at each grows, the number of individuals i satisfying this condition is likely to be quite small, even for relatively large n. As a consequence, the estimator can be very unstable and exhibit large sampling variability. Thus, the estimator is realistic for use in practice only if K and the numbers of options at each decision point are modest; performance beyond $K = 2$ or 3 is likely to be poor. Even when $K = 2$ or 3 at most and the estimator is feasibly implemented, it is inefficient, often substantially so, because it disregards the data from all individuals whose treatments received through all K decisions are not consistent with those that would be selected by d.

An alternative estimator that, although still based on data only from individuals i for whom $\mathcal{C}_{d,i} = 1$, can exhibit substantially smaller sampling variability than $\widehat{\mathcal{V}}_{IPW}(d)$ in (5.64) is, analogous to (3.25),

$$\widehat{\mathcal{V}}_{IPW^*}(d) = \left[\sum_{i=1}^{n} \frac{\mathcal{C}_{d,i}}{\left\{\prod_{k=2}^{K} \pi_{d,k}(\overline{X}_{ki}; \widehat{\gamma}_k)\right\} \pi_{d,1}(X_{1i}; \widehat{\gamma}_1)}\right]^{-1}$$

$$\times \sum_{i=1}^{n} \frac{\mathcal{C}_{d,i} Y_i}{\left\{\prod_{k=2}^{K} \pi_{d,k}(\overline{X}_{ki}; \widehat{\gamma}_k)\right\} \pi_{d,1}(X_{1i}; \widehat{\gamma}_1)},$$

(5.67)

which has the form of a weighted average of the observed Y_i. It can be shown by an argument similar to that above that a summand in the first term on the right-hand side of (5.67) has expectation equal to one when the true $\pi_{d,k}(\overline{X}_{ki})$, $k = 1, \ldots, K$, are substituted, so that n^{-1} times the term in brackets converges in probability to one and the estimator is consistent for the true value $\mathcal{V}(d)$. Although we have presented simple inverse probability weighting in the multiple decision case in the context of (5.64) for ease of exposition, if estimation of $\mathcal{V}(d)$ is to be based on a simple inverse weighted estimator in practice, it is strongly recommended that this be accomplished using (5.67) rather than (5.64).

As in the single decision case, the counterintuitive result noted in the remark at the end Section 3.3.2 extends to this setting. It can be shown that, even if the propensities in (5.60) or (5.65) are known for $k = 1, \ldots, K$, given correctly specified models $\pi_k(h_k; \gamma_k)$ or $\omega_k(h_k, a_k; \gamma_k)$, $k = 1, \ldots, K$, for them, estimating the parameters γ_k by maximum likelihood and substituting the fitted models in the estimators (5.64) and (5.67) is preferable on efficiency grounds to using the known propensities.

Alternative forms of $\widehat{\mathcal{V}}_{IPW}(d)$ and $\widehat{\mathcal{V}}_{IPW*}(d)$ that may be somewhat easier to implement can be deduced by analogy to (3.26) in the single decision case. When $\mathcal{C}_d = 1$, $A_1 = d_1(X_1)$, and $A_k = d_k\{\overline{X}_k, \overline{d}_{k-1}(\overline{X}_{k-1})\}$, $k = 2, \ldots, K$, almost surely, so that $\mathcal{C}_d$ can be expressed equivalently as

$$\mathcal{C}_d = \mathrm{I}\{A_1 = d_1(H_1), \ldots, A_k = d_k(H_k), \ldots, A_K = d_K(H_K)\}. \quad (5.68)$$

Moreover, when $\mathcal{C}_d = 1$, it is straightforward to see that, in the summands for each i, the denominator

$$\left\{ \prod_{k=2}^{K} \pi_{d,k}(\overline{X}_{ki}) \right\} \pi_{d,1}(X_{1i})$$

can be replaced by

$$\prod_{k=1}^{K} p_{A_k|\overline{X}_k, \overline{A}_{k-1}}(A_{ki}|\overline{X}_{ki}, \overline{A}_{k-1,i}) = \prod_{k=1}^{K} p_{A_k|H_k}(A_{ki}|H_{ki}) \quad (5.69)$$

without altering the value of the estimator. Thus, equivalent expressions for these estimators are obtained by substituting a model for (5.69) in the denominators of (5.64) or (5.67). For example, considering $\widehat{\mathcal{V}}_{IPW}(d)$ with two options at each decision point and fitted logistic propensity models, (5.64) is unchanged if, for each i, the denominator of the summand,

$$\left\{ \prod_{k=2}^{K} \pi_{d,k}(\overline{X}_{ki}; \widehat{\gamma}_k) \right\} \pi_{d,1}(X_{1i}; \widehat{\gamma}_1),$$

is replaced by

$$\prod_{k=1}^{K} \pi_k(H_{ki}; \widehat{\gamma}_k)^{A_{ki}} \{1 - \pi_k(H_{ki}; \widehat{\gamma}_k)\}^{1-A_{ki}}. \qquad (5.70)$$

As in the single decision case in Section 3.3.3, it is natural to wonder if further improvement over (5.67) can be achieved through the addition of an appropriate "augmentation term." It is indeed possible to appeal to the theory of semiparametrics (Robins et al., 1994; Tsiatis, 2006) to characterize the class of augmented inverse probability weighted estimators for $\mathcal{V}(d)$ and identify the efficient estimator in the class. As shown by Zhang et al. (2013), this is accomplished by casting the multiple decision situation as a "dropout" problem. Specifically, an individual for whom the treatment options actually received through Decision $k - 1$ coincide with those that would be selected by the rules $d_1, \ldots, d_{k-1}$ for that individual's evolving history but for whom the option received at Decision k is not consistent with that dictated by d_k can be viewed from a missing data perspective as having "dropped out" at Decision k. For such an individual, his observed outcome Y does not reflect $Y^*(d)$, but he contributes partial information on d through Decision k in the sense that, by SUTVA, $\overline{X}_k = \overline{X}_k^*(\overline{d}_{k-1})$. The augmentation term seeks to recover this information to improve efficiency over the simple inverse weighted estimators. The development is considerably more complex than that for $K = 1$ and is deferred to Section 6.4.4.

Other approaches to estimation of the value of a fixed, multistage regime $d \in \mathcal{D}$ have been proposed in addition to those based on the inverse probability weighting and the g-computation algorithm discussed in this and the previous section. We review these in Section 6.4.

5.6 Characterization of an Optimal Regime

As discussed in Section 5.3, assuming that larger outcomes are more beneficial, an optimal multiple decision regime $d^{opt} \in \mathcal{D}$ achieves the maximum value among all $d \in \mathcal{D}$; that is, as in (5.12), satisfies

$$E\{Y^*(d^{opt})\} \geq E\{Y^*(d)\} \text{ for all } d \in \mathcal{D}.$$

As in the single decision setting, identification and estimation of an optimal regime is of central interest. Not surprisingly, derivation of the form of an optimal regime is more involved than in the single decision case. We now present an informal sketch of how the principle of *backward induction* is used to characterize an optimal multiple decision regime. Backward induction may be familiar to readers acquainted with Bayesian approaches to clinical trial design; e.g., see Carlin et al. (2010).

Because we seek to maximize the value $E\{Y^*(d)\}$, which is a quantity involving potential outcomes, the formal, precise characterization of an optimal regime is in terms of the distribution of X_1 and W^* in (5.9). As in the single decision case, estimation of an optimal regime based on observed data (5.16),

$$(X_{1i}, A_{1i}, \ldots, X_{Ki}, A_{Ki}, Y_i) \quad i = 1, \ldots, n,$$

requires that an optimal regime be expressed equivalently in terms of these data.

The formal argument characterizing an optimal multiple decision regime in terms of potential outcomes can be challenging for those encountering the principle of backward induction for the first time. Accordingly, to introduce the reasoning without the complication of thinking in terms of potential outcomes, in this section we demonstrate informally how backward induction is used to define an optimal regime in terms of the observed data. The characterization in terms of potential outcomes is given in Section 7.2.2, and a formal proof that the regime so defined is indeed optimal is presented in Section 7.2.3. In Section 7.2.4, we show that, under SUTVA (5.17), the SRA (5.18), and the positivity assumption (5.20), an optimal regime can be reexpressed in terms of the observed data, as presented here. The formal account given in those sections may be more intuitive after review of the development here.

K = 2 Decisions

For simplicity, we first take $K = 2$, which suffices to demonstrate the reasoning. The backward inductive argument starts at the final, in this case second, decision. The reader can compare this argument to that in terms of potential outcomes in Section 7.2.2.

Consider a randomly chosen individual who has reached Decision 2. At Decision 2, her past history $H_2 = (X_1, A_1, X_2)$ is already determined. Thus, at this point, having started with baseline information $H_1 = X_1$, she has already received treatment option A_1 and achieved subsequent intervening information X_2. Given that H_2 "is what it is" at this point, intuitively, the optimal decision that can be made now, at Decision 2, is to choose $a_2 \in \mathcal{A}_2$ to maximize her expected outcome given that she has achieved this history. Indeed, with the history H_2 already determined, this situation is analogous to that of a single decision, $K = 1$, with H_2 playing the role of "baseline" information.

Specifically, if the realized value of her history is $h_2 = (\overline{x}_2, a_1) = (x_1, x_2, a_1)$, her expected outcome given this history and if she now receives option $a_2 \in \mathcal{A}_2$ is

$$Q_2(h_2, a_2) = E(Y \mid H_2 = h_2, A_2 = a_2),$$

which is the regression of Y on history and Decision 2 treatment. This suggests that $a_2 \in \mathcal{A}_2$ should be chosen to maximize $Q_2(h_2, a_2)$, so that an optimal rule at Decision 2 is of the form

$$d_2^{opt}(h_2) = d_2^{opt}(\overline{x}_2, a_1) = \arg\max_{a_2 \in \mathcal{A}_2} Q_2(h_2, a_2). \qquad (5.71)$$

In the case where $\mathcal{A}_2 = \{0, 1\}$ and option 0 is the default, this reduces to

$$d_2^{opt}(h_2) = I\{Q_2(h_2, 1) > Q_2(h_2, 0)\}.$$

Thus, an optimal rule at the final decision is in the same spirit as that in the single decision case in Section 3.4; compare to (3.39) and (3.40).

Note that we can write equivalently

$$Q_2(h_2, a_2) = Q_2(\overline{x}_2, \overline{a}_2) = E(Y \mid \overline{X}_2 = \overline{x}_2, \overline{A}_2 = \overline{a}_2),$$

where, for brevity, $E(Y \mid \overline{X}_2 = \overline{x}_2, \overline{A}_2 = \overline{a}_2) = E(Y \mid \overline{X} = \overline{x}, \overline{A} = \overline{a})$ using the convention in Section 5.2. The rule (5.71) chooses the treatment option $a_2 \in \mathcal{A}_2$ that maximizes $Q_2(h_2, a_2)$, and the corresponding maximum expected outcome given history to Decision 2 is

$$V_2(h_2) = V_2(\overline{x}_2, a_1) = \max_{a_2 \in \mathcal{A}_2} Q_2(h_2, a_2) = \max_{a_2 \in \mathcal{A}_2} Q_2(\overline{x}_2, a_1, a_2). \quad (5.72)$$

In the case of $\mathcal{A}_2 = \{0, 1\}$, (5.72) is simply

$$V_2(h_2) = V_2(\overline{x}_2, a_1) = \max\{Q_2(h_2, 1), Q_2(h_2, 0)\}.$$

Intuitively, $V_2(h_2)$ is the maximum expected outcome for an individual with history h_2 who then follows rule $d_2^{opt}(h_2)$ in (5.71) at Decision 2.

Now step back to Decision 1. If a randomly chosen individual presents with baseline information/history $H_1 = X_1$, we wish to make an optimal decision on treatment at this stage acknowledging that she also *will receive* treatment at Decision 2 in the future by following the rule d_2^{opt} in (5.71). Consider, then, a randomly chosen patient with baseline information H_1, and suppose he receives treatment option A_1 in $\mathcal{A}_1$ at Decision 1. He will go on to achieve intervening information X_2, and, based on the history he will then have at Decision 2, $H_2 = (X_1, A_1, X_2)$, he will receive a treatment option in $\mathcal{A}_2$ at Decision 2 chosen according to the rule d_2^{opt}. From above, the option chosen by d_2^{opt} maximizes his expected outcome given his history at this point, so that it follows from (5.72) that his (maximized) expected outcome will be

$$V_2(H_2) = V_2(\overline{X}_2, A_1) = V_2(X_1, X_2, A_1). \qquad (5.73)$$

Note that, for a given realized history $H_1 = h_1 = x_1$ and specific option

$a_1 \in \mathcal{A}_1$, $V_2(x_1, X_2, a_1)$ is a function of the yet-to-be realized intervening information X_2, which accordingly is represented as a random variable.

Suppose then that a patient with realized baseline history h_1 receives option $a_1 \in \mathcal{A}_1$. Given this history and this Decision 1 treatment, the expected value of the maximized expected outcome he will have if he receives treatment at Decision 2 following d_2^{opt} is thus, from (5.73),

$$Q_1(h_1, a_1) = E\{V_2(H_2) \mid H_1 = h_1, A_1 = a_1\}$$
$$= E\{V_2(x_1, X_2, a_1) \mid X_1 = x_1, A_1 = a_1\}. \qquad (5.74)$$

It is intuitive that $a_1 \in \mathcal{A}_1$ should be chosen to make (5.74) as large as possible. This suggests that an optimal rule at Decision 1 should satisfy

$$d_1^{opt}(h_1) = d_1^{opt}(x_1) = \arg\max_{a_1 \in \mathcal{A}_1} Q_1(h_1, a_1), \qquad (5.75)$$

which reduces to

$$d_1^{opt}(h_1) = I\{Q_1(h_1, 1) > Q_1(h_1, 0)\}$$

when $\mathcal{A}_1 = \{0, 1\}$. It is critical to recognize that the definition of $Q_1(h_1, a_1)$ in (5.74) is different from the definition in the single decision case in Chapter 3.

The corresponding maximum expected value (of the maximum expected outcome) is then

$$V_1(h_1) = V_1(x_1) = \max_{a_1 \in \mathcal{A}_1} Q_1(h_1, a_1). \qquad (5.76)$$

That is, using the above definitions,

$$V_1(h_1) = V_1(x_1)$$

$$= \max_{a_1 \in \mathcal{A}_1} E\left\{ \max_{a_2 \in \mathcal{A}_2} E(Y \mid X_1 = x_1, X_2, \overline{A}_2 = \overline{a}_2) \,\middle|\, X_1 = x_1, A_1 = a_1 \right\}.$$

This quantity has the interpretation as the maximum expected outcome that an individual presenting with baseline information $h_1 = x_1$ would achieve if the rules d_1^{opt} and d_2^{opt} in (5.75) and (5.71), respectively, were to be used to select treatment at each decision point.

It is clear that $d^{opt} = (d_1^{opt}, d_2^{opt})$ defined in (5.71) and (5.75) is a treatment regime, as it comprises a set of rules, each corresponding to a decision point, taking an individual's history as input and selecting a treatment option from those available. The foregoing reasoning suggests that d^{opt} is an optimal regime; this is demonstrated formally in Sections 7.2.2–7.2.4.

With H_1 the baseline information of a randomly chosen individual, the random variable $V_1(H_1)$ takes on values across all possible $h_1 \in \mathcal{H}_1$. Intuitively, then,

$$E\{V_1(H_1)\}$$

is the (unconditional) expected outcome (average across all individuals in the population) if all individuals were to receive treatment according to the rules d_1^{opt} and d_2^{opt}. This suggests that $E\{V_1(H_1)\}$ is the value of d^{opt} and that in fact

$$E\{Y^*(d^{opt})\} = E\{V_1(H_1)\} \geq E\{Y^*(d)\} \quad \text{for all } d \in \mathcal{D}; \quad (5.77)$$

this is shown formally in Section 7.2.3.

$K > 2$ Decisions

This backward reasoning extends to $K > 2$ decisions. At Decision K, define for any $h_K = (\overline{x}_K, \overline{a}_{K-1})$

$$Q_K(h_K, a_K) = Q_K(\overline{x}_K, \overline{a}_K) = Q_K(\overline{x}, \overline{a}) = E(Y|\overline{X} = \overline{x}, \overline{A} = \overline{a}). \tag{5.78}$$

Then, analogous to (5.71) and (5.72), define

$$d_K^{opt}(h_K) = d_K^{opt}(\overline{x}_K, \overline{a}_{K-1}) = \arg\max_{a_K \in \mathcal{A}_K} Q_K(h_K, a_K), \tag{5.79}$$

and

$$V_K(h_K) = V_K(\overline{x}_K, \overline{a}_{K-1}) = \max_{a_K \in \mathcal{A}_K} Q_K(h_K, a_K). \tag{5.80}$$

That is, at the final, Kth decision point, the optimal decision is to choose the option in $\mathcal{A}_K$ that maximizes expected outcome given Decision K treatment and the accrued history over all previous decisions (which is already determined).

Now step back to Decision $K - 1$. Let

$$Q_{K-1}(h_{K-1}, a_{K-1}) = Q_{K-1}(\overline{x}_{K-1}, \overline{a}_{K-1})$$
$$= E\{V_K(\overline{x}_{K-1}, X_K, \overline{a}_{K-1})|\overline{X}_{K-1} = \overline{x}_{K-1}, \overline{A}_{K-1} = \overline{a}_{K-1}\}.$$

Then by the same reasoning for Decision 1 in the case $K = 2$ above, the rule at Decision $K - 1$ is

$$d_{K-1}^{opt}(h_{K-1}) = d_{K-1}^{opt}(\overline{x}_{K-1}, \overline{a}_{K-2}) = \arg\max_{a_{K-1} \in \mathcal{A}_{K-1}} Q_{K-1}(h_{K-1}, a_{K-1}),$$

and define

$$V_{K-1}(h_{K-1}) = V_{K-1}(\overline{x}_{K-1}, \overline{a}_{K-2}) = \max_{a_{K-1} \in \mathcal{A}_{K-1}} Q_{K-1}(h_{K-1}, a_{K-1}).$$

Intuitively, we can apply this same reasoning recursively as we move backward through earlier decisions. For $k = K - 1, \ldots, 1$ and any $h_k = (\overline{x}_k, \overline{a}_{k-1})$, defining

$$Q_k(h_k, a_k) = Q_k(\overline{x}_k, \overline{a}_k) = E\{V_{k+1}(\overline{x}_k, X_{k+1}, \overline{a}_k) | \overline{X}_k = \overline{x}_k, \overline{A}_k = \overline{a}_k\}, \tag{5.81}$$

we have that

$$d_k^{opt}(h_k) = d_k^{opt}(\overline{x}_k, \overline{a}_{k-1}) = \arg\max_{a_k \in \mathcal{A}_k} Q_k(h_k, a_k), \tag{5.82}$$

and

$$V_k(h_k) = V_k(\overline{x}_k, \overline{a}_{k-1}) = \max_{a_k \in \mathcal{A}_k} Q_k(h_k, a_k). \tag{5.83}$$

As we show in Section 7.2.4, the positivity assumption guarantees that the conditional expectations in (5.78) and (5.81) are well defined.

As for the case $K = 2$, it is clear that $d^{opt} = (d_1^{opt}, \ldots, d_K^{opt})$ is a treatment regime, and it is shown to be an optimal regime, expressed in terms of the observed data, in Sections 7.2.2–7.2.4. Analogous to (5.77), it is also shown that the value of an optimal regime is then given by

$$\mathcal{V}(d^{opt}) = E\{Y^*(d^{opt})\} = E\{V_1(H_1)\} = E\{V_1(X_1)\}. \tag{5.84}$$

Conceptually, each rule d_k^{opt}, $k = K - 1, \ldots, 1$, chooses the option from $\mathcal{A}_k$ that maximizes the expected value of the maximum expected outcome, given Decision k treatment and the current history, that would be attained if rules $d_{k+1}^{opt}, \ldots, d_K^{opt}$ are used in the future, in the same spirit as for Decision 1 in the case $K = 2$. This is calculated at each decision point in a backward recursive fashion as more future rules are taken into account. When all rules have been applied, by virtue of the "maximization of the expected maximum" with each, intuitively, the maximum unconditional expected outcome (average over the population) if all individuals were to follow the rules d_k^{opt}, $k = 1, \ldots, K$, should be achieved.

The $Q_k(h_k, a_k) = Q_k(\overline{x}_k, \overline{a}_k)$, $k = 1, \ldots, K$, in (5.78) and (5.81) are referred to as *Q-functions* in the literature on dynamic treatment regimes. This term arises from the computer science literature on reinforcement learning methods for sequential decision making and in particular that of *Q-learning* introduced by Watkins and Dayan (1992). In Section 5.7.1, we describe the Q-learning method for estimation of an optimal regime based on the characterization of d^{opt} in (5.79)–(5.83).

As noted in Section 3.4, $V_k(h_k)$, $k = 1, \ldots, K$, are referred to as *value functions*. Intuitively, at Decision k, the value function reflects the expected outcome ("value") that will result from following optimal rules now and in the future (at Decisions $k, \ldots, K$), given past history to

Decision k. For $k = 1$, as shown in (5.84), the expectation of the value function is the value of an optimal regime in $\mathcal{D}$.

As discussed in Section 3.4 for a single decision, at any decision point $k = 1, \ldots, K$, it is possible that more than one treatment option in $\mathcal{A}_k$ achieves the maximum in (5.80) or (5.83) for some value of the history h_k. If this is the case at Decision k, then there is more than one possible rule d_k^{opt}, with different versions selecting different options that achieve the maximum for such an h_k. Different optimal regimes can thus be formulated by traversing all combinations of rules selecting different such options, showing that there can be more than one optimal regime. As in the single decision case, one of the options at each decision point can be designated as the default when more than one option achieves the maximum for a given history to achieve a unique representation of an optimal regime. In the more precise presentation of these results in Sections 7.2.2–7.2.4), we define all of these quantities carefully in terms of the feasible sets of treatment options at each decision point.

Remark. It is common upon being exposed to the backward induction argument for the first time to ask why it is not possible to define d^{opt} in a *forward* fashion, starting from Decision 1. It is certainly true that implementation of the rules $d_1^{opt}, \ldots, d_K^{opt}$ to select treatment options at each of the K decision points for a given individual takes place in a forward manner. However, *derivation* of the rules is another matter.

Consider Decision 1. When a treatment decision is made at this first decision point, the expected outcome that would be attained after all K decisions depends on future decisions. If those decisions have not yet been carried out, it is impossible to guarantee that the treatment option being selected at Decision 1 is the best choice. That is, the ultimate outcome associated with any regime d and thus its associated value depend on what is done at all K decisions. Accordingly, maximizing expected outcome over the options at Decision 1 only, without regard to future decisions, cannot possibly lead to the maximum possible expected outcome.

5.7   Estimation of an Optimal Regime

We review two classes of methods for estimation of an optimal multiple decision regime suggested by the developments in Sections 5.5.2 and 5.6. In Chapter 7, additional approaches are presented.

5.7.1   Q-learning

The characterization of an optimal multiple decision regime in terms of the observed data given in Section 5.6 immediately suggests the method for estimation of $d^{opt} \in \mathcal{D}$ referred to as *Q-learning*. Q-learning can be viewed as a generalization of regression-based estimation of a single decision optimal regime discussed in Section 3.5.1.

From Section 5.6, an optimal regime is represented in terms of the Q-functions in (5.78) and (5.81); namely,

$$Q_K(h_K, a_K) = Q_K(\overline{x}_K, \overline{a}_K) = Q_K(\overline{x}, \overline{a}) = E(Y|\overline{X} = \overline{x}, \overline{A} = \overline{a}),$$
$$(5.85)$$

and, for $k = K - 1, \ldots, 1$,

$$Q_k(h_k, a_k) = Q_k(\overline{x}_k, \overline{a}_k) = E\{V_{k+1}(\overline{x}_k, X_{k+1}, \overline{a}_k)|\overline{X}_k = \overline{x}_k, \overline{A}_k = \overline{a}_k\},$$
$$(5.86)$$

where, for $k = 1, \ldots, K$,

$$V_k(h_k) = V_k(\overline{x}_k, \overline{a}_{k-1}) = \max_{a_k \in \mathcal{A}_k} Q_k(h_k, a_k). \qquad (5.87)$$

Q-learning is based on direct modeling and fitting of the Q-functions (5.85) and (5.86).

Specifically, in the standard Q-learning approach, one posits parametric models

$$Q_k(h_k, a_k; \beta_k) = Q_k(\overline{x}_k, \overline{a}_k; \beta_k), \quad k = K, K - 1, \ldots, 1, \qquad (5.88)$$

say, each depending on a finite-dimensional parameter β_k. The posited models can be linear or nonlinear in β_k and include main effects of and interactions among the elements of $\overline{x}_k$ and $\overline{a}_k$; linear models are popular in practice. In applications, the β_k usually are taken not to share common components across k, so are distinct for $k = 1, \ldots, K$; we adopt this convention here.

From (5.85), development of the model $Q_K(h_K, a_K; \beta_K)$ is a conventional regression modeling exercise, as $E(Y|\overline{X} = \overline{x}, \overline{A} = \overline{a})$ is the regression of observed outcome on an individual's full accrued intervening information and treatments received over the K decisions. Note from (5.86) that $Q_k(h_k, a_k; \beta_k)$ for $k = K - 1, \ldots, 1$ is a model for the conditional expectation of $V_{k+1}(H_{k+1})$ defined in (5.87); thus, it is not a model for a directly observed outcome as in a conventional regression setting. We discuss this further below.

Given models (5.88), estimators $\widehat{\beta}_k$ for β_k are obtained in a backward iterative fashion for $k = K, K-1, \ldots, 1$ by solving suitable M-estimating equations, such as those corresponding to OLS or WLS. For definiteness and greater generality, we present the Q-learning approach in the case of the latter.

Remark. In some accounts of Q-learning in the applied literature, particularly in the behavioral sciences, Q-learning is taken by definition to involve the use of OLS. However, as we demonstrate here, the estimation method for the β_k need not be restricted to OLS.

The Q-learning algorithm begins at Decision K. Based on (5.85), given a posited model $Q_K(h_K, a_K; \beta_K) = Q_K(\overline{x}_K, \overline{a}_K; \beta_K)$ for $E(Y|\overline{X} = \overline{x}, \overline{A} = \overline{a})$, $\widehat{\beta}_K$ is found by solving

$$\sum_{i=1}^{n} \frac{\partial Q_K(H_{Ki}, A_{Ki}; \beta_K)}{\partial \beta_K} \Sigma_K^{-1}(H_{Ki}, A_{Ki})\{Y_i - Q_K(H_{Ki}, A_{Ki}; \beta_K)\} = 0$$
(5.89)

in β_K, where $\Sigma_K(h_K, a_K)$ is a working variance model for

$$\mathrm{var}(Y|H_K = h_K, A_K = a_K) = \mathrm{var}(Y|\overline{X} = \overline{x}, \overline{A} = \overline{a}),$$

which is taken to be equal to 1 if homoscedasticity is assumed, so that the estimating equations (5.89) reduce to those of OLS. If Y is binary, maximum likelihood leads to WLS with the form of $\Sigma_K^{-1}(h_K, a_K)$ determined by the variance of a Bernoulli distribution.

Substituting $Q_K(h_K, a_K; \beta_K)$ in (5.79) defining $d_K^{opt}(h_K) = d_K^{opt}(\overline{x}_K, \overline{a}_{K-1})$, we obtain the estimator

$$\widehat{d}_{Q,K}^{opt}(h_K) = d_K^{opt}(h_K; \widehat{\beta}_K) = \arg\max_{a_K \in \mathcal{A}_K} Q_K(h_K, a_K; \widehat{\beta}_K). \qquad (5.90)$$

Now move to Decision $K - 1$. Based on (5.87), form the *pseudo outcomes*

$$\widetilde{V}_{Ki} = \max_{a_K \in \mathcal{A}_K} Q_K(H_{Ki}, a_K; \widehat{\beta}_K), \quad i = 1, \ldots, n. \qquad (5.91)$$

The pseudo outcomes (5.91) can be regarded as "predicted values" based on the assumed Decision K model for the maximum expected outcome for each individual if d_K^{opt} were used to select treatment at Decision K.

Given a posited model

$$Q_{K-1}(h_{K-1}, a_{K-1}; \beta_{K-1}) = Q_{K-1}(\overline{x}_{K-1}, \overline{a}_{K-1}; \beta_{K-1})$$

for

$$E\{V_K(\overline{x}_{K-1}, X_K, \overline{a}_{K-1})|\overline{X}_{K-1} = \overline{x}_{K-1}, \overline{A}_{K-1} = \overline{a}_{K-1}\}$$

as in (5.86), the estimator $\widehat{\beta}_{K-1}$ for β_{K-1} is found by solving in β_{K-1}

$$\sum_{i=1}^{n} \frac{\partial Q_{K-1}(H_{K-1,i}, A_{K-1,i}; \beta_{K-1})}{\partial \beta_{K-1}} \Sigma_{K-1}^{-1}(H_{K-1,i}, A_{K-1,i})$$

$$\times \{\widetilde{V}_{Ki} - Q_{K-1}(H_{K-1,i}, A_{K-1,i}; \beta_{K-1})\} = 0, \qquad (5.92)$$

where, again, $\Sigma_{K-1}(h_{K-1}, a_{K-1})$ is a working variance model. In (5.92), the pseudo outcomes $\widetilde{V}_{Ki}$ are treated as if they are genuine, observed outcomes, so that, strictly speaking, solution of (5.92) is a nonstandard estimation problem. We discuss the implications of this below.

The resulting estimator for $d_{K-1}^{opt}(h_{K-1}) = d_{K-1}^{opt}(\overline{x}_{K-1}, \overline{a}_{K-2})$ is then

$$\widehat{d}_{Q,K-1}^{opt}(h_{K-1}) = d_{K-1}^{opt}(h_{K-1}; \widehat{\beta}_{K-1})$$

$$= \underset{a_{K-1} \in \mathcal{A}_{K-1}}{\arg\max} \; Q_{K-1}(h_{K-1}, a_{K-1}; \widehat{\beta}_{K-1}). \qquad (5.93)$$

This process continues in the obvious fashion for $k = K - 2, \ldots, 1$. At Decision k, form the pseudo outcomes

$$\widetilde{V}_{k+1,i} = \underset{a_{k+1} \in \mathcal{A}_{k+1}}{\max} \; Q_{k+1}(H_{k+1,i}, a_{k+1}; \widehat{\beta}_{k+1}) \qquad (5.94)$$

for $i = 1, \ldots, n$. Then, given a posited model $Q_k(h_k, a_k; \beta_k) = Q_k(\overline{x}_k, \overline{a}_k; \beta_k)$ for

$$E\{V_{k+1}(\overline{x}_k, X_{k+1}, \overline{a}_k) | \overline{X}_k = \overline{x}_k, \overline{A}_k = \overline{a}_k\},$$

solve

$$\sum_{i=1}^{n} \frac{\partial Q_k(H_{ki}, A_{ki}; \beta_k)}{\partial \beta_k} \Sigma_k^{-1}(H_{ki}, A_{ki}) \{\widetilde{V}_{k+1,i} - Q_k(H_{ki}, A_{ki}; \beta_k)\} = 0$$

$$(5.95)$$

in β_k to obtain $\widehat{\beta}_k$ and the corresponding estimated rule

$$\widehat{d}_{Q,k}^{opt}(h_k) = d_k^{opt}(h_k; \widehat{\beta}_k) = \arg\max_{a_k \in \mathcal{A}_k} Q_k(h_k, a_k; \widehat{\beta}_k). \qquad (5.96)$$

Finally, once $\widehat{\beta}_1$ is obtained, form the pseudo outcomes

$$\widetilde{V}_{1i} = \max_{a_1 \in \mathcal{A}_1} Q_1(H_{1i}, a_1; \widehat{\beta}_1), \quad i = 1, \ldots, n.$$

Summarizing, the Q-learning algorithm involves solving for $k = K, K - 1, \ldots, 1$ appropriate estimating equations as in (5.89), (5.92), and (5.95) to obtain estimators $\widehat{\beta}_k$, and then forming estimated optimal rules as in (5.90), (5.93), and (5.96) by substitution. Denote the estimated optimal regime resulting from this procedure as

$$\widehat{d}_Q^{opt} = \{\widehat{d}_{Q,1}^{opt}(h_1), \ldots, \widehat{d}_{Q,K}^{opt}(h_K)\}. \qquad (5.97)$$

Based on (5.84), an estimator for the value $\mathcal{V}(d^{opt})$ is

$$\widehat{\mathcal{V}}_Q(d^{opt}) = n^{-1} \sum_{i=1}^{n} \widetilde{V}_{1i} = n^{-1} \sum_{i=1}^{n} \max_{a_1 \in \mathcal{A}_1} Q_1(H_{1i}, a_1; \widehat{\beta}_1). \qquad (5.98)$$

Analogous to the discussion at the end of Section 3.5.1, it should come as no surprise that $\widehat{V}_Q(d^{opt})$ in (5.98) is a nonregular estimator, so that inference on the true value $V(d^{opt})$ achieved by an optimal regime $d \in \mathcal{D}$ is challenging. This is discussed in detail in Chapter 10.

Remark. When $K = 1$, the Q-learning algorithm involves the single step in which a model for $Q_1(h_1, a_1) = Q_1(x_1, a_1) = E(Y | H_1 = h_1, A_1 = a_1) = E(Y | X_1 = x_1, A_1 = a_1)$ is posited and fitted. Thus, it is evident that in the single decision case Q-learning reduces to the regression-based estimation method presented in Section 3.5.1.

We have presented the estimating equations (5.89), (5.92), and (5.95) in the conventional WLS form, with leading term in the summand for each $k = 1, \ldots, K$ given by

$$\frac{\partial Q_k(H_{ki}, A_{ki}; \beta_k)}{\partial \beta_k} \Sigma_k^{-1}(H_{ki}, A_{ki}), \tag{5.99}$$

where taking $\Sigma_k(\,\cdot\,)$ to be a constant yields OLS. At the Kth decision, with actual observed responses Y_i, standard theory for generalized estimating equations implies that (5.99) is the optimal leading term when, in truth,

$$\text{var}(Y | \overline{X}_K = \overline{x}_K, \overline{A}_K = \overline{a}_K) = \Sigma_K(h_K, a_K),$$

in the sense that solving the estimating equation leads to the asymptotically efficient estimator for β_K. However, for $k < K$, with the estimating equation based on treating the pseudo outcomes $\widetilde{V}_{k+1,i}$ as genuine, observed outcomes, this theory may no longer apply, so that the estimators $\widehat{\beta}_k$, $k = 1, \ldots, K - 1$, may not be efficient. It is apparent that deriving the optimal leading term corresponding to the efficient estimating equations for $k < K$ would involve considerable complication.

Demonstration of Q-learning for $K = 2$

We demonstrate the Q-learning algorithm for $K = 2$ when there are two treatment options at each decision point coded as 0 and 1, both of which are feasible for all individuals regardless of their histories, so that $\mathcal{A}_1 = \{0, 1\}$ and $\mathcal{A}_2 = \{0, 1\}$. As is popular in many contexts and certainly when the observed outcome Y is continuous, we consider adopting linear models for the Q-functions at both decision points. For definiteness, let

$$\widetilde{h}_1 = (1, h_1^T)^T = (1, x_1^T)^T, \qquad \widetilde{h}_2 = (1, h_2^T)^T = (1, x_1^T, a_1, x_2^T)^T,$$

and define $\widetilde{H}_1$ and $\widetilde{H}_2$ analogously.

At Decision 2, suppose we posit the linear model for $Q_2(h_2, a_2) = Q_2(\overline{x}_2, \overline{a}_2) = E(Y|\overline{X}_2 = \overline{x}_2, \overline{A}_2 = \overline{a}_2)$ given by

$$Q_2(h_2, a_2; \beta_2) = \widetilde{h}_2^T \beta_{21} + a_2(\widetilde{h}_2^T \beta_{22}), \qquad \beta_2 = (\beta_{21}^T, \beta_{22}^T)^T. \tag{5.100}$$

As discussed above, this is a conventional regression modeling problem involving an observed outcome, so that standard diagnostic and variable selection techniques can be used to evaluate the suitability of (5.100) and assumptions such as homoscedasticity. Suppose that, following such evaluation, the assumption that $\mathrm{var}(Y|\overline{X}_2 = \overline{x}_2, \overline{A}_2 = \overline{a}_2)$ is constant is adopted and, accordingly, (5.100) is fitted via OLS to obtain the estimator $\widehat{\beta}_2 = (\widehat{\beta}_{21}^T, \widehat{\beta}_{22}^T)^T$.

It is straightforward to deduce that, under the model (5.100),

$$V_2(h_2; \beta_2) = \max_{a_2 \in \{0,1\}} Q_2(h_2, a_2; \beta_2) = \widetilde{h}_2^T \beta_{21} + (\widetilde{h}_2^T \beta_{22}) \mathrm{I}(\widetilde{h}_2^T \beta_{22} > 0).$$

It follows from (5.79) with $K = 2$ that, under model (5.100), the optimal rule at Decision 2 is

$$d_2^{opt}(h_2) = d_2^{opt}(\overline{x}_2, a_1) = \mathrm{I}(\widetilde{h}_2^T \beta_{22} > 0),$$

which, from (5.90), can be estimated by

$$\widehat{d}_{Q,2}^{opt}(h_2) = d_{Q,2}^{opt}(h_2; \widehat{\beta}_2) = \mathrm{I}(\widetilde{h}_2^T \widehat{\beta}_{22} > 0). \tag{5.101}$$

From (5.91) or (5.94), form the pseudo outcomes

$$\widetilde{V}_{2i} = \widetilde{H}_{2i}^T \widehat{\beta}_{21} + (\widetilde{H}_{2i}^T \widehat{\beta}_{22}) \mathrm{I}(\widetilde{H}_{2i}^T \widehat{\beta}_{22} > 0), \quad i = 1, \ldots, n.$$

At Decision 1, we must specify a model for

$$Q_1(h_1, a_1) = Q_1(x_1, a_1) = E\{V_2(x_1, X_2, a_1)|X_1 = x_1, A_1 = a_1\}$$

in (5.81) with $k = 1$. We adopt the linear model

$$Q_1(h_1, a_1; \beta_1) = \widetilde{h}_1^T \beta_{11} + a_1(\widetilde{h}_1^T \beta_{12}), \qquad \beta_1 = (\beta_{11}^T, \beta_{12}^T)^T. \tag{5.102}$$

Treating the pseudo outcomes $\widetilde{V}_{2i}$, $i = 1, \ldots, n$, as conventional observed outcomes and assuming homoscedasticity, the model (5.102) can be fitted using OLS, yielding the estimator $\widehat{\beta}_1 = (\widehat{\beta}_{11}^T, \widehat{\beta}_{12}^T)^T$.

As above, it follows from (5.82) with $k = 1$ that, under (5.102), the optimal rule at Decision 1 is of the form

$$d_1^{opt}(h_1) = d_1^{opt}(x_1) = \mathrm{I}(\widetilde{h}_1^T \beta_{12} > 0),$$

which can be estimated as

$$\widehat{d}_{Q,1}^{opt}(h_1) = d_{Q,1}^{opt}(x_1; \widehat{\beta}_1) = \mathrm{I}(\widetilde{h}_1^T \widehat{\beta}_{12} > 0). \tag{5.103}$$

The estimated optimal regime under the models (5.102) and (5.100) is then $\hat{d}_Q^{opt} = (\hat{d}_{Q,1}^{opt}, \hat{d}_{Q,2}^{opt})$, where $\hat{d}_{Q,2}^{opt}$ and $\hat{d}_{Q,1}^{opt}$ are given in (5.101) and (5.103), respectively.

Under (5.102),

$$V_1(h_1; \beta_1) = \max_{a_1 \in \{0,1\}} Q_1(h_1, a_1; \beta_1) = \tilde{h}_1^T \beta_{11} + (\tilde{h}_1^T \beta_{12}) I(\tilde{h}_1^T \beta_{12} > 0),$$

from which we can form pseudo outcomes

$$\tilde{V}_{1i} = \tilde{H}_{1i}^T \hat{\beta}_{11} + (\tilde{H}_{1i}^T \hat{\beta}_{12}) I(\tilde{H}_{1i}^T \hat{\beta}_{12} > 0), \quad i = 1, \dots, n.$$

By (5.98), the value of d^{opt} can be estimated by

$$\hat{\mathcal{V}}_Q(d^{opt}) = n^{-1} \sum_{i=1}^{n} \tilde{V}_{1i}.$$

This simple setting with $K = 2$ suffices to illustrate the potential for almost certain misspecification of the Q-function models for $k = K-1, \dots, 1$ noted above. In (5.102) above, $Q_1(h_1, a_1; \beta_1)$ is a model for the conditional expectation of $V_2(H_2)$ given $(X_1 = x_1, A_1 = a_1)$, where

$$V_2(h_2) = \max_{a_2 \in \{0,1\}} E(Y | \overline{X}_2 = \overline{x}_2, A_1 = a_1, A_2 = a_2).$$

Suppose that, in truth, for scalar x_1 and x_2,

$$Q_2(h_2, a_2) = E(Y | \overline{X}_2 = \overline{x}_2, \overline{A}_2 = \overline{a}_2) = -x_1 + a_2(0.5a_1 + x_2),$$

so that a linear model $Q_2(h_2, a_2; \beta_2)$ like that in (5.100) is in fact correctly specified. Suppose further that the distribution of X_2 given $(X_1 = x_1, A_1 = a_1)$ is normal with mean δx_1 and variance σ^2. Then it can be shown that the true conditional expectation

$$
\begin{aligned}
Q_1(h_1, a_1) &= E\{V_2(x_1, X_2, a_1) \mid X_1 = x_1, A_1 = a_1\} \\
&= -x_1 + \frac{\sigma}{\sqrt{2\pi}} \exp\{-(0.5a_1 + \delta x_1)^2/(2\sigma^2)\} \\
&\quad + (0.5a_1 + \delta x_1)\Phi\{(0.5a_1 + \delta x_1)/\sigma\},
\end{aligned}
\tag{5.104}
$$

where, as in Chapter 3, $\Phi(\cdot)$ is the cumulative distribution function of the standard normal distribution; see Section 5.3 and the supplemental material of Schulte et al. (2014) for details of the derivation of (5.104). Clearly, the true relationship $Q_1(h_1, a_1)$ in (5.104) is unlikely to be well approximated by a linear model like that in (5.102). Thus, even though the true relationship $Q_2(h_2, a_2)$ is represented faithfully by a linear model, the conditional expectation of its maximum, $Q_1(h_1, a_1)$ cannot be.

It is clear that, for $K > 2$, such misspecification propagates through the models for the Q-functions at all of Decisions $K - 1, \ldots, 1$. Thus, even if a linear model is appropriate at Decision K, linear models for the Q-functions at all other decisions would almost certainly not be.

We discuss implementation of Q-learning further in Section 5.7.4.

5.7.2 Value Search Estimation

As discussed for $K = 1$ in Section 3.5.3, in Q-learning for multiple decisions, the posited Q-function models at each decision point determine the forms of the decision rules and thereby induce a class of regimes indexed by the K sets of parameters involved in these models. Thus, in Q-learning, the estimated optimal regime is restricted to be contained in this class. Of course, as in Section 3.5.3, a true optimal regime d^{opt} in the class $\mathcal{D}$ of all possible regimes need not be in this restricted class. Given that misspecification of the Q-functions for $k < K$ is highly likely, there is the potential for the estimated optimal regime via Q-learning to be a poor estimator for d^{opt}.

Analogous to the perspective taken in Section 3.5.3 in the single decision case, it may be appealing instead to restrict deliberately to a class of multiple decision regimes $\mathcal{D}_\eta$, indexed by a parameter η, and to focus on estimation of an optimal regime within this restricted class.

For example, one might restrict attention to regimes involving thresholds for values of the components in the h_k, $k = 1, \ldots, K$, analogous to (3.83). For definiteness, suppose $K = 3$, $\mathcal{A}_k = \{0, 1\}$, $k = 1, 2, 3$; $h_1 = x_1 = (x_{11}, x_{12})^T$; $x_2 = (x_{21}, x_{22})^T$, so that $h_2 = (x_{11}, x_{12}, x_{21}, x_{22}, a_1)$; and $x_3 = (x_{31}, x_{32})^T$, so that $h_3 = (x_{11}, x_{12}, x_{21}, x_{22}, x_{31}, x_{32}, \bar{a}_2)$, where x_{k1} and x_{k2} are scalar covariates, $k = 1, 2, 3$. Then $\mathcal{D}_\eta$ might be taken to comprise regimes characterized by rules

$$d_1(h_1; \eta_1) = \mathrm{I}(x_{11} < \eta_{11}, x_{12} < \eta_{12}), \quad \eta_1 = (\eta_{11}, \eta_{12})^T,$$
$$d_2(h_2; \eta_2) = \mathrm{I}(x_{11} < \eta_{21}, x_{21} < \eta_{22}, x_{22} < \eta_{23}), \quad \eta_2 = (\eta_{21}, \eta_{22}, \eta_{23})^T,$$
$$d_3(h_3; \eta_3) = \mathrm{I}(x_{31} < \eta_{31})\mathrm{I}(a_2 = 0) + \mathrm{I}(x_{32} > \eta_{32})\mathrm{I}(a_2 = 1),$$
$$\eta_3 = (\eta_{31}, \eta_{32})^T,$$

so that $\mathcal{D}_\eta$ has elements

$$d_\eta = \{d_1(h_1; \eta_1), d_2(h_2; \eta_2), d_3(h_3; \eta_3)\}, \quad \eta = (\eta_1^T, \eta_2^T, \eta_3^T)^T.$$

In general, the form of the rules for each decision point characterizing regimes d_η in the class $\mathcal{D}_\eta$ can be motivated by subject matter and practical considerations such as cost, ease of implementation, and interpretability. For K decisions, if $\mathcal{D}_\eta$ has elements

$$d_\eta = \{d_1(h_1; \eta_1), \dots, d_K(h_K; \eta_K)\}, \quad \eta = (\eta_1^T, \dots, \eta_K^T)^T,$$

then it is of interest to estimate an optimal restricted regime d_η^{opt} in $\mathcal{D}_\eta$ characterized by

$$
\begin{aligned}
d_\eta^{opt} &= \{d_1(h_1; \eta_1^{opt}), \dots, d_K(h_K; \eta_K^{opt})\}, \\
\eta^{opt} &= (\eta_1^{opt\, T}, \dots, \eta_K^{opt\, T})^T = \arg\max_\eta \mathcal{V}(d_\eta).
\end{aligned}
\tag{5.105}
$$

That is, as in the single decision case, an optimal restricted regime in $\mathcal{D}_\eta$ achieves the maximum value among all regimes d_η in $\mathcal{D}_\eta$, which corresponds to $\eta = \eta^{opt}$. Thus, estimation of d_η^{opt} is equivalent to estimating η^{opt} satisfying (5.105).

As in the single decision case, (5.105) suggests maximizing an estimator for the value of a fixed regime, evaluated at d_η, in η. That is, estimate η^{opt} by

$$\widehat{\eta}^{opt} = (\widehat{\eta}_1^{opt\, T}, \dots, \widehat{\eta}_K^{opt\, T})^T = \arg\max_\eta \widehat{\mathcal{V}}(d_\eta),$$

where $\widehat{\mathcal{V}}(d)$ is an estimator for the value of a fixed regime, to obtain the estimator

$$\widehat{d}_\eta^{opt} = \{d_1(h_1, \widehat{\eta}_1^{opt}), \dots, d_K(h_K, \widehat{\eta}_K^{opt})\}.
\tag{5.106}$$

By analogy to the single decision case, we refer to $\widehat{d}_\eta^{opt}$ in (5.106) as a *value search estimator*, also known as a direct or policy search estimator.

Here, we discuss value search estimation of d_η^{opt} based on the inverse probability weighted estimator (5.64). For any regime $d_\eta \in \mathcal{D}_\eta$, so equivalently for any fixed η, write for brevity

$$d_{\eta,k}(h_k) = d_k(h_k; \eta_k), \quad k = 1, \dots, K.$$

Then, with $d_{\eta,1}(h_1) = d_{\eta,1}(x_1)$, as in (5.6), define recursively for $k = 2, \dots, K$

$$\overline{d}_{\eta,k}(\overline{x}_k) = [d_{\eta,1}(x_1), d_{\eta,2}\{\overline{x}_2, d_{\eta,1}(x_1)\}, \dots, d_{\eta,k}\{\overline{x}_k, \overline{d}_{\eta,k-1}(\overline{x}_{k-1})\}],$$

and let

$$\overline{d}_\eta(\overline{x}) = \overline{d}_{\eta,K}(\overline{x}_K).$$

Then, as in (5.55) in Section 5.5.2, for any fixed η corresponding to a fixed regime d_η in $\mathcal{D}_\eta$,

$$\mathcal{C}_{d_\eta} = I\{\overline{A} = \overline{d}_\eta(\overline{X})\}.$$

As in Section 5.5.2, $\mathcal{C}_{d_\eta}$ is the indicator of whether or not the treatment options actually received by an individual coincide with those that would be selected by the rules in d_η for all K decisions.

From (5.56), let

$$\pi_{d_\eta,1}(X_1; \eta_1, \gamma_1)$$

be a model for $p_{A_1|X_1}\{d_{\eta,1}(X_1)|X_1\}$ and

$$\pi_{d_\eta,k}(\overline{X}_k; \eta_k, \gamma_k), \quad k = 2, \ldots, K,$$

be models for

$$p_{A_k|\overline{X}_k, \overline{A}_{k-1}}[d_{\eta,k}\{\overline{X}_k, \overline{d}_{\eta,k-1}(\overline{X}_{k-1})\}|\overline{X}_k, \overline{d}_{\eta,k-1}(\overline{X}_{k-1})], \quad k = 2, \ldots, K.$$

For example, in the case of two options at each decision point, with $\pi_k(h_k)$ defined as in (5.60) and represented via logistic regression models $\pi_k(h_k; \gamma_k)$, $k = 1, \ldots, K$, from (5.63), the induced models are

$$\pi_{d_\eta,1}(X_1; \eta_1, \gamma_1) = \pi_1(X_1; \gamma_1)^{d_{\eta,1}(X_1)}\{1 - \pi_1(X_1; \gamma_1)\}^{1-d_{\eta,1}(X_1)}$$

$$\pi_{d_\eta,k}(\overline{X}_k; \eta_k, \gamma_k) = \pi_k\{\overline{X}_k, \overline{d}_{\eta,k-1}(\overline{X}_{k-1}); \gamma_k\}^{d_{\eta,k}\{\overline{X}_k, \overline{d}_{\eta,k-1}(\overline{X}_{k-1})\}}$$

$$\times [1 - \pi_k\{\overline{X}_k, \overline{d}_{\eta,k-1}(\overline{X}_{k-1}); \gamma_k\}]^{1-d_{\eta,k}\{\overline{X}_k, \overline{d}_{\eta,k-1}(\overline{X}_{k-1})\}},$$
$$k = 2, \ldots, K.$$

A similar formulation is possible when there are more than two options, as in Section 5.5.2.

The inverse probability weighted estimator for $\mathcal{V}(d_\eta)$ for fixed η is

$$\widehat{\mathcal{V}}_{IPW}(d_\eta) = n^{-1} \sum_{i=1}^{n} \frac{\mathcal{C}_{d_\eta,i} Y_i}{\left\{\prod_{k=2}^{K} \pi_{d_\eta,k}(\overline{X}_{ki}; \eta_k, \widehat{\gamma}_k)\right\} \pi_{d_\eta,1}(X_{1i}; \eta_1, \widehat{\gamma}_1)},$$
$$(5.107)$$

where $\widehat{\gamma}_k$ are estimators for γ_K, $k = 1, \ldots, K$; e.g., with two options at each decision, obtained by maximizing (5.62). As in Section 5.5.2, under SUTVA, the SRA, and the positivity assumption, if the propensity models $\pi_k(h_k; \gamma_k)$ or $\omega_k(h_k, a_k; \gamma_k)$ are correctly specified for $k = 1, \ldots, K$, so that the induced models $\pi_{d_\eta,k}(\overline{X}_k; \gamma_k)$, $k = 1, \ldots, K$, are also correct, then (5.107) is a consistent estimator for the true value $\mathcal{V}(d_\eta)$ for fixed η. This is true by default if the data are from a SMART because then the propensities are known. The same holds true for the alternative inverse probability weighted estimator based on (5.67),

$$\widehat{\mathcal{V}}_{IPW^*}(d_\eta) = \left[\sum_{i=1}^{n} \frac{\mathcal{C}_{d_\eta,i}}{\left\{\prod_{k=2}^{K} \pi_{d_\eta,k}(\overline{X}_{ki}; \eta_k, \widehat{\gamma}_k)\right\} \pi_{d_\eta,1}(X_{1i}; \eta_1, \widehat{\gamma}_1)}\right]^{-1}$$

$$\times \sum_{i=1}^{n} \frac{\mathcal{C}_{d_\eta,i} Y_i}{\left\{\prod_{k=2}^{K} \pi_{d_\eta,k}(\overline{X}_{ki}; \eta_k, \widehat{\gamma}_k)\right\} \pi_{d_\eta,1}(X_{1i}; \eta_1, \widehat{\gamma}_1)}. \quad (5.108)$$

As in the single decision case, maximize (5.107) in η to obtain

$$\widehat{\eta}_{IPW}^{opt} = (\widehat{\eta}_{1,IPW}^{opt\,T}, \ldots, \widehat{\eta}_{K,IPW}^{opt\,T})^T.$$

The value search estimator for an optimal regime $d_\eta^{opt} \in \mathcal{D}_\eta$ is then

$$\widehat{d}_{\eta,IPW}^{opt} = \{d_1(h_1, \widehat{\eta}_{1,IPW}^{opt}), \ldots, d_K(h_K, \widehat{\eta}_{K,IPW}^{opt})\}.$$

Similarly, using (5.108),

$$\widehat{\eta}_{IPW*}^{opt} = (\widehat{\eta}_{1,IPW*}^{opt\,T}, \ldots, \widehat{\eta}_{K,IPW*}^{opt\,T})^T$$

$$\widehat{d}_{\eta,IPW*}^{opt} = \{d_1(h_1, \widehat{\eta}_{1,IPW*}^{opt}), \ldots, d_K(h_K, \widehat{\eta}_{K,IPW*}^{opt})\}.$$

The value achieved by d_η^{opt}, $\mathcal{V}(d_\eta^{opt})$, can be estimated by substituting $\widehat{\eta}_{IPW}^{opt}$ or $\widehat{\eta}_{IPW*}^{opt}$ in (5.107) or (5.108), respectively. As with the estimator for $\mathcal{V}(d^{opt})$ based on Q-learning, these estimators are nonregular, so that inference on the value of an optimal restricted regime $d_\eta^{opt} \in \mathcal{D}_\eta$ is again challenging.

Value search estimation based on augmented inverse probability weighted estimators is discussed in Section 7.4.3.

5.7.3 Backward Iterative Implementation of Value Search Estimation

Although conceptually straightforward, value search estimation of an optimal regime via maximization in η of $\widehat{\mathcal{V}}_{IPW}(d_\eta)$ in (5.107) or of any other estimator for $\mathcal{V}(d_\eta)$, such as (5.108) or an augmented inverse probability weighted estimator as discussed at the end of Section 5.5.2, can be challenging. One major obstacle is that, because η comprises parameters characterizing all of the K rules, even if η_k is of relatively low dimension for each $k = 1, \ldots, K$, $\eta = (\eta_1^T, \ldots, \eta_K^T)^T$ can be of sufficiently high dimension to make direct optimization of the value estimator untenable. This dimensionality issue is discussed in greater depth in Section 7.4.3.

An approach to circumventing this challenge exploits a backward iterative strategy first described by Zhao et al. (2015a), who proposed it in extending the outcome weighted learning approach for a single decision outlined in Section 4.3 to multistage problems, a method they refer to as backward outcome weighted learning (BOWL); see also Zhang and Zhang (2018a). We sketch the intuition underlying this approach, focusing on the inverse probability weighted estimator (5.107). A more formal, detailed, and general account of the backward iterative strategy is given in Section 7.4.4.

For definiteness, consider $\widehat{\mathcal{V}}_{IPW}(d_\eta)$ in (5.107) in the case where there are $m_k \geq 2$ treatment options in $\mathcal{A}_k$, $k = 1, \ldots, K$, and the propensities at each decision point are represented by models $\omega_k(h_k, a_k; \gamma_k)$. As noted in (5.69) at the end of Section 5.5.2, because $A_1 = d_{\eta,1}(X_1)$ and $A_k = d_{\eta,k}\{\overline{X}_k, \overline{d}_{\eta,k-1}(\overline{X}_{k-1})\}$ when $\mathcal{C}_{d_\eta} = 1$, it is straightforward that (5.107) is unaltered by replacing the denominator

$$\left\{ \prod_{k=2}^{K} \pi_{d_\eta,k}(\overline{X}_{ki}; \eta_k, \widehat{\gamma}_k) \right\} \pi_{d_\eta,1}(X_{1i}; \eta_1, \widehat{\gamma}_1)$$

by

$$\underline{\omega}_{1,K}(H_{Ki}, A_{Ki}; \underline{\widehat{\gamma}}_1),$$

where

$$\underline{\omega}_{k,K}(h_K, a_K; \underline{\gamma}_k) = \prod_{j=k}^{K} \omega_j(h_j, a_j; \gamma_j), \quad k = 1, \ldots, K; \qquad (5.109)$$

and $\underline{\gamma}_k = (\gamma_k^T, \ldots, \gamma_K^T)^T$, $k = 1, \ldots, K$, with $\underline{\widehat{\gamma}}_k$ defined similarly. In (5.109) and in (5.112) below, double subscripting by k and K may seem redundant but is used for consistency with the more general presentation in Section 7.4.4. This yields the equivalent representation for (5.107) given by

$$\widehat{\mathcal{V}}_{IPW}(d_\eta) = n^{-1} \sum_{i=1}^{n} \frac{\mathcal{C}_{d_\eta,i} Y_i}{\underline{\omega}_{1,K}(H_{Ki}, A_{Ki}; \underline{\widehat{\gamma}}_1)}, \qquad (5.110)$$

on which we focus henceforth.

Define for $k = 1, \ldots, K$

$$\underline{d}_{\eta,k} = (d_{\eta,k}, d_{\eta,k+1}, \ldots, d_{\eta,K}), \qquad (5.111)$$

so that $\underline{d}_{\eta,k}$ comprises the last $K - k - 1$ rules in d_η, and $\underline{d}_{\eta,1} = d_\eta$. Let

$$\mathfrak{C}_{d_\eta,k,K} = I\{A_k = d_{\eta,k}(H_k), \ldots, A_K = d_{\eta,K}(H_K)\} \qquad (5.112)$$

be the indicator of whether or not the treatment options actually received at the kth through Kth decision points are consistent with those selected by the corresponding rules in d_η. Note that, from (5.68), $\mathcal{C}_{d_\eta} = \mathfrak{C}_{d_\eta,1,K}$.

With these definitions, for $k = 1, \ldots, K$, let

$$\mathcal{G}_{IPW,k}(\underline{d}_{\eta,k}; \underline{\gamma}_k) = \frac{\mathfrak{C}_{d_\eta,k,K} Y}{\underline{\omega}_{k,K}(H_K, A_K; \underline{\gamma}_k)}, \qquad (5.113)$$

where dependence of the left-hand side of (5.113) on (H_K, A_K, Y) for all $k = 1, \ldots, K$ is suppressed in the notation for brevity. From (5.110), it is immediate that

$$\widehat{\mathcal{V}}_{IPW}(d_\eta) = n^{-1} \sum_{i=1}^{n} \mathcal{G}_{IPW,1i}(\underline{d}_{\eta,1}; \underline{\widehat{\gamma}}_1), \qquad (5.114)$$

where, for $k = 1, \ldots, K$, $\mathcal{G}_{IPW,ki}(\underline{d}_{\eta,1}; \underline{\gamma}_1)$ denotes evaluation at (H_{Ki}, A_{Ki}, Y_i).

The backward iterative strategy we now describe is based on the principle of backward induction that underlies characterization of an optimal regime and the method of Q-learning. At Decision K, an individual has already achieved history H_K, so, as in Section 5.6, selection of a Decision K treatment option is analogous to a single decision problem in which an individual presents with "baseline" information H_K. Let

$$\widehat{\mathcal{V}}_{IPW}^{(K)}(d_{\eta,K}) = n^{-1} \sum_{i=1}^{n} \mathcal{G}_{IPW,Ki}(d_{\eta,K}; \widehat{\gamma}_K)$$

$$= n^{-1} \sum_{i=1}^{n} \frac{\mathrm{I}\{A_{Ki} = d_{\eta,K}(H_{Ki})\} Y_i}{\omega_K(H_{Ki}, A_{Ki}; \widehat{\gamma}_K)}, \tag{5.115}$$

where in (5.115) we have used the facts that $\underline{\omega}_{K,K}(h_K, a_K; \underline{\gamma}_K) = \omega_K(h_K, a_K; \gamma_K)$ and $\mathfrak{C}_{d_{\eta,K},K} = \mathrm{I}\{A_K = d_{\eta,K}(H_K)\}$ from (5.109) and (5.112). From Sections 3.5.3 and 3.5.5, (5.115) has the form of an inverse probability weighted estimator for a single decision problem, with Decision K and $d_{\eta,K}$ playing the roles of the single decision point and the corresponding single decision rule, respectively. As introduced more formally in Sections 6.4.2 and 7.2.3, let

$$Y^*(\overline{a}_{k-1}, d_{\eta,k}, \ldots, d_{\eta,K}) = Y^*(\overline{a}_{k-1}, \underline{d}_{\eta,k}), \quad k = 1, \ldots, K,$$

be the potential outcome an individual would achieve if she were to receive options $a_1, \ldots, a_{k-1}$ at Decisions 1 to $k-1$ and then be treated according to the rules $d_{\eta,k}, \ldots, d_{\eta,K}$ at Decisions k to K. Then, as argued in Section 7.4.4, with the propensity model $\omega_K(h_K, a_K; \gamma_K)$ correctly specified, $\widehat{\mathcal{V}}_{IPW}^{(K)}(d_{\eta,K})$ can be viewed as a consistent estimator for

$$E\{Y^*(\overline{A}_{K-1}, d_{\eta,K})\}, \tag{5.116}$$

where now $Y^*(\overline{A}_{K-1}, d_{\eta,K})$ is the potential outcome above for an individual who is observed to receive options $\overline{A}_{K-1}$ at the first $K-1$ decision points. Intuitively, (5.116) can be interpreted as the "value" of the "single decision regime" with rule $d_{\eta,K}$, where $\overline{A}_{K-1}$ is part of the "baseline" information H_K.

Note that the estimator (5.115) and the "value" (5.116) depend on η only through η_K. The first step of the backward algorithm is thus to maximize $\widehat{\mathcal{V}}_{IPW}^{(K)}(d_{\eta,K})$ in (5.115) in η_K to obtain $\widehat{\eta}_{K,B,IPW}^{opt}$ and thus to estimate $d_{\eta,K}^{opt}$ by

$$\widehat{d}_{\eta,K,B}^{opt}(h_K) = d_K(h_K; \widehat{\eta}_{K,B,IPW}^{opt}). \tag{5.117}$$

Here, the subscript "B" emphasizes that $\widehat{\eta}^{opt}_{K,B,IPW}$ and thus (5.117) are obtained via the backward strategy. A little thought reveals that $\widehat{\eta}^{opt}_{K,B,IPW}$ maximizing (5.115) is not likely to be the same as $\widehat{\eta}^{opt}_{K,IPW}$ globally maximizing (5.107) in all of $\eta_1, \ldots, \eta_K$, so jointly with $\widehat{\eta}^{opt}_{1,IPW}, \ldots, \widehat{\eta}^{opt}_{K-1,IPW}$. We return to this point shortly.

Now consider Decision $K - 1$, and let

$$
\widehat{\mathcal{V}}^{(K-1)}_{IPW}(\underline{d}_{\eta,K-1}) = n^{-1} \sum_{i=1}^{n} \mathcal{G}_{IPW,K-1,i}(\underline{d}_{\eta,K-1}; \widehat{\underline{\gamma}}_{K-1})
$$

$$
= n^{-1} \sum_{i=1}^{n} \mathcal{G}_{IPW,K-1,i}(d_{\eta,K-1}, d_{\eta,K}; \widehat{\underline{\gamma}}_{K-1}) \tag{5.118}
$$

$$
= n^{-1} \sum_{i=1}^{n} \frac{\text{I}\{A_{K-1,i} = d_{\eta,K-1}(H_{K-1,i}), A_{Ki} = d_{\eta,K}(H_{Ki})Y_i}{\underline{\omega}_{K-1,K}(H_{Ki}, A_{Ki}; \widehat{\underline{\gamma}}_{K-1})}.
$$

Inspection of (5.118) shows that it has the form of a value estimator for a two-decision problem, with Decisions $K - 1$ and K playing the roles of Decisions 1 and 2, $d_{\eta,K-1}$ and $d_{\eta,K}$ playing the roles of the corresponding decision rules, and H_{K-1} playing the role of "baseline" information. By reasoning analogous to that for (5.116), with the propensity models $\omega_{K-1}(h_{K-1}, a_{K-1}; \gamma_{K-1})$ and $\omega_K(h_K, a_K; \gamma_K)$ correctly specified, (5.118) can be viewed as a consistent estimator for the "value"

$$
E\{Y^*(\overline{A}_{K-2}, d_{\eta,K-1}, d_{\eta,K})\},
$$

where $\overline{A}_{K-2}$ is part of the "baseline" information H_{K-1}.

With the estimator $\widehat{d}^{opt}_{\eta,K,B}$ in (5.117) for $d^{opt}_{\eta,K}$ already in hand, an obvious approach is to substitute this estimator in (5.118) and, holding $d_{\eta,K}$ fixed at $\widehat{d}^{opt}_{\eta,K,B}$, maximize the resulting quantity $\widehat{\mathcal{V}}^{(K-1)}_{IPW}(d_{\eta,K-1}, \widehat{d}^{opt}_{\eta,K,B})$ in η_{K-1} to obtain $\widehat{\eta}^{opt}_{K-1,B,IPW}$ and

$$
\widehat{d}^{opt}_{\eta,K-1,B}(h_{K-1}) = d_{K-1}(h_{K-1}; \widehat{\eta}^{opt}_{K-1,B,IPW}). \tag{5.119}
$$

As for (5.117), $\widehat{\eta}^{opt}_{K-1,B,IPW}$ is almost certainly not the same as $\widehat{\eta}^{opt}_{K-1,IPW}$ globally maximizing (5.107) in all of $\eta_1, \ldots, \eta_K$.

Continuing in this fashion for $k = K - 2, \ldots, 1$, at Decision k, define

$$
\widehat{\mathcal{V}}^{(k)}_{IPW}(\underline{d}_{\eta,k}) = n^{-1} \sum_{i=1}^{n} \mathcal{G}_{IPW,ki}(\underline{d}_{\eta,k}; \widehat{\underline{\gamma}}_k)
$$

$$
= n^{-1} \sum_{i=1}^{n} \mathcal{G}_{IPW,ki}(d_{\eta,k}, \underline{d}_{\eta,k+1}; \widehat{\underline{\gamma}}_k). \tag{5.120}
$$

As for (5.115) and (5.118), with correct propensity models, (5.120) can be viewed as a consistent estimator for the "value"

$$E\{Y^*(\overline{A}_{k-1}, \underline{d}_{\eta,k})\} = E\{Y^*(\overline{A}_{k-1}, d_{\eta,k}, \underline{d}_{\eta,k+1})\}.$$

With $\widehat{\underline{d}}_{\eta,k+1,B}^{opt} = (\widehat{d}_{\eta,k+1,B}^{opt}, \ldots, \widehat{d}_{\eta,K,B}^{opt})$ already in hand, substituting in (5.120) to obtain

$$\widehat{\mathcal{V}}_{IPW}^{(k)}(d_{\eta,k}, \widehat{\underline{d}}_{\eta,k+1,B}^{opt})$$

and treating $\widehat{\underline{d}}_{\eta,k+1,B}^{opt}$ as fixed, maximize in η_k to obtain $\widehat{\eta}_{k,B,IPW}^{opt}$ and

$$\widehat{d}_{\eta,k,B}^{opt}(h_k) = d_k(h_k; \widehat{\eta}_{k,B,IPW}^{opt}). \tag{5.121}$$

As above, $\widehat{\eta}_{k,B,IPW}^{opt}$ need not be the same as $\widehat{\eta}_{k,IPW}^{opt}$ globally maximizing (5.107).

At the end of this algorithm, from (5.117), (5.119), and (5.121), the estimator for d_η^{opt} is given by

$$\widehat{d}_{\eta,B,IPW}^{opt} = \{d_1(h_1; \widehat{\eta}_{1,B,IPW}^{opt}), \ldots, d_K(h_K; \widehat{\eta}_{K,B,IPW}^{opt})\}, \tag{5.122}$$

and the corresponding estimator $\widehat{\mathcal{V}}_{B,IPW}(d_\eta^{opt})$, say, for $\mathcal{V}(d_\eta^{opt})$ is found by substituting (5.122) in $\widehat{\mathcal{V}}_{IPW}(d_\eta)$ in (5.107) or, equivalently, (5.110). The appeal of this strategy is clear: direct, global, and almost certainly high-dimensional maximization of (5.107) in all of $\eta = (\eta_1^T, \ldots, \eta_K^T)^T$ is replaced by a recursive series of lower-dimensional maximizations in each of $\eta_K, \ldots, \eta_1$.

As emphasized above, however, (5.122) is clearly not the same as the estimator $\widehat{d}_{\eta,IPW}^{opt}$ that results from maximizing the full inverse probability weighted estimator (5.107), or equivalently (5.110), jointly in all of $\eta = (\eta_1^T, \ldots, \eta_K^T)^T$ to obtain $\widehat{\eta}_{IPW}^{opt} = (\widehat{\eta}_{1,IPW}^{opt~T}, \ldots, \widehat{\eta}_{K,IPW}^{opt~T})^T$. Thus, intuitively, it is not necessarily the case that $\widehat{d}_{\eta,B,IPW}^{opt}$ in (5.122) is a valid estimator for an optimal restricted regime $d_\eta^{opt} \in \mathcal{D}_\eta$ defined in (5.105). In Section 7.4.4, we present an argument that $\widehat{d}_{\eta,B,IPW}^{opt}$ and other estimators obtained by analogous backward iterative algorithms are valid estimators for an optimal restricted regime d_η^{opt} if in fact a true global optimal regime d^{opt} is contained in the restricted class $\mathcal{D}_\eta$, in which case d^{opt} and d_η^{opt} are equivalent. However, this need not be the case otherwise.

Backward Outcome Weighted Learning (BOWL)

At the kth step of the backward algorithm, a "value" estimator is maximized in the parameter η_k characterizing a single (the kth) decision rule. It follows that, when each set of possible treatment options $\mathcal{A}_k$ involves two options that are feasible for all individuals, the maximization at each step can be likened to a weighted classification problem by manipulations analogous to those in Section 4.2.2. This is the foundation of the original proposal of Zhao et al. (2015a). In particular, Zhao et al. (2015a) advocate maximization of each of $\widehat{\mathcal{V}}_{IPW}^{(K)}(d_{\eta,K})$ in η_K and $\widehat{\mathcal{V}}_{IPW}^{(k)}(d_{\eta,k}, \widehat{\underline{d}}_{\eta,k+1,B}^{opt})$ in η_k, $k = K-1, \ldots, 1$, by recasting it as a weighted classification problem in a manner similar to that used for OWL in Section 4.3. Specifically, coding the treatment options at each decision point as $\{-1, 1\}$, writing each decision rule in terms of a decision function as in (4.33) and taking the restricted class of regimes $\mathcal{D}_\eta$ to be induced by a richly parameterized set of decision functions, they replace the resulting nonconvex 0-1 loss function at each step by the convex "surrogate" hinge loss function (4.35) and add a penalty term to control overfitting as in (4.36). The resulting method, referred to by the authors as BOWL, is reviewed in more detail in Section 7.4.5.

5.7.4 Implementation and Practical Performance

Q-learning

Implementation of Q-learning is in principle straightforward, as each step of the procedure requires positing regression models that can then be fitted using established methods and software. However, as noted in Section 5.7.1, development of models for $k = K-1, \ldots, 1$ is not a standard regression exercise, as these are models for pseudo, rather than observed, outcomes. As demonstrated in that section, this leads to almost certain model misspecification. Intuitively, the estimated optimal regime $\widehat{d}_Q^{opt}$ in (5.97) and the value estimator $\widehat{\mathcal{V}}_Q(d^{opt})$ in (5.98) could be far from an optimal regime $d^{opt} \in \mathcal{D}$ and the true value $\mathcal{V}(d^{opt})$, respectively, when the models for the Q-functions are incorrectly specified. In fact, because K models are now involved, $K-1$ of which are unconventional, the consequences of such misspecification could be more dramatic than those in the single decision case discussed in Section 3.5.4.

To address this difficulty, as noted for the single decision case in Section 4.5, some authors (Qian and Murphy, 2011; Zhao et al., 2011; Moodie et al., 2014) have advocated representing the Q-functions using flexible nonparametric regression modeling techniques. As noted by Schulte et al. (2014), many nonparametric approaches require tuning; e.g., via cross validation, to balance bias and variance, and the resulting final models may be complex and difficult to interpret, leading to "black box" rules that clinicians may view with skepticism relative to the simpler rules that arise from parsimonious parametric models.

Even with parametric models, when the number of decision points K is large, the number of parameters that must be estimated is considerable. In this case, postulating models that share parameters across decisions has been advocated (e.g., Robins, 2004; Robins et al., 2008; Chakraborty et al., 2016).

Despite the potential drawbacks of Q-learning highlighted here and in Section 5.7.1, this approach is popular in practice, as it can be implemented using familiar methods and readily available software. Although model misspecification has the potential to lead to poor performance, simulation evidence suggests that, in some circumstances, the Q-learning estimator $\widehat{d}_Q^{opt}$ can achieve reasonable performance with possibly misspecified parametric models. In particular, its value, $\mathcal{V}(\widehat{d}_Q^{opt})$, the expected outcome if the estimated regime were used to select treatment options in the population, when evaluated numerically by simulation as described in the single decision case in Section 3.5.4, can approach that of a true optimal regime $d^{opt} \in \mathcal{D}$. Schulte et al. (2014) present a suite of simulation studies demonstrating this phenomenon for $K = 2$. The extent to which the Q-learning estimator performs well despite model misspecification is problem-specific. In any case, it is important that the analyst be aware of these features and take a pragmatic view of the results of such analyses.

Value Search Estimation

Global maximization of $\widehat{\mathcal{V}}_{IPW}(d_\eta)$ or $\widehat{\mathcal{V}}_{IPW*}(d_\eta)$ in η can be more challenging than for the single decision case discussed in Section 3.5.4. As for $K = 1$, this is a nonsmooth optimization problem; Zhang et al. (2013) describe use of a genetic algorithm due to Goldberg (1989) for this purpose, implemented in the R package rgenoud (Mebane and Sekhon, 2011). Moreover, as noted in Section 5.7.3, because η comprises parameters characterizing all of the K rules, even if η_k is of low dimension for each $k = 1, \ldots, K$, η can be of sufficiently high dimension to make this optimization more formidable, and a direct grid search is generally not feasible. The backward iterative strategy presented in Section 5.7.3 is a practical approach to circumventing the dimensionality issue when each η_k is of low dimension. This approach is also especially appealing because the reduction of the global optimization problem to a series of maximizations in the parameter for a single decision rule facilitates recasting each step as a weighted classification problem and exploiting the developments for single decision regimes in Sections 4.2.2 and 4.3. As sketched at the end of Section 5.7.3, this was the original motivation underlying the BOWL approach of Zhao et al. (2015a). These authors and others who have adapted this approach demonstrate that, although this method need not in principle yield a valid estimator for an optimal restricted regime, estimated regimes so obtained often achieve good performance approaching that of a true optimal regime in practice.

As discussed in the remark in Section 5.5.2, because for each fixed η simple inverse probability weighted estimators for the value involve data only from individuals for whom $\mathcal{C}_{d_\eta} = 1$, so for whom the treatment options actually received at all K decisions coincide with those dictated by d_η, they can be an unstable, inefficient estimators for $\mathcal{V}(d_\eta)$. As shown in simulation studies with $\widehat{\mathcal{V}}_{IPW}(d_\eta)$ reported by Zhang et al. (2013), this translates into poor performance of the estimated optimal restricted regime $\widehat{d}_{\eta,IPW}^{opt}$. In general, regardless of implementation, this approach is likely to suffer degradation of performance beyond $K = 2$ or 3.

Zhang et al. (2013) propose basing value search estimation instead on augmented inverse probability weighted estimators for $\mathcal{V}(d_\eta)$ for fixed η, as noted at the end of Section 5.5.2, which yield considerably improved performance, with the value of the resulting estimated regimes comparable to that of a true optimal regime. We present details of value search estimation based on augmented inverse probability weighted estimators in Section 7.4.3.

Implementation and performance of the additional approaches to estimation of an optimal multiple decision regime presented in Chapter 7 are discussed in Section 7.4.9.

5.8 Application

Implementations of estimators for the value of a fixed regime and for an optimal multiple decision treatment regime introduced in this chapter are demonstrated on the book's companion website given in the Preface. All codes used to generate simulated data and to implement each method are available on the website.

Chapter 6

Multiple Decision Treatment Regimes: Formal Framework

6.1 Introduction

Chapter 5 provides a high-level introduction to the statistical framework for the multiple decision problem and to fundamental concepts and results underlying methods for estimation of the value of a fixed multiple decision treatment regime and for characterization and estimation of an optimal multiple decision regime and its value. The presentation deliberately sidesteps technical details and proofs so as to emphasize the main ideas. Chapter 5 provides sufficient coverage for readers interested primarily in an overview of this area.

In this chapter and Chapter 7, we provide a more rigorous account of the multiple decision problem for readers interested in the technical underpinnings. This includes proofs of results presented without proof in Chapter 5 and additional approaches not covered in that chapter.

We first present in this chapter a precise description of the potential outcomes framework and the identifiability assumptions introduced in Section 5.3. This is based on a formal definition of the sets of treatment options that are feasible for patients with a given history at each decision point and implies a formal definition of regimes themselves, an explicit statement of which is suppressed in Chapter 5. We then reiterate the main identifiability result that the distribution of potential outcomes associated with a fixed regime can be identified from observed data within this framework and provide a formal proof. The rest of this chapter is devoted to an account of methods for estimation of the value of a fixed regime, including several not introduced in Chapter 5.

Within the framework established in this chapter involving the notion of feasible sets of treatment options, Chapter 7 provides a more formal account of characterization and estimation of an optimal treatment regime, including via methods not discussed in Chapter 5.

The reader should review Chapter 5 before proceeding with this and the next chapter, as these chapters are meant to augment the material in Chapter 5 rather than to stand alone. We do not restate the definition of a treatment regime involving K decisions and the notation in Section 5.2 here. Although we do revisit some definitions and results presented in

Chapter 5 for continuity and convenience, we refer the reader to that chapter for fuller discussion, particularly of practical considerations.

6.2   Statistical Framework

6.2.1   Potential Outcomes for K Decisions

We assume that there is an outcome of interest for which larger values are preferred, which is ascertained either following Decision K or is defined in terms of the intervening information arising between decision points and following Decision K, as discussed in Section 5.3.1. As defined in that section, for a particular set of treatment options $\bar{a} = \bar{a}_K = (a_1, \ldots, a_K) \in \overline{\mathcal{A}}_K = \overline{\mathcal{A}}$ and baseline information X_1, the associated potential outcomes are

$$\{X_1, X_2^*(a_1), X_3^*(\bar{a}_2), \ldots, X_K^*(\bar{a}_{K-1}), Y^*(\bar{a})\}. \tag{6.1}$$

As in Section 5.3.1, the random variables

$$X_k^*(\bar{a}_{k-1}), \quad k = 2, \ldots, K, \tag{6.2}$$

represent the intervening information that would be achieved by a randomly chosen individual between Decisions $k-1$ and k if he were administered options $\bar{a}_{k-1}$ through Decision $k-1$. Likewise, $Y^*(\bar{a})$ is the final outcome of interest an individual would achieve if he were administered the full set of K options $\bar{a}$ through Decision K, which as above would be ascertained subsequent to Decision K or be defined in terms of components of the potential intervening variables in (6.2) and other information that would arise after Decision K. The variables in (6.1), with or without the baseline information X_1, are referred to collectively as potential outcomes. For convenience, write

$$\overline{X}_k^*(\bar{a}_{k-1}) = \{X_1, X_2^*(a_1), X_3(\bar{a}_2), \ldots, X_k^*(\bar{a}_{k-1})\}, \quad k = 1, \ldots, K.$$

Note that this formulation assumes implicitly that the potential intervening variables (6.2) between Decisions $k-1$ and k depend only on the treatment options administered through Decision $k-1$ and are not affected by future treatments. This is intuitively sensible, as is the embedded assumption that the baseline information X_1 is not affected by any of the future treatment assignments.

As emphasized in previous chapters, this potential outcomes framework provides a formal basis for comparisons of outcomes associated with different sequences $\bar{a}$ with a causal interpretation. For a given individual, the "best" sequence is obviously

$$\arg\max_{\bar{a} \in \overline{\mathcal{A}}} Y^*(\bar{a}); \tag{6.3}$$

that is, the particular sequence associated with the largest potential final outcome that could be achieved by the individual. As in the point exposure setting of Chapter 2, ordinarily, for a given individual, it is possible to observe the final potential outcome $Y^*(\cdot)$ for only a single treatment sequence; specifically, the sequence comprising the options actually received by the individual over the K decision points. Thus, analogous to the situation in Section 2.3, it is impossible to determine an optimal sequence at the individual level.

This fundamental challenge of causal inference leads to consideration of causal interpretations at the population level. For example, the comparison of two treatment sequences $\bar{a} = (a_1, \ldots, a_K)$ and $\bar{a}' = (a'_1, \ldots, a'_K)$ is based ordinarily on the difference between $E\{Y^*(\bar{a})\}$ and $E\{Y^*(\bar{a}')\}$; that is, the difference between the average outcome that would be achieved if all individuals in the population were administered the sequence $\bar{a}$ over all K decisions and that if all individuals were administered $\bar{a}'$. Because $E\{Y^*(\bar{a})\}$ and $E\{Y^*(\bar{a}')\}$ are the values associated with $\bar{a}$ and $\bar{a}'$, this is the difference in values for the two sequences.

As in (5.9), we define the set of all possible potential outcomes as

$$
W^* = \Big\{ X_2^*(a_1), X_3^*(\bar{a}_2), \ldots, X_K^*(\bar{a}_{K-1}), Y^*(\bar{a}),
$$

$$
\text{for } a_1 \in \mathcal{A}_1, \bar{a}_2 \in \overline{\mathcal{A}}_2, \ldots, \bar{a}_{K-1} \in \overline{\mathcal{A}}_{K-1}, \bar{a} \in \overline{\mathcal{A}} \Big\}. \tag{6.4}
$$

In the literature, the baseline information X_1 may or may not be included in the definition of W^* as proves convenient for the specific situation. The elements of W^* represent potential intervening information and final outcome under all treatment sequences $\bar{a}$.

Remarks. (i) In Chapter 5 and the above formulation, we have noted that the outcome of interest is either ascertained following Decision K or defined in terms of intervening information between decision points and additional information arising after Decision K. In some accounts in the literature, the latter situation is made explicit, using a formulation underlying reinforcement learning in computer science, as follows.

For each $k = 2, \ldots, K$, variables derived from the intervening information that are involved in the definition of the final outcome are denoted separately, and $X_k^*(\bar{a}_{k-1})$ is taken to refer to intervening information that is not directly involved in defining the final outcome. Specifically, define $R_k^*(\bar{a}_{k-1})$, $k = 2, \ldots, K$, to be variables that would arise between Decisions $k - 1$ and k and are used to define the final outcome, and let $R_{K+1}^*(\bar{a})$ denote information that would arise after Decision K used for this purpose. Then, for a particular set of treatment options $\bar{a} = (a_1, \ldots, a_K) \in \overline{\mathcal{A}}_K = \overline{\mathcal{A}}$, the potential outcomes can be defined as

$$\Big[X_1, \{X_2^*(a_1), R_2^*(a_1)\}, \{X_3^*(\overline{a}_2), R_3^*(\overline{a}_2)\}, \dots,$$

$$\{X_K^*(\overline{a}_{K-1}), R_K^*(\overline{a}_{K-1})\}, R_{K+1}^*(\overline{a}), Y^*(\overline{a})\Big], \qquad (6.5)$$

where, as in (6.1), we include the baseline information X_1 for completeness. Following the convention in the reinforcement learning literature, the $R_k^*(\overline{a}_{k-1})$, $k = 2, \dots, K+1$, are referred to as *rewards*. Ordinarily, the potential final outcome of interest under $\overline{a}$ is taken to be

$$Y^*(\overline{a}) = \sum_{k=2}^{K+1} R_k^*(\overline{a}_{k-1}). \qquad (6.6)$$

For example, recall the situation of HIV-infected patients discussed in Sections 1.2.3 and 5.3.1, in which the final outcome is the number of clinic visits following initiation of treatment, including a final visit subsequent to the Kth decision point, at which CD4 T cell count is above 200 cells/mm^3. Here, $R_k^*(\overline{a}_{k-1})$ is the indicator of whether or not the CD4 count ascertained immediately prior to Decision k, $k = 2, \dots, K$, is greater than 200; $R_{K+1}^*(\overline{a})$ is the indicator of whether or not the final CD4 measure taken following Decision K is greater than 200; and thus $Y^*(\overline{a})$ in (6.6) is the total number of visits at which CD4 count exceeds 200.

If we take all rewards but the final potential reward under $\overline{a}$, $R_{K+1}^*(\overline{a})$, to be null, from (6.6), $Y^*(\overline{a})$ and $R_{K+1}^*(\overline{a})$ are one in the same, and (6.5) reduces to (6.1). This reflects the setting in which the final outcome is ascertained after the Kth decision point.

Regardless of whether or not components of each $X_k^*(\overline{a}_{k-1})$, $k = 2, \dots, K$, are used in defining the final outcome, it is clear that subsuming the rewards for $k = 2, \dots, K$ in the intervening information causes no conceptual difficulty. Accordingly, we continue to denote the potential outcomes as in (6.1), so that any intervening information that is used to define the final outcome is included implicitly in the $X_k^*(\overline{a}_{k-1})$, $k = 2, \dots, K$, and any additional information ascertained after Decision K is subsumed in $Y^*(\overline{a})$. An analogous convention applies when we discuss the corresponding observed data.

(ii). In the development so far here and in Chapter 5, the definitions of the potential outcomes imply that the dimension of each of $X_k^*(\overline{a}_{k-1})$ is the same for all $\overline{a}_{k-1}$, $k = 2, \dots, K$. If we view $X_k^*(\overline{a}_{k-1})$ as containing all intervening information that could be collected between Decisions $k-1$ and k, it may be that certain components of this information would not be ascertained depending on the treatment options in $\overline{a}_{k-1}$. For example, in the acute leukemia setting in Section 1.2.1, if induction chemotherapy option a_1 at Decision 1 were to lead to nonresponse, making the patient eligible only for salvage therapy options at Decision 2, then, immediately prior to Decision 2, it would not be necessary to measure a variable that is used only to assist in the choice of a maintenance option for responders.

To avoid cumbersome notation, we do not make this explicit. In such circumstances, the relevant components of $X_k^*(\overline{a}_{k-1})$ are taken to be null, and we allow the corresponding components of realized values x_k to take on the null value as well. Under this convention, the set $\mathcal{X}_k$ is understood to include such x_k.

As in Section 5.3.1, we require a definition of potential outcomes associated with dynamic treatment regimes. Before we give a precise definition of a treatment regime and the associated potential outcomes, we define the notion of feasible sets of treatment options.

6.2.2 Feasible Sets and Classes of Treatment Regimes

As discussed in Section 5.2, at any decision point k, $k = 1, \ldots, K$, not all treatment options in the set $\mathcal{A}_k$ of all available options need be feasible for all individuals. For individuals with certain histories, some options may be inappropriate, unethical, or inconsistent with the intended implementation of a regime. This is true in the acute leukemia example in Section 1.2.1, where there are four options at Decision 2: two maintenance therapies, which are appropriate, and thus feasible, only for patients who respond to the induction therapy administered at Decision 1; and two salvage therapies, which are feasible only for patients who do not respond to induction therapy. Response status is ascertained between Decisions 1 and 2 and may be either an explicit component or function of an individual's history h_2; thus, the set of feasible treatment options for any individual is predicated on her history h_2 at the time of Decision 2. Similarly, as in the HIV treatment example in Section 1.2.3, if an HIV-infected patient's virus has been established to have become resistant to a certain antiretroviral agent, it would be inappropriate, and indeed unethical, to continue that individual on that agent, so that whether or not the agent is feasible at any decision point depends on his current resistance status, which would be contained in his history to that point. In a health policy context where interest is in regimes for use in resource limited settings, the feasible options at each decision point may be restricted deliberately to those that are less costly unless an individual's condition, as reflected in her history, is especially serious.

From this perspective, the definition of a treatment regime $d = (d_1, \ldots, d_K)$ and of $\mathcal{D}$ must be predicated on a formal specification of the sets of feasible treatment options at each decision point $k = 1, \ldots, K$

for an individual with a particular realized history $h_k = (\overline{x}_k, \overline{a}_{k-1}) \in \mathcal{H}_k = \overline{\mathcal{X}}_k \times \overline{\mathcal{A}}_{k-1}$ to that point. As in Chapter 5, in what follows, we use the notation h_k and $\mathcal{H}_k$ and $(\overline{x}_k, \overline{a}_{k-1})$ and $\overline{\mathcal{X}}_k \times \overline{\mathcal{A}}_{k-1}$ interchangeably. For any history $h_k = (\overline{x}_k, \overline{a}_{k-1}) \in \mathcal{H}_k$ at Decision k, $k = 1, \ldots, K$, we represent the set of feasible treatment options at Decision k as

$$\Psi_k(h_k) = \Psi_k(\overline{x}_k, \overline{a}_{k-1}) \subseteq \mathcal{A}_k, \quad k = 1, \ldots, K, \tag{6.7}$$

where, as noted in Section 5.3.3, a_0 is taken to be null, so that when $k = 1$, (6.7) is interpreted as

$$\Psi_1(h_1) = \Psi_1(x_1) \subseteq \mathcal{A}_1.$$

Thus, for Decision k, $\Psi_k(h_k)$ is the set of options in $\mathcal{A}_k$ that are feasible for an individual with history h_k and may comprise a strict subset of $\mathcal{A}_k$ or all of $\mathcal{A}_k$, depending on h_k. For each $k = 1, \ldots, K$, $\Psi_k(h_k)$ can be thought of as a function mapping $\mathcal{H}_k$ to the set of all possible subsets of $\mathcal{A}_k$. For the K-decision setting, we refer to the K feasible sets collectively as

$$\Psi = (\Psi_1, \ldots, \Psi_K).$$

As an example, consider again the setting of acute leukemia in Section 1.2.1. Suppose that both induction chemotherapy options C_1 and C_2 are feasible for all individuals at Decision 1 regardless of baseline information. Then, with $\mathcal{A}_1 = \{C_1, C_2\}$, $\Psi_1(h_1) = \mathcal{A}_1$ for all h_1. With $\mathcal{A}_2 = \{M_1, M_2, S_1, S_2\}$, so comprising the two maintenance and two salvage options, at Decision 2, if h_2 indicates that an individual responded to induction therapy, so that only maintenance options are feasible, then $\Psi_2(h_2) = \{M_1, M_2\} \subset \mathcal{A}_2$ for all such h_2; if h_2 shows an individual is a nonresponder, then for such h_2, $\Psi_2(h_2) = \{S_1, S_2\} \subset \mathcal{A}_2$.

An alternative, more complex specification of these sets would take into account additional information. For instance, if C_1 is contraindicated for patients with renal impairment, and if h_1 includes information on renal function, then $\Psi_1(h_1) = \mathcal{A}_1$ for individuals whose h_1 indicates normal function and $\Psi_1(h_1) = \{C_2\}$ for those for whom it indicates impairment. Similarly, specification of $\Psi_2(h_2)$ can take into account information in h_2 beyond response status; e.g., if S_1 is known to increase the risk of adverse events in nonresponding patients with low white blood cell count, it might be prudent to define $\Psi_2(h_2) = \{S_1, S_2\}$ for h_2 indicating nonresponse and Decision 2 white blood cell count WBC_2 exceeding some threshold and $\Psi_2(h_2) = \{S_2\}$ for h_2 showing nonresponse and WBC_2 less than or equal to the threshold.

Remark. Ideally, specification of the sets $\Psi_k(h_k)$, $k = 1, \ldots, K$, is dictated by the disease/disorder context, the treatment options at each decision point, the patient population, and so on, and thus is based on scientific considerations. From a practical perspective, specification of the feasible sets should incorporate only information in h_k that is critical to selection of treatment. Ordinarily, even if h_k is high dimensional, then, this would involve a low-dimensional subset or function of the components of h_k. For example, in the leukemia setting, the feasible sets involve the single component of h_2 "response status" (remission or not); in the ADHD example in Section 1.2.2, the feasible sets may involve "response status" determined by an ADHD severity score that is a function of components of h_2. We discuss conception of these sets in light of the limitations of the available data in Section 6.2.4.

It should be clear that, given specified feasible sets Ψ, a treatment regime $d = (d_1, \ldots, d_K)$ whose rules select treatment options at each decision point k for individuals with history h_k from among the options in $\Psi_k(h_k)$ is defined in terms of Ψ. Thus, treatment regimes are Ψ-specific, and, given a particular Ψ, the set of all possible regimes $\mathcal{D}$ is dependent on Ψ. Accordingly, an optimal regime is understood to be optimal within the class of all Ψ-specific regimes. Henceforth, then, we assume that a particular fixed Ψ has been specified, but we suppress dependence on Ψ in the notation for brevity and continue to use d and $\mathcal{D}$ without explicit reference to Ψ.

As above, because only a few components or functions of h_k may determine the feasible sets, there is usually a small number ℓ_k, say, of distinct subsets of $\mathcal{A}_k$ that are feasible sets at Decision k for all h_k. For example, in the leukemia setting, $\ell_2 = 2$, as $\Psi_2(h_2) = \{M_1, M_2\}$ for h_2 indicating response and $\Psi_2(h_2) = \{S_1, S_2\}$ for h_2 indicating nonresponse. It is reasonable to expect that the form of the Ψ_2-specific rule $d_2(h_2)$ might be different for responders and nonresponders, as the rule selects from different sets of options depending on response status, and it may be that different components of h_2 are important in selecting maintenance versus salvage therapy. Letting r_2 be the component of h_2 indicating response, we can represent $d_2(h_2)$ as

$$d_2(h_2) = \mathrm{I}(r_2 = 1)\, d_{2,1}(h_2) + \mathrm{I}(r_2 = 0)\, d_{2,2}(h_2),$$

where $d_{2,1}(h_2)$ and $d_{2,2}(h_2)$ are rules selecting maintenance therapy for responders and salvage therapy for nonresponders, respectively.

In the leukemia example, the subsets that are feasible sets are nonoverlapping, but this is not required. For example, suppose that $\mathcal{A}_2$ includes an additional option N, corresponding to "no further treatment," which might be considered by some patients and physicians in practice regardless of response status. Then the set of feasible options for responders is $\{M_1, M_2, N\}$ and that for nonresponders is $\{S_1, S_2, N\}$.

In general, with ℓ_k distinct subsets $\mathcal{A}_{k,l} \subseteq \mathcal{A}_k$, $l = 1, \ldots, \ell_k$, say, as feasible sets at Decision k, $k = 1, \ldots, K$, let $s_k(h_k)$ take on values $1, \ldots, \ell_k$ according to which of these subsets $\Psi_k(h_k)$ corresponds for given h_k. Then, letting $d_{k,l}(h_k)$ denote the rule corresponding to the lth subset $\mathcal{A}_{k,l}$,

$$d_k(h_k) = \sum_{l=1}^{\ell_k} \mathrm{I}\{s_k(h_k) = l\}\, d_{k,l}(h_k). \tag{6.8}$$

In the sequel, it is understood that the rule $d_k(h_k)$ may be expressed as in (6.8) where appropriate.

In fact, this discussion highlights that, depending on the scientific context, a class $\mathcal{D}$ of Ψ-specific regimes of interest may or may not contain static regimes. As in Section 5.2, a regime d is static if all of its rules $d_k(h_k)$, $k = 1, \ldots, K$, do not use any of the information in h_k to assign treatment, so that $d_k(h_k)$ returns the same option in $\Psi_k(h_k)$ regardless of h_k for all $k = 1, \ldots, K$. In the acute leukemia example, with $\ell_2 = 2$, because $\Psi_2(h_2) = \{M_1, M_2\} = \mathcal{A}_{2,1}$, say, for h_2 indicating response and $\Psi_2(h_2) = \{S_1, S_2\} = \mathcal{A}_{2,2}$ for h_2 indicating nonresponse, there is no option at Decision 2 that is feasible for all possible histories h_2 that could be seen at that point. Thus, a static rule at Decision 2 is not possible, so that there are no static regimes in the Ψ-specific class $\mathcal{D}$. In contrast, if $\Psi_2(h_2) = \{M_1, M_2, N\}$ for responders and $\Psi_2(h_2) = \{S_1, S_2, N\}$ for nonresponders, then, assuming both chemotherapeutic options at Decision 1, $\{C_1, C_2\}$, are feasible for all individuals regardless of baseline history, there are two feasible static regimes, "Give C_1 followed by N (regardless of response status)" and "Give C_2 followed by N (regardless of response status)." Nonetheless, in the context of clinical practice and precision medicine, it is unlikely that a regime that takes into account none of a patient's history, and at the very least response status, in the decision to administer no further treatment would be of interest.

Remark. The concept of feasible sets of treatment options is deliberately sidestepped in the discussion of single decision regimes in Chapters 3 and 4. In most practical situations involving a single decision point, that decision corresponds to the point at which selection of an initial intervention is to take place; e.g., the time of diagnosis of a disease or disorder. Ordinarily, interest in this context is in a fixed set of treatment options that are feasible for all individuals in a given patient population; if there are other options that are feasible only for a subpopulation of patients, they are often studied separately. Often, there are exactly two competing such options, so that much of the literature and certainly the classification-based approaches reviewed in Chapter 4 restrict to this situation. Accordingly, the notion of feasible sets of treatment options is suppressed in work on single decision regimes.

In the multiple decision case, however, although all available options at Decision 1 may be feasible for all individuals, at subsequent decision points, acknowledging the existence of sets of treatment options that are feasible only for individuals with certain histories is almost always required. As the acute leukemia example illustrates, following administration of an initial treatment, how an individual's disease or disorder evolves dictates how she should be treated subsequently, as with response status in this setting. Similarly, in the ADHD example, whether or not a child responds to the initial intervention determines if that intervention is continued or modified by intensification or augmentation. Interestingly, formal acknowledgment of feasible sets is often downplayed in the literature on methods for multiple decision regimes.

For any Ψ-specific regime $d = (d_1, \ldots, d_K)$, at Decision k, the rule $d_k(h_k) = d_k(\overline{x}_k, \overline{a}_{k-1})$ returns only options in $\Psi_k(h_k) = \Psi_k(\overline{x}_k, \overline{a}_{k-1})$; that is,

$$d_k(h_k) = d_k(\overline{x}_k, \overline{a}_{k-1}) \in \Psi_k(h_k) \subseteq \mathcal{A}_k.$$

This suggests that d_k need map only a subset of $\mathcal{H}_k = \overline{\mathcal{X}}_k \times \overline{\mathcal{A}}_{k-1}$ to $\mathcal{A}_k$. In Section 6.2.4, we formalize this notion and discuss considerations for the study of Ψ-specific regimes based on data.

Remark. We define feasible sets in (6.7) for all $h_k \in \mathcal{H}_k$ for each $k = 1, \ldots, K$, even though implementation of a Ψ-specific regime restricts the possible values of h_k, $k = 2, \ldots, K$, to lie in a subset of $\mathcal{H}_k$. For example, in the HIV treatment setting, at any decision point k, $\mathcal{A}_k$ contains two options, administer antiretroviral therapy or not. For a patient who is on therapy at Decision $k - 1$ and whose virus becomes resistant between Decisions $k - 1$ and k, so that h_k includes positive resistance status at Decision k, for such h_k, Ψ would likely involve $\Psi_k(h_k)$ comprising the single option "do not administer therapy." Accordingly, for a patient following any Ψ-specific regime, $d_k(h_k)$ would assign this option, and, as a consequence, possible realizations of $h_{k+1} = (\overline{x}_{k+1}, \overline{a}_k)$ for such a patient exclude those involving $a_k =$ "administer therapy." This suggests limiting the definition of $\Psi_k(h_k)$ to h_k in subsets of $\mathcal{H}_k$ determined by such considerations. However, we allow the broader definition for all $h_k \in \mathcal{H}_k$ to accommodate other possible treatment assignment mechanisms. A patient with this same history h_k and thus positive resistance status at Decision k being treated in routine clinical practice could possibly insist on continuing therapy nonetheless and be assigned to $a_k =$ "administer therapy" at Decision k. Thus, possible realizations of h_{k+1} for such a patient include configurations that would not occur under implementation of a Ψ-specific regime. In (6.7), we thus adopt the perspective that specification of feasible sets should be for all possible histories, even if some histories are superfluous in the context of Ψ-specific regimes. This proves convenient in the discussion in Section 7.3 of regimes for patients presenting at decision points subsequent to the first.

6.2.3 Potential Outcomes for a Fixed K-Decision Regime

In Section 5.3.1, for a regime $d \in \mathcal{D}$, we define informally in (5.10) the potential intervening information and final outcome that would arise if a randomly chosen individual were to receive treatment options at Decisions 1 to K by following the rules in d. Namely, including baseline information, these potential outcomes are

$$\{X_1, X_2^*(d_1), X_3^*(\overline{d}_2), \ldots, X_K^*(\overline{d}_{K-1}), Y^*(d)\}, \tag{6.9}$$

where $\overline{d}_k$, $k = 1, \ldots, K$, refers to the first k rules in d as defined in (5.5). We now give a more precise definition of these potential outcomes in terms of the set of all potential outcomes W^* in (6.4).

Imagine that there is a superpopulation of individuals, denoted by Ω, where we can view an element $\omega \in \Omega$ as an individual from this population. That is, Ω is the sample space relevant to the baseline information and potential outcomes in W^*. Thus, for every $\omega \in \Omega$, we have $X_1(\omega)$; $X_k^*(\overline{a}_{k-1})(\omega)$, $k = 2, \ldots, K$; and $Y^*(\overline{a})(\omega)$ for all sequences $\overline{a} \in \overline{\mathcal{A}}$. Then $X_1(\omega)$ maps from the sample space Ω to $\mathcal{X}_1$; and, for any $\overline{a} \in \overline{\mathcal{A}}$, $X_k^*(\overline{a}_{k-1})(\omega)$ maps from Ω to $\mathcal{X}_k$, $k = 2, \ldots, K$, and $Y^*(\overline{a})(\omega)$ maps from Ω to the appropriate space for the final outcome; e.g., $\mathbb{R}$ for a continuous outcome.

For any $d \in \mathcal{D}$, $d = (d_1, \ldots, d_K)$, we define the potential outcomes in (6.9) recursively as follows. For any $\omega \in \Omega$, let

$$X_1(\omega) = x_1,$$
$$d_1(x_1) = a_1,$$

where a_1 is an option in $\Psi_1(x_1)$. Then define

$$X_2^*(d_1)(\omega) = X_2^*(a_1)(\omega) = x_2,$$
$$d_2(\overline{x}_2, a_1) = a_2,$$

$$\vdots \tag{6.10}$$

$$d_{K-1}(\overline{x}_{K-1}, \overline{a}_{K-2}) = a_{K-1},$$
$$X_K^*(\overline{d}_{K-1})(\omega) = X_K^*(\overline{a}_{K-1})(\omega) = x_K,$$
$$d_K(\overline{x}_K, a_{K-1}) = a_K,$$
$$Y^*(d)(\omega) = Y^*(\overline{a})(\omega) = y,$$

where a_k are options in $\Psi_k(\overline{x}_k, \overline{a}_{k-1})$, $k = 2, \ldots, K$. That is, $X_k^*(\overline{d}_{k-1})(\omega)$ represents the covariate information that would arise between Decisions $k-1$ and k were individual ω to receive the treatments sequentially dictated by the first $k-1$ rules in d. Similarly, $Y^*(d)(\omega)$ is the final response that ω would experience if she were to receive the K treatments dictated by d. From (6.10), $X_k^*(\overline{d}_{k-1})$, $k = 2, \ldots, K$ and $Y^*(d)$ are seen to be functions of the potential outcomes W^*.

We summarize using the following streamlined notation. We can write

$$X_2^*(d_1) = \sum_{a_1 \in \mathcal{A}_1} X_2^*(a_1) \mathrm{I}\{d_1(X_1) = a_1\},$$

$$X_k^*(\overline{d}_{k-1}) = \sum_{\overline{a}_{k-1} \in \overline{\mathcal{A}}_{k-1}} X_k^*(\overline{a}_{k-1}) \prod_{j=1}^{k-1} \mathrm{I}\left[d_j\{\overline{X}_j^*(\overline{a}_{j-1}), \overline{a}_{j-1}\} = a_j\right], \quad (6.11)$$

$$k = 3, \ldots, K$$

$$Y^*(d) = \sum_{\overline{a} \in \overline{\mathcal{A}}} Y^*(\overline{a}) \prod_{j=1}^{K} \mathrm{I}\left[d_j\{\overline{X}_j^*(\overline{a}_{j-1}), \overline{a}_{j-1}\} = a_j\right].$$

We discuss the representation (6.11) further in Section 6.2.4. As in Section 5.5.2, define

$$\overline{X}_k^*(\overline{d}_{k-1}) = \{X_1, X_2^*(d_1), X_3^*(\overline{d}_2), \ldots, X_k^*(\overline{d}_{k-1})\}, \quad k = 2, \ldots, K.$$

As in Section 5.3.1, with $Y^*(d)$ so defined for regime $d \in \mathcal{D}$, the value of d is

$$\mathcal{V}(d) = E\{Y^*(d)\}, \tag{6.12}$$

the expected outcome if all individuals in the population were to receive treatment according to the rules in d. An optimal regime $d^{opt} \in \mathcal{D}$ maximizes the value (6.12) and thus satisfies

$$E\{Y^*(d^{opt})\} \geq E\{Y^*(d)\} \text{ for all } d \in \mathcal{D}, \tag{6.13}$$

or, equivalently,

$$d^{opt} = \arg\max_{d \in \mathcal{D}} E\{Y^*(d)\} = \arg\max_{d \in \mathcal{D}} \mathcal{V}(d).$$

As discussed in Section 3.4 in the single decision case, an optimal regime need not lead to the optimal sequence of treatment options for a randomly chosen individual. An optimal sequence of treatments for an individual is that corresponding to the largest final potential outcome that can be achieved by the individual; that is, as in (6.3),

$$\arg\max_{\overline{a} \in \overline{\mathcal{A}}} Y^*(\overline{a}).$$

From the definition of $Y^*(d)$ in (6.11) above, it is straightforward that

$$Y^*(d) \leq \max_{\bar{a} \in \bar{\mathcal{A}}} Y^*(\bar{a}) \text{ for all } d \in \mathcal{D},$$

which implies that

$$Y^*(d^{opt}) \leq \max_{\bar{a} \in \bar{\mathcal{A}}} Y^*(\bar{a})$$

almost surely, and

$$E\{Y^*(d^{opt})\} \leq E\left\{\max_{\bar{a} \in \bar{\mathcal{A}}} Y^*(\bar{a})\right\}.$$

Thus, an optimal multiple decision regime may not necessarily select the "best" sequence of treatment options for a given individual over all K decisions. Instead, an optimal regime leads to the "best" sequence of decisions that can be made based on the available information on the individual.

Under the assumptions discussed next, methods for estimation of the value (6.12) of a regime $d \in \mathcal{D}$ based on observed data are reviewed in Section 6.4. A precise characterization of an optimal regime satisfying (6.13) and accounts of several methods for estimation of an optimal regime based on observed data are given in Chapter 7.

6.2.4   Identifiability Assumptions

We assume henceforth that the data on a randomly chosen individual from the population are

$$(X_1, A_1, X_2, A_2, \ldots, X_K, A_K, Y) \tag{6.14}$$

and that the observed data available for inference on a fixed or optimal regime are i.i.d.

$$(X_{1i}, A_{1i}, \ldots, X_{Ki}, A_{Ki}, Y_i), \quad i = 1, \ldots, n, \tag{6.15}$$

from n participants in a longitudinal study; e.g., from an existing observational database, a prospective observational study, or a SMART. As in Section 5.3.2, X_1 is baseline information at Decision 1, taking values in $\mathcal{X}_1$; A_k, $k = 1, \ldots, K$, taking values in $\mathcal{A}_k$, $k = 1, \ldots, K$, respectively, are the treatment options actually received; and X_k, $k = 2, \ldots, K$, taking values in $\mathcal{X}_k$, $k = 2, \ldots, K$, are the collections of intervening information ascertained between Decisions $k-1$ and k. The observed outcome Y can be defined in terms of components of the intervening information X_k, $k = 2, \ldots, K$, and additional information collected after Decision K or is ascertained entirely after Decision K. Section 5.3.2 presents a detailed account of the challenge of time-dependent confounding posed by observational data and the advantages of data derived from a SMART.

Remark. Analogous to the discussion in Remark (i) in Section 6.2.1 in the context of potential outcomes, in some literature accounts, the components of the intervening information that are used to define Y are represented as rewards separately from the information that is not part of the final outcome. That is, letting the rewards R_k, $k = 2, \ldots, K$, and R_{K+1} be the variables arising between Decisions $k - 1$ and k and after Decision K, respectively, used to define Y, and letting X_k be the remaining information, $k = 2, \ldots, K$, as in (6.5), the observed data are represented as

$$\{X_1, A_1, (X_2, R_2), A_2, \ldots, (X_K, R_K), A_K, R_{K+1}, Y\}.$$

As with the potential outcomes (6.5), we subsume the rewards into the intervening information and final outcome and write the observed data as in (6.14).

The objective is to use the observed data (6.15) to make inference on the value of a fixed regime and on an optimal regime, quantities that are defined in terms of the potential outcomes in (6.9). This requires that it be possible to identify the distribution of these potential outcomes from that of the observed data (6.14). As discussed in Section 5.3.3, this identifiability holds under SUTVA, the SRA, and the positivity assumption and will be shown formally in Section 6.3. For completeness, we restate the first two assumptions as given in Section 5.3.3, and then present a precise statement of the positivity assumption for a given specification of feasible sets $\Psi = (\Psi_1, \ldots, \Psi_K)$. This statement arises through a careful description of the subsets of $\mathcal{H}_k = \overline{\mathcal{X}}_k \times \overline{\mathcal{A}}_{k-1}$, $k = 1, \ldots, K$, consisting of possible realizations of histories $h_k = (x_k, a_{k-1})$ that are consistent with having followed a Ψ-specific regime up to Decision k.

SUTVA (Consistency Assumption)

SUTVA states that the observed intervening information between decision points and the final observed outcome are those that potentially would be seen under the treatments actually received and are the same, or consistent, regardless of how the treatments are administered; namely,

$$X_k = X_k^*(\overline{A}_{k-1}) = \sum_{\overline{a}_{k-1} \in \overline{\mathcal{A}}_{k-1}} X_k^*(\overline{a}_{k-1}) \mathrm{I}(\overline{A}_{k-1} = \overline{a}_{k-1}), \quad k = 2, \ldots, K,$$

$$(6.16)$$

$$Y = Y^*(\overline{A}) = \sum_{\overline{a} \in \overline{\mathcal{A}}} Y^*(\overline{a}) \mathrm{I}(\overline{A} = \overline{a}).$$

Sequential Randomization Assumption

The strongest version of the SRA states that

$$W^* \perp\!\!\!\perp A_k | \overline{X}_k, \overline{A}_{k-1}, \quad k = 1, \dots, K, \quad \text{where } A_0 \text{ is null,} \qquad (6.17)$$

written equivalently as

$$W^* \perp\!\!\!\perp A_k | H_k, \quad k = 1, \dots, K.$$

Detailed considerations for the SRA are given in Section 5.3.3; most notable is that this assumption cannot be verified from the observed data, so that it must be adopted based on domain expertise and conviction that the information that was used by clinicians and patients to select the observed treatment options at each decision point is included in the observed $X_1, \dots, X_K$ and is thus available to the data analyst. For a given specification of feasible sets Ψ, it is clear that the SRA will hold by design in a SMART if participants are randomized to all of the options in $\Psi_k(h_k) = \Psi_k(\overline{x}_k, \overline{a}_{k-1})$ at each decision point $k = 1, \dots, K$ with probabilities that can depend on $h_k = (\overline{x}_k, \overline{a}_{k-1})$. This observation follows formally from the discussion of the positivity assumption next.

Positivity Assumption

Whether or not it is possible to deduce the distribution of the potential outcomes (6.9),

$$\{X_1, X_2^*(d_1), X_3^*(\overline{d}_2), \dots, X_K^*(\overline{d}_{K-1}), Y^*(d)\},$$

from the distribution of the observed data (6.14),

$$(X_1, A_1, X_2, A_2, \dots, X_K, A_k, Y),$$

for all $d \in \mathcal{D}$ is predicated on all treatment options in the feasible sets $\Psi_k(h_k) = \Psi_k(\overline{x}_k, \overline{a}_{k-1})$, $k = 1, \dots, K$, being represented in the observed data. By "represented in the data" we mean that, at each decision point k, there are individuals who received each of the options in $\Psi_k(h_k)$ in accordance with their histories h_k. For example, consider the acute leukemia setting with $\Psi_1(h_1) = \mathcal{A}_1 = \{C_1, C_2\}$ for all h_1 and $\Psi_2(h_2) = \{M_1, M_2\}$ for h_2 indicating response and $\Psi_2(h_2) = \{S_1, S_2\}$ for h_2 indicating nonresponse. There must be individuals in the data who received C_1 or C_2 at Decision 1 and responders who received either M_1 or M_2 and nonresponders who received either S_1 or S_2 at Decision 2. If, say, all nonresponding individuals in the data received S_1, this condition would not be satisfied.

This intuitive requirement is reflected in the following formulation,

through which the positivity assumption arises. As noted at the end of
Section 5.3.3, to avoid measure theoretic considerations that can distract from the development, here and subsequently, we treat all random
variables as discrete. Thus, for example, one can view expressions such
as

$$P\{X_k^*(\overline{a}_{k-1}) = x_k \mid \overline{X}_{k-1}^*(\overline{a}_{k-2}) = \overline{x}_{k-1}\}$$

and

$$P(X_k = x_k \mid \overline{X}_{k-1} = \overline{x}_{k-1}, \overline{A}_{k-1} = \overline{a}_{k-1})$$

in (6.21) and (6.22) below as conditional densities when some components of the potential or observed information are not discrete.

At Decision 1, define

$$\Gamma_1 = \{x_1 \in \mathcal{X}_1 \text{ satisfying } P(X_1 = x_1) > 0\},$$

the set of all possible realizations of baseline information $h_1 = x_1$; and

$$\Lambda_1 = \{(x_1, a_1) \text{ such that } x_1 = h_1 \in \Gamma_1, \ a_1 \in \Psi_1(h_1)\},$$

the set of all possible pairs of baseline histories and associated treatment
options in $\Psi_1(h_1) = \Psi_1(x_1)$. As above, all treatment options in Λ_1 must
be represented in the observed data. To ensure this, we thus require that

$$P(A_1 = a_1 | X_1 = x_1) = P(A_1 = a_1 | H_1 = h_1) > 0 \quad \text{for all} \ (h_1, a_1) \in \Lambda_1.$$
$$(6.18)$$

The condition (6.18) is the first component of the positivity assumption.
Now consider Decision 2 and define

$$\Gamma_2 = \Big[(\overline{x}_2, a_1) \in \overline{\mathcal{X}}_2 \times \mathcal{A}_1 \text{ satisfying } (x_1, a_1) \in \Lambda_1 \text{ and}$$

$$P\{X_2^*(a_1) = x_2 \mid X_1 = x_1\} > 0\Big]. \qquad (6.19)$$

The set $\Gamma_2 \subseteq \mathcal{H}_2$ contains all possible histories $h_2 = (\overline{x}_2, a_1)$ that are
consistent with having followed a Ψ-specific regime at Decision 1. Under
SUTVA (6.16) and the SRA (6.17), Γ_2 can be written equivalently in
terms of the observed data as

$$\Gamma_2 = \Big[(\overline{x}_2, a_1) \in \overline{\mathcal{X}}_2 \times \mathcal{A}_1 \text{ satisfying } (x_1, a_1) \in \Lambda_1 \text{ and}$$

$$P(X_2 = x_2 \mid X_1 = x_1, A_1 = a_1) > 0\Big]. \qquad (6.20)$$

This equivalence of (6.19) and (6.20) follows because the first component
of the positivity assumption (6.18) implies that $P(X_1 = x_1, A_1 = a_1) > 0$ for $(x_1, a_1) \in \Lambda_1$, so that the probability in (6.20) is well defined. Then

$$P(X_2 = x_2 \mid X_1 = x_1, A_1 = a_1) = P\{X_2^*(a_1) = x_2 \mid X_1 = x_1, A_1 = a_1\}$$

$$= P\{X_2^*(a_1) = x_2 \mid X_1 = x_1\},$$

as was demonstrated in (5.29) using SUTVA and the SRA.

Now let

$$\Lambda_2 = \{(\overline{x}_2, \overline{a}_2) \text{ such that } (\overline{x}_2, a_1) = h_2 \in \Gamma_2, \ a_2 \in \Psi_2(h_2)\}$$

be the set of all possible histories h_2 and associated treatment options in $\Psi_2(h_2)$. To ensure that all options are represented in the observed data, we require that

$$P(A_2 = a_2 \mid H_2 = h_2) > 0 \quad \text{for all} \ (h_2, a_2) \in \Lambda_2,$$

which is the second component of the positivity assumption.

Continuing in this fashion, at Decision k, define recursively

$$\Gamma_k = \Big[(\overline{x}_k, \overline{a}_{k-1}) \in \overline{\mathcal{X}}_k \times \overline{\mathcal{A}}_{k-1} \text{ satisfying } (\overline{x}_{k-1}, \overline{a}_{k-1}) \in \Lambda_{k-1} \text{ and}$$

$$P\{X_k^*(\overline{a}_{k-1}) = x_k \mid \overline{X}_{k-1}^*(\overline{a}_{k-2}) = \overline{x}_{k-1}\} > 0 \Big], \qquad (6.21)$$

where, as above, $\Gamma_k \subseteq \mathcal{H}_k$ contains all possible histories h_k that are consistent with having followed a Ψ-specific regime through Decision $k - 1$. We demonstrate shortly that Γ_k can be written equivalently as

$$\Gamma_k = \Big[(\overline{x}_k, \overline{a}_{k-1}) \in \overline{\mathcal{X}}_k \times \overline{\mathcal{A}}_{k-1} \text{ satisfying } (\overline{x}_{k-1}, \overline{a}_{k-1}) \in \Lambda_{k-1} \text{ and}$$

$$P(X_k = x_k \mid \overline{X}_{k-1} = \overline{x}_{k-1}, \overline{A}_{k-1} = \overline{a}_{k-1}) > 0 \Big]. \qquad (6.22)$$

Define

$$\Lambda_k = \{(\overline{x}_k, \overline{a}_k) \text{ such that } (\overline{x}_k, \overline{a}_{k-1}) = h_k \in \Gamma_k, \ a_k \in \Psi_k(h_k)\},$$

the set of all possible histories h_k and associated treatment options in $\Psi_k(h_k)$. To ensure that all options in $\Psi_k(h_k)$ are represented in the observed data, we require that

$$P(A_k = a_k \mid H_k = h_k) > 0 \quad \text{for all} \ (h_k, a_k) \in \Lambda_k,$$

the kth component of the positivity assumption.

Through this recursive construction for $k = 1, \ldots, K$, using the definition of Λ_k, the positivity assumption arises as

$$P(A_k = a_k | H_k = h_k) = P(A_k = a_k | \overline{X}_k = \overline{x}_k, \overline{A}_{k-1} = \overline{a}_{k-1}) > 0$$
$$\text{for } h_k = (\overline{x}_k, \overline{a}_{k-1}) \in \Gamma_k, \ \text{and} \ a_k \in \Psi_k(h_k) = \Psi_k(\overline{x}_k, \overline{a}_{k-1}),$$
$$k = 1, \ldots, K. \qquad (6.23)$$

We can now give more precise definitions of a Ψ-specific treatment regime and the class $\mathcal{D}$. A Ψ-specific regime $d = (d_1, \ldots, d_K)$ comprises rules d_k, where, for $k = 1, \ldots, K$, d_k is a mapping from the subset $\Gamma_k \subseteq \mathcal{H}_k$ into $\mathcal{A}_k$ satisfying $d_k(h_k) \in \Psi_k(h_k)$ for every $h_k \in \Gamma_k$. The class $\mathcal{D}$ of Ψ-specific regimes is the set of all such d.

Remark. For the positivity assumption (6.23) to be fulfilled in practice, there must be some individuals in the data who received each option in each $\Psi_k(h_k)$, $k = 1, \ldots, K$. In a SMART, as long as there are subjects with history h_k randomized to all options in $\Psi_k(h_k)$ for each Decision $k = 1, \ldots, K$, the positivity assumption holds by design. Indeed, this is a fundamental design principle for SMARTs. If the data arise from an observational study, there is no guarantee that (6.23) need hold. We discuss further implications for observational studies below.

It remains to show for general $k = 1, \ldots, K$ that Γ_k in (6.21) can be represented equivalently in terms of the observed data as in (6.22). This is of course trivially true for $k = 1$ and is shown above for $k = 2$. Before we present the argument, we state a simple lemma that is used repeatedly in the proof.

Lemma 6.2.1. *Let A and H be random variables, assume that the potential outcomes $W^* \perp\!\!\!\perp A|H$, and consider two functions $\mathfrak{f}_1(W^*)$ and $\mathfrak{f}_2(W^*)$ of W^*. If the event $\{\mathfrak{f}_2(W^*) = f_2, H = h, A = a\}$ has positive probability, then*

$$P\{\mathfrak{f}_1(W^*) = f_1 | \mathfrak{f}_2(W^*) = f_2, H = h, A = a\}$$
$$= P\{\mathfrak{f}_1(W^*) = f_1 | \mathfrak{f}_2(W^*) = f_2, H = h\}. \quad (6.24)$$

Proof. $W^* \perp\!\!\!\perp A|H$ implies that $\{\mathfrak{f}_1(W^*), \mathfrak{f}_2(W^*)\} \perp\!\!\!\perp A|H$. The left-hand side of (6.24) can be written as

$$\frac{P\{\mathfrak{f}_1(W^*) = f_1, \mathfrak{f}_2(W^*) = f_2 | H = h, A = a\}}{P\{\mathfrak{f}_2(W^*) = f_2 | H = h, A = a\}}. \quad (6.25)$$

Because the event $(H = h, A = a)$ has positive probability and by the conditional independence assumption, (6.25) is equal to

$$\frac{P\{\mathfrak{f}_1(W^*) = f_1, \mathfrak{f}_2(W^*) = f_2 | H = h\}}{P\{\mathfrak{f}_2(W^*) = f_2 | H = h\}}$$
$$= P\{\mathfrak{f}_1(W^*) = f_1 | \mathfrak{f}_2(W^*) = f_2, H = h\},$$

completing the proof. $\square$

Equivalence of (6.21) and (6.22)

We wish to show that, for any $h_k = (\overline{x}_k, \overline{a}_{k-1}) \in \Gamma_k$ in (6.21),

$$P(X_k = x_k \mid \overline{X}_{k-1} = \overline{x}_{k-1}, \overline{A}_{k-1} = \overline{a}_{k-1})$$
$$= P\{X_k^*(\overline{a}_{k-1}) = x_k \mid \overline{X}_{k-1}^*(\overline{a}_{k-2}) = \overline{x}_{k-1}\}. \qquad (6.26)$$

Proof. We need to show first that

$$P(\overline{X}_{k-1} = \overline{x}_{k-1}, \overline{A}_{k-1} = \overline{a}_{k-1}) > 0, \qquad (6.27)$$

so that $P(X_k = x_k \mid \overline{X}_{k-1} = \overline{x}_{k-1}, \overline{A}_{k-1} = \overline{a}_{k-1})$ in (6.22) is well defined, and then show the equality (6.26). Because we have already demonstrated these results for $k = 1, 2$, the proof is by induction.

Accordingly, assume that these results hold for $h_{k-1} = (\overline{x}_{k-1}, \overline{a}_{k-2}) \in \Gamma_{k-1}$, so that

$$P(\overline{X}_{k-2} = \overline{x}_{k-2}, \overline{A}_{k-2} = \overline{a}_{k-2}) > 0, \qquad (6.28)$$

and

$$P(X_{k-1} = x_{k-1} \mid \overline{X}_{k-2} = \overline{x}_{k-2}, \overline{A}_{k-2} = \overline{a}_{k-2})$$
$$= P\{X_{k-1}^*(\overline{a}_{k-2}) = x_{k-1} \mid \overline{X}_{k-2}^*(\overline{a}_{k-3}) = \overline{x}_{k-2}\} > 0. \quad (6.29)$$

It follows by taking the product of (6.28) and the left-hand side of (6.29) that

$$P(\overline{X}_{k-1} = \overline{x}_{k-1}, \overline{A}_{k-2} = \overline{a}_{k-2}) > 0. \qquad (6.30)$$

Because $h_{k-1} = (\overline{x}_{k-1}, \overline{a}_{k-2}) \in \Gamma_{k-1}$, by the positivity assumption,

$$P(A_{k-1} = a_{k-1} \mid \overline{X}_{k-1} = \overline{x}_{k-1}, \overline{A}_{k-2} = \overline{a}_{k-2}) > 0, \qquad (6.31)$$

as $a_{k-1} \in \Psi_{k-1}(\overline{x}_{k-1}, \overline{a}_{k-2})$. It follows from the product of (6.30) and (6.31) that (6.27) holds.

We now show (6.26), which is accomplished by repeated application of Lemma 6.2.1. By SUTVA (6.16), the left-hand side of (6.26) is equal to

$$P\{X_k^*(\overline{a}_{k-1}) = x_k \mid \overline{X}_{k-1} = \overline{x}_{k-1}, \overline{A}_{k-2} = \overline{a}_{k-2}, A_{k-1} = a_{k-1}\}$$
$$= P\{X_k^*(\overline{a}_{k-1}) = x_k \mid \overline{X}_{k-1} = \overline{x}_{k-1}, \overline{A}_{k-2} = \overline{a}_{k-2}\} \qquad (6.32)$$
$$= P\{X_k^*(\overline{a}_{k-1}) = x_k \mid \overline{X}_{k-2} = \overline{x}_{k-2}, X_{k-1}^*(\overline{a}_{k-2}) = x_{k-1}, \overline{A}_{k-2} = \overline{a}_{k-2}\} \qquad (6.33)$$

$$= P\{X_k^*(\overline{a}_{k-1}) = x_k \mid \overline{X}_{k-2} = \overline{x}_{k-2}, X_{k-1}^*(\overline{a}_{k-2}) = x_{k-1},$$
$$\overline{A}_{k-3} = \overline{a}_{k-3}, A_{k-2} = a_{k-2}\}, \qquad (6.34)$$

where (6.32) follows by the SRA (6.17), which implies that $X_k^*(\overline{a}_{k-1}) \perp\!\!\!\perp A_{k-1} \mid \overline{X}_{k-1}, \overline{A}_{k-2}$; and (6.33) follows by SUTVA. In Lemma 6.2.1, identify $\mathfrak{f}_1(W^*) = X_k^*(\overline{a}_{k-1})$, $\mathfrak{f}_2(W^*) = X_{k-1}^*(\overline{a}_{k-2})$, $A = A_{k-2}$, and $H = (\overline{X}_{k-2}, \overline{A}_{k-3})$. Then, by Lemma 6.2.1, because $W^* \perp\!\!\!\perp A \mid H$ by the SRA, (6.34) is equal to

$$P\{X_k^*(\overline{a}_{k-1}) = x_k \mid \overline{X}_{k-2} = \overline{x}_{k-2}, X_{k-1}^*(\overline{a}_{k-2}) = x_{k-1}, \overline{A}_{k-3} = \overline{a}_{k-3}\}$$
$$= P\{X_k^*(\overline{a}_{k-1}) = x_k \mid \overline{X}_{k-3} = \overline{x}_{k-3}, X_{k-2}^*(\overline{a}_{k-3}) = x_{k-2},$$
$$X_{k-1}^*(\overline{a}_{k-2}) = x_{k-1}, \overline{A}_{k-4} = \overline{a}_{k-4}, A_{k-3} = a_{k-3}\} \quad (6.35)$$

by SUTVA.

Now use Lemma 6.2.1 again, identifying $\mathfrak{f}_1(W^*) = X_k^*(\overline{a}_{k-1})$, $\mathfrak{f}_2(W^*) = \{X_{k-2}^*(\overline{a}_{k-3}), X_{k-1}^*(\overline{a}_{k-2})\}$, $A = A_{k-3}$, and $H = (\overline{X}_{k-3}, \overline{A}_{k-4})$, to show that (6.35) is equal to

$$P\{X_k^*(\overline{a}_{k-1}) = x_k \mid \overline{X}_{k-3} = \overline{x}_{k-3}, X_{k-2}^*(\overline{a}_{k-3}) = x_{k-2},$$
$$X_{k-1}^*(\overline{a}_{k-2}) = x_{k-1}, \overline{A}_{k-4} = \overline{a}_{k-4}\}.$$

Continuing in this fashion and applying Lemma 6.2.1 repeatedly leads to the left-hand side of (6.26) being equal to

$$P\{X_k^*(\overline{a}_{k-1}) = x_k \mid \overline{X}_{k-1}^*(\overline{a}_{k-2}) = \overline{x}_{k-1}\}. \quad (6.36)$$

Because $h_k = (\overline{x}_k, \overline{a}_{k-1}) \in \Gamma_k$, (6.36) is greater than zero. We have thus demonstrated the equality (6.26) and that

$$P(X_k = x_k \mid \overline{X}_{k-1} = \overline{x}_{k-1}, \overline{A}_{k-1} = \overline{a}_{k-1}) > 0$$

for $h_k = (\overline{x}_k, \overline{a}_{k-1}) \in \Gamma_k$. Because we have already shown (6.26) and (6.27) for $k = 2$, the induction argument is complete. $\qquad \square$

Remark. The representation (6.11) of $X_2^*(d_1), X_3^*(\overline{d}_2), \ldots, X_K^*(\overline{d}_{K-1})$, and $Y^*(d)$ in terms of W^* involves products of the form

$$\prod_{j=1}^k \mathrm{I}\left[d_j\{\overline{X}_j^*(\overline{a}_{j-1}), \overline{a}_{j-1}\} = a_j\right], \quad k = 2, \ldots, K.$$

Recall that for a Ψ-specific regime d, the jth rule d_j maps from Γ_j to $\mathcal{A}_j$. It is possible that there are realizations $(\overline{x}_j, \overline{a}_{j-1})$ for which

$$P\{\overline{X}_j^*(\overline{a}_{j-1}) = \overline{x}_j\} > 0$$

but $(\overline{x}_j, \overline{a}_{j-1}) \notin \Gamma_j$. We adopt the convention that, for such realizations,

$$\mathrm{I}\{d_j(\overline{x}_j, \overline{a}_{j-1}) = a_j\} = 0$$

for any a_j. Thus, such realizations make no contribution to the summations over $\overline{a}_k \in \overline{\mathcal{A}}_k$, $k = 2, \ldots, K$, in (6.11).

We close this section by returning to specification of the feasible sets $\Psi_k(h_k)$, $k = 1, \ldots, K$. As noted in Section 6.2.2, ideally, the Ψ_k are specified based on scientific considerations and thus without reference to data. Clearly, a prospectively designed study, such as a SMART, which ensures that all options in each predetermined $\Psi_k(h_k)$ at each decision point $k = 1, \ldots, K$ are represented in the resulting data, would form the ideal basis for estimation of the value of a fixed regime $d \in \mathcal{D}$ or of an optimal regime in $\mathcal{D}$.

In practice, however, interest in formulation and evaluation of regimes may be predicated on an existing observational database. Here, with retrospectively collected data, for a given specification of feasible sets Ψ, it cannot be guaranteed that all options in each $\Psi_k(h_k)$, $k = 1, \ldots, K$, are represented in the data. Viewing such data as n i.i.d. copies of $(X_1, A_1, \ldots, X_K, A_K, Y)$, define

$$\Gamma_1^{max} = \{x_1 \in \mathcal{X}_1 \text{ satisfying } P(X_1 = x_1) > 0\},$$
$$\Psi_1^{max}(x_1) = \{a_1 \in \mathcal{A}_1 \text{ satisfying } P(A_1 = a_1 | H_1 = h_1) > 0$$
$$\text{for all } h_1 = x_1 \in \Gamma_1^{max}\},$$
$$\Lambda_1^{max} = \{(x_1, a_1) \text{ such that } x_1 = h_1 \in \Gamma_1^{max}, \ a_1 \in \Psi_1^{max}(h_1)\};$$

and, for $k = 2, \ldots, K$,

$$\Gamma_k^{max} = \Big[(\overline{x}_k, \overline{a}_{k-1}) \in \overline{\mathcal{X}}_k \times \overline{\mathcal{A}}_{k-1} \text{ satisfying } (\overline{x}_{k-1}, \overline{a}_{k-1}) \in \Lambda_{k-1}^{max}$$
$$\text{and } P(X_k = x_k \mid \overline{X}_{k-1} = \overline{x}_{k-1}, \overline{A}_{k-1} = \overline{a}_{k-1}) > 0 \Big],$$
$$\Psi_k^{max}(h_k) = \{a_k \in \mathcal{A}_k \text{ satisfying } P(A_k = a_k | H_k = h_k) > 0$$
$$\text{for all } h_k = (\overline{x}_k, \overline{a}_{k-1}) \in \Gamma_k^{max}\},$$
$$\Lambda_k^{max} = \{(\overline{x}_k, \overline{a}_k) \text{ such that } (\overline{x}_k, \overline{a}_{k-1}) = h_k \in \Gamma_k^{max}, \ a_k \in \Psi_k^{max}(h_k)\}.$$

Intuitively, the class of regimes dictated by $\Psi^{max} = (\Psi_1^{max}, \ldots, \Psi_K^{max})$ is the largest class of treatment regimes that can be considered based on these available data. Robins (2004) has referred to this largest class as the class of "feasible regimes." If interest focuses on evaluation of Ψ-specific regimes for a particular choice $\Psi = (\Psi_1, \ldots, \Psi_K)$ based on these observed data, it may not be possible to estimate the value of a given Ψ-specific regime or to estimate an optimal regime in the associated class $\mathcal{D}$. This will be possible if

$$\Psi_k(\overline{x}_k, \overline{a}_{k-1}) \subseteq \Psi_k^{max}(\overline{x}_k, \overline{a}_{k-1}), \ \ k = 1, \ldots, K,$$

for all $(\overline{x}_k, \overline{a}_{k-1}) \in \Gamma_k \subseteq \Gamma_k^{max}$.

6.3 The g-Computation Algorithm

As discussed in Section 5.4, the g-computation algorithm shows that, under SUTVA, the SRA, and the positivity assumption, it is possible to identify the distribution of the potential outcomes associated with a fixed treatment regime from that of the observed data. We now return to this fundamental result and provide a proof that, for a particular specification of feasible sets $\Psi = (\Psi_1, \ldots, \Psi_K)$ and a Ψ-specific regime $d \in \mathcal{D}$, the distribution of the potential outcomes (6.9),

$$\{X_1, X_2^*(d_1), X_3^*(\overline{d}_2), \ldots, X_K^*(\overline{d}_{K-1}), Y^*(d)\},$$

can be represented in terms of that of the observed data (6.14),

$$(X_1, A_1, X_2, A_2, \ldots, X_K, A_k, Y).$$

As in the last section, we treat all random variables as discrete.

We first revisit the basic form of the g-computation algorithm for a treatment sequence $\overline{a}$ given in (5.24). In Section 5.4, we stated that, under SUTVA, the SRA, and the positivity assumption, the joint density of the potential outcomes corresponding to $\overline{a}$,

$$\{X_1, X_2^*(a_1), X_3^*(\overline{a}_2), \ldots, X_K^*(\overline{a}_{K-1}), Y^*(\overline{a})\},$$

can be expressed in terms of that of the observed data. In Chapter 5, we downplayed the concept of feasible sets of treatment options. Although all of $X_2^*(a_1), X_3^*(\overline{a}_2), \ldots, X_K^*(\overline{a}_{K-1}), Y^*(\overline{a})$ are well-defined for any $\overline{a}$, for specified feasible sets $\Psi = (\Psi_1, \ldots, \Psi_K)$, unless $\Psi_k(h_k) = \mathcal{A}_k$ for all h_k, $k = 1, \ldots, K$, there may be certain sequences $\overline{a}$ that can never occur under any Ψ-specific regime. Thus, this identifiability result, although of theoretical interest, is of less practical relevance than the g-computation algorithm corresponding to a fixed Ψ-specific regime $d \in \mathcal{D}$.

Accordingly, for a Ψ-specific regime $d \in \mathcal{D}$, we focus attention on demonstrating a result analogous to that in (5.40) and (5.41) when SUTVA (6.16), the SRA (6.17), and the positivity assumption (6.23) hold. In particular, recall the recursive representation $\overline{d}_k(\overline{x}_k)$ of the treatment options selected by d through Decision k for $k = 2, \ldots, K$ given in (5.6) introduced at the end of Section 5.2. This formulation makes explicit that the options selected at each decision point depend only on the realizations of baseline and evolving intervening information $x_1, \ldots, x_K$. Under these conditions, the g-computation algorithm states that the joint density of the potential outcomes $\{X_1, X_2^*(d_1), X_3^*(\overline{d}_2), \ldots, X_K^*(\overline{d}_{K-1}), Y^*(d)\}$ can be obtained as

$$p_{X_1, X_2^*(d_1), X_3^*(\overline{d}_2), \ldots, X_K^*(\overline{d}_{K-1}), Y^*(d)}(x_1, \ldots, x_K, y) \qquad (6.37)$$
$$= p_{Y|\overline{X}, \overline{A}}\{y | \overline{x}, \overline{d}(\overline{x})\}$$

$$\times p_{X_K | \overline{X}_{K-1}, \overline{A}_{K-1}} \{ x_K | \overline{x}_{K-1}, \overline{d}_{K-1}(\overline{x}_{K-1}) \}$$

$$\vdots \tag{6.38}$$

$$\times p_{X_2 | X_1, A_1} \{ x_2 | x_1, d_1(x_1) \}$$
$$\times p_{X_1}(x_1),$$

for any realization $(x_1, x_2, \ldots, x_K, y)$ for which (6.37) is positive. That is, for such realizations, the joint density of the potential outcomes (6.37) can be expressed in terms of that of the observed data as in (6.38).

In the argument presented next demonstrating this result, the realizations $(x_1, x_2, \ldots, x_K, y)$ for which this equivalence is satisfied are determined by the nature of the feasible sets. To this end, assuming that the potential outcome $Y^*(\overline{a})$ and observed outcome Y take values $y \in \mathcal{Y}$, and, analogous to the definition of (6.21), let

$$\Gamma_{K+1} = \Big[(\overline{x}, \overline{a}, y) \in \overline{\mathcal{X}} \times \overline{\mathcal{A}} \times \mathcal{Y} \text{ satisfying } (\overline{x}, \overline{a}) \in \Lambda_K \text{ and}$$

$$P\{ Y^*(\overline{a}) = y \mid \overline{X}_K^*(\overline{a}_{K-1}) = \overline{x}_K \} > 0 \Big]. \tag{6.39}$$

By regarding $Y^*(\overline{a})$ as $\overline{X}_{K+1}^*(\overline{a})$ and Y as X_{K+1}, it should be clear that, by an extension of the induction argument in the previous section to $k = 1, \ldots, K+1$, Γ_{K+1} in (6.39) can be expressed equivalently as

$$\Gamma_{K+1} = \Big[(\overline{x}, \overline{a}, y) \in \overline{\mathcal{X}} \times \overline{\mathcal{A}} \times \mathcal{Y} \text{ satisfying } (\overline{x}, \overline{a}) \in \Lambda_K \text{ and}$$

$$P(Y = y \mid \overline{X} = \overline{x}, \overline{A}_K = \overline{a}_K) > 0 \Big].$$

We now present the proof of the equivalence of (6.37) and (6.38) under SUTVA, the SRA, and the positivity assumption.

g-Computation Algorithm for Fixed $d \in \mathcal{D}$

Taking all random variables to be discrete as above for simplicity, (6.37) and (6.38) become

$$P\{ X_1 = x_1, X_2^*(d_1) = x_2, \ldots, X_K^*(\overline{d}_{K-1}) = x_K, Y^*(d) = y \} \tag{6.40}$$
$$= P\{ Y = y \mid \overline{X}_K = \overline{x}_K, \overline{A}_K = \overline{d}_K(\overline{x}_{K-1}) \}$$
$$\times P(X_K = x_K \mid \overline{X}_{K-1} = \overline{x}_{K-1}, \overline{A}_{K-1} = \overline{d}_{K-1}(\overline{x}_{K-2}) \}$$

$$\vdots \tag{6.41}$$

$$\times P\{ X_2 = x_2 \mid X_1 = x_1, A_1 = d_1(x_1) \}$$
$$\times P(X_1 = x_1),$$

for any realization $(x_1, x_2, \ldots, x_K, y)$ such that

$$P\{X_1 = x_1, X_2^*(d_1) = x_2, \ldots, X_K^*(\overline{d}_{K-1}) = x_K, Y^*(d) = y\} > 0.$$

We thus want to demonstrate that (6.40) can be written as the product (6.41).

Proof. The proof is almost immediate because it follows directly from the demonstration of the equivalence of (6.21) and (6.22).

Now (6.40) can be factorized as

$$\begin{aligned}
P\{X_1 &= x_1, X_2^*(d_1) = x_2, \ldots, X_K^*(\overline{d}_{K-1}) = x_K, Y^*(d) = y\} \\
&= P\{Y^*(d) = y \mid \overline{X}_K^*(\overline{d}_{K-1}) = \overline{x}_K\} \\
&\quad \times P\{X_K^*(\overline{d}_{K-1}) = x_K \mid \overline{X}_{K-1}^*(\overline{d}_{K-2}) = \overline{x}_{K-1}\} \\
&\qquad \vdots \\
&\quad \times P\{X_2^*(d_1) = x_2 \mid X_1 = x_1\} \\
&\quad \times P(X_1 = x_1),
\end{aligned} \tag{6.42}$$

and, because (6.40) is positive, all components of the product in (6.42) are positive. Thus, comparing (6.41) to (6.42), it suffices to show that

$$\begin{aligned}
P\{Y^*(d) = y \mid \overline{X}_K^*(\overline{d}_{K-1}) = \overline{x}_K\} \\
= P\{Y = y \mid \overline{X}_K = \overline{x}_K, \overline{A}_K = \overline{d}_K(\overline{x}_{K-1})\},
\end{aligned} \tag{6.43}$$

where

$$P\{Y = y \mid \overline{X}_K = \overline{x}_K, \overline{A}_K = \overline{d}_K(\overline{x}_{K-1})\} > 0;$$

and, for $k = 2, \ldots, K$,

$$\begin{aligned}
P\{X_k^*(\overline{d}_{k-1}) = x_k \mid \overline{X}_{k-1}^*(\overline{d}_{k-2}) = \overline{x}_{k-1}\} \\
= P(X_k = x_k \mid \overline{X}_{k-1} = \overline{x}_{k-1}, \overline{A}_{k-1} = \overline{d}_{k-1}(\overline{x}_{k-2})\},
\end{aligned} \tag{6.44}$$

where

$$P(X_k = x_k \mid \overline{X}_{k-1} = \overline{x}_{k-1}, \overline{A}_{k-1} = \overline{d}_{k-1}(\overline{x}_{k-2})\} > 0.$$

Note that these results follow immediately if we can show that

$$\{\overline{x}_k, \overline{d}_{k-1}(\overline{x}_{k-1})\} \in \Gamma_k, \quad k = 2, \ldots, K+1, \tag{6.45}$$

where, as above, we regard $Y^*(d)$ as $\overline{X}_{K+1}^*(d)$. In particular, if (6.45) is true, then by the equivalence of the representations (6.21) and (6.22) of Γ_k for $k = 1, \ldots, K+1$, (6.43) and (6.44) must hold.

The proof is by induction. Consider $k = 2$. Because $P(X_1 = x_1) > 0$,

$x_1 \in \Gamma_1$, and because d is a Ψ-specific regime, $d_1(x_1) \in \Psi_1(h_1)$, so that $\{x_1, d_1(x_1)\} \in \Lambda_1$. From above, because (6.40) is positive,

$$P\{X_2^*(d_1) = x_2 \mid X_1 = x_1\} > 0;$$

thus, it follows that $\{\overline{x}_2, d_1(x_1)\} \in \Gamma_2$.

Now suppose that we have already shown that

$$\{\overline{x}_{k-1}, \overline{d}_{k-2}(\overline{x}_{k-2})\} \in \Gamma_{k-1}.$$

We now argue that this implies (6.45). Because d is a Ψ-specific regime, $d_{k-1}(\overline{x}_{k-1}) \in \Psi_{k-1}(h_k)$, and thus

$$\{\overline{x}_{k-1}, \overline{d}_{k-1}(\overline{x}_{k-1})\} \in \Lambda_{k-1}.$$

Moreover, because (6.40) is positive,

$$P\{X_k^*(\overline{d}_{k-1}) = x_k \mid \overline{X}_{k-1}^*(\overline{d}_{k-2}) = \overline{x}_{k-1}\} > 0.$$

Combining these results, it follows that

$$\{\overline{x}_k, \overline{d}_{k-1}(\overline{x}_{k-1})\} \in \Gamma_k,$$

which is (6.45). The induction proof is complete because we have already shown (6.45) for $k = 2$. $\qquad\square$

As in Section 5.4, the general result (6.38), which can be expressed compactly as in (5.41) as

$$
\begin{aligned}
p_{X_1, X_2^*(d_1), X_3^*(\overline{d}_2), \ldots, X_K^*(\overline{d}_{K-1}), Y^*(d)} & (x_1, \ldots, x_K, y) \\
= p_{Y|\overline{X}, \overline{A}} & \{y|\overline{x}, \overline{d}_K(\overline{x})\} \qquad (6.46) \\
\times \left[\prod_{k=2}^{K} p_{X_k|\overline{X}_{k-1}, \overline{A}_{k-1}} \right. & \left. \{x_k|\overline{x}_{k-1}, \overline{d}_{k-1}(\overline{x}_{k-1})\} \right] p_{X_1}(x_1),
\end{aligned}
$$

leads to the expression for the marginal density of $Y^*(d)$,

$$
\begin{aligned}
p_{Y^*(d)}(y) = \int_{\overline{X}} \Bigg(& \; p_{Y|\overline{X}, \overline{A}}\{y|\overline{x}, \overline{d}(\overline{x})\} \qquad (6.47) \\
\times \left[\prod_{k=2}^{K} p_{X_k|\overline{X}_{k-1}, \overline{A}_{k-1}} \right. & \left. \{x_k|\overline{x}_{k-1}, \overline{d}_{k-1}(\overline{x}_{k-1})\} \right] p_{X_1}(x_1) \Bigg) \\
\times d\nu_K(x_K) & \cdots d\nu_1(x_1),
\end{aligned}
$$

given in (5.42), where $d\nu_K(x_K) \cdots d\nu_1(x_1)$ is the dominating measure; and to the expression for the value of d,

$$E\{Y^*(d)\} = \int_{\overline{\mathcal{X}}} \left(\quad E\{Y|\overline{X} = \overline{x}, \overline{A} = \overline{d}(\overline{x})\} \right. \tag{6.48}$$

$$\left. \times \left[\prod_{k=2}^{K} p_{X_k|\overline{X}_{k-1},\overline{A}_{k-1}}\{x_k|\overline{x}_{k-1}, \overline{d}_{k-1}(\overline{x}_{k-1})\} \right] p_{X_1}(x_1) \right)$$

$$\times d\nu_K(x_K) \cdots d\nu_1(x_1),$$

given in (5.43) and the analogous expression (5.44) when all random variables are discrete.

6.4 Estimation of the Value a Fixed Regime

The g-computation algorithm for a fixed Ψ-specific regime $d \in \mathcal{D}$ implies that, under SUTVA (6.16), the SRA (6.17), and the positivity assumption (6.23), it is possible to estimate the value $\mathcal{V}(d) = E\{Y^*(d)\}$ based on the observed data (6.15),

$$(X_{1i}, A_{1i}, \ldots, X_{Ki}, A_{Ki}, Y_i), \quad i = 1, \ldots, n.$$

We now discuss several approaches to this task. Two of these, using the g-formula directly and using inverse probability weighting, are presented in Section 5.5. Here, we briefly review these two approaches and consider three additional methods.

Throughout the rest of this chapter, we take SUTVA (6.16), the SRA (6.17), and the positivity assumption (6.23) to hold.

6.4.1 Estimation via g-Computation

The expressions for the marginal density and expectation of $Y^*(d)$ in terms of the observed data given in (6.47) and (6.48) at the end of the previous section can, in principle, form the basis for estimation of the value of a fixed Ψ-specific regime $d \in \mathcal{D}$. As discussed in Section 5.5.1, for example, the analyst can posit, fit based on the observed data, and substitute in either expression parametric models for each component. This approach and the practical challenges it presents are covered in detail in Section 5.5.1.

6.4.2 Regression-based Estimation

In the single decision case, as demonstrated in Section 3.3.1, under simpler versions of SUTVA, the SRA, and the positivity assumption, estimation of the value of a fixed regime can be based on a model for the regression of outcome on baseline history and treatment received. We now discuss how regression modeling can be used to estimate $\mathcal{V}(d)$ for a fixed, multiple decision Ψ-specific regime $d \in \mathcal{D}$. We consider two approaches.

Backward Induction Approach

The first approach uses the principle of backward induction, which underlies characterization of an optimal multiple decision regime, as discussed in Section 5.6 and Chapter 7. Specifically, this approach is based on the following recursive formulation.

For $(h_K, a_K) = (\overline{x}_K, \overline{a}_K) \in \Lambda_K$, so that $h_K \in \Gamma_K$ and $a_K \in \Psi_K(h_K)$, define

$$Q_K^d(h_K, a_K) = E(Y | H_K = h_K, A_K = a_K), \qquad (6.49)$$

and let

$$V_K^d(h_K) = Q_K^d\{h_K, d_K(h_K)\}, \qquad (6.50)$$

which is (6.49) evaluated at $a_K = d_K(h_K)$. Here, because d is a Ψ-specific regime, $d_K(h_K) \in \Psi_K(h_K)$. Then for each $k = K - 1, K - 2, \ldots, 1$, for $(h_k, a_k) = (\overline{x}_k, \overline{a}_k) \in \Lambda_k$, so that $h_k \in \Gamma_k$ and $a_k \in \Psi_k(h_k)$, define

$$Q_k^d(h_k, a_k) = E\{V_{k+1}^d(H_{k+1}) \mid H_k = h_k, A_k = a_k\} \qquad (6.51)$$

and

$$V_k^d(h_k) = Q_k^d\{h_k, d_k(h_k)\}, \qquad (6.52)$$

where, as above, $d_k(h_k) \in \Psi_k(h_k)$.

Remark. With the exception of $Q_K^d(h_K, a_K)$ in (6.49), which is the same as $Q_K(h_K, a_K)$ defined in (5.45), the quantities $Q_k^d(h_k, a_k)$ are different from the Q-functions $Q_k(h_k, a_k)$, $k = 1, \ldots, K - 1$, as defined in Section 5.6; and similarly for $V_k^d(h_k)$, $k = 1, \ldots, K$, and the value functions $V_k(h_k)$. The superscript d here emphasizes dependence on the fixed regime d rather than maximization over options to obtain d^{opt}.

Representation of the Value

We now demonstrate that, with these definitions, the value of $d \in \mathcal{D}$ satisfies

$$\mathcal{V}(d) = E\{Y^*(d)\} = E\{V_1^d(H_1)\}. \qquad (6.53)$$

The result (6.53) and the equality (6.54) below that is central to its proof motivate the estimation method discussed following this argument.

Proof. To show (6.53), we prove that, for $k = 1, \ldots, K$,

$$V_k^d(h_k) = E\{Y^*(\overline{a}_{k-1}, d_k, \ldots, d_K) \mid H_k = h_k\} \quad \text{for } h_k \in \Gamma_k. \quad (6.54)$$

By definition, for all $h_k = (\overline{x}_k, \overline{a}_{k-1}) \in \Gamma_k$, the left-hand side of (6.54) is well defined. We first argue that the right-hand side is also well defined. Here, as introduced in Section 5.7.3, $Y^*(\overline{a}_{k-1}, d_k, \ldots, d_K)$ is the potential outcome if an individual were to receive options $a_1, \ldots, a_{k-1}$ at Decisions 1 to $k - 1$ and then be treated according to the rules $d_k(h_k), d_{k+1}(h_{k+1}), \ldots, d_K(h_K)$ at the remaining decision points. Because the right-hand side of (6.54) involves conditioning on $H_k = h_k \in \Gamma_k$, $a_1 \in \Psi_1(h_1), \ldots, a_{k-1} \in \Psi_{k-1}(h_{k-1})$. We show below that $Y^*(\overline{a}_{k-1}, d_k, \ldots, d_K)$ can be represented in terms of W^* as in (6.11). If (6.54) is true, then, taking $k = 1$,

$$V_1^d(h_1) = E\{Y^*(\overline{d}_K) \mid H_1 = h_1\} = E\{Y^*(d) \mid H_1 = h_1\},$$

from which it follows immediately that (6.53) holds, as required.

The proof of (6.54) is by induction. We first show that (6.54) holds for $k = K$. Here, from (6.49) and (6.50), for $h_K \in (\overline{x}_K, \overline{a}_{K-1}) \in \Gamma_K$,

$$\begin{aligned} V_K^d(h_K) &= E\{Y \mid H_K = h_K, A_K = d_K(h_K)\} \\ &= E\{Y^*(\overline{a}_{K-1}, d_K) \mid H_K = h_K, A_K = d_K(h_K)\} \quad (6.55) \\ &= E\{Y^*(\overline{a}_{K-1}, d_K) \mid H_K = h_K\}, \quad (6.56) \end{aligned}$$

where (6.55) follows by SUTVA and (6.56) follows by the SRA, which is (6.54) for $k = K$.

The induction proof is completed by showing, for given $k = K - 1, \ldots, 1$, if

$$V_{k+1}^d(h_{k+1}) = E\{Y^*(\overline{a}_k, d_{k+1}, \ldots, d_K) \mid H_{k+1} = h_{k+1}\} \text{ for } h_{k+1} \in \Gamma_{k+1}, \quad (6.57)$$

then

$$V_k^d(h_k) = E\{Y^*(\overline{a}_{k-1}, d_k, \ldots, d_K) \mid H_k = h_k\} \quad \text{for } h_k \in \Gamma_k,$$

so that, because (6.54) holds for $k = K$, it holds by induction for all $k = K, \ldots, 1$.

By definition from (6.52) and the fact that (6.57) holds, recalling that $H_{k+1} = (\overline{X}_{k+1}, \overline{A}_k)$,

$$\begin{aligned} V_k^d(h_k) &= E\{V_{k+1}^d(H_{k+1}) \mid H_k = h_k, A_k = d_k(h_k)\} \\ &= E\left[E\{Y^*(\overline{A}_k, d_{k+1}, \ldots, d_K) \mid H_{k+1}\} \Big| H_k = h_k, A_k = d_k(h_k) \right] \\ &= E\{Y^*(\overline{A}_k, d_{k+1}, \ldots, d_K) \mid H_k = h_k, A_k = d_k(h_k)\} \quad (6.58) \end{aligned}$$

$$= E\{Y^*(\overline{a}_{k-1}, d_k, \ldots, d_K) \mid H_k = h_k, A_k = d_k(h_k)\} \qquad (6.59)$$
$$= E\{Y^*(\overline{a}_{k-1}, d_k, \ldots, d_K) \mid H_k = h_k\},$$

the desired result. Here, (6.58) follows by standard properties of conditional expectation, and the equality in (6.59) is intuitive because $\overline{A}_k = (\overline{A}_{k-1}, A_k)$ and $H_k = (\overline{X}_k, \overline{A}_{k-1}) = (\overline{x}_k, \overline{a}_{k-1})$. The final equality then follows by the SRA. We have thus demonstrated (6.54). □

Equality of (6.58) and (6.59)

The equality of (6.58) and (6.59) central to this result, namely,

$$E\{Y^*(\overline{A}_k, d_{k+1}, \ldots, d_K) \mid H_k = h_k, A_k = d_k(h_k)\}$$
$$= E\{Y^*(\overline{a}_{k-1}, d_k, \ldots, d_K) \mid H_k = h_k, A_k = d_k(h_k)\},$$

is seemingly obvious. However, it is instructive to prove formally that it holds. The argument is based on representation of the potential outcomes in these expressions in terms of W^*. The following proof is rather involved and can be skipped without loss of continuity by readers uninterested in this level of technical detail.

Proof. For brevity, define for $k = 1, \ldots, K$,

$$\underline{a}_k = (a_k, \ldots, a_K),$$

and $\underline{A}_k$ similarly. Note that, when $H_k = h_k = (\overline{x}_k, \overline{a}_{k-1})$, $A_k = d_k(h_k)$,

$$Y^*(\overline{A}_k, d_{k+1}, \ldots, d_K) = \sum_{\underline{a}_{k+1} \in \underline{A}_{k+1}} \left\{ Y^*\{\overline{a}_{k-1}, d_k(h_k), \underline{a}_{k+1}\} \right.$$
$$\times \mathrm{I}\left(d_{k+1}\left[\overline{x}_k, X_{k+1}^*\{\overline{a}_{k-1}, d_k(h_k)\}, \overline{a}_{k-1}, d_k(h_k)\right] = a_{k+1}\right) \qquad (6.60)$$
$$\times \prod_{j=k+2}^{K} \mathrm{I}\left(d_j\left[\mathcal{U}_{j,k}\{d_k(h_k)\}, \overline{a}_{k-1}, d_k(h_k), a_{k+1}, \ldots, a_{j-1}\right] = a_j\right) \left. \right\},$$

where, for $j > k+1$ and $u \in A_k$,

$$\mathcal{U}_{j,k}(u) = \{\overline{x}_k, X_{k+1}^*(\overline{a}_{k-1}, u), \ldots, X_j^*(\overline{a}_{k-1}, u, a_{k+1}, \ldots, a_{j-1})\}.$$

In (6.60), we have used the fact that, as discussed in Section 5.2, after the kth decision point, the treatment options dictated by d are recursively defined in terms of $\overline{x}_k$ and $\overline{a}_k$. Thus, in obvious shorthand notation, we can write (6.58) as

$$E\{(6.60)|H_k = h_k, A_k = d_k(h_k)\}.$$

Now consider (6.59). It is straightforward that

$$Y^*(\overline{a}_{k-1}, d_k, \ldots, d_K) \tag{6.61}$$

$$= \sum_{\underline{a}_k \in \underline{\mathcal{A}}_k} \left\{ Y^*(\overline{a}_{k-1}, \underline{a}_k) \prod_{j=k}^{K} \mathrm{I}\left[d_j\{\overline{X}_j^*(\overline{a}_{j-1}), \overline{a}_{j-1}\} = a_j \right] \right\}.$$

Under SUTVA, when $H_k = h_k$, $A_k = d_k(h_k)$, $\overline{X}_{k-1}^*(\overline{a}_{k-2}) = \overline{x}_{k-1}$ and $X_k^*(\overline{a}_{k-1}) = x_k$. Consequently, (6.61) can be written as

$$Y^*(\overline{a}_{k-1}, d_k, \ldots, d_K) = \sum_{\underline{a}_k \in \underline{\mathcal{A}}_k} \left(Y^*(\overline{a}_{k-1}, a_k, \underline{a}_{k+1}) \, \mathrm{I}\{d_k(\overline{x}_k, \overline{a}_{k-1}) = a_k\} \right.$$

$$\left. \times \mathrm{I}\{d_{k+1}(\overline{x}_{k+1}, \overline{a}_k) = a_{k+1}\} \prod_{j=k+2}^{K} \mathrm{I}\left[d_j\{\mathcal{U}_{j,k}(a_k), \overline{a}_{j-1}\} = a_j \right] \right),$$

which, using $h_k = (\overline{x}_k, \overline{a}_{k-1})$, can be reexpressed as

$$Y^*(\overline{a}_{k-1}, d_k, \ldots, d_K)$$

$$= \sum_{\underline{a}_{k+1} \in \underline{\mathcal{A}}_{k+1}} \left\{ Y^*\{\overline{a}_{k-1}, d_k(h_k), \underline{a}_{k+1}\} \right.$$

$$\times \mathrm{I}\left(d_{k+1}\left[\overline{x}_k, X_{k+1}^*\{\overline{a}_{k-1}, d_k(h_k)\}, \overline{a}_{k-1}, d_k(h_k) \right] = a_{k+1} \right) \tag{6.62}$$

$$\left. \times \prod_{j=k+2}^{K} \mathrm{I}\left(d_j\left[\mathcal{U}_{j,k}\{d_k(h_k)\}, \overline{a}_{k-1}, d_k(h_k), a_{k+1}, \ldots, a_{j-1} \right] = a_j \right) \right\}.$$

Thus, (6.59) is given by

$$E\{(6.62)|H_k = h_k, A_k = d_k(h_k)\}.$$

Comparison of (6.60) to (6.62) shows that they are identical, thus demonstrating that (6.58) and (6.59) are the same. □

The foregoing developments suggest a strategy for estimation of the value of $d \in \mathcal{D}$ using the observed data (6.15) based on positing models for $Q_k^d(h_k, a_k) = Q_k^d(\overline{x}_k, \overline{a}_k)$, $k = 1, \ldots, K$. The approach is similar in spirit to the method of Q-learning used to estimate an optimal multiple decision regime discussed in Section 5.7.1. Start at Decision K, and, from (6.49), posit a model

$$Q_K^d(h_K, a_K; \beta_K), \tag{6.63}$$

say, for $Q_K^d(h_K, a_K) = E(Y|H_K = h_K, A_K = a_K)$ in terms of a parameter β_K. As this is a conventional regression model involving an observed outcome, standard techniques can be used to develop this model. Estimate β_K by $\widehat{\beta}_K$ solving a suitable M-estimating equation as in Section 2.5; e.g., the OLS estimating equation

$$\sum_{i=1}^{n} \frac{\partial Q_K^d(H_{Ki}, A_{Ki}; \beta_K)}{\partial \beta_K} \{Y_i - Q_K^d(H_{Ki}, A_{Ki}; \beta_K)\} = 0 \qquad (6.64)$$

or a WLS estimating equation incorporating a working model for $\text{var}(Y|H_K = h_K, A_K = a_K)$. Form pseudo outcomes

$$\widetilde{V}_{Ki}^d = Q_K^d\{H_{Ki}, d_K(H_{Ki}); \widehat{\beta}_K\}, \quad i = 1, \ldots, n,$$

which are the predicted outcomes based on the fitted model if each individual were to have received treatment according to rule d_K at Decision K based on his history to that point.

Now consider Decision $K-1$, and, from (6.51) with $k = K-1$, posit a parametric model

$$Q_{K-1}^d(h_{K-1}, a_{K-1}; \beta_{K-1}) \qquad (6.65)$$

for

$$E\{V_K^d(H_K) \mid H_{K-1} = h_{K-1}, A_{K-1} = a_{K-1}\}.$$

This suggests obtaining the estimator $\widehat{\beta}_{K-1}$ for β_{K-1} by solving a suitable M-estimating equation; e.g., the OLS estimating equation

$$\sum_{i=1}^{n} \frac{\partial Q_{K-1}^d(H_{K-1,i}, A_{K-1,i}; \beta_{K-1})}{\partial \beta_{K-1}} \qquad (6.66)$$

$$\times \{\widetilde{V}_{Ki}^d - Q_{K-1}^d(H_{K-1,i}, A_{K-1,i}; \beta_{K-1})\} = 0$$

or a WLS estimating equation. This is a nonstandard modeling and estimation problem; see below. Obtain the pseudo outcomes

$$\widetilde{V}_{K-1,i}^d = Q_{K-1}^d\{H_{K-1,i}, d_{K-1}(H_{K-1,i}); \widehat{\beta}_{K-1}\}, \quad i = 1, \ldots, n.$$

Continuing in this fashion, for each $k = K-2, \ldots, 1$, based on (6.51), posit a model

$$Q_k^d(h_k, a_k; \beta_k) \qquad (6.67)$$

for

$$E\{V_{k+1}^d(H_{k+1}) \mid H_k = h_k, A_k = a_k\},$$

obtain the estimator $\widehat{\beta}_k$ for β_k by solving an M-estimating equation such as the OLS equation

$$\sum_{i=1}^{n} \frac{\partial Q_k^d(H_{ki}, A_{ki}; \beta_k)}{\partial \beta_k} \{\widetilde{V}_{k+1,i}^d - Q_k^d(H_{ki}, A_{ki}; \beta_k)\} = 0 \qquad (6.68)$$

or WLS including a working variance model. Again, this is not a conventional modeling and estimation problem and is discussed further momentarily. Construct pseudo outcomes

$$\widetilde{V}_{ki}^d = Q_k^d\{H_{ki}, d_k(H_{ki}); \widehat{\beta}_k\}, \quad i = 1, \ldots, n.$$

Finally, based on (6.53), the estimator for the value $\mathcal{V}(d)$ is

$$\widehat{\mathcal{V}}_Q(d) = n^{-1} \sum_{i=1}^n \widetilde{V}_{1i}^d. \tag{6.69}$$

It is straightforward to observe that, as long as the model $Q_K^d(h_K, a_K; \beta_K)$ is correctly specified, so that there exists $\beta_{K,0}$ such that $Q_K^d(h_K, a_K; \beta_{K,0}) = E(Y|H_K = h_K, A_K = a_K)$, the OLS equation (6.64) is an unbiased estimating equation, and, from (6.50), we can write $V_K^d(h_K; \beta_{K,0}) = Q_K^d\{h_K, d_K(h_K); \beta_{K,0}\}$, say. Then, from (6.52), if the models $Q_k^d(h_k, a_k; \beta_k)$ are correctly specified, $k = K - 1, \ldots, 1$, there are true values $\beta_{k,0}$ such that

$$Q_k^d(h_k, a_k; \beta_{k,0}) = E\{V_{k+1}^d(H_{k+1}) \mid H_k = h_k, A_k = a_k\},$$

and it follows from (6.51) and (6.52) that

$$V_{k+1}^d(h_{k+1}; \beta_{k+1,0}) = Q_{k+1}^d\{h_{k+1}, d_{k+1}(h_{k+1}); \beta_{k+1,0}\}.$$

Replacing $\widetilde{V}_{k+1}^d$ by $V_{k+1}^d(H_{k+1}; \beta_{k+1})$, $k = K - 1, \ldots, 1$ in (6.66) and (6.68), it can then be shown that these estimating equations are unbiased in that the estimating function

$$\frac{\partial Q_k^d(H_k, A_k; \beta_k)}{\partial \beta_k}\{V_{k+1}^d(H_{k+1}; \beta_{k+1}) - Q_k^d(H_k, A_k; \beta_k)\}$$

evaluated at $\beta_{k,0}$ and $\beta_{k+1,0}$, can be shown to have mean zero for $k = 1, \ldots, K - 1$. Namely, writing for brevity

$$Q_{\beta,k,0}^d = \frac{\partial Q_k^d(H_k, A_k; \beta_{k,0})}{\partial \beta_k},$$

$$E\left[Q_{\beta,k,0}^d\{V_{k+1}^d(H_{k+1}; \beta_{k+1,0}) - Q_k^d(H_k, A_k; \beta_{k,0})\}\right]$$

$$= E\left(E\left[Q_{\beta,k,0}^d\{V_{k+1}^d(H_{k+1}; \beta_{k+1,0}) - Q_k^d(H_k, A_k; \beta_{k,0})\} \mid H_k, A_k\right]\right)$$

$$= E\left(Q_{\beta,k,0}^d\left[E\{V_{k+1}^d(H_{k+1}; \beta_{k+1,0}) \mid H_k, A_k\} - Q_k^d(H_k, A_k; \beta_{k,0})\right]\right)$$

$$= 0.$$

Analogous arguments show that WLS estimating equations incorporating working variance models similarly are unbiased.

Thus, as long as all posited models are correctly specified, this approach is expected to lead to consistent estimators for the true values $\beta_{k,0}$ and thus for the true value $\mathcal{V}(d)$ of d.

Remarks. (i) As for Q-learning in Section 5.7.1, except for $k = K$, development and fitting of the models $Q_k^d(h_k, a_k; \beta_k)$, $k = K - 1, \ldots, 1$, in (6.65) and (6.67) is a nonstandard statistical problem, as these are models for

$$E\{V_{k+1}^d(H_{k+1}) \mid H_k = h_k, A_k = a_k\}, \quad k = K - 1, \ldots, 1, \qquad (6.70)$$

for a given $d \in \mathcal{D}$. In practice, one would posit ordinary linear or nonlinear regression models $Q_k^d(h_k, a_k; \beta_k)$ for (6.70) involving, for example, main effect and interaction terms in components of h_k and a_k. As for Q-learning, these models are almost certain to be misspecified, so that the same caveats as for estimation of an optimal regime via Q-learning apply here. Moreover, because from (6.70) the $Q_k^d(h_k, a_k; \beta_k)$ are models for the regression of the d-dependent quantity $V_{k+1}^d(H_{k+1})$ on H_k and A_k, for each fixed d, although not involving d explicitly, these models are d-dependent. Thus, even if models of the same form are used for different fixed d, the fits will be different because the pseudo outcomes at each step are d-dependent.

(ii) The estimator (6.69) for the value of a fixed Ψ-specific regime $d \in \mathcal{D}$ uses the data from all n individuals in the observed data at each step of the backward recursion to estimate the parameters $\beta_K, \beta_{K-1}, \ldots, \beta_1$ in the posited models, which is not the case for the competing regression method we discuss next. This feature is a consequence of regarding the rules $d_k(h_k) = d_k(\overline{x}_k, \overline{a}_{k-1})$, $k = 1, \ldots, K$, as defined in terms of h_k, and thus in terms of both $\overline{x}_k$ and $\overline{a}_{k-1}$. However, as discussed in Section 5.2, from the point of view of an individual following its K rules, a fixed regime d can be represented solely in terms of the baseline and evolving intervening information $x_1, \ldots, x_K$, as in (5.6). Thus, the representation in terms of h_k is redundant. This is illustrated in the example at the end of Section 5.2, where it is shown for $K = 2$ that defining rules $d_k(h_k)$ in terms of h_k results in possibly multiple superfluous configurations that could never occur in the implementation of d.

Thus, in estimating the value of a fixed regime $d \in \mathcal{D}$ using the backward recursive algorithm leading to (6.69), it would be possible to use any redundant representation of d. Theoretically, if all the models $Q_k^d(h_k, a_k; \beta_k)$, $k = 1, \ldots, K$, are correctly specified, any such redundant representation leads to the same result. However, as in Remark (i), misspecification of these models is almost certain to be the case in practice.

Thus, given the need to model pseudo outcomes, which depend on the particular representation chosen, under misspecification, different representations can yield different estimates using the same observed data.

Moreover, if one wishes to estimate the values associated with each of several fixed regimes in $\mathcal{D}$, estimation for each would involve positing and fitting a different set of models for $k = K-1, \ldots, 1$, as in Remark (i). In contrast, as discussed in Section 5.5.1, estimation of the value for any regime $d \in \mathcal{D}$ using the g-computation algorithm can be based on a single set of models for the conditional densities $p_{X_k | \overline{X}_{k-1}, \overline{A}_{k-1}}(x_k | \overline{x}_{k-1}, \overline{a}_{k-1})$, $k = 1, \ldots, K$, and $p_{Y | \overline{X}, \overline{A}}(y | \overline{x}, \overline{a})$. Of course, disadvantages of value estimation based on the g-computation algorithm relative to the method here are the need to develop models for entire distributions rather than for means and the required high-dimensional integration.

(iii) Specification of the models $Q_k^d(h_k, a_k; \beta_k)$, $k = 1, \ldots, K$, also requires careful consideration depending on the nature of the feasible sets. If $\Psi_k(h_k)$ comprises the same treatment options in $\mathcal{A}_k$ for all h_k at Decision k, $k = 1, \ldots, K$, e.g., $\Psi_k(h_k) = \mathcal{A}_k$, then development of these models is straightforward, as in Remark (i). However, modeling can be more complicated when the $\Psi_k(h_k)$ comprise different subsets of options depending on h_k for any k.

As discussed in Section 6.2.2, in most practical situations, although h_k may be high dimensional, only a few components or functions of h_k determine the feasible sets, so that there is a small number ℓ_k of distinct subsets of $\mathcal{A}_k$ that are feasible sets at Decision k for all h_k. Recall again Decision 2 in the acute leukemia setting, where $\ell_2 = 2$, and the binary indicator r_2, response status, determines $\Psi_2(h_2) = \{M_1, M_2\}$ for $r_2 = 1$ indicating response and $\Psi_2(h_2) = \{S_1, S_2\}$ for $r_2 = 0$. In this case, it is natural to develop separate models for responders and nonresponders. That is, the model $Q_2^d(h_2, a_2; \beta_2)$ might be formulated as

$$Q_2^d(h_2, a_2; \beta_2) = I(r_2 = 0)Q_{2,1}^d(h_2, a_2; \beta_{21}) + I(r_2 = 1)Q_{2,2}^d(h_2, a_2; \beta_{22}),$$

$\beta_2 = (\beta_{21}^T, \beta_{22}^T)^T$, where $Q_{2,1}^d(h_2, a_2; \beta_{21})$ and $Q_{2,2}^d(h_2, a_2; \beta_{22})$ are separate models for nonresponders and responders, respectively; and it is understood that the argument a_2 takes on values in the relevant distinct subset as $r_2 = 0$ or 1. Here, the distinct subsets are nonoverlapping in that no treatment option appears in more than one subset, but the same reasoning applies even if they do overlap. For example, if $\mathcal{A}_k$ comprises three options coded as $\{1, 2, 3\}$ and the distinct but overlapping subsets are $\{1, 2\}$, $\{2, 3\}$, and $\{1, 2, 3\}$, so $\ell_k = 3$, it is most straightforward for the analyst to posit three separate models. In these situations, each model can be fitted using the data from individuals whose histories coincide with each subset. More complex modeling and estimation strategies taking into account overlap of the distinct subsets can be developed on a case by case basis.

In general, as in Section 6.2.2 with ℓ_k distinct subsets $\mathcal{A}_{k,l} \subseteq \mathcal{A}_k$, $l = 1, \ldots, \ell_k$, as feasible sets at Decision k, each involving two or more treatment options in $\mathcal{A}_k$, with $s_k(h_k) = 1, \ldots, \ell_k$ according to which of these subsets corresponds to $\Psi_k(h_k)$ for given h_k, one can posit ℓ_k separate models and take

$$Q_k^d(h_k, a_k; \beta_k) = \sum_{l=1}^{\ell_k} \mathrm{I}\{s_k(h_k) = l\} Q_{k,l}^d(h_k, a_k; \beta_{kl}). \qquad (6.71)$$

(iv) As illustrated in Section 1.2.2 in the setting of ADHD with $K = 2$, it is common in the context of behavioral and mental health disorders for $\Psi_k(h_k)$ to consist of a single option in $\mathcal{A}_k$ for some h_k. Here, with two decision points, following selection of an initial intervention at Decision 1, with two options, medication or low intensity behavioral modification therapy, individuals are evaluated for response status. At Decision 2, responders, for whom the current intervention is apparently effective, have a single option, to continue the initial intervention, C; for nonresponders, the two options are to augment, A, or intensify, I, the current intervention. Thus, $\mathcal{A}_2 = \{\mathsf{C}, \mathsf{A}, \mathsf{I}\}$, and, with r_2 depending on h_2 indicating response status, $\ell_2 = 2$, with $\Psi_2(h_2) = \{\mathsf{C}\}$ if $r_2 = 1$ and $\Psi_2(h_2) = \{\mathsf{A}, \mathsf{I}\}$ if $r_2 = 0$. For responding individuals, effectively, there is no decision to be made, as C is always selected.

Here, with $\ell_2 = 2$ subsets, one of which has a single option, intuitively, the model corresponding to this subset should be taken to depend only on the history h_2 and not on Decision 2 treatment. In fact, as we now argue, rather than relying on this model to yield pseudo outcomes $\widetilde{V}_{2i}^d$ for individuals i for whom $\Psi_2(H_{2i}) = \{\mathsf{C}\}$ in the above estimation strategy, it is sensible to take instead $\widetilde{V}_{2i}^d = Y_i$ for such individuals. To see this, note that, by definition,

$$V_2^d(H_2) = E\{Y \mid H_2, A_2 = d_2(H_2)\}.$$

For h_2 such that $\Psi_2(h_2)$ has a single element, $d_2(h_2)$ takes on this single value, so that the events

$$\{H_2 = h_2, A_2 = d_2(h_2)\} \quad \text{and} \quad \{H_2 = h_2\}$$

are the same, yielding

$$V_2^d(H_2) = E(Y \mid H_2).$$

Letting $M_2(h_2)$ denote the number of options in $\Psi_2(h_2)$, define

$$V_2^{d*}(Y, H_2) = V_2^d(H_2)\,\mathrm{I}\{M_2(H_2) > 1\} + Y\mathrm{I}\{M_2(H_2) = 1\}.$$

Then it is straightforward that

$$
\begin{aligned}
E\{V_2^{d*}(Y, H_2) \mid H_1, A_1\} &= E[V_2^d(H_2)\mathrm{I}\{M_2(H_2) > 1\} \mid H_1, A_1] \\
&\quad + E[E(Y \mid H_2)\mathrm{I}\{M_2(H_2) = 1\} \mid H_1, A_1] \\
&= E[V_2^d(H_2)\mathrm{I}\{M_2(H_2) > 1\} + V_2^d(H_2)\mathrm{I}\{M_2(H_2) = 1\} \mid H_1, A_1] \\
&= E\{V_2^d(H_2) \mid H_1, A_1\} = Q_1^d(H_1, A_1). \qquad (6.72)
\end{aligned}
$$

The result (6.72) confirms that, for individuals for whom $\Psi_2(H_2)$ contains a single option, the observed outcome can be "carried backward" in fitting of the model corresponding to Decision 1. Accordingly, this practice is generally recommended over obtaining pseudo outcomes from a fitted model for such individuals, given the possibility of model misspecification.

. For $K > 2$, this result generalizes via a similar argument. At Decision $k = 1, \ldots, K - 1$, suppose there are ℓ_k possible subsets, and let $M_k(h_k)$ denote the number of options in $\Psi_k(h_k)$. By definition, from (6.51) and (6.52) and using $h_{k+1} = (\overline{x}_{k+1}, \overline{a}_{k-1}, a_k)$,

$$
\begin{aligned}
V_k^d(H_k) &= E[V_{k+1}^d\{\overline{X}_{k+1}, \overline{A}_{k-1}, d_k(H_k)\} \mid H_k, A_k = d_k(H_k)] \\
&= E[V_{k+1}^d\{X_{k+1}, H_k, d_k(H_k)\} \mid H_k, A_k = d_k(H_k)].
\end{aligned}
$$

If $M_k(H_k) = 1$, the events

$$
\{H_k = h_k, A_k = d_k(h_k)\} \quad \text{and} \quad \{H_k = h_k\}
$$

are the same, so that

$$
V_k^d(H_k) = E[V_{k+1}^d\{X_{k+1}, H_k, d_k(H_k)\} \mid H_k]. \qquad (6.73)
$$

Thus, defining

$$
\begin{aligned}
V_k^{d*}(X_{k+1}, H_k) &= V_k^d(H_k)\,\mathrm{I}\{M_k(H_k) > 1\} \\
&\quad + V_{k+1}^d\{X_{k+1}, H_k, d_k(H_k)\}\,\mathrm{I}\{M_k(H_k) = 1\},
\end{aligned}
$$

$$
\begin{aligned}
&E\{V_k^{d*}(X_{k+1}, H_k) \mid H_{k-1}, A_{k-1}\} \\
&= E\left[E\{V_k^{d*}(X_{k+1}, H_k) \mid H_k\} \big| H_{k-1}, A_{k-1})\right] \\
&= E\Big(V_k^d(H_k)\,\mathrm{I}\{M_k(H_k) > 1\} \\
&\quad + E\left[V_{k+1}^d\{X_{k+1}, H_k, d_k(H_k)\} \mid H_k\right]\mathrm{I}\{M_k(H_k) = 1\}\big| H_{k-1}, A_{k-1}\Big) \\
&= E\left[V_k^d(H_k)\,\mathrm{I}\{M_k(H_k) > 1\} + V_k^d(H_k)\,\mathrm{I}\{M_k(H_k) = 1\} \mid H_{k-1}, A_{k-1}\right] \\
&= E\{V_k^d(H_k) \mid H_{k-1}, A_{k-1}\},
\end{aligned}
$$

where the second to last equality follows from (6.73). Thus, from (6.51),

$$E\{V_k^{d*}(X_{k+1}, H_k) \mid H_{k-1}, A_{k-1}\} = Q_{k-1}^d(H_{k-1}, A_{k-1}),$$

generalizing (6.72). This shows that, at Decision k, for individuals for whom $M_k(H_k) > 1$ and $M_{k+1}(H_{k+1}) = 1$, $\tilde{V}_{k+2}^d$ can be "carried backward" and substituted for $\tilde{V}_{k+1}^d$ in (6.68).

Monotone Coarsening Approach

We now consider a second approach, which is based on an analogy to the situation of *monotone coarsening*, to be discussed further in Section 6.4.4.

For a fixed regime $d \in \mathcal{D}$, taking $\overline{X}_{K+1}^*(d) = Y^*(d)$ as in Section 6.3, consider the quantities

$$E\{Y^*(d) | X_1, X_2^*(d_1), \ldots, X_k^*(\overline{d}_{k-1})\} = E\{Y^*(d) \mid \overline{X}_k^*(\overline{d}_{k-1})\},$$

for $k = 1, \ldots, K + 1$, and let

$$\mu_k^d(\overline{x}_k) = E\{Y^*(d) \mid \overline{X}_k^*(\overline{d}_{k-1}) = \overline{x}_k\}, \quad k = 1, \ldots, K + 1. \qquad (6.74)$$

Of course, for $k = K + 1$, (6.74) yields $\mu_{K+1}^d\{\overline{X}_{K+1}^*(d)\} = Y^*(d)$; and for $k = 1$, (6.74) gives

$$\mu_1^d(X_1) = E\{Y^*(d) | X_1\}$$

almost surely. Thus, the value of d can be written as

$$\mathcal{V}(d) = E\{Y^*(d)\} = E\{\mu_1^d(X_1)\}. \qquad (6.75)$$

The approach we now discuss is based on positing models for $\mu_k^d(\overline{x}_k)$ · in (6.74) in terms of parameters β_k, namely,

$$\mu_k^d(\overline{x}_k; \beta_k), \quad k = 1, \ldots, K, \qquad (6.76)$$

say, and fitting them recursively for $k = K, K - 1, \ldots, 1$ to obtain estimators $\widehat{\beta}_k$. Considerations for positing these models are discussed in the remark below. An estimator for the value based on (6.75) is then obtained as

$$\widehat{\mathcal{V}}_\mu(d) = n^{-1} \sum_{i=1}^n \mu_1^d(X_{1i}; \widehat{\beta}_1). \qquad (6.77)$$

By standard properties of conditional expectation,

$$E\{Y^*(d) \mid \overline{X}_k^*(\overline{d}_{k-1})\} = E\left[E\{Y^*(d) \mid \overline{X}_{k+1}^*(\overline{d}_k)\} \,\middle|\, \overline{X}_k^*(\overline{d}_{k-1})\right],$$

so that, for $k = 1, \ldots, K$,

$$\mu_k^d\{\overline{X}_k^*(\overline{d}_{k-1})\} = E\left[\mu_{k+1}^d\{\overline{X}_{k+1}^*(\overline{d}_k)\}\,\Big|\,\overline{X}_k^*(\overline{d}_{k-1})\right]. \tag{6.78}$$

Using SUTVA, the SRA, and the positivity assumption, it follows by the equivalence of (6.43) and (6.44) that, for $k = 1, \ldots, K$ and any function $f(\cdot)$,

$$E\{f(\overline{X}_{k+1}) \mid \overline{X}_k, \overline{A}_k = \overline{d}_k(\overline{X}_k)\} = E\left[f\{\overline{X}_{k+1}^*(\overline{d}_k)\}\,\Big|\,\overline{X}_k^*(\overline{d}_{k-1})\right], \tag{6.79}$$

taking $X_{K+1} = Y$ as before.

These developments motivate estimators for β_k, $k = 1, \ldots, K$, that can be obtained in a backward recursive fashion as follows. Consider $k = K$. Here, by (6.74) and using (6.79),

$$\mu_K^d(\overline{x}_K) = E\{Y^*(d) \mid \overline{X}_K^*(\overline{d}_{K-1}) = \overline{x}_K\} \tag{6.80}$$
$$= E\{Y|\overline{X}_K = \overline{x}_K, \overline{A}_K = \overline{d}_K(\overline{x}_K)\} = E\{Y|\overline{X}_K = \overline{x}_K, \overline{A} = \overline{d}(\overline{x})\}.$$

The equality (6.80) suggests estimating β_K using the data from individuals for whom $\overline{A} = \overline{d}(\overline{X})$, so, as discussed in Section 5.5.2, for whom the treatment options actually received coincide with those selected by d for all K decisions. Defining

$$\mathcal{C}_d = \mathcal{C}_{\overline{d}_K} = I\{\overline{A} = \overline{d}(\overline{X})\} \tag{6.81}$$

as in (5.55), this can be accomplished by solving in β_K a suitable M-estimating equation as in Section 2.5, such as the OLS equation

$$\sum_{i=1}^{n} \mathcal{C}_{\overline{d}_K, i}\frac{\partial \mu_K^d(\overline{X}_{Ki}; \beta_K)}{\partial \beta_K}\{Y_i - \mu_K^d(\overline{X}_{Ki}; \beta_K)\} = 0 \tag{6.82}$$

or the WLS estimating equation incorporating a working variance model for $\mathrm{var}(Y|\overline{H}_K = \overline{h}_K, A_K = a_K)$, to obtain $\widehat{\beta}_K$.

Similarly, for $k = K - 1, \ldots, 1$, (6.78) and (6.79) imply that

$$\mu_k^d(\overline{x}_k) = E\left[\mu_{k+1}^d\{\overline{X}_{k+1}^*(\overline{d}_k)\}\,\Big|\,\overline{X}_k^*(\overline{d}_{k-1}) = \overline{x}_k\right]$$
$$= E\{\mu_{k+1}^d(\overline{X}_{k+1}) \mid \overline{X}_k = \overline{x}_k, \overline{A}_k = \overline{d}_k(\overline{x}_k)\},$$

which suggests estimating β_k using the data from all individuals for whom $\overline{A}_k = \overline{d}_k(\overline{X}_k)$; that is, with

$$[A_1 = d_1(X_1), A_2 = d_2\{X_2, d_1(X_1)\}, \ldots, A_k = d_k\{\overline{X}_k, \overline{d}_{k-1}(\overline{X}_{k-1})\}],$$

so whose treatments actually received are consistent with those selected by d through the first k decisions. Analogous to (6.81), define

$$\mathcal{C}_{\overline{d}_k} = I\{\overline{A}_k = \overline{d}_k(\overline{X}_k)\}. \tag{6.83}$$

Then find $\widehat{\beta}_k$ as the solution to an M-estimating equation, such as the OLS equation

$$\sum_{i=1}^{n} \mathcal{C}_{\overline{d}_k,i} \frac{\partial \mu_k^d(\overline{X}_{ki}; \beta_k)}{\partial \beta_k} \{\mu_{k+1}^d(\overline{X}_{k+1,i}; \widehat{\beta}_{k+1}) - \mu_k^d(\overline{X}_{ki}; \beta_k)\} = 0. \quad (6.84)$$

At $k = 1$, the fitted model is then used to estimate the value as in (6.77).

As for the estimating equations involved in the backward induction approach, it is straightforward to demonstrate that the OLS estimating equations (6.82) and (6.84) and analogous WLS equations are unbiased if the models $\mu_k^d(\overline{x}_k; \beta_k)$ are correctly specified for $k = 1, \ldots, K$, so that there are true values $\beta_{k,0}$. For example, for OLS, this follows by showing using a similar conditioning argument that the estimating functions

$$\mathcal{C}_{\overline{d}_k} \frac{\partial \mu_k^d(\overline{X}_k; \beta_k)}{\partial \beta_k} \{\mu_{k+1}^d(\overline{X}_{k+1}; \beta_{k+1}) - \mu_k^d(\overline{X}_k; \beta_k)\}$$

have mean zero when evaluated at $\beta_{k,0}$. Thus, under these conditions, (6.77) is a consistent estimator for the true value $\mathcal{V}(d)$.

Remark. Of course, as with the backward induction approach, correct specification of all K posited models is a significant challenge. From (6.80), the model $\mu_K^d(\overline{x}_K; \beta_K)$ should depend only on $\overline{x}_K$ and can be developed using standard modeling techniques, independently of d. The models $\mu_k^d(\overline{x}_k; \beta_k)$ for

$$\mu_k^d(\overline{x}_k) = E\{\mu_{k+1}^d(\overline{X}_{k+1}) \mid \overline{X}_k = \overline{x}_k, \overline{A}_k = \overline{d}_k(\overline{x}_k)\},$$

$k = K-1, \ldots, 1$ should also depend on $\overline{x}_k$ only; and, as for the backward induction approach, would be taken in practice to be ordinary linear or nonlinear models in $\overline{x}_k$ for each k, so are very likely to be misspecified. Moreover, as in Remark (i) in the discussion of the backward induction approach, because they are models for the regression of the d-dependent quantity $\mu_{k+1}^d(\overline{X}_{k+1})$ on $\overline{X}_k$, a different set of models must be posited for each fixed $d \in \mathcal{D}$. Finally, analogous to the considerations discussed in Remark (iii), development of the models $\mu_k^d(\overline{x}_k; \beta_k)$ must also respect the nature of the feasible sets at each decision point.

Relative to the backward induction approach, this method has the advantage that, because the required models involve only the baseline and intervening information $\overline{x}_k$, $k = 1, \ldots, K$, and not the treatments received, the issue of redundant representations is not relevant. Nonetheless, a major disadvantage is that each estimating equation uses data only from individuals i for whom the treatments actually received through Decision k are consistent with those dictated by regime d for $k = 1, \ldots, K$. For larger k, the number of individuals satisfying this condition will be small, especially for large K, leading to unstable if not untenable estimators for the parameters β_k.

For either of the foregoing approaches, in principle, one can view $\widehat{V}_Q(d)$ in (6.69) or $\widehat{V}_\mu(d)$ (6.77) as arising from solution of a system of stacked estimating equations and appeal to the theory of M-estimation to derive an approximate sampling distribution for the estimator. However, it is evident that an analytical derivation of such a result would be prohibitive if not impossible. Accordingly, approximate standard errors, confidence intervals, and so on can be obtained via a nonparametric bootstrap.

6.4.3 Inverse Probability Weighted Estimator

As discussed in Section 5.5.2, an alternative approach to estimation of the value of a fixed Ψ-specific regime $d \in \mathcal{D}$ is based on inverse probability weighting. This approach is motivated by a representation of $E\{Y^*(d)\}$ in terms of the observed data that is different from that arising through the g-computation algorithm in (5.43), depending on the densities of treatment received given past history in (5.54); namely,

$$
\begin{aligned}
p_{A_1|H_1}(a_1|h_1) &= p_{A_1|X_1}(a_1|x_1), & &\text{(6.85)}\\
p_{A_k|H_k}(a_k|h_k) &= p_{A_k|\overline{X}_k,\overline{A}_{k-1}}(a_k|\overline{x}_k,\overline{a}_{k-1}) & &k = 2,\ldots,K,
\end{aligned}
$$

involved in the positivity assumption (6.23).

As in Section 5.5.2, let

$$
\begin{aligned}
\pi_{d,1}(X_1) &= p_{A_1|X_1}\{d_1(X_1)|X_1\}, & &\text{(6.86)}\\
\pi_{d,k}(\overline{X}_k) &= p_{A_k|\overline{X}_k,\overline{A}_{k-1}}[d_k\{\overline{X}_k,\overline{d}_{k-1}(\overline{X}_{k-1})\}|\overline{X}_k,\overline{d}_{k-1}(\overline{X}_{k-1})],\\
& \qquad\qquad k = 2,\ldots,K,
\end{aligned}
$$

be the densities in (6.85) evaluated at $d_1(X_1)$ and $d_k\{\overline{X}_k,\overline{d}_{k-1}(\overline{X}_{k-1})\}$, respectively; and, as in (5.55) and (6.81), let

$$
\mathcal{C}_d = \mathcal{C}_{\overline{d}_K} = \mathrm{I}\{\overline{A} = \overline{d}(\overline{X})\}
$$

be the indicator of whether or not the treatment options actually received by an individual are the same as those selected by d for all K decisions.

With these definitions, the inverse probability weighted estimator of the value $\mathcal{V}(d) = E\{Y^*(d)\}$ in (5.57) given by

$$
\widehat{V}_{IPW}(d) = n^{-1}\sum_{i=1}^{n}\frac{\mathcal{C}_{d,i}Y_i}{\left\{\prod_{k=2}^{K}\pi_{d,k}(\overline{X}_{ki})\right\}\pi_{d,1}(X_{1i})} \tag{6.87}
$$

is an unbiased estimator for $\mathcal{V}(d)$. This follows from the fact that, under SUTVA (6.16), the SRA (6.17) and the positivity assumption (6.23), it can be shown that

$$E\left[\frac{\mathcal{C}_d Y}{\left\{\prod_{k=2}^{K} \pi_{d,k}(\overline{X}_k)\right\} \pi_{d,1}(X_1)}\right] = E\{Y^*(d)\}, \qquad (6.88)$$

so that $\widehat{\mathcal{V}}_{IPW}(d)$ converges in probability to $E\{Y^*(d)\}$. A sketch of the argument leading to (6.88) is presented in Section 5.5.2; we now provide a more rigorous proof of a somewhat more general result.

Demonstration of (6.88)

We show that, for some function $f(\overline{x}, y)$,

$$E\left[\frac{\mathcal{C}_d f(\overline{X}, Y)}{\left\{\prod_{k=2}^{K} \pi_{d,k}(\overline{X}_k)\right\} \pi_{d,1}(X_1)}\right] = E[f\{\overline{X}_K^*(\overline{d}_{K-1}), Y^*(d)\}], \quad (6.89)$$

so that (6.88) follows by taking $f(\overline{x}, y) = y$.

Proof. Analogous to Section 5.5.2, with W^* as defined in (6.4),

$$E\left[\frac{\mathcal{C}_d f(\overline{X}, Y)}{\left\{\prod_{k=2}^{K} \pi_{d,k}(\overline{X}_k)\right\} \pi_{d,1}(X_1)}\right]$$

$$= E\left(\frac{\mathcal{C}_d f\{\overline{X}_K^*(\overline{d}_{K-1}), Y^*(d)\}}{\left\{\prod_{k=2}^{K} \pi_{d,k}\{\overline{X}_k^*(\overline{d}_{k-1})\}\right] \pi_{d,1}(X_1)}\right)$$

$$= E\left\{E\left(\frac{I\{\overline{A} = \overline{d}(\overline{X})\}f\{\overline{X}_K^*(\overline{d}_{K-1}), Y^*(d)\}}{\left[\prod_{k=2}^{K} \pi_{d,k}\{\overline{X}_k^*(\overline{d}_{k-1})\}\right] \pi_{d,1}(X_1)}\middle| X_1, W^*\right)\right\},$$

$$= E\left(\frac{P\{\overline{A} = \overline{d}(\overline{X})|X_1, W^*\}f\{\overline{X}_K^*(\overline{d}_{K-1}), Y^*(d)\}}{\left[\prod_{k=2}^{K} \pi_{d,k}\{\overline{X}_k^*(\overline{d}_{k-1})\}\right] \pi_{d,1}(X_1)}\right), \qquad (6.90)$$

using SUTVA and the fact that, from the formal representations of $X_k^*(\overline{d}_{k-1})$, $k = 2, \ldots, K$, and $Y^*(d)$ in (6.11), $f\{\overline{X}_K^*(\overline{d}_{K-1}), Y^*(d)\}$ and the denominator of (6.90) are functions of $\{X_1, W^*\}$. The key step is to demonstrate that

$$\left[\prod_{k=2}^{K} \pi_{d,k}\{\overline{X}_k^*(\overline{d}_{k-1})\}\right] \pi_{d,1}(X_1) = P\{\overline{A} = \overline{d}(\overline{X})|X_1, W^*\} > 0 \quad (6.91)$$

almost surely. If (6.91) holds, then the desired result (6.89) follows immediately.

To show (6.91), we first argue that, for (x_1, w) such that

$$P(X_1 = x_1, W^* = w) > 0,$$

$$P\{\overline{A} = \overline{d}(\overline{X})|X_1 = x_1, W^* = w\} > 0. \tag{6.92}$$

Because from (6.11) $\{X_2^*(d_1), \ldots, X_K^*(\overline{d}_{K-1})\}$ are functions of W^*, there are corresponding $x_2, \ldots, x_K$ with

$$P\{X_1 = x_1, X_2^*(d_1) = x_2, \ldots, X_k^*(\overline{d}_{k-1}) = x_k\}$$
$$= P\{\overline{X}_k^*(\overline{d}_{k-1}) = \overline{x}_k\} > 0, \tag{6.93}$$

$k = 2, \ldots, K$. By SUTVA, we can write (6.92) equivalently as

$$P[\overline{A} = \overline{d}\{\overline{X}_K^*(\overline{d}_{K-1})\}|X_1 = x_1, W^* = w]$$
$$= P\{A_1 = d_1(x_1)|X_1 = x_1, W^* = w\} \tag{6.94}$$
$$\times \prod_{k=2}^{K} P[A_k = d_k\{\overline{x}_k, \overline{d}_{k-1}(\overline{x}_{k-1})\}|\overline{A}_{k-1} = \overline{d}_{k-1}(\overline{x}_{k-1}), X_1 = x_1, W^* = w].$$

The factorization in (6.94) is well defined if each of the terms in the product is positive or, equivalently, if

$$P\{\overline{A}_k = \overline{d}_k(\overline{x}_k), X_1 = x_1, W^* = w\} > 0 \tag{6.95}$$

for $k = 1, \ldots, K$, from whence it follows that (6.92) holds.

We demonstrate (6.95) by induction. First take $k = 1$, in which case (6.95) is

$$P\{A_1 = d_1(x_1), X_1 = x_1, W^* = w\}$$
$$= P\{A_1 = d_1(x_1) \mid X_1 = x_1, W^* = w\}P(X_1 = x_1, W^* = w),$$

which is positive if

$$P\{A_1 = d_1(x_1) \mid X_1 = x_1, W^* = w\} > 0.$$

Because $P(X_1 = x_1) > 0$, so that $x_1 \in \Gamma_1$, and because d is a Ψ-specific regime, so that $d_1(x_1) \in \Psi_1(x_1)$, it follows by the positivity assumption that

$$P\{A_1 = d_1(x_1) \mid X_1 = x_1, W^* = w\} = P\{A_1 = d_1(x_1) \mid X_1 = x_1\} > 0, \tag{6.96}$$

where the first equality is due to the SRA. Thus, (6.95) holds for $k = 1$.

Now assume that we have shown that (6.95) is true. To complete the induction proof, we must demonstrate that

$$P\{\overline{A}_{k+1} = \overline{d}_{k+1}(\overline{x}_{k+1}), X_1 = x_1, W^* = w\} > 0. \qquad (6.97)$$

Because $\overline{X}_k^*(\overline{d}_{k-1})$ includes X_1 by definition and by the above construction, $(X_1 = x_1, W^* = w)$ and $\{\overline{X}_{k+1}^*(d) = \overline{x}_{k+1}, W^* = w\}$ are equivalent. Thus, we can write (6.97) as

$$
\begin{aligned}
&P\{\overline{A}_{k+1} = \overline{d}_{k+1}(\overline{x}_{k+1}), X_1 = x_1, W^* = w\} \\
&= P[A_{k+1} = d_{k+1}\{\overline{x}_{k+1}, \overline{d}_k(\overline{x}_k)\} \\
&\qquad | \overline{A}_k = \overline{d}_k(\overline{x}_k), \overline{X}_{k+1}^*(\overline{d}_k) = \overline{x}_{k+1}, W^* = w] \\
&\quad \times P\{\overline{A}_k = \overline{d}_k(\overline{x}_k), X_1 = x_1, W^* = w\},
\end{aligned}
$$

and we must show that the first term on the right-hand side is positive. This term satisfies

$$
\begin{aligned}
&P[A_{k+1} = d_{k+1}\{\overline{x}_{k+1}, \overline{d}_k(\overline{x}_k)\} | \overline{A}_k = \overline{d}_k(\overline{x}_k), \overline{X}_{k+1}^*(\overline{d}_k) = \overline{x}_{k+1}, W^* = w] \\
&= P[A_{k+1} = d_{k+1}\{\overline{x}_{k+1}, \overline{d}_k(\overline{x}_k)\} | \overline{X}_{k+1} = \overline{x}_{k+1}, \overline{A}_k = \overline{d}_k(\overline{x}_k), W^* = w] \\
&= P[A_{k+1} = d_{k+1}\{\overline{x}_{k+1}, \overline{d}_k(\overline{x}_k)\} | \overline{X}_{k+1} = \overline{x}_{k+1}, \overline{A}_k = \overline{d}_k(\overline{x}_k)], \quad (6.98)
\end{aligned}
$$

where the first equality holds by SUTVA and the second by the SRA. Because from above $\{x_1, d_1(x_1)\} \in \Lambda_1$ and because (6.93) holds, the argument leading to (6.45) yields $\{\overline{x}_{k+1}, \overline{d}_k(\overline{x}_k)\} \in \Gamma_{k+1}$, and $d_{k+1}\{\overline{x}_{k+1}, \overline{d}_k(\overline{x}_k)\} \in \Psi_{k+1}(h_{k+1})$ because d is a Ψ-specific regime. It thus follows by the positivity assumption (6.23) that (6.98) is positive, and (6.97) follows.

The proof of (6.91) is complete by applying (6.96) and (6.98) to (6.94) to obtain

$$
\begin{aligned}
P\{\overline{A} = \overline{d}(\overline{X}) | X_1, W^*\} &= p_{A_1|X_1}\{d_1(X_1)|X_1\} \\
&\quad \times \left(\prod_{k=2}^{K} p_{A_k|\overline{X}_k, \overline{A}_{k-1}}[d_k\{\overline{X}_k, \overline{d}_{k-1}(\overline{X}_{k-1})\} | \overline{X}_k, \overline{d}_{k-1}(\overline{X}_{k-1})] \right) \\
&= \pi_{d,1}(X_1) \left[\prod_{k=2}^{K} \pi_{d,k}\{\overline{X}_k^*(\overline{d}_{k-1})\} \right]
\end{aligned}
$$

almost surely using the definitions in (6.86).   □

As noted above, (6.88) is obtained by taking $f(\overline{x}, y) = y$, demonstrating not only that the inverse probability weighted estimator $\widehat{\mathcal{V}}_{IPW}(d)$ in (6.87) is a consistent estimator for the true value $\mathcal{V}(d)$ for fixed $d \in \mathcal{D}$ but that $E\{Y^*(d)\}$ can be represented in terms of the observed data in this way. The representation of $E\{Y^*(d)\}$ in (6.88) is thus an alternative to that in (5.43) obtained via the g-computation algorithm.

In fact, (6.89) can be used to derive a representation of the joint density of X_1 and the potential outcomes corresponding to a fixed $d \in \mathcal{D}$, $\{X_1, X_2^*(d_1), \ldots, X_K^*(\bar{d}_{K-1}), Y^*(d)\}$, in terms of the observed data that is an alternative to that from the g-computation algorithm in (6.46). For fixed realization $(x_1, \bar{x}_2, \ldots, \bar{x}_K, y)$, treating all random variables as discrete and taking

$$f\{\overline{X}_K^*(\bar{d}_{K-1}), Y^*(d)\}$$
$$= I\{X_1 = x_1, X_2^*(d_1) = x_2, \ldots, X_K^*(\bar{d}_{K-1}) = x_K, Y^*(d) = y\},$$

(6.89) yields

$$P\{X_1 = x_1, X_2^*(d_1) = x_2, \ldots, X_K^*(\bar{d}_{K-1}) = x_K, Y^*(d) = y\}$$
$$= p_{X_1, X_2^*(d_1), X_3^*(\bar{d}_2), \ldots, X_K^*(\bar{d}_{K-1}), Y^*(d)}(x_1, \ldots, x_K, y)$$
$$= E\left[\frac{\mathcal{C}_d\, I(X_1 = x_1, X_2 = x_2, \ldots, X_K = x_K, Y = y)}{\left\{\prod_{k=2}^K \pi_{d,k}(\overline{X}_k)\right\}\pi_{d,1}(X_1)}\right].$$

This suggests estimating the joint density by

$$n^{-1}\sum_{i=1}^n \frac{\mathcal{C}_{d,i}\, I(X_{1i} = x_1, X_{2i} = x_2, \ldots, X_{Ki} = x_K, Y_i = y)}{\left\{\prod_{k=2}^K \pi_{d,k}(\overline{X}_{ki})\right\}\pi_{d,1}(X_{1i})}.$$

Similarly, a representation in terms of the observed data of the joint distribution function of $\{X_1, X_2^*(d_1), \ldots, X_K^*(\bar{d}_{K-1}), Y^*(d)\}$ follows from choosing

$$f\{\overline{X}_K^*(\bar{d}_{K-1}), Y^*(d)\}$$
$$= I\{X_1 \leq x_1, X_2^*(d_1) \leq x_2, \ldots, X_K^*(\bar{d}_{K-1}) \leq x_K, Y^*(d) \leq y\},$$

and a representation of the marginal density of $Y^*(d)$ in terms of the observed data different from that in (6.47) is obtained with

$$f\{\overline{X}_K^*(\bar{d}_{K-1}), Y^*(d)\} = I\{Y^*(d) = y\}.$$

These expressions suggest corresponding estimators analogous to that for the joint density. In what follows, we focus on estimation of the value $\mathcal{V}(d)$.

As noted in Section 5.5.2, the expression

$$\left\{\prod_{k=2}^K \pi_{d,k}(\overline{X}_k)\right\}\pi_{d,1}(X_1)$$

in the denominators of $\widehat{\mathcal{V}}_{IPW}(d)$ in (6.87) and these other estimators can be interpreted as the propensity for receiving treatment consistent with regime d through all K decisions, given the observed history. From (6.86), this depends on the propensities of treatment given past history,

$$p_{A_k|H_k}(a_k|h_k) = P(A_k = a_k \mid H_k = h_k), \quad k = 1, \ldots, K, \qquad (6.99)$$

involved in the positivity assumption (6.23). As in Sections 5.5.2 and 5.7.2, models for the propensities are posited and fitted in practice. As for regression modeling in Section 6.4.2, specification and fitting of such models must respect the nature of the feasible sets; we defer discussion of the considerations involved to the end of this section.

Supposing that the propensity model at Decision k depends on a parameter γ_k, substituting the posited models in (6.86) induces models $\pi_{d,1}(X_1; \gamma_1)$ and $\pi_{d,k}(\overline{X}_k; \gamma_k)$, as exemplified in the case of two options at each decision point in (5.63). Given estimators $\widehat{\gamma}_k$, $k = 1, \ldots, K$, from (6.87), the inverse probability weighted estimator for the value is then given by

$$\widehat{\mathcal{V}}_{IPW}(d) = n^{-1} \sum_{i=1}^{n} \frac{\mathcal{C}_{d,i} Y_i}{\left\{ \prod_{k=2}^{K} \pi_{d,k}(\overline{X}_{ki}; \widehat{\gamma}_k) \right\} \pi_{d,1}(X_{1i}; \widehat{\gamma}_1)} \qquad (6.100)$$

as in (5.64).

From (5.67), the alternative estimator

$$\widehat{\mathcal{V}}_{IPW^*}(d) = \left[\sum_{i=1}^{n} \frac{\mathcal{C}_{d,i}}{\left\{ \prod_{k=2}^{K} \pi_{d,k}(\overline{X}_{ki}; \widehat{\gamma}_k) \right\} \pi_{d,1}(X_{1i}; \widehat{\gamma}_1)} \right]^{-1}$$
$$\times \sum_{i=1}^{n} \frac{\mathcal{C}_{d,i} Y_i}{\left\{ \prod_{k=2}^{K} \pi_{d,k}(\overline{X}_{ki}; \widehat{\gamma}_k) \right\} \pi_{d,1}(X_{1i}; \widehat{\gamma}_1)} \qquad (6.101)$$

for the value $\mathcal{V}(d)$, which is in the form of a weighted average of the observed Y_i, often enjoys substantially smaller sampling variation than (6.100). It is straightforward that, as long as the models for the propensities in (6.99) are all correctly specified, taking $f(\cdot, \cdot) \equiv 1$, from (6.89), n^{-1} times the first term in brackets on the right-hand side of (6.101) converges in probability to one, demonstrating formally that $\widehat{\mathcal{V}}_{IPW^*}(d)$ is a consistent estimator for the true value.

As in Section 5.5.2, because when $\mathcal{C}_d = 1$, $A_1 = d_1(X_1)$, and $A_k = d_k\{\overline{X}_k, \overline{d}_{k-1}(\overline{X}_{k-1})\}$, $k = 2, \ldots, K$, from (5.68), $\mathcal{C}_d$ can be expressed equivalently as

$$\mathcal{C}_d = \mathrm{I}\{A_1 = d_1(H_1), \ldots, A_k = d_k(H_k), \ldots, A_K = d_K(H_K)\}; \quad (6.102)$$

and from (5.69), the denominator in the summands in $\widehat{\mathcal{V}}_{IPW}(d)$ and $\widehat{\mathcal{V}}_{IPW*}(d)$,

$$\left\{ \prod_{k=2}^{K} \pi_{d,k}(\overline{X}_{ki}; \widehat{\gamma}_k) \right\} \pi_{d,1}(X_{1i}; \widehat{\gamma}_1),$$

can be replaced by the fitted model for

$$\prod_{k=1}^{K} p_{A_k | H_k}(A_{ki} | H_{ki}) \qquad (6.103)$$

without altering the values of the estimators, as demonstrated in (5.70) and (5.110) for two and greater than two options at each decision point, respectively.

As noted in Section 5.5.2, even if the propensities in (6.99) are known, it is preferable on efficiency grounds to adopt models containing the true propensities and estimate the parameters in these via maximum likelihood. Large sample approximations to the sampling distribution of these estimators can be obtained by appealing to standard M-estimation theory; alternatively, standard errors and other measures of uncertainty can be obtained via a nonparametric bootstrap. Further discussion of the value estimators (6.100) and (6.101) and practical considerations regarding their use is presented in Section 5.5.2.

Considerations for Propensity Modeling

We close this section by discussing tactics for modeling the propensities (6.99).

First consider data from a SMART, in which case the propensities are known, so that $\pi_{d,1}(X_1)$ and $\pi_{d,k}(\overline{X}_k)$, $k = 2, \ldots, K$, in the denominator of (6.100) are known for each individual. Although the estimator $\widehat{\mathcal{V}}_{IPW}(d)$ in (6.87) can be used as is in this case, as noted above, it is preferable to estimate the propensities nonetheless by appropriate sample proportions. In a SMART, the positivity assumption holds, and thus, for $k = 1, \ldots, K$, $h_k \in \Gamma_k$ and $a_k \in \Psi_k(h_k)$. Accordingly, the sample proportions must respect the nature of the feasible sets, as follows.

As discussed in Remark (iii) in Section 6.4.2, because in most situations one or only a few components or functions of h_k determine the feasible sets, there is a small number ℓ_k of distinct subsets $\mathcal{A}_{k,l} \subseteq \mathcal{A}_k$, $l = 1, \ldots, \ell_k$, that are feasible sets for all $h_k \in \Gamma_k$. Thus, to estimate $P(A_k = a_k \mid H_k = h_k)$ in a SMART, these sample proportions are based on the data from individuals whose histories dictate one of these distinct subsets. For example, in the acute leukemia setting in Section 1.2.1, if data are available from a SMART as in Figure 5.1, from Remark (iii), at Decision 2, $\ell_2 = 2$, and, letting r_2 depending on h_2 indicate response, $\Psi_2(h_2) = \{M_1, M_2\} = \mathcal{A}_{2,1}$ for $r_2 = 1$, and $\Psi_2(h_2) = \{S_1, S_2\} = \mathcal{A}_{2,2}$ for $r_2 = 0$. It follows that, for each $a_2 \in \mathcal{A}_{2,1}$, $P(A_2 = a_2 \mid H_2 = h_2)$ can be estimated by

$$\left(\sum_{i=1}^{n} I(R_{2i} = 1) \right)^{-1} \sum_{i=1}^{n} I(R_{2i} = 1) I(A_{2i} = a_2),$$

and for $a_2 \in \mathcal{A}_{2,2}$ by

$$\left(\sum_{i=1}^{n} I(R_{2i} = 0) \right)^{-1} \sum_{i=1}^{n} I(R_{2i} = 0) I(A_{2i} = a_2).$$

In SMARTs where there may be a single feasible option for some histories at a decision point, as for responders at Decision 2 in the ADHD setting of Section 1.2.2 and also discussed in Remark (iii), again letting r_2 depending on h_2 indicate response, when $r_2 = 1$, so that the corresponding feasible set comprises a single element a_2, $P(A_2 = a_2 \mid H_2 = h_2) = 1$, and no estimation is required. These considerations generalize in the obvious way to SMARTs with $K \geq 2$ decision points and distinct subsets with more than two options; see below.

When the data are from an observational study, as in Section 5.5.2, models must be posited and fitted for the propensities in (6.99) for each $k = 1, \ldots, K$. As above, for Decision k, with $\mathcal{A}_{k,l} \subseteq \mathcal{A}_k$, $l = 1, \ldots, \ell_k$, the distinct subsets of $\mathcal{A}_k$ that are feasible sets, a separate model is specified for each distinct subset. Using again the acute leukemia setting as an example, with $\ell_2 = 2$ at Decision 2, let as above $\mathcal{A}_{2,1} = \{M_1, M_2\}$ denote the subset corresponding to h_2 with $r_2 = 1$. Then coding the two options as $\{0, 1\}$, a logistic regression model depending on h_2 (except for r_2 if it is an explicit component of h_2) for $\pi_{2,1}(h_2) = P(A_2 = 1 \mid H_2 = h_2)$ for such h_2, $\pi_{2,1}(h_2; \gamma_{21})$, say, can be posited as in Section 5.5.2 and fitted using the data (H_{2i}, A_{2i}) for individuals i for whom $R_{2i} = 1$ (so $l = 1$). Likewise, letting $\mathcal{A}_{2,2} = \{S_1, S_2\}$ denote the subset for h_2 with $r_2 = 0$ and coding the two options as $\{0, 1\}$, a logistic regression model depending on h_2 for $\pi_{2,2}(h_2) = P(A_2 = 1 \mid H_2 = h_2)$ for such h_2, $\pi_{2,2}(h_2; \gamma_{22})$, can be fitted to the data for individuals i with $R_{2i} = 0$.

In general, as in Section 6.2.2, at Decision k, for ℓ_k distinct subsets $\mathcal{A}_{k,l}$, $l = 1, \ldots, \ell_k$, each involving two or more options in $\mathcal{A}_k$, for the lth subset, involving $m_{kl} \geq 2$ options, say, with $s_k(h_k) = l$ according to which of these subsets is relevant for given h_k, one can posit ℓ_k separate logistic or multinomial (polytomous) logistic regression models as appropriate. For the latter, which subsumes the former, coding the m_{kl} options in $\mathcal{A}_{k,l}$ as $\{1, \ldots, m_{kl}\}$, for $a_k \in \{1, \ldots, m_{kl}\}$, as in (5.65) and

(5.66), let

$$\omega_{k,l}(h_k, a_k) = P(A_k = a_k | H_k = h_k), \quad k = 1, \ldots, K,$$

$$\omega_{k,l}(h_k, m_{kl}) = 1 - \sum_{a_k=1}^{m_{kl}-1} \omega_{k,l}(h_k, a_k). \tag{6.104}$$

One would posit models

$$\omega_{k,l}(h_k, a_k; \gamma_{kl}), \quad l = 1, \ldots, \ell_k, \tag{6.105}$$

for finite-dimensional parameter γ_{kl}, where $a_k \in \mathcal{A}_{k,l}$. For each $l = 1, \ldots, \ell_k$, the model can be fitted by maximum likelihood based on the data from individuals for whom $s_k(h_k) = l$. Then, analogous to (6.71) in the case of regression modeling, take

$$\omega_k(h_k, a_k; \gamma_k) = \sum_{l=1}^{\ell_k} I\{s_k(h_k) = l\} \omega_{k,l}(h_k, a_k; \gamma_{kl}),$$

$$\gamma_k = (\gamma_{k1}^T, \ldots, \gamma_{k\ell_k}^T)^T, \tag{6.106}$$

where it is understood that the argument a_k takes on values in the relevant distinct subset. Specification of separate models for each l is required when the subsets are nonoverlapping, so that no option appears in more than one subset, but for simplicity one would ordinarily posit separate models even if they do overlap. As above, if for certain h_k a subset comprises a single option a_k, then $P(A_k = a_k \mid H_k = h_k) = 1$, and no model need be posited and fitted.

Of course, if the data are from a SMART, for the lth subset, the required sample proportions for each option can be estimated by positing and fitting a logistic (two options) or multinomial logistic (more than two options) models involving only treatment indicators to the data on individuals with realized h_k corresponding to the lth subset, so with $s_k(h_k) = l$.

The separate propensities corresponding to each of the ℓ_k distinct feasible sets at Decision k, $k = 1, \ldots, K$, as in (6.104), and the resulting need for separate models for these for each $l = 1, \ldots \ell_k$ as in (6.105) and (6.106) has implications for the form of the expression

$$\left\{ \prod_{k=2}^{K} \pi_{d,k}(\overline{X}_k) \right\} \pi_{d,1}(X_1)$$

in the denominators of the inverse probability weighted estimators. In particular, it straightforward to observe that (6.86) can be written as

$$\pi_{d,1}(X_1) = \sum_{l=1}^{\ell_1} I\{s_1(h_1) = l\} \prod_{a_1=1}^{m_{1l}} \omega_{1,l}(X_1, a_1)^{I\{d_1(X_1)=a_1\}}$$

$$\pi_{d,k}(\overline{X}_k) = \sum_{l=1}^{\ell_k} \mathrm{I}\{s_k(h_k) = l\} \tag{6.107}$$

$$\times \prod_{a_k=1}^{m_{kl}} \omega_{k,l}\{\overline{X}_k, \overline{d}_{k-1}(\overline{X}_{k-1}), a_k\}^{\mathrm{I}[d_k\{\overline{X}_k,\overline{d}_{k-1}(\overline{X}_{k-1})\}=a_k)]},$$

$$k = 2,\ldots,K.$$

From (6.107), the induced models $\pi_{d,1}(X_1; \gamma_1)$ and $\pi_{d,k}(\overline{X}_k; \gamma_k)$ are then found by substituting the models (6.105); namely,

$$\pi_{d,1}(X_1; \gamma_1) = \sum_{l=1}^{\ell_1} \mathrm{I}\{s_1(h_1) = l\} \prod_{a_1=1}^{m_{1l}} \omega_{1,l}(X_1, a_1; \gamma_{1l})^{\mathrm{I}\{d_1(X_1)=a_1\}}$$

$$\pi_{d,k}(\overline{X}_k; \gamma_k) = \sum_{l=1}^{\ell_k} \mathrm{I}\{s_k(h_k) = l\} \tag{6.108}$$

$$\times \prod_{a_k=1}^{m_{kl}} \omega_{k,l}\{\overline{X}_k, \overline{d}_{k-1}(\overline{X}_{k-1}), a_k; \gamma_{kl}\}^{\mathrm{I}[d_k\{\overline{X}_k,\overline{d}_{k-1}(\overline{X}_{k-1})\}=a_k)]},$$

$$k = 2,\ldots,K.$$

6.4.4 Augmented Inverse Probability Weighted Estimator

As noted at the end of Section 5.5.2, it is possible to improve considerably on the simple inverse probability weighted value estimators in the previous section by using the theory of semiparametrics (Robins et al., 1994; Tsiatis, 2006) to characterize the class of augmented inverse probability weighted estimators for $\mathcal{V}(d)$ for fixed $d \in \mathcal{D}$ and to identify the efficient estimator in the class. Zhang et al. (2013) obtain the form of estimators in this class and the efficient estimator within it by casting the problem of estimation of the value of a K-decision regime as involving data subject to *monotone coarsening* (Tsiatis, 2006, Chapter 7), a special case of which is the familiar setting of "dropout," as follows.

An individual whose treatment options received through Decision $k - 1$ are consistent with those that would be selected by the rules $d_1,\ldots,d_{k-1}$ under his evolving history, so with

$$A_1 = d_1(X_1),\ldots, A_{k-1} = d_{k-1}\{\overline{X}_{k-1}, \overline{d}_{k-2}(\overline{X}_{k-2})\},$$

but whose treatment option received at Decision k is not consistent with that selected by d_k, so with $A_k \neq d_k\{\overline{X}_k, \overline{d}_{k-1}(\overline{X}_{k-1})\}$, has, under SUTVA, observed

$$X_2 = X_2^*(d_1),\ldots, X_k = X_k^*(\overline{d}_{k-1});$$

i.e., $\overline{X}_k = \overline{X}_k^*(\overline{d}_{k-1})$. However, this individual's observed $X_{k+1}, \ldots, X_K$ and Y do not reflect the potential outcomes he would have if he were to continue to follow the rules $d_k, \ldots, d_K$.

Thus, from the perspective of information on $\{X_1, \overline{X}_K^*(\overline{d}_{K-1}), Y^*(d)\}$, and in particular on $Y^*(d)$, for this individual, $\overline{X}_k^*(\overline{d}_{k-1})$ is observed, but $X_{k+1}^*(\overline{d}_k), \ldots, X_K^*(\overline{d}_{K-1}), Y^*(d)$ are "missing," and, effectively, in terms of receiving treatment consistent with d, he has "dropped out" at Decision k. Because the information on the potential outcomes available from an individual who "drops out" at Decision k is contained in the information that would be available if she instead were to "drop out" at Decision $k+1$, the missingness, or "coarsening," of the information is monotone.

Under SUTVA (6.16) and the SRA (6.17), Zhang et al. (2013) demonstrate that, from a coarsened data perspective, the "dropout" in this context is according to a missing (or coarsening) at random mechanism; see Section 3 of the supplementary material to Zhang et al. (2013) for a detailed argument. Under these conditions, the positivity assumption (6.23), and the assumption that the densities

$$p_{A_1|H_1}(a_1|h_1) = p_{A_1|X_1}(a_1|x_1),$$
$$p_{A_k|H_k}(a_k|h_k) = p_{A_k|\overline{X}_k, \overline{A}_{k-1}}(a_k|\overline{x}_k, \overline{a}_{k-1}), \quad k = 2, \ldots, K,$$

in (6.85) are known or can be modeled correctly, a correspondence to the general formulation in Chapters 7 and 9 of Tsiatis (2006) for estimation under monotone coarsening at random can then be made to derive the class of all consistent and asymptotically normal estimators for $\mathcal{V}(d)$.

The form of estimators in this class that we present here is different from, but equivalent to, that of Zhang et al. (2013), as we demonstrate shortly. Define as in (6.81) and (6.83)

$$\mathcal{C}_{\overline{d}_k} = \mathrm{I}\{\overline{A}_k = \overline{d}_k(\overline{X}_k)\}, \quad k = 1, \ldots, K,$$

the indicator that the treatment options received through Decision k are consistent with those dictated by the first k rules in d. Note that, for $k < K$, $\mathcal{C}_{\overline{d}_k} = 1$ implies nothing about the consistency of treatment options received subsequent to Decision k with those that would be selected by the rules $d_{k+1}, \ldots, d_K$. As before, $\mathcal{C}_d = \mathcal{C}_{\overline{d}_K}$ is the indicator that all K treatments received are consistent with those dictated by d. Define $\mathcal{C}_{d_0} \equiv 1$; let

$$\pi_{d,1}(X_1) = p_{A_1|X_1}\{d_1(X_1)|X_1\}, \tag{6.109}$$
$$\pi_{d,k}(\overline{X}_k) = p_{A_k|\overline{X}_k, \overline{A}_{k-1}}[d_k\{\overline{X}_k, \overline{d}_{k-1}(\overline{X}_{k-1})\}|\overline{X}_k, \overline{d}_{k-1}(\overline{X}_{k-1})],$$
$$k = 2, \ldots, K,$$

as in (6.86); and, for brevity, let $\overline{\pi}_{d,1}(X_1) = \pi_{d,1}(X_1)$ and

$$\overline{\pi}_{d,k}(\overline{X}_k) = \left\{ \prod_{j=2}^{k} \pi_{d,j}(\overline{X}_j) \right\} \pi_{d,1}(X_1), \quad k = 2, \ldots, K, \qquad (6.110)$$

with $\overline{\pi}_{d,0} \equiv 1$. As in Section 6.4.3, positing models for the propensities

$$p_{A_k|H_k}(a_k|h_k) = P(A_k = a_k \mid H_k = h_k), \quad k = 1, \ldots, K, \qquad (6.111)$$

in terms of parameters γ_k and substituting these in (6.109) leads to models $\pi_{d,1}(X_1; \gamma_1)$ and $\pi_{d,k}(\overline{X}_k; \gamma_k)$ and thus, from (6.110), to models $\overline{\pi}_{d,k}(\overline{X}_k; \overline{\gamma}_k)$, $k = 1, \ldots, K$, where $\overline{\gamma}_k = (\gamma_1^T, \ldots, \gamma_k^T)^T$.

Given estimators $\widehat{\gamma}_k$ for γ_k, $k = 1, \ldots, K$, obtained as discussed in Sections 5.5.2 and 6.4.3, if the propensity models are all correctly specified, it follows from the semiparametric theory that all consistent and asymptotically normal estimators for $\mathcal{V}(d)$ are asymptotically equivalent to an estimator of the augmented inverse probability weighted form

$$\widehat{\mathcal{V}}_{AIPW}(d) = n^{-1} \sum_{i=1}^{n} \left[\frac{\mathcal{C}_{d,i} Y_i}{\left\{ \prod_{k=2}^{K} \overline{\pi}_{d,k}(\overline{X}_{ki}; \widehat{\gamma}_k) \right\} \pi_{d,1}(X_{1i}; \widehat{\gamma}_1)} \right. \qquad (6.112)$$

$$\left. + \sum_{k=1}^{K} \left\{ \frac{\mathcal{C}_{\overline{d}_{k-1},i}}{\overline{\pi}_{d,k-1}(\overline{X}_{k-1,i}; \widehat{\overline{\gamma}}_{k-1})} - \frac{\mathcal{C}_{\overline{d}_k,i}}{\overline{\pi}_{d,k}(\overline{X}_{ki}, \widehat{\overline{\gamma}}_k)} \right\} L_k(\overline{X}_{ki}) \right],$$

where $L_k(\overline{x}_k)$ are arbitrary functions of $\overline{x}_k$; and $\widehat{\overline{\gamma}}_k = (\widehat{\gamma}_1^T, \ldots, \widehat{\gamma}_k^T)^T$, $k = 1, \ldots, K$. Clearly, taking $L_k(\overline{x}_k) \equiv 0$, $k = 1, \ldots, K$, yields the simple inverse probability weighted estimator (6.100). It is straightforward to observe that, when $K = 1$, because $\mathcal{C}_{d_0} \equiv 1$, $\overline{\pi}_{d,0} \equiv 1$ and $X_1 = H_1$, the estimator (6.112) reduces to the augmented inverse probability weighted estimator (3.27) in the single decision case in Section 3.3.3.

As for (3.27), if all K models for the propensities (6.111) are correctly specified, so that there are true values $\gamma_{k,0}$ of the model parameters, $k = 1, \ldots, K$, yielding the true propensities, it can be shown that the second "augmentation term" in (6.112) evaluated at $\gamma_{k,0}$, $k = 1, \ldots, K$, converges in probability to zero for arbitrary $L_k(\overline{x}_k)$, $k = 1, \ldots, K$. Thus, the estimator (6.112) is a consistent estimator for $\mathcal{V}(d)$. However, the asymptotic variance of $\widehat{\mathcal{V}}_{AIPW}(d)$ depends on this term and thus on the choice of $L_k(\overline{x}_k)$. The "augmentation term" involves data from individuals whose observed treatments are not consistent with those dictated by d at all K decisions. As discussed next, under judicious specification of $L_k(\overline{x}_k)$, $k = 1, \ldots, K$, this term can serve to increase efficiency over the simple inverse weighted estimator by exploiting the information in these data.

Remark. As in the Remark following (3.30) in Section 3.3.3 for the single decision case, the augmented inverse probability weighted estimator (6.112) can be expressed equivalently by replacing the denominators of the leading and augmentation terms by quantities analogous to (6.103). Also, the $\mathcal{C}_{\overline{a}_k,i}$, $k = 1, \ldots, K$, can be replaced by terms analogous to (6.102). See Section 7.4.4 for an explicit demonstration.

From semiparametric theory, the optimal choice of the $L_k(\overline{x}_k)$ leading to the estimator with smallest asymptotic variance among all estimators in the class (6.112) is

$$L_k(\overline{x}_k) = E\{Y^*(d) \mid \overline{X}_k^*(\overline{d}_{k-1}) = \overline{x}_k\}, \quad k = 1, \ldots, K. \qquad (6.113)$$

Of course, the conditional expectations $E\{Y^*(d) \mid \overline{X}_k^*(\overline{d}_{k-1})\}$, as functionals of the joint distribution of $\{X_1, X_2^*(d_1), \ldots, X_k^*(\overline{d}_{k-1}), Y^*(d)\}$, are unknown in practice. This suggests positing and fitting models for $E\{Y^*(d) \mid \overline{X}_k^*(\overline{d}_{k-1}) = \overline{x}_k\}$, $k = 1, \ldots, K$, and then substituting the fitted models in (6.112).

In fact, in Section 6.4.2, we have already discussed approaches to this task. In particular, inspection of the optimal $L_k(\overline{x}_k)$ in (6.113) shows that it is identical to $\mu_k^d(\overline{x}_k)$ defined in (6.74) in Section 6.4.2. This suggests positing models

$$\mu_k^d(\overline{x}_k; \beta_k), \quad k = 1, \ldots, K,$$

as in (6.76) and fitting them using the backward recursive "monotone coarsening" approach presented in that section. That is, obtain estimators $\widehat{\beta}_k$, $k = K, K-1, \ldots, 1$, by solving the estimating equations (6.82) and (6.84) for $k = K-1, \ldots, 1$, and then take

$$L_k(\overline{X}_{ki}) = \mu_k^d(\overline{X}_{ki}; \widehat{\beta}_k), \quad k = 1, \ldots, K, \qquad (6.114)$$

for each $i = 1, \ldots, n$ in (6.112).

An alternative strategy is to exploit the regression modeling approach based on backward induction in Section 6.4.2. In that section, with $V_k^d(h_k)$, $k = 1, \ldots, K$, defined as in (6.50) and (6.52), namely,

$$V_k^d(h_k) = Q_k^d\{h_k, d_k(h_k)\}, \quad k = 1, \ldots, K,$$

where $Q_K^d(h_K, a_K) = E(Y \mid H_K = h_K, A_K = a_K)$, and

$$Q_k^d(h_k, a_k) = E\{V_{k+1}^d(H_{k+1}) \mid H_k = h_k, A_k = a_k\},$$

we proved (6.54),

$$V_k^d(h_k) = E\{Y^*(\overline{a}_{k-1}, d_k, \ldots, d_K) \mid H_k = h_k\} \quad \text{for } h_k \in \Gamma_k.$$

Under SUTVA (6.16) and the SRA (6.17), by manipulations analogous to those leading to (6.26), it can be shown that

$$V_k^d\{\overline{x}_k, \overline{d}_{k-1}(\overline{x}_{k-1})\} = E\{Y^*(d) \mid \overline{X}_k = \overline{x}_k, \overline{A}_{k-1} = \overline{d}_{k-1}(\overline{x}_{k-1})\}$$
$$= E\{Y^*(d) \mid \overline{X}_k^*(\overline{d}_{k-1}) = \overline{x}_k\}. \tag{6.115}$$

This suggests positing models $Q_k^d(h_k, a_k; \beta_k)$, $k = K, K-1, \ldots, 1$, as in (6.63), (6.65), and (6.67); fitting these via the backward algorithm to obtain $\widehat{\beta}_k$, $k = K, K-1, \ldots, 1$; and, with

$$V_k^d\{\overline{x}_k, \overline{d}_{k-1}(\overline{x}_{k-1}); \beta_k\} = Q_k^d\{\overline{x}_k, \overline{d}_k(\overline{x}_k); \beta_k\},$$

taking

$$L_k(\overline{X}_{ki}) = V_k^d\{\overline{X}_{ki}, \overline{d}_{k-1}(\overline{X}_{k-1,i}); \widehat{\beta}_k\}, \quad k = 1, \ldots, K, \tag{6.116}$$

for $i = 1, \ldots, n$ in (6.112).

In either case, specification of the models $\mu_k^d(\overline{x}_k; \beta_k)$ or $Q_k^d(h_k, a_k; \beta_k)$, $k = 1, \ldots, K$, involves the considerations discussed in the remarks in Section 6.4.2. With the backward induction approach, when one of the distinct subsets of $\mathcal{A}_k$ that is a feasible set comprises a single treatment option, "carrying backward" $V_{k+1}^d\{\overline{X}_{k+1,i}, \overline{d}_k(\overline{X}_{k,i}); \widehat{\beta}_{k+1}\}$ as $L_k(\overline{X}_{k,i})$ for relevant individuals i is problematic, as the latter depends only on $\overline{X}_{k,i}$. However, it can be shown that the difference in braces in the augmentation term in (6.112) is equal to zero for such individuals, rendering this issue moot.

Yet another approach is to appeal to the g-computation algorithm to estimate $E\{Y^*(d) \mid \overline{X}_k^*(\overline{d}_{k-1}) = \overline{x}_k\}$, $k = 1, \ldots, K$, via Monte Carlo integration, exploiting the developments in Section 5.4. Posit models for the conditional densities $p_{Y|\overline{X},\overline{A}}(y|\overline{x}, \overline{a})$, $p_{X_k|\overline{X}_{k-1},\overline{A}_{k-1}}(x_k|\overline{x}_{k-1}, \overline{a}_{k-1})$, $k = 2, \ldots, K$, and $p_{X_1}(x_1)$ as in (5.46); namely,

$$p_{Y|\overline{X},\overline{A}}(y|\overline{x}, \overline{a}; \beta_{K+1}),$$
$$p_{X_k|\overline{X}_{k-1},\overline{A}_{k-1}}(x_k|\overline{x}_{k-1}, \overline{a}_{k-1}; \beta_k), \quad k = 2, \ldots, K, \tag{6.117}$$
$$p_{X_1}(x_1; \beta_1),$$

where in (6.117) we use $\beta = (\beta_1^T, \ldots, \beta_{K+1}^T)^T$ to denote the parameters involved. The estimator $\widehat{\beta} = (\widehat{\beta}_1^T, \ldots, \widehat{\beta}_{K+1}^T)^T$ can be obtained by maximizing the partial likelihood (5.47).

For each individual i, $i = 1, \ldots, n$, if $\overline{X}_{ki} = \overline{x}_k$, we wish to estimate $E\{Y^*(d) \mid \overline{X}_k^*(\overline{d}_{k-1}) = \overline{x}_k\}$. This can be accomplished by generating a random sample of M replicates from the distribution of $Y^*(d)$ given $\overline{X}_k^*(\overline{d}_k) = \overline{x}_k$ by carrying out the following steps for $r = 1, \ldots, M$:

1. Generate $x_{k+1,r}$ from

$$p_{X_{k+1}|\overline{X}_k, \overline{A}_k}\{x_{k+1} \mid \overline{x}_k, \overline{d}_k(\overline{x}_k); \widehat{\beta}_{k+1}\}.$$

2. Continue in this fashion and generate $x_{k+j,r}$ from

$$p_{X_{k+j}|\overline{X}_{k+j-1}, \overline{A}_{k+j-1}}\{x_{k+j} \mid \overline{x}_k, x_{k+1,r}, \ldots, x_{k+j-1,r},$$
$$\overline{d}_{k+j-1}(\overline{x}_k, x_{k+1,r}, \ldots, x_{k+j-1,r}); \widehat{\beta}_{k+j}\},$$

for $j = 2, \ldots, K - k$.

3. Generate random y_r from

$$p_{Y|\overline{X}, \overline{A}}\{y|\overline{x}_k, x_{k+1,r}, \ldots, x_{K,r}, \overline{d}_K(\overline{x}_k, x_{k+1,r}, \ldots, x_{K,r}); \widehat{\beta}_{K+1}\}.$$

Obtain M replicates $y_1, \ldots, y_M$ for each $k = 1, \ldots, K$. Then take

$$L_k(\overline{X}_{ki}) = M^{-1} \sum_{r=1}^{M} y_r, \quad k = 1, \ldots, K, \tag{6.118}$$

in (6.112). This strategy involves the same significant practical challenges of development of the required models and computational intensity associated with implementation of the g-computation algorithm for direct estimation of $\mathcal{V}(d)$ discussed in Section 5.4.

Analogous to (3.29) in the single decision case, let

$$\mathcal{Q}_{d,k}(\overline{x}_k; \beta_k), \quad k = 1, \ldots, K, \tag{6.119}$$

be the models for $E\{Y^*(d) \mid \overline{X}_k^*(\overline{d}_k) = \overline{x}_k\}$ in terms of parameters β_k, $k = 1, \ldots, K$, implied by any of the foregoing three approaches. The models (6.119) resulting from the simulation-based g-computation approach are induced by the models for the densities in (6.117) and are clearly not available in a closed form. Given estimators $\widehat{\beta}_k$, $k = 1, \ldots, K$, obtained as described above and substituting the fitted models (6.114), (6.116), or (6.118) for $L_k(\overline{X}_k)$ in (6.112) leads to the estimator

$$\widehat{\mathcal{V}}_{AIPW}(d) = n^{-1} \sum_{i=1}^{n} \left[\frac{\mathcal{C}_{d,i} Y_i}{\left\{\prod_{k=2}^{K} \pi_{d,k}(\overline{X}_{ki}; \widehat{\gamma}_k)\right\} \pi_{d,1}(X_{1i}; \widehat{\gamma}_1)} \right. \tag{6.120}$$
$$\left. + \sum_{k=1}^{K} \left\{ \frac{\mathcal{C}_{\overline{d}_{k-1},i}}{\overline{\pi}_{d,k-1}(\overline{X}_{k-1,i}; \widehat{\gamma}_{k-1})} - \frac{\mathcal{C}_{\overline{d}_k,i}}{\overline{\pi}_{d,k}(\overline{X}_{k,i}, \widehat{\gamma}_k)} \right\} \mathcal{Q}_{d,k}(\overline{X}_{ki}; \widehat{\beta}_k) \right].$$

It follows from the semiparametric theory and can be verified via an argument in the spirit of that in Section 2.7 that the augmented inverse probability weighted estimator (6.120) is doubly robust; see Section 4 of the supplementary material to Zhang et al. (2013) and Tsiatis (2006, Chapter 10). That is, $\widehat{\mathcal{V}}_{AIPW}(d)$ is a consistent and asymptotically normal estimator for the true value $\mathcal{V}(d)$ if, for all $k = 1, \ldots, K$, either the models for the propensities (6.111) and thus for $\pi_{d,1}(x_1)$ and $\pi_{d,k}(\overline{x}_k)$, $k = 2, \ldots, K$, in (6.109) or the models for $E\{Y^*(d) \mid \overline{X}_k^*(\overline{d}_k) = \overline{x}_k\}$ in (6.119) are correctly specified. Thus, in principle, as in the single decision case, the estimator $\widehat{\mathcal{V}}_{AIPW}(d)$ offers protection against misspecification of these models. Of course, as discussed in Sections 6.4.1 and 6.4.2, development of these models is considerably more complicated than in the single decision case, and model misspecification is likely. If the observed data are from a SMART, in which case the propensities (6.111) and thus the forms of $\pi_{d,1}(x_1)$ and $\pi_{d,k}(\overline{x}_k)$, $k = 2, \ldots, K$, are known, $\widehat{\mathcal{V}}_{AIPW}(d)$ is guaranteed to be consistent regardless of whether or not the models $\mathcal{Q}_{d,k}(\overline{x}_k; \beta_k)$, $k = 1, \ldots, K$, in (6.119) are correctly specified.

If all of the models are correctly specified, so that the augmented inverse probability weighted estimator (6.120) is constructed using the optimal choice of $L_k(\overline{X}_k)$, $k = 1, \ldots, K$, then $\widehat{\mathcal{V}}_{AIPW}(d)$ is efficient, achieving the smallest asymptotic variance among estimators in the class (6.120). In particular, $\widehat{\mathcal{V}}_{AIPW}(d)$ can exhibit considerably less sampling variation than the simple inverse probability weighted estimators (6.100) and (6.101), which are based only on data from individuals for whom the treatment options actually received are consistent with those selected by d at all K decisions. As above, because the models $\mathcal{Q}_{d,k}(\overline{x}_k; \beta_k)$ in (6.119) are highly likely to be misspecified, full efficiency may not be achieved in practice; however, even in this case, the "augmentation term" can recover substantial information from other individuals for whom the treatments received are consistent with d only through some Decision $k < K$.

As for the simple inverse probability weighted estimators, in principle, (6.120) can be cast as an M-estimator solving an estimating equation jointly with estimating equations for $\widehat{\gamma}_k$ and $\widehat{\beta}_k$, $k = 1, \ldots, K$, and the theory for M-estimation in Section 2.5 can be used to derive an approximate large sample distribution of $\widehat{\mathcal{V}}_{AIPW}(d)$, although this can be rather involved.

Zhang et al. (2013) present the estimator (6.120) in an equivalent form that follows directly from the generic presentation in Chapters 7–10 of Tsiatis (2006). We sketch this alternative formulation here. Let D take on the values $1, \ldots, K, \infty$, where $D = 1$ if $A_1 \neq d_1(X_1)$; $D = k$ if $\overline{A}_{k-1} = \overline{d}_{k-1}(\overline{X}_{k-1})$ and $A_k \neq d_k\{X_k, \overline{d}_{k-1}(\overline{X}_{k-1})\}$, $k = 2, \ldots, K$; and $D = \infty$ if $\overline{A} = \overline{d}(\overline{X})$. Thus, D can be viewed as recording the decision point at which "dropout" occurs; i.e., $D = 1$ if an individual's actual treatment option at the first decision point is not consistent with that selected by d, $D = k$ if the treatments received are consistent with

d through Decision $k - 1$ and then deviate from d at Decision k, and $D = \infty$ indicates that the options received by the individual are the same as those selected by d for all K decisions. Define the discrete hazard of "dropout" (coarsening) given baseline information and all potential outcomes as

$$P\{D = k \mid D \geq k, X_1, W^*\}, \quad k = 1, \ldots, K.$$

Under SUTVA (6.16), the SRA (6.17) and the positivity assumption (6.23), by manipulations similar to those involved in demonstrating (6.88), it can be shown that the hazard depends on $\{X_1, W^*\}$ only through X_1 for $k = 1$ and through $\overline{X}_k^*(\overline{d}_{k-1}) = \overline{X}_k$ if $D = k$, $k = 2, \ldots, K$, so on the information observed up to the point of "dropout," and

$$P\{D = 1 \mid D \geq 1, X_1, W^*\}$$
$$= P\{A_1 \neq d_1(X_1) \mid X_1\} = \lambda_1(X_1) = 1 - \pi_{d,1}(X_1), \quad (6.121)$$
$$P\{D = k \mid D \geq k, X_k, W^*\}$$
$$= P[A_k \neq d_k\{\overline{X}_k, \overline{d}_{k-1}(\overline{X}_{k-1})\} \mid \overline{X}_k, \overline{A}_{k-1} = \overline{d}_{k-1}(\overline{X}_{k-1})]$$
$$= \lambda_k(\overline{X}_k) = 1 - \pi_{d,k}(\overline{X}_k), \quad k = 2, \ldots, K. \quad (6.122)$$

It follows using (6.110) that

$$P(D > k \mid X_1, W^*) = P(\mathcal{C}_{\overline{d}_k} = 1 \mid X_1, W^*) = \overline{\pi}_{d,k}(\overline{X}_k), \quad k = 1, \ldots, K.$$

Then the augmented inverse probability weighted estimator (6.120) can be expressed equivalently as

$$\widehat{\mathcal{V}}_{AIPW}(d) = n^{-1} \sum_{i=1}^{n} \left[\frac{I(D_i = \infty)Y_i}{\overline{\pi}_{d,K}(\overline{X}_{K,i}, \widehat{\overline{\gamma}}_K)} \right. \quad (6.123)$$

$$\left. + \sum_{k=1}^{K} \left\{ \frac{I(D_i = k) - \lambda_k(\overline{X}_{ki}; \widehat{\gamma}_k) I(D_i \geq k)}{\overline{\pi}_{d,k}(\overline{X}_{k,i}, \widehat{\overline{\gamma}}_k)} \right\} \mathcal{Q}_{d,k}(\overline{X}_{ki}; \widehat{\beta}_k) \right],$$

where $\lambda_k(\overline{X}_{ki}; \widehat{\gamma}_k) = 1 - \pi_{d,k}(\overline{X}_k; \widehat{\gamma}_k)$, $k = 1, \ldots, K$, from (6.121) and (6.122); compare (6.123) to (6) of Zhang et al. (2013), which takes $\mathcal{Q}_{d,k}(\overline{x}_k; \beta_k)$ to be based on (6.114). It is straightforward using the above definitions to demonstrate that (6.123) and (6.120) are the same.

6.4.5 Estimation via Marginal Structural Models

We close this chapter with a brief discussion of an alternative strategy for estimation of the value of a fixed regime that is appropriate when scientific interest focuses on regimes comprising simple rules that can be represented in terms of a (low-dimensional) parameter η. Suppose that attention is restricted to a subset of regimes $\mathcal{D}_\eta \subset \mathcal{D}$ with elements

$$d_\eta = \{d_1(h_1; \eta_1), \ldots, d_K(h_K; \eta_K)\}, \quad \eta = (\eta_1^T, \ldots, \eta_K^T)^T,$$

and we wish to estimate the value of a fixed regime d_{η^*} corresponding to a particular η^*, $\mathcal{V}(d_{\eta^*}) = E\{Y^*(d_{\eta^*})\}$. As in the following example, the class $\mathcal{D}_\eta$ may often be even simpler, such that $\eta = \eta_1 = \cdots = \eta_K$.

As a concrete context, consider the setting of treatment of HIV-infected patients in Sections 1.2.3 and 5.3.1. Here, patients visit the clinic monthly, at which times decisions on whether or not to administer antiretroviral therapy for the next month are made on the basis of a patient's current immunologic and virologic status, which includes CD4 T cell count (cells/mm^3), where lower CD4 counts reflect poorer immunologic status. For simplicity, we disregard the possibility of resistant virus and take the two feasible treatment options at each visit to be (i) take antiretroviral therapy for the next month, coded as 1; and (ii) do not take antiretroviral therapy for the next month, coded as 0. Suppose that interest focuses on regimes with K rules corresponding to K monthly clinic visits, which involve a common threshold η below which antiretroviral therapy is administered and above which it is not; that is,

$$d_k(h_k; \eta) = \mathrm{I}(\mathsf{CD4}_k \leq \eta), \quad k = 1, \ldots, K, \tag{6.124}$$

where $\mathsf{CD4}_k$ is the patient's CD4 T cell count (cells/mm^3) immediately prior to Decision k. Thus, the class $\mathcal{D}_\eta$ comprises regimes d_η with rules of the form (6.124) for scalar threshold η. A measure by which to assess benefit of such regimes for HIV treatment may be the patient's viral load, the concentration of viral RNA present in the blood (viral RNA copies/ml), ascertained one month after the final, Kth visit, where lower values are desirable. Thus, let the outcome of interest be negative viral load following Decision K, so that $Y^*(d_\eta)$ is a patient's negative viral load if he were to be administered antiretroviral therapy at all K decision points according to regime d_η, and larger values of $Y^*(d_\eta)$ are preferred.

Suppose we are interested in the value of regime d_{η^*} with rules of the form (6.124) for a particular threshold η^*, $\mathcal{V}(d_{\eta^*})$. If data are available from a dedicated study in which participants were assigned to receive treatment at each decision point according to the rules in d_{η^*} and negative viral load following Decision K was ascertained, it is straightforward to estimate $\mathcal{V}(d_{\eta^*})$ based on the observed data. However, it is likely that no such study would have been conducted and that the data available for this task are observational, involving n patients who visited the clinic monthly for whom, at each of K such visits, the information X_k, $k = 1, \ldots, K$, collected at baseline ($k = 1$) and in the intervening periods between visits includes $CD4_k$; and the options A_k actually received at visits $k = 1, \ldots, K$ and final viral load measured one month after visit K are recorded. Because patients will have received antiretroviral therapy (1) or not (0) at each visit at the discretion of clinicians, there may be a paucity of patients in the data whose actual treatment experience is consistent with having followed regime d_{η^*}.

A strategy for using such data to estimate $\mathcal{V}(d_{\eta^*})$ can be based on the work of Orellana et al. (2010a,b), who proposed adopting a parsimonious model for $\mathcal{V}(d_\eta)$ as a function of η depending on a parameter α, which can be estimated from the observed data. Estimation of $\mathcal{V}(d_{\eta^*})$ is then accomplished by substituting η^* in the fitted model. Specifically, if, in truth, $\mathcal{V}(d_\eta) = E\{Y^*(d_\eta)\} = \mu(\eta)$ for some function $\mu(\cdot)$, posit a parametric model for $\mu(\eta)$ in terms of a finite-dimensional parameter α,

$$\mu(\eta; \alpha), \tag{6.125}$$

referred to as a *marginal structural model*. For example, in the HIV setting, we might specify a model quadratic in the threshold η,

$$\mu(\eta; \alpha) = \alpha_1 + \alpha_2 \eta + \alpha_3 \eta^2, \quad \alpha = (\alpha_1, \alpha_2, \alpha_3)^T. \tag{6.126}$$

By analogy to a standard regression model, in (6.125), η plays the role of the "covariate." If we fit the structural model (6.125) based on observed data to obtain an estimator $\widehat{\alpha}$ for α by suitable methods discussed next, then, for a specific threshold η^* of interest, the value of d_{η^*} can be estimated by

$$\widehat{\mathcal{V}}_{MSM}(d_{\eta^*}) = \mu(\eta^*; \widehat{\alpha}),$$

analogous to a "predicted value" at a particular setting of interest of the "covariate" in standard regression. The hope is that the structural model is a correct specification of the true relationship $\mu(\eta)$ between the value $\mathcal{V}(d_\eta)$ and η across a plausible range of thresholds of interest, in which case $\widehat{\mathcal{V}}_{MSM}(d_{\eta^*})$ should be a reliable estimator for $\mathcal{V}(d_{\eta^*})$.

We now describe an approach to estimation of α from observational data as above. In such observed data, some individuals will have realized treatments received consistent with more than one value of η, and some may have experience that is not consistent with any threshold η. To appreciate this, consider $K = 2$. An individual for whom $CD4_1=300$ with $A_1 = 1$ and $CD4_2=400$ with $A_2 = 0$ has realized treatment experience consistent with regimes d_η with η equal to any value in the interval $[300, 400)$. Likewise, an individual with $CD4_1=300$ with $A_1 = 1$ and $CD4_2=400$ with $A_2 = 1$ has treatment experience consistent with $\eta \geq 400$, and an individual with $CD4_1=300$ with $A_1 = 0$ and $CD4_2=400$ with $A_2 = 0$ has actual treatments received consistent with $\eta < 300$.

The treatment experience for an individual for whom $CD4_1 = 300$ with $A_1 = 0$ and $CD4_2 = 400$ with $A_2 = 1$ is not consistent with following any regime d_η of the form (6.124).

An estimator $\widehat{\alpha}$ for α based on these data can be found as the solution to

$$\sum_{i=1}^{n} \int_{\mathcal{D}_\eta} \left[\frac{\mathcal{C}_{d_\eta, i}}{\left\{ \prod_{k=2}^{K} \pi_{d_\eta, k}(\overline{X}_{ki}; \widehat{\gamma}_k) \right\} \pi_{d_\eta, 1}(X_{1i}; \widehat{\gamma}_1)} \right.$$
$$\left. \times \frac{\partial \mu(\eta; \alpha)}{\partial \alpha} w(\eta) \{ Y_i - \mu(\eta; \alpha) \} \right] d\nu(d_\eta) = 0, \qquad (6.127)$$

where $d\nu(d_\eta)$ is some appropriate dominating measure placed on $d_\eta \in \mathcal{D}_\eta$. As an example, if interest focuses on thresholds in the range $[100, 500]$, for a specified finite partition of this range $\eta_{(j)}$, $j = 1, \ldots, m$, say $\eta_{(j)} = 100 + 400(j-1)/(m-1)$, taking $d\nu(d_\eta)$ to place point mass on the $\eta_{(j)}$, (6.127) becomes

$$\sum_{i=1}^{n} \sum_{j=1}^{m} \left[\frac{\mathcal{C}_{d_{\eta_{(j)}}, i}}{\left\{ \prod_{k=2}^{K} \pi_{d_{\eta_{(j)}}, k}(\overline{X}_{ki}; \widehat{\gamma}_k) \right\} \pi_{d_{\eta_{(j)}}, 1}(X_{1i}; \widehat{\gamma}_1)} \right.$$
$$\left. \times \frac{\partial \mu(\eta_{(j)}; \alpha)}{\partial \alpha} w(\eta_{(j)}) \{ Y_i - \mu(\eta_{(j)}; \alpha) \} \right] = 0. \qquad (6.128)$$

In (6.127) and (6.128), a given individual i can contribute information on multiple thresholds in the range of interest or none at all, and each of his contributions is weighted by the reciprocal of an estimator for the propensity of receiving treatment consistent with d_η or $d_{\eta_{(j)}}$ given observed history, as for the inverse probability weighted estimator (6.100).

Under SUTVA (6.16), the SRA (6.17), and the positivity assumption (6.23), and assuming that the marginal structural model $\mu(\eta; \alpha)$ and the models for the propensities (6.111) and thus for $\pi_{d,1}(x_1)$ and $\pi_{d,k}(\overline{x}_k)$, $k = 2, \ldots, K$, are all correctly specified, by manipulations analogous to those leading to (6.89), it can be shown that (6.127) is an unbiased estimating equation for the true value of α. In the context of (6.128), as long as the data involve a sufficient number of individuals who received treatment consistent with at least one $\eta_{(j)}$, $j = 1, \ldots, m$, the estimator $\widehat{\alpha}$ should be reasonable in practice.

In particular, under these conditions, the estimators for α found by solving (6.127) or (6.128) jointly with estimating equations leading to the estimator $\widehat{\gamma}_k$, $k = 1, \ldots, K$, are M-estimators. Accordingly, $\widehat{\alpha}$ so obtained is consistent and asymptotically normal, and an approximate large sample sampling distribution for the estimator $\widehat{\mathcal{V}}_{MSM}(d_{\eta^*}) = \mu(\eta^*; \widehat{\alpha})$, can be obtained using standard theory for M-estimation.

These estimating equations are based on simple inverse probability weighting. It is possible by appealing to semiparametric theory to derive augmented inverse probability weighted estimating equations for estimation of α and to identify that leading to the efficient estimator. This is rather involved and is not presented here; see Orellana et al. (2010a,b).

In general, as $\mathcal{D}$ is Ψ-specific for some feasible sets Ψ, regimes in the class $\mathcal{D}_\eta$ must be Ψ-specific. If estimation is to be based on observational data, the regimes d_η must also be feasible regimes in the sense described at the end of Section 6.2.4.

Remark. Marginal structural models were first introduced to represent the value for a specified static treatment regime (e.g. Mark and Robins, 1993; Robins, 1997, 1999a,b; Hernán et al., 2000; Robins et al., 2000). As discussed in Section 6.2.2, static regimes are of little interest in precision medicine. Moreover, there may be no or only a few static regimes in $\mathcal{D}$; such regimes must comprise options at each decision point that are feasible for all possible histories. Accordingly, we do not review this early work involving static regimes. This work does provide the foundation for the approach to value estimation based on marginal structural models for dynamic regimes presented here.

6.5 Application

Implementations of estimators for the value of a fixed regime introduced in this chapter are demonstrated on the book's companion website given in the Preface. All codes used to generate simulated data and to implement each method are available on the website.

Chapter 7

Optimal Multiple Decision Treatment Regimes

7.1 Introduction

In this chapter, we build on the developments in Chapter 6 and present a rigorous exposition of optimal Ψ-specific multiple (K) decision treatment regimes within the class of Ψ-specific regimes $\mathcal{D}$ for a given specification $\Psi = (\Psi_1, \ldots, \Psi_K)$ of feasible sets. The reader should review Chapters 5 and 6 before approaching this material, as the notation and definitions introduced in these chapters are used here for the most part without comment. Chapter 5 provides a less formal discussion of optimal multiple decision regimes that serves as a prelude to the account here, and Chapter 6 establishes the framework involving feasible sets and the assumptions required.

We first give a careful characterization of an optimal regime d^{opt} in terms of potential outcomes using the principle of backward induction and demonstrate that a regime so characterized is indeed optimal; that is, satisfies

$$E\{Y^*(d^{opt})\} \geq E\{Y^*(d)\} \text{ for all } d \in \mathcal{D}$$

as in (6.13). Under the identifiability assumptions presented in Chapter 6 in the context of the class $\mathcal{D}$ of Ψ-specific regimes, we then show that an optimal regime characterized in terms of potential outcomes can be expressed equivalently in terms of the observed data.

In this development, an optimal regime comprises K decision rules corresponding to K decision points, and the implicit goal is to implement it in patients who start following the rules at the outset, so at Decision 1. However, in routine clinical practice, a patient may present at a decision point subsequent to the first having already received treatment options at prior decision points according to a mechanism different from that dictated by the corresponding rules in an optimal regime in $\mathcal{D}$. Of natural interest in this situation is how to treat such a patient optimally henceforth. We discuss formulation of an optimal regime for treating patients who present "midstream" in the sequence of K decisions.

The rest of the chapter provides an account of methods for estimation of an optimal Ψ-specific regime, both those introduced in Chapter 5 and additional approaches not discussed in that chapter. As in Chapters 5 and 6, we focus mostly on the use of parametric models, although more flexible models are discussed in Sections 7.4.4, 7.4.6, and 7.4.8.

7.2 Characterization of an Optimal Regime

7.2.1 Ψ-Specific Regimes

For convenience, we summarize the definitions of a Ψ-specific regime d and the class $\mathcal{D}$ for a given specification of feasible sets $\Psi = (\Psi_1, \ldots, \Psi_K)$. As in Section 6.2.4, define

$$\Gamma_1 = \{x_1 \in \mathcal{X}_1 \text{ satisfying } P(X_1 = x_1) > 0\}, \tag{7.1}$$

$$\Lambda_1 = \{(x_1, a_1) \text{ such that } x_1 = h_1 \in \Gamma_1, \ a_1 \in \Psi_1(h_1)\};$$

and, for $k = 2, \ldots, K$, define

$$\Gamma_k = \Big[h_k = (\overline{x}_k, \overline{a}_{k-1}) \in \overline{\mathcal{X}}_k \times \overline{\mathcal{A}}_{k-1} \text{ satisfying } (\overline{x}_{k-1}, \overline{a}_{k-1}) \in \Lambda_{k-1}$$

$$\text{and } P\{X_k^*(\overline{a}_{k-1}) = x_k \mid \overline{X}_{k-1}^*(\overline{a}_{k-2}) = \overline{x}_{k-1}\} > 0 \Big] \tag{7.2}$$

as in (6.21) and

$$\Lambda_k = \{(\overline{x}_k, \overline{a}_k) \text{ such that } (\overline{x}_k, \overline{a}_{k-1}) = h_k \in \Gamma_k, \ a_k \in \Psi_k(h_k)\}.$$

For $k = 2, \ldots, K$, $\Gamma_k \subseteq \mathcal{H}_k$ contains all possible histories h_k that are consistent with having followed a Ψ-specific regime through Decision $k - 1$, and Λ_k is the set of all possible histories $h_k \in \Gamma_k$ and associated treatment options in $\Psi_k(h_k)$ at Decision k, $k = 1, \ldots, K$. As in Section 6.3, assume also that the potential outcome $Y^*(\overline{a})$ and observed outcome Y take values $y \in \mathcal{Y}$, and let

$$\Gamma_{K+1} = \Big[(\overline{x}, \overline{a}, y) \in \overline{\mathcal{X}} \times \overline{\mathcal{A}} \times \mathcal{Y} \text{ satisfying } (\overline{x}, \overline{a}) \in \Lambda_K \text{ and}$$

$$P\{Y^*(\overline{a}) = y \mid \overline{X}_K^*(\overline{a}_{K-1}) = \overline{x}_K\} > 0 \Big] \tag{7.3}$$

as in (6.39).

With these definitions, a Ψ-specific regime $d = (d_1, \ldots, d_K)$ consists of rules $d_k(h_k)$ such that d_k maps from the sets Γ_k in (7.1) and (7.2) to $\mathcal{A}_k$; that is,

$$d_k : \ \Gamma_k \to \mathcal{A}_k,$$

satisfying $d_k(h_k) \in \Psi_k(h_k)$ for every $h_k \in \Gamma_k$, $k = 1, \ldots, K$. The class $\mathcal{D}$ of all Ψ-specific regimes is the set of all such K-decision regimes $d = (d_1, \ldots, d_K)$. As in Chapter 6, the dependence on Ψ is suppressed in the notation, but it is critical to recognize that these definitions are Ψ-specific.

As discussed in Section 6.2.2, if there are ℓ_k distinct subsets $\mathcal{A}_{k,l} \subseteq \mathcal{A}_k$, $l = 1, \ldots, \ell_k$, that are feasible sets at Decision k, $d_k(h_k)$ may be a collection of rules $d_{k,l}(h_k)$ for $\mathcal{A}_{k,l}$, where $d_{k,l}$ maps from a set $\Gamma_{k,l} \subseteq \Gamma_k$ to $\mathcal{A}_{k,l}$ and thus $\mathcal{A}_k$, and $d_{k,l}(h_k) \in \Psi_k(h_k)$. With $s_k(h_k) = 1, \ldots, \ell_k$ indicating which of these distinct subsets corresponds to $\Psi_k(h_k)$ for given h_k, from (6.8),

$$d_k(h_k) = \sum_{l=1}^{\ell_k} \mathrm{I}\{s_k(h_k) = l\} d_{k,l}(h_k). \tag{7.4}$$

The goal is to characterize an optimal regime $d^{opt} \in \mathcal{D}$ such that

$$E\{Y^*(d^{opt})\} \geq E\{Y^*(d)\} \quad \text{for all } d \in \mathcal{D} \tag{7.5}$$

and to estimate d^{opt} from observed data.

The foregoing framework and definitions of regimes $d \in \mathcal{D}$ and of an optimal regime are in terms of potential outcomes, as is the characterization of an optimal regime in $\mathcal{D}$ in Section 7.2.2, presented next. Estimation of an optimal regime is predicated on an equivalent characterization in terms of observed data

$$(X_1, A_1, X_2, A_2, \ldots, X_K, A_K, Y). \tag{7.6}$$

As demonstrated in Section 6.2.4, under SUTVA (6.16), the SRA (6.17), and the positivity assumption (6.23) given by

$$P(A_k = a_k | H_k = h_k) = P(A_k = a_k | \overline{X}_k = \overline{x}_k, \overline{A}_{k-1} = \overline{a}_{k-1}) > 0$$
$$\text{for } h_k = (\overline{x}_k, \overline{a}_{k-1}) \in \Gamma_k, \quad \text{and} \quad a_k \in \Psi_k(h_k) = \Psi_k(\overline{x}_k, \overline{a}_{k-1}),$$
$$k = 1, \ldots, K, \tag{7.7}$$

(7.2) and (7.3) can be written equivalently as

$$\Gamma_k = \Big[h_k = (\overline{x}_k, \overline{a}_{k-1}) \in \overline{\mathcal{X}}_k \times \overline{\mathcal{A}}_{k-1} \text{ satisfying } (\overline{x}_{k-1}, \overline{a}_{k-1}) \in \Lambda_{k-1}$$
$$\text{and } P(X_k = x_k \mid \overline{X}_{k-1} = \overline{x}_{k-1}, \overline{A}_{k-1} = \overline{a}_{k-1}) > 0 \Big] \tag{7.8}$$

for $k = 2, \ldots, K$ and

$$\Gamma_{K+1} = \Big[(\overline{x}, \overline{a}, y) \in \overline{\mathcal{X}} \times \overline{\mathcal{A}} \times \mathcal{Y} \text{ satisfying } (\overline{x}, \overline{a}) \in \Lambda_K \text{ and}$$
$$P(Y = y \mid \overline{X} = \overline{x}, \overline{A} = \overline{a}) > 0 \Big]. \tag{7.9}$$

In Section 7.2.4, under these assumptions, we use (7.8) and (7.9) to derive this equivalent characterization of an optimal regime.

7.2.2   Characterization in Terms of Potential Outcomes

We now describe formally how an optimal K-decision treatment regime is characterized based on the principle of backward induction. As noted in Section 5.6, because an optimal regime $d^{opt} \in \mathcal{D}$ maximizes the value $\mathcal{V}(d) = E\{Y^*(d)\}$ and thus satisfies (7.5), it is natural that this characterization is in terms of X_1 and the potential outcomes

$$W^* = \Big\{ X_2^*(a_1), X_3^*(\overline{a}_2), \ldots, X_K^*(\overline{a}_{K-1}), Y^*(\overline{a}),$$

$$\text{for } a_1 \in \mathcal{A}_1, \overline{a}_2 \in \overline{\mathcal{A}}_2, \ldots, \overline{a}_{K-1} \in \overline{\mathcal{A}}_{K-1}, \overline{a} \in \overline{\mathcal{A}} \Big\},$$

given in (6.4). In the next section, we provide a formal proof that a regime so characterized is an optimal regime in that it satisfies (7.5).

$K = 2$ Decisions

As in Section 5.6, we first present the reasoning in detail for $K = 2$ decisions and then discuss the general case.

Consider a randomly chosen individual. At the final decision point, Decision 2, if she started with realized baseline information $X_1 = x_1 = h_1 \in \Gamma_1$ and received option $a_1 \in \Psi_1(x_1) = \Psi_1(h_1)$ at Decision 1, she will have already achieved intervening information $X_2^*(a_1)$. Thus, the optimal decision that can be made now, at Decision 2, with the Decision 1 option a_1 and $\overline{X}_2^*(a_1) = \{X_1, X_2^*(a_1)\}$ already determined and having realized value $\overline{x}_2 = (x_1, x_2)$, $h_2 = (\overline{x}_2, a_1) \in \Gamma_2$, is to choose the option $a_2 \in \Psi_2(h_2)$ that would result in the largest expected outcome given that she is at this point. The outcome that the individual would achieve under option $a_2 \in \Psi_2(h_2)$, having already received a_1 at Decision 1, is $Y^*(a_1, a_2)$. Accordingly, her expected outcome given where she is now is

$$E\{Y^*(a_1, a_2)|\overline{X}_2^*(a_1) = \overline{x}_2\}. \tag{7.10}$$

Now $(\overline{x}_2, \overline{a}_2) = (\overline{x}, \overline{a}) \in \Lambda_2$, so, assuming that $Y^*(\overline{a}_2)$ takes values $y \in \mathcal{Y}$ so that $(\overline{x}, \overline{a}, y) \in \Gamma_3$ as in (7.3) with $K = 2$, (7.10) is well defined.

This suggests that an optimal Ψ-specific rule at Decision 2 should select $a_2 \in \Psi_2(h_2)$ to maximize (7.10); that is, an optimal rule should be of the form

$$d_2^{opt}(h_2) = d_2^{opt}(\overline{x}_2, a_1) = \underset{a_2 \in \Psi_2(h_2)}{\arg\max} \; E\{Y^*(a_1, a_2)|\overline{X}_2^*(a_1) = \overline{x}_2\}. \tag{7.11}$$

An optimal Decision 2 rule (7.11) thus takes as input an individual's history $h_2 = (\overline{x}_2, a_1) = (x_1, x_2, a_1) \in \Gamma_2$ and chooses the treatment option in $\Psi_2(h_2)$ that maximizes expected outcome given this history.

From (7.11), this maximum expected outcome is

$$V_2(h_2) = V_2(\overline{x}_2, a_1) = \max_{a_2 \in \Psi_2(h_2)} E\{Y^*(a_1, a_2) | \overline{X}_2^*(a_1) = \overline{x}_2\}. \quad (7.12)$$

Now consider Decision 1. If a randomly chosen individual presents with baseline information $X_1 = x_1 = h_1 \in \Gamma_1$, the optimal decision that can be made at this point is to choose the option $a_1 \in \Psi_1(h_1)$ that maximizes her expected outcome given $X_1 = x_1$, taking into account that she will receive treatment at Decision 2 by following the optimal rule d_2^{opt} in (7.11). If option $a_1 \in \Psi_1(h_1)$ is selected at Decision 1, the individual will present at Decision 2 with information $\overline{X}_2^*(a_1) = \{x_1, X_2^*(a_1)\}$; we represent the intervening information $X_2^*(a_1)$ between Decisions 1 and 2 as a random variable, as it is yet to be determined at Decision 1. Upon receiving treatment in the feasible set $\Psi_2\{x_1, X_2^*(a_1), a_1\}$ according to d_2^{opt}, she will have expected outcome given this information equal to

$$V_2\{x_1, X_2^*(a_1), a_1\} = \max_{a_2 \in \Psi_2\{x_1, X_2^*(a_1), a_1\}} E\{Y^*(a_1, a_2) | X_2^*(a_1), X_1 = x_1\}$$

in (7.12).

This implies that $a_1 \in \Psi_1(h_1)$ should be chosen so as to make the expected value of $V_2\{x_1, X_2^*(a_1), a_1\}$, given X_1 evaluated at $X_1 = x_1$, as large as possible. That is, if the realized value of $X_1 = x_1$, an optimal rule at Decision 1 should be of the form

$$d_1^{opt}(h_1) = d_1^{opt}(x_1) = \arg\max_{a_1 \in \Psi_1(h_1)} E[V_2\{x_1, X_2^*(a_1), a_1\} | X_1 = x_1], \quad (7.13)$$

where the conditional expectation in (7.13) is well defined because $(x_1, a_1) \in \Lambda_1$ and $X_2^*(a_1)$ takes values in Γ_2. The Decision 1 rule in (7.13) thus selects $a_1 \in \Psi_1(h_1)$ to maximize the maximum expected outcome that would result from choosing the feasible treatment option at Decision 2 optimally given the history available at that point. The resulting maximum of the maximum expected outcome that an individual presenting with realized baseline information x_1 would achieve if rules d_1^{opt} and d_2^{opt} are used to select treatment options at Decisions 1 and 2 is then

$$V_1(h_1) = V_1(x_1) = \max_{a_1 \in \Psi_1(h_1)} E[V_2\{x_1, X_2^*(a_1), a_1\} | X_1 = x_1]$$

$$= \max_{a_1 \in \Psi_1(h_1)} E\left[\max_{a_2 \in \Psi_2\{x_1, X_2^*(a_1), a_1\}} E\{Y^*(a_1, a_2) | X_2^*(a_1), X_1 = x_1\} \middle| X_1 = x_1 \right].$$

Clearly, $d^{opt} = (d_1^{opt}, d_2^{opt})$ defined by (7.11) and (7.13) is a set of rules, each corresponding to a decision point and mapping an individual's history to feasible treatment options. Intuition suggests that d^{opt}

is in fact an optimal regime. We prove this formally for general K shortly.

Remark. As discussed in Section 7.2.1, if there are ℓ_k distinct subsets $\mathcal{A}_{k,l}$ of $\mathcal{A}_k$, $l = 1, \ldots, \ell_k$, that are feasible sets at Decision k, $k = 1, 2$, a rule d_k for $d \in \mathcal{D}$ can comprise different rules corresponding to each subset. Consistent with this, the rules d_2^{opt} and d_1^{opt} defined in (7.11) and (7.13) can be composed of several rules, as follows. For definiteness, consider Decision 2 and the acute leukemia setting of Section 1.2.1. Here, there are two distinct subsets of $\mathcal{A}_2$ that are feasible sets, corresponding to the options for which a patient is eligible depending on her response status; and, as in Section 7.2.1, any decision rule d_2 would naturally involve separate rules for responders and nonresponders as in (7.4). The definition (7.11) leads straightforwardly to such a d_2^{opt}. If h_2 indicates response, maximization is over $\Psi_2(h_2) = \{\mathsf{M}_1, \mathsf{M}_2\}$, defining a rule for such h_2 that chooses between these two options. Likewise, if h_2 indicates nonresponse, maximization is over $\Psi_2(h_2) = \{\mathsf{S}_1, \mathsf{S}_2\}$ so defines a rule for such h_2 selecting one of the salvage options. This of course extends to the general case of K decisions presented next. We discuss this further in the context of estimation of an optimal regime in Section 7.4.

K Decisions

The foregoing backward inductive reasoning extends to the general K decision case. A randomly chosen individual at the final, Kth decision point presenting at baseline with information $X_1 = x_1 = h_1 \in \Gamma_1$ has already received options $a_k \in \Psi_k(h_k)$, $k = 1, \ldots, K - 1$, on the basis of achieved intervening information $\overline{X}_{K-1}^*(\overline{a}_{K-2}) = \{X_1, X_2^*(a_1), \ldots, X_{K-1}^*(\overline{a}_{K-2})\}$ and has additional information $X_K^*(\overline{a}_{K-1})$ that has accrued since Decision $K - 1$. Thus, the optimal decision at Decision K, with $\overline{a}_{K-1}$ and $\overline{X}_K^*(\overline{a}_{K-1})$ already determined with realized value $\overline{x}_K = (x_1, \ldots, x_K)$, so that $h_K = (\overline{x}_K, \overline{a}_{K-1}) \in \Gamma_K$, is to choose $a_K \in \Psi_K(h_K)$ such that his expected outcome given he is at this point is largest; that is, to maximize in a_K

$$E\{Y^*(\overline{a}_{K-1}, a_K) \mid \overline{X}_K^*(\overline{a}_{K-1}) = \overline{x}_K\}.$$

Thus, for any $\overline{x}_K \in \overline{\mathcal{X}}_K$, $\overline{a}_{K-1} \in \overline{\mathcal{A}}_{K-1}$ for which $h_K = (\overline{x}_K, \overline{a}_{K-1}) \in \Gamma_K$, define

$$d_K^{(1)opt}(h_K) = \underset{a_K \in \Psi_K(h_K)}{\arg\max} \ E\{Y^*(\overline{a}_{K-1}, a_K) | \overline{X}_K^*(\overline{a}_{K-1}) = \overline{x}_K\}, \quad (7.14)$$

and define the maximum expected outcome achieved as

$$V_K^{(1)}(h_K) = \underset{a_K \in \Psi_K(h_K)}{\max} \ E\{Y^*(\overline{a}_{K-1}, a_K) | \overline{X}_K^*(\overline{a}_{K-1}) = \overline{x}_K\}. \quad (7.15)$$

In (7.14) and (7.15) and in analogous expressions for $k = 1, \ldots, K - 1$ below, the superscript "(1)" is meant to indicate explicitly that the rules pertain to a patient presenting at Decision 1, to distinguish this situation from that in which a patient presents at a subsequent decision point, discussed in Section 7.3.

Stepping back to Decision $K - 1$, an individual will present at this decision point with intervening information $\overline{X}^*_{K-1}(\overline{a}_{K-2})$ already determined following administration of options $a_k \in \Psi_k(h_k)$, $k = 1, \ldots, K-2$, with realized value $\overline{x}_{K-1} \in \mathcal{X}_{K-1}$, such that $h_{K-1} = (\overline{x}_{K-1}, \overline{a}_{K-2}) \in \Gamma_{K-1}$. We wish now to select an option in $\Psi_{K-1}(h_{K-1})$ to maximize his expected outcome given that he already has this history and acknowledging that he will go on to receive treatment at Decision K by following the rule $d^{(1)opt}_K$ in (7.14). Analogous to Decision 1 in the case $K = 2$ above, if option $a_{K-1} \in \Psi_{K-1}(h_{K-1})$ is selected now at Decision $K - 1$, the individual will present at Decision K with information $\overline{X}^*_K(\overline{a}_{K-1}) = \{\overline{x}_{K-1}, X^*_K(\overline{a}_{K-1})\}$, and, upon receiving an option in the feasible set $\Psi_K\{\overline{x}_{K-1}, X^*_K(\overline{a}_{K-1}), \overline{a}_{K-1}\}$ dictated by $d^{(1)opt}_K$, will have expected outcome given this information equal to, from (7.15),

$$V^{(1)}_K\{\overline{x}_{K-1}, X^*_K(\overline{a}_{K-1}), \overline{a}_{K-1}\}$$
$$= \max_{\substack{a_K \in \\ \Psi_K\{\overline{x}_{K-1}, X^*_K(\overline{a}_{K-1}), \overline{a}_{K-1}\}}} E\{Y^*(\overline{a}_{K-1}, a_K) | X^*_K(\overline{a}_{K-1}), \overline{X}^*_{K-1}(\overline{a}_{K-2}) = \overline{x}_{K-1}\}.$$

This suggests that $a_{K-1} \in \Psi_{K-1}(h_{K-1})$ should be chosen to make the expected value of $V^{(1)}_K\{\overline{x}_{K-1}, X^*_K(\overline{a}_{K-1}), \overline{a}_{K-1}\}$ given $\overline{X}^*_{K-1}(\overline{a}_{K-2}) = \overline{x}_{K-1}$ as large as possible, leading to the rule

$$d^{(1)opt}_{K-1}(h_{K-1}) \tag{7.16}$$
$$= \operatorname*{arg\,max}_{a_{K-1} \in \Psi_{K-1}(h_{K-1})} E[V^{(1)}_K\{\overline{x}_{K-1}, X^*_K(\overline{a}_{K-2}, a_{K-1}), \overline{a}_{K-2}, a_{K-1}\}$$
$$| \overline{X}^*_{K-1}(\overline{a}_{K-2}) = \overline{x}_{K-1}]$$

and maximum expected outcome achieved

$$V^{(1)}_{K-1}(h_{K-1})$$
$$= \max_{a_{K-1} \in \Psi_{K-1}(h_{K-1})} E[V^{(1)}_K\{\overline{x}_{K-1}, X^*_K(\overline{a}_{K-2}, a_{K-1}), \overline{a}_{K-2}, a_{K-1}\}$$
$$| \overline{X}^*_{K-1}(\overline{a}_{K-2}) = \overline{x}_{K-1}].$$

Continuing with this reasoning, for $k = K-2, \ldots, 2$ and any $\overline{x}_k \in \overline{\mathcal{X}}_k$, $\overline{a}_{k-1} \in \overline{\mathcal{A}}_{k-1}$ for which $h_k = (\overline{x}_k, \overline{a}_{k-1}) \in \Gamma_k$, let

$$d^{(1)opt}_k(h_k) \tag{7.17}$$
$$= \operatorname*{arg\,max}_{a_k \in \Psi_k(h_k)} E[V^{(1)}_{k+1}\{\overline{x}_k, X^*_{k+1}(\overline{a}_{k-1}, a_k), \overline{a}_{k-1}, a_k\} | \overline{X}^*_k(\overline{a}_{k-1}) = \overline{x}_k]$$

and

$$V_k^{(1)}(h_k) = \max_{a_k \in \Psi_k(h_k)} E[V_{k+1}^{(1)}\{\overline{x}_k, X_{k+1}^*(\overline{a}_{k-1}, a_k), \overline{a}_{k-1}, a_k\}|\overline{X}_k^*(\overline{a}_{k-1}) = \overline{x}_k].$$

(7.18)

Finally, for $k = 1$,

$$d_1^{(1)opt}(x_1) = \arg\max_{a_1 \in \Psi_1(h_1)} E[V_2^{(1)}\{x_1, X_2^*(a_1), a_1\}|X_1 = x_1]$$ (7.19)

and

$$V_1^{(1)}(x_1) = \max_{a_1 \in \Psi_1(h_1)} E[V_2^{(1)}\{x_1, X_2^*(a_1), a_1\}|X_1 = x_1].$$ (7.20)

As in the case $K = 2$ above, all of the conditional expectations in (7.14)–(7.20) are well defined because $h_k \in \Gamma_k$, $k = 1, \ldots, K$.

By the definition of $d_K^{(1)opt}(h_K)$ in (7.14), $d_K^{(1)opt}(h_K)$ is the element of $\Psi_K(h_K)$ at which the maximum in (7.15) is achieved, and thus $V_K^{(1)}(h_K)$ in (7.15) can be written equivalently as

$$V_K^{(1)}(h_K) = E[Y^*\{\overline{a}_{K-1}, d_K^{(1)opt}(h_K)\}|\overline{X}_K^*(\overline{a}_{K-1}) = \overline{x}_K].$$

Similarly, by the definition of $d_k^{(1)opt}(h_k)$ in (7.17), $k = K - 1, \ldots, 2$, $V_k^{(1)}(h_k)$ in (7.18) can be written as

$$V_k^{(1)}(h_k) = E\left(V_{k+1}^{(1)}\left[\overline{x}_k, X_{k+1}^*\{\overline{a}_{k-1}, d_k^{(1)opt}(h_k)\}, \overline{a}_{k-1}, d_k^{(1)opt}(h_k)\right]\right|$$
$$\overline{X}_k^*(\overline{a}_{k-1}) = \overline{x}_k\Bigg),$$

and

$$V_1^{(1)}(h_1) = E\left(V_2^{(1)}\left[x_1, X_2^*\{d_1^{(1)opt}(h_1)\}, d_1^{(1)opt}(h_1)\right]\bigg| X_1 = x_1\right).$$

It is clear that $d^{(1)opt} = (d_1^{(1)opt}, \ldots, d_K^{(1)opt})$ defined above is a treatment regime in $\mathcal{D}$, as it comprises a set of rules, each of which uses patient information accrued to each decision point to assign treatment from among the possible options in Ψ. By the backward recursive construction, each rule in $d^{(1)opt}$ selects the treatment from among the feasible options that maximizes the expected potential outcome given prior potential information accrued to that point that would be achieved if subsequent optimal rules were to be followed henceforth. Intuition suggests that this should lead to the maximum achievable expected potential outcome and thus that $d^{(1)opt}$ is an optimal regime.

Remark. As discussed in Section 5.6, at any decision point $k = 1, \ldots, K$, for some $h_k \in \Gamma_k$, it is possible that more than one treatment option in $\Psi_k(h_k)$ achieves the maximum in (7.15), (7.18), or (7.20). If so, there is more than one possible rule $d_k^{(1)opt}$, each selecting a different option that leads to the maximum for such an h_k, so that an optimal regime need not be unique. A unique representation can be defined by choosing one of these options in $\Psi_k(h_k)$ as the default. We downplay this issue in the sequel and assume without comment that such a default has been specified in discussions where a unique representation is implicit.

7.2.3 Justification

In this section, we confirm the intuition that $d^{(1)opt} \in \mathcal{D}$ defined by (7.14), (7.16), (7.17) for $k = K - 2, \ldots, 2$, and (7.19), is an optimal regime via an explicit "brute force" argument.

Optimality of $d^{(1)opt} \in \mathcal{D}$

We show that

$$E\{Y^*(d^{(1)opt})\} \geq E\{Y^*(d)\} \quad \text{for all } d \in \mathcal{D} \tag{7.21}$$

as in (7.5).

Proof. From (6.11) in Section 6.2.3, recall that, for any d in the class $\mathcal{D}$ of Ψ-specific regimes, $Y^*(d)$ is defined formally in terms of W^* as

$$Y^*(d) = \sum_{\bar{a} \in \bar{\mathcal{A}}} Y^*(\bar{a}) \prod_{j=1}^{K} \mathrm{I}\left[d_j\{\overline{X}_j^*(\bar{a}_{j-1}), \bar{a}_{j-1}\} = a_j\right], \tag{7.22}$$

where, by the remark near the end of Section 6.2.4, the product in (7.22) is zero for realizations $(\bar{x}_K, \bar{a}_{K-1}) \notin \Gamma_K$. The expression (7.22) can be written equivalently as

$$Y^*(d) = \sum_{\bar{a}_{K-1} \in \bar{\mathcal{A}}_{K-1}} \left(\prod_{j=1}^{K-1} \mathrm{I}\left[d_j\{\overline{X}_j^*(\bar{a}_{j-1}), \bar{a}_{j-1}\} = a_j\right] \right.$$
$$\left. \times Y^*\left[\bar{a}_{K-1}, d_K\{\overline{X}_K^*(\bar{a}_{K-1}), \bar{a}_{K-1}\}\right] \right). \tag{7.23}$$

By $Y^*\left[\bar{a}_{K-1}, d_K\{\overline{X}_K^*(\bar{a}_{K-1}), \bar{a}_{K-1}\}\right]$ in (7.23), we mean the potential outcome if an individual were to receive options $\bar{a}_{K-1} = (a_1, \ldots, a_{K-1})$ at the first $K - 1$ decisions and then receive the option at Decision K dictated by d_K for this treatment history and the associated intervening information $\overline{X}_K^*(\overline{a}_{K-1})$ up to Decision K. From (7.23), it follows that, for any $d \in \mathcal{D}$,

$$
E\{Y^*(d)\} = \sum_{\overline{a}_{K-1} \in \overline{\mathcal{A}}_{K-1}} E\left\{ \prod_{j=1}^{K-1} \mathrm{I}\left[d_j\{\overline{X}_j^*(\overline{a}_{j-1}), \overline{a}_{j-1}\} = a_j\right] \right.
$$
$$
\left. \times E\left(Y^*\left[\overline{a}_{K-1}, d_K\{\overline{X}_K^*(\overline{a}_{K-1}), \overline{a}_{K-1}\}\right] \middle| \overline{X}_K^*(\overline{a}_{K-1})\right) \right\}. \quad (7.24)
$$

Because d and $d^{(1)opt}$ are regimes in $\mathcal{D}$, the set of rules $(\overline{d}_{K-1}, d_K^{(1)opt})$ is also a regime in $\mathcal{D}$. Thus, from (7.24),

$$
E\{Y^*(\overline{d}_{K-1}, d_K^{(1)opt})\} = \sum_{\overline{a}_{K-1} \in \overline{\mathcal{A}}_{K-1}} E\left\{ \prod_{j=1}^{K-1} \mathrm{I}\left[d_j\{\overline{X}_j^*(\overline{a}_{j-1}), \overline{a}_{j-1}\} = a_j\right] \right.
$$
$$
\left. \times E\left(Y^*\left[\overline{a}_{K-1}, d_K^{(1)opt}\{\overline{X}_K^*(\overline{a}_{K-1}), \overline{a}_{K-1}\}\right] \middle| \overline{X}_K^*(\overline{a}_{K-1})\right) \right\}. \quad (7.25)
$$

Conditional on $\overline{X}_K^*(\overline{a}_{K-1}) = \overline{x}_K$ for any realization $(\overline{x}_K, \overline{a}_{K-1}) \in \Gamma_K$, $d_K(\overline{x}_K, \overline{a}_{K-1}) \in \Psi_K(h_K)$. Then, by the definition of $d_K^{(1)opt}(h_K) = d_K^{(1)opt}(\overline{x}_K, \overline{a}_{K-1})$ in (7.14),

$$
E\left[Y^*\{\overline{a}_{K-1}, d_K(\overline{x}_K, \overline{a}_{K-1})\} \middle| \overline{X}_K^*(\overline{a}_{K-1}) = \overline{x}_K\right]
$$
$$
\leq E\left[Y^*\{\overline{a}_{K-1}, d_K^{(1)opt}(\overline{x}_K, \overline{a}_{K-1})\} \middle| \overline{X}_K^*(\overline{a}_{K-1}) = \overline{x}_K\right],
$$

so, comparing (7.25) to (7.24), it follows that

$$
E\{Y^*(d)\} \leq E\{Y^*(\overline{d}_{K-1}, d_K^{(1)opt})\}. \quad (7.26)
$$

Moreover, using the definition of $V_K^{(1)}(h_K)$ in (7.15), (7.25) can be written as

$$
E\{Y^*(\overline{d}_{K-1}, d_K^{(1)opt})\} \qquad\qquad\qquad\qquad (7.27)
$$
$$
= \sum_{\overline{a}_{K-1} \in \overline{\mathcal{A}}_{K-1}} E\left(\prod_{j=1}^{K-1} \mathrm{I}\left[d_j\{\overline{X}_j^*(\overline{a}_{j-1}), \overline{a}_{j-1}\} = a_j\right] V_K^{(1)}\{\overline{X}_K^*(\overline{a}_{K-1}), \overline{a}_{K-1}\} \right).
$$

To streamline the notation henceforth, define

$$
\mathcal{J}_k^d = \prod_{j=1}^{k} \mathrm{I}\left[d_j\{\overline{X}_j^*(\overline{a}_{j-1}), \overline{a}_{j-1}\} = a_j\right], \quad k = 1, \ldots, K;
$$

and let

$$\mathcal{K}_k(d_{k-1}) = \left[\overline{a}_{k-2}, d_{k-1}\{\overline{X}^*_{k-1}(\overline{a}_{k-2}), \overline{a}_{k-2}\}\right], \quad k = K, \ldots, 3,$$

$$\mathcal{K}_2(d_1) = d_1(X_1).$$

Analogous to (7.24) and using this notation, (7.27) can be written as

$$E\{Y^*(\overline{d}_{K-1}, d_K^{(1)opt})\} = \sum_{\overline{a}_{K-2} \in \overline{A}_{K-2}} E\left\{\mathcal{J}^d_{K-2}\right.$$

$$\left. \times E\left(V_K^{(1)}\left[\overline{X}^*_K\{\mathcal{K}_K(d_{K-1})\}, \mathcal{K}_K(d_{K-1})\right]\middle|\overline{X}^*_{K-1}(\overline{a}_{K-2})\right)\right\}. \quad (7.28)$$

Because d and $d^{(1)opt}$ are regimes in $\mathcal{D}$, $(\overline{d}_{K-2}, d_{K-1}^{(1)opt}, d_K^{(1)opt})$ is also a regime in $\mathcal{D}$, and, from (7.28),

$$E\{Y^*(\overline{d}_{K-2}, d_{K-1}^{(1)opt}, d_K^{(1)opt})\} = \sum_{\overline{a}_{K-2} \in \overline{A}_{K-2}} E\left\{\mathcal{J}^d_{K-2}\right.$$

$$\left. \times E\left(V_K^{(1)}\left[\overline{X}^*_K\{\mathcal{K}_K(d_{K-1}^{(1)opt})\}, \mathcal{K}_K(d_{K-1}^{(1)opt})\right]\middle|\overline{X}^*_{K-1}(\overline{a}_{K-2})\right)\right\}. \quad (7.29)$$

Conditional on $\overline{X}^*_{K-1}(\overline{a}_{K-2}) = \overline{x}_{K-1}$ for any realization $(\overline{x}_{K-1}, \overline{a}_{K-2}) \in \Gamma_{K-1}$, $d_{K-1}(\overline{x}_{K-1}, \overline{a}_{K-2}) \in \Psi_{K-1}(h_{K-1})$. Then, by the definition of $d_{K-1}^{(1)opt}(h_{K-1})$ in (7.16) and reasoning analogous to that above, comparing (7.29) to (7.28) and from (7.26),

$$E\{Y^*(d)\} \le E\{Y^*(\overline{d}_{K-1}, d_K^{(1)opt})\} \le E\{Y^*(\overline{d}_{K-2}, d_{K-1}^{(1)opt}, d_K^{(1)opt})\}. \quad (7.30)$$

From (7.18) with $k = K - 1$, (7.29) can be written as

$$E\{Y^*(\overline{d}_{K-2}, d_{K-1}^{(1)opt}, d_K^{(1)opt})\}$$

$$= \sum_{\overline{a}_{K-2} \in \overline{A}_{K-2}} E\left[\mathcal{J}^d_{K-2}V_{K-1}^{(1)}\{\overline{X}^*_{K-1}(\overline{a}_{K-2}), \overline{a}_{K-2}\}\right]$$

$$= \sum_{\overline{a}_{K-3} \in \overline{A}_{K-3}} E\left\{\mathcal{J}^d_{K-3}\right. \qquad (7.31)$$

$$\left. \times E\left(V_{K-1}^{(1)}\left[\overline{X}^*_{K-1}\{\mathcal{K}_{K-1}(d_{K-2})\}, \mathcal{K}_{K-1}(d_{K-2})\right]\middle|\overline{X}^*_{K-2}(\overline{a}_{K-3})\right)\right\},$$

and, because $(\overline{d}_{K-3}, d_{K-2}^{(1)opt}, d_{K-1}^{(1)opt}, d_K^{(1)opt}) \in \mathcal{D}$, it follows that

$$E\{Y^*(\overline{d}_{K-3}, d_{K-2}^{(1)opt}, d_{K-1}^{(1)opt}, d_K^{(1)opt})\} = \sum_{\overline{a}_{K-3} \in \overline{A}_{K-3}} E\left\{\mathcal{J}^d_{K-3}\right. \qquad (7.32)$$

$$\left. \times E\left(V_{K-1}^{(1)}\left[\overline{X}^*_{K-1}\{\mathcal{K}_{K-1}(d_{K-2}^{(1)opt})\}, \mathcal{K}_{K-1}(d_{K-2}^{(1)opt})\right]\middle|\overline{X}^*_{K-2}(\overline{a}_{K-3})\right)\right\}.$$

As above, using (7.17) with $k = K - 2$, comparing (7.32) to (7.31), and appealing to (7.30), we obtain

$$E\{Y^*(d)\} \leq E\{Y^*(\bar{d}_{K-1}, d_K^{(1)opt})\} \leq E\{Y^*(\bar{d}_{K-2}, d_{K-1}^{(1)opt}, d_K^{(1)opt})\}$$
$$\leq E\{Y^*(\bar{d}_{K-3}, d_{K-2}^{(1)opt}, d_{K-1}^{(1)opt}, d_K^{(1)opt})\}.$$

Continuing in this backward recursive fashion, it is straightforward to observe that the final step yields

$$E\{Y^*(d^{(1)opt})\} = E\left\{E\left(V_2^{(1)}\left[\overline{X}_2^*\{d_1^{(1)opt}(X_1)\}, d_1^{(1)opt}(X_1)\right]\bigg| X_1\right)\right\}$$
$$= E\{V_1^{(1)}(X_1)\} \tag{7.33}$$

from (7.20). Thus, defining $\underline{d}_k^{(1)opt} = (d_k^{(1)opt}, d_{k+1}^{(1)opt}, \ldots, d_K^{(1)opt})$, $k = 1, \ldots, K$, similar to (5.111), we can conclude that, for any $d \in \mathcal{D}$,

$$E\{Y^*(d)\} \leq \cdots \leq E\{Y^*(\bar{d}_{k-1}, \underline{d}_k^{(1)opt})\} \leq \cdots \leq E\{Y^*(d^{(1)opt})\},$$

which demonstrates that $d^{(1)opt}$ satisfies (7.21) and thus is an optimal regime. Moreover, (7.33) yields the expression for the value of an optimal regime $d^{(1)opt}$ given in (5.84). □

7.2.4 Characterization in Terms of Observed Data

We now show that, under SUTVA (6.16), the SRA (6.17) and the positivity assumption (7.7), an optimal regime as characterized in Section 7.2.2 can be expressed equivalently in terms of the observed data (7.6). This result is immediate, following from the equivalent representations under these assumptions of Γ_k, $k = 1, \ldots, K + 1$, in terms of potential outcomes as in (7.2) and (7.3) and in terms of the observed data as in (7.8) and (7.9).

Define for $h_K = (\overline{x}_K, \overline{a}_{K-1}) \in \Gamma_K$ as in (7.8) with $k = K$

$$Q_K(h_K, a_K) = Q_K(\overline{x}_K, \overline{a}_K) = E(Y|\overline{X} = \overline{x}, \overline{A} = \overline{a}), \tag{7.34}$$

$$d_K^{opt}(h_K) = d_K^{opt}(\overline{x}_K, \overline{a}_{K-1}) = \operatorname*{arg\,max}_{a_K \in \Psi_K(h_K)} Q_K(h_K, a_K), \tag{7.35}$$

$$V_K(h_K) = V_K(\overline{x}_K, \overline{a}_{K-1}) = \max_{a_K \in \Psi_K(h_K)} Q_K(h_K, a_K). \tag{7.36}$$

The definitions (7.34)–(7.36) are analogous to those in (5.78)–(5.80) in Section 5.6; here, however, attention is restricted to the class $\mathcal{D}$ of Ψ-specific regimes, so that (7.34)–(7.36) apply to $h_K \in \Gamma_K$, and maximization is over the options in the feasible set $\Psi_K(h_K)$. Assuming that Y takes values in $\mathcal{Y}$, so that realizations of $(\overline{X}, \overline{A}, Y)$ are in Γ_{K+1} in (7.9), $Q_K(h_K, a_K)$ is well defined.

Similarly, for $k = K - 1, \ldots, 2$ and $h_k = (\overline{x}_k, \overline{a}_{k-1}) \in \Gamma_k$ in (7.8), define

$$
\begin{aligned}
Q_k(h_k, a_k) &= Q_k(\overline{x}_k, \overline{a}_k) \\
&= E\{V_{k+1}(\overline{x}_k, X_{k+1}, \overline{a}_k) | \overline{X}_k = \overline{x}_k, \overline{A}_k = \overline{a}_k\}, \qquad (7.37)
\end{aligned}
$$

$$
d_k^{opt}(h_k) = d_k^{opt}(\overline{x}_k, \overline{a}_{k-1}) = \operatorname*{arg\,max}_{a_k \in \Psi_k(h_k)} Q_k(h_k, a_k), \qquad (7.38)
$$

$$
V_k(h_k) = V_k(\overline{x}_k, \overline{a}_{k-1}) = \max_{a_k \in \Psi_k(h_k)} Q_k(h_k, a_k); \qquad (7.39)
$$

and, for $h_1 = x_1 \in \Gamma_1$ in (7.1),

$$
Q_1(h_1, a_1) = Q_1(x_1, a_1) = E\{V_2(x_1, X_2, a_1) | X_1 = x_1, A_1 = a_1\}, \quad (7.40)
$$

$$
d_1^{opt}(h_1) = d_1^{opt}(x_1) = \operatorname*{arg\,max}_{a_1 \in \Psi_1(h_1)} Q_1(h_1, a_1), \qquad (7.41)
$$

$$
V_1(h_1) = V_1(x_1) = \max_{a_1 \in \Psi_1(h_1)} Q_1(h_1, a_1), \qquad (7.42)
$$

analogous to (5.81)–(5.83), $k = K - 1, \ldots, 1$. Because $h_k \in \Gamma_k$ for $k = 1, \ldots, K$, all of the conditional expectations in these expressions are well defined.

Comparison of $d_K^{opt}(h_K)$ and $V_K(h_K)$ in (7.35) and (7.36), which are defined for $h_K \in \Gamma_K$ in (7.2), $k = K$, to $d_K^{(1)opt}(h_K)$ and $V_K^{(1)}(h_K)$ in (7.14) and (7.15) shows that

$$
d_K^{(1)opt}(h_K) = d_K^{opt}(h_K), \quad V_K^{(1)}(h_K) = V_K(h_K)
$$

if

$$
E\{Y^*(\overline{a}) \mid \overline{X}_K^*(\overline{a}_{K-1}) = \overline{x}_K\} = E(Y \mid \overline{X} = \overline{x}, \overline{A} = \overline{a}). \qquad (7.43)
$$

Likewise, comparison of $d_k^{opt}(h_k)$ and $V_k(h_k)$ in (7.38) and (7.39), $k = K - 1, \ldots, 2$, to $d_k^{(1)opt}(h_k)$ and $V_k^{(1)}(h_k)$ in (7.17) and (7.18) shows that

$$
d_k^{(1)opt}(h_k) = d_k^{opt}(h_k), \quad V_k^{(1)}(h_k) = V_k(h_k)
$$

if

$$
\begin{aligned}
E[V_{k+1}^{(1)}\{\overline{x}_k, X_{k+1}^*(\overline{a}_k), \overline{a}_k\} \mid \overline{X}_k^*(\overline{a}_{k-1}) = \overline{x}_k] \\
= E\{V_{k+1}(\overline{x}_k, X_{k+1}, \overline{a}_k) \mid \overline{X}_k = \overline{x}_k, \overline{A}_k = \overline{a}_k\}. \qquad (7.44)
\end{aligned}
$$

Finally, from the expressions for $d_1^{opt}(h_1)$ and $V_1(h_1)$ in (7.41) and (7.42) and those for $d_1^{(1)opt}(h_1)$ and $V_1^{(1)}(h_1)$ in (7.19) and (7.20),

$$
d_1^{(1)opt}(h_1) = d_1^{opt}(h_1), \quad V_1^{(1)}(h_1) = V_1(h_1)
$$

if

$$E[V_2^{(1)}\{x_1, X_2^*(a_1), a_1\} \mid X_1 = x_1]$$
$$= E\{V_2(x_1, X_2, a_1) \mid X_1 = x_1, A_1 = a_1\}. \tag{7.45}$$

The expressions on the left-hand sides of (7.43), (7.44), and (7.45) involve the conditional distributions of $Y^*(\overline{a})$ given $\overline{X}_K^*(\overline{a}_{K-1})$, of $X_{k+1}^*(\overline{a}_k)$ given $\overline{X}_k^*(\overline{a}_{k-1})$, and of $X_2^*(a_1)$ given X_1, respectively, as in the definitions of Γ_k, $k = 1, \ldots, K+1$, in (7.2) and (7.3) in terms of potential outcomes. The right-hand sides involve the conditional distributions of Y given $\overline{X}$ and $\overline{A}$, of X_{k+1} given $\overline{X}_k$ and $\overline{A}_k$, and of X_2 given X_1 and A_1, respectively, as in the definitions of Γ_k, $k = 1, \ldots, K+1$ in (7.8) and (7.9) in terms of the observed data. As shown in Section 6.2.4 in the demonstration of the equivalence of (6.21) and (6.22) and as evident in the resulting equivalent expressions for the sets Γ_k, $k = 1, \ldots, K+1$, under SUTVA, the SRA, and the positivity assumption, these corresponding conditional distributions are the same. It thus follows immediately from the above that, for $h_k = (\overline{x}_k, \overline{a}_{k-1}) \in \Gamma_k$,

$$d_k^{(1)opt}(h_k) = d_k^{opt}(h_k), \quad V_k^{(1)}(h_k) = V_k(h_k), \quad k = 1, \ldots, K, \tag{7.46}$$

confirming that an optimal regime can be expressed equivalently in terms of the observed data.

Moreover, it follows from (7.33) and (7.45) that

$$\mathcal{V}(d^{opt}) = E\{Y^*(d^{opt})\} = E\{V_1(H_1)\} = E\{V_1(X_1)\}. \tag{7.47}$$

7.3   Optimal "Midstream" Regimes

The topic of this section is a bit specialized and can be skipped on first reading without loss of continuity.

We have defined an optimal Ψ-specific treatment regime comprising K decision rules. Implicit in this development is that such a regime is to be implemented in patients from a population of interest who start following its rules at Decision 1 and continue through all K decision points. In routine clinical practice, however, a patient may be encountered for the first time at one of the decision points subsequent to Decision 1. For definiteness, suppose such a patient presents "midstream," immediately prior to the ℓth decision point, $\ell = 2, \ldots, K$. A natural question is how to select treatment options from the feasible sets optimally for this patient henceforth, so at Decisions $\ell, \ell+1, \ldots, K$.

For such a midstream patient, the first $\ell - 1$ treatment decisions presumably have been made according to routine practice. When the patient presents at Decision ℓ, then, he will have a realized past history that can be viewed as a realization of random variables $(X_1, A_1^{(p)}, \ldots, X_{\ell-1}^{(p)}, A_{\ell-1}^{(p)}, X_\ell^{(p)})$, say. The $A_k^{(p)}$, $k = 1, \ldots, \ell-1$, are the treatments received by such a patient according to the treatment assignment mechanism governing routine clinical practice, where we assume that $A_k^{(p)}$ takes values $a_k \in \mathcal{A}_k$, $k = 1, \ldots \ell - 1$. The $X_k^{(p)}$, $k = 2, \ldots, \ell$, denote the resulting intervening information collected between Decisions $k-1$ and k, $k = 2, \ldots, \ell$, and X_1 denotes the information with which such a patient from the population would present at Decision 1 as before. We distinguish $A_k^{(p)}$, $k = 1, \ldots, \ell - 1$, and $X_k^{(p)}$, $k = 2, \ldots, \ell$, from A_k and X_k to allow the possibility that the treatment assignment mechanism for observed data that might be used to estimate an optimal regime is different from that in routine clinical practice, as would be the case if the observed data are from a SMART.

Implicit in the definition of $X_k^{(p)}$, $k = 2, \ldots, \ell$, is that the components of $X_k^{(p)}$ are the same variables that enter into the first ℓ rules in Ψ-specific treatment regimes, stated formally as the consistency assumption

$$X_k^{(p)} = X_k^*(\overline{A}_{k-1}^{(p)}), \quad k = 2, \ldots, \ell. \tag{7.48}$$

The assumption (7.48) further clarifies that patients who might present at Decision 1 and those presenting midstream are from the same population of interest.

For given $\ell = 2, \ldots, K$, define

$$\overline{X}_\ell^{(p)} = (X_1, X_2^{(p)}, \ldots, X_\ell^{(p)}) \text{ and } \overline{A}_{\ell-1}^{(p)} = (A_1^{(p)}, \ldots, A_{\ell-1}^{(p)}).$$

We thus seek the form of rules $d_k^{(\ell)opt}(h_k)$, $k = \ell, \ell + 1, \ldots, K$, say, that dictate how to treat optimally such a midstream patient presenting at Decision ℓ with realized past history $(\overline{X}_\ell^{(p)}, \overline{A}_{\ell-1}^{(p)}) = (\overline{x}_\ell, \overline{a}_{\ell-1}) = h_\ell$. Recall that, from the remark at the end of Section 6.2.2, h_ℓ need not be consistent with having followed a Ψ-specific regime through Decision $\ell - 1$. To this end, write

$$d^{(\ell)} = (d_\ell^{(\ell)}, d_{\ell+1}^{(\ell)} \ldots, d_K^{(\ell)})$$

to denote Ψ-specific regimes starting at the ℓth decision consisting of rules $d_k^{(\ell)}(h_k)$ that map from sets $\Gamma_k^{(\ell)}$ defined below to $\mathcal{A}_k$ and satisfy $d_k^{(\ell)}(h_k) \in \Psi_k(h_k)$ for every $h_k \in \Gamma_k^{(\ell)}$. Define $\mathcal{D}^{(\ell)}$ to be the class of all such regimes.

Because at Decision ℓ a midstream patient presents with realized history $(\overline{X}_\ell^{(p)}, \overline{A}_{\ell-1}^{(p)}) = (\overline{x}_\ell, \overline{a}_{\ell-1}) = h_\ell$, intuitively, from the point of view of treating the patient henceforth, this situation is analogous to that in which a patient presents at Decision 1 with realized baseline history $X_1 = x_1$. Accordingly, define the sets

$$\Gamma_\ell^{(\ell)} = \Big[(\overline{x}_\ell, \overline{a}_{\ell-1}) \in \overline{\mathcal{X}}_\ell \times \overline{\mathcal{A}}_{\ell-1} \quad \text{satisfying} \tag{7.49}$$
$$P\{(\overline{X}_\ell^{(p)} = \overline{x}_\ell, \overline{A}_{\ell-1}^{(p)} = \overline{a}_{\ell-1}) = (\overline{x}_\ell, \overline{a}_{\ell-1})\} > 0\Big],$$

$$\Lambda_\ell^{(\ell)} = \Big\{(\overline{x}_\ell, \overline{a}_\ell) \quad \text{such that} \quad (\overline{x}_\ell, \overline{a}_{\ell-1}) = h_\ell \in \Gamma_\ell^{(\ell)}, a_\ell \in \Psi_\ell(h_\ell)\Big\};$$

and, with

$$\mathcal{W}_{\ell,\ell} = (\overline{X}_\ell^{(p)} = \overline{x}_\ell, \overline{A}_{\ell-1}^{(p)} = \overline{a}_{\ell-1}),$$

$$\mathcal{W}_{\ell,j} = \{\overline{X}_\ell^{(p)} = \overline{x}_\ell, \overline{A}_{\ell-1}^{(p)} = \overline{a}_{\ell-1}, X_{\ell+1}^*(\overline{a}_\ell) = x_{\ell+1}, \dots, X_j^*(\overline{a}_{j-1}) = x_j\},$$
$$j = \ell+1, \dots, K,$$

define for $k = \ell+1, \dots, K$

$$\Gamma_k^{(\ell)} = \Big[h_k = (\overline{x}_k, \overline{a}_{k-1}) \in \overline{\mathcal{X}}_k \times \overline{\mathcal{A}}_{k-1} \text{ satisfying } (\overline{x}_{k-1}, \overline{a}_{k-1}) \in \Lambda_{k-1}^{(\ell)}$$
$$\text{and } P\{X_k^*(\overline{a}_{k-1}) = x_k \mid \mathcal{W}_{\ell,k-1}\} > 0\Big], \tag{7.50}$$

$$\Lambda_k^{(\ell)} = \{(\overline{x}_k, \overline{a}_k) \quad \text{such that} \quad (\overline{x}_k, \overline{a}_{k-1}) = h_k \in \Gamma_k^{(\ell)}, \ a_k \in \Psi_k(h_k)\},$$

and

$$\Gamma_{K+1}^{(\ell)} = \Big[(\overline{x}, \overline{a}, y) \in \overline{\mathcal{X}} \times \overline{\mathcal{A}} \times \mathcal{Y} \text{ satisfying } (\overline{x}, \overline{a}) \in \Lambda_K^{(\ell)} \text{ and}$$
$$P\{Y^*(\overline{a}) = y \mid \mathcal{W}_{\ell,K}\} > 0\Big]. \tag{7.51}$$

Note that, when $\ell = 1$, the definitions of $\Gamma_\ell^{(\ell)}$ and $\Gamma_k^{(\ell)}$, $k = \ell+1, \dots, K+1$, in (7.49)–(7.51) coincide with those of Γ_1 and Γ_k, $k = 2, \dots, K+1$, in (7.1)–(7.3), where as in previous chapters $A_0^{(p)}$ and a_0 are null.

Thus, viewing this as a problem of making $K - \ell + 1$ decisions at decision points $\ell, \ell+1, \dots, K$ with initial state $(\overline{X}_\ell^{(p)} = \overline{x}_\ell, \overline{A}_{\ell-1}^{(p)} = \overline{a}_{\ell-1})$, by a backward induction argument analogous to that in Section 7.2.2 for $\ell = 1$ with initial state $X_1 = x_1$, define

$$d_K^{(\ell)opt}(h_K) = \underset{a_K \in \Psi_K(h_K)}{\arg\max} \ E\{Y^*(\overline{a}_{K-1}, a_K) | \mathcal{W}_{\ell,K}\}, \tag{7.52}$$

$$V_K^{(\ell)}(h_K) = \underset{a_K \in \Psi_K(h_K)}{\max} \ E\{Y^*(\overline{a}_{K-1}, a_K) | \mathcal{W}_{\ell,K}\} \tag{7.53}$$

for any $\overline{x}_K \in \overline{\mathcal{X}}_K$, $\overline{a}_{K-1} \in \overline{\mathcal{A}}_{K-1}$ for which $h_K = (\overline{x}_K, \overline{a}_{K-1}) \in \Gamma_K^{(\ell)}$.

Then, for $k = K - 1, \ldots, \ell + 1$ and any $\overline{x}_k \in \overline{\mathcal{X}}_k$, $\overline{a}_{k-1} \in \overline{\mathcal{A}}_{k-1}$ for which $h_k = (\overline{x}_k, \overline{a}_{k-1}) \in \Gamma_k^{(\ell)}$, define

$$d_k^{(\ell)opt}(h_k) \tag{7.54}$$
$$= \underset{a_k \in \Psi_k(h_k)}{\arg\max} \, E[V_{k+1}^{(\ell)}\{\overline{x}_k, X_{k+1}^*(\overline{a}_{k-1}, a_k), \overline{a}_{k-1}, a_k\}|\mathcal{W}_{\ell,k}],$$

$$V_k^{(\ell)}(h_k) = \underset{a_k \in \Psi_k(h_k)}{\max} \, E[V_{k+1}^{(\ell)}\{\overline{x}_k, X_{k+1}^*(\overline{a}_{k-1}, a_k), \overline{a}_{k-1}, a_k\}|\mathcal{W}_{\ell,k}].$$
$$\tag{7.55}$$

Finally, using the definition of $\mathcal{W}_{\ell,\ell}$,

$$d_\ell^{(\ell)opt}(h_\ell) \tag{7.56}$$
$$= \underset{a_\ell \in \Psi_\ell(h_\ell)}{\arg\max} \, E[V_{\ell+1}^{(\ell)}\{\overline{x}_\ell, X_{\ell+1}^*(\overline{a}_{\ell-1}, a_\ell), \overline{a}_{\ell-1}, a_\ell\}|\overline{X}_\ell^{(p)} = \overline{x}_\ell, \overline{A}_{\ell-1}^{(p)} = \overline{a}_{\ell-1}],$$

$$V_\ell^{(\ell)}(h_\ell) \tag{7.57}$$
$$= \underset{a_\ell \in \Psi_\ell(h_\ell)}{\max} \, E[V_{\ell+1}^{(\ell)}\{\overline{x}_\ell, X_{\ell+1}^*(\overline{a}_{\ell-1}, a_\ell), \overline{a}_{\ell-1}, a_\ell\}|\overline{X}_\ell^{(p)} = \overline{x}_\ell, \overline{A}_{\ell-1}^{(p)} = \overline{a}_{\ell-1}].$$

By an argument similar to that in Section 7.2.3, which is omitted here for brevity, it can be shown that

$$d^{(\ell)opt} = (d_\ell^{(\ell)opt}, d_{\ell+1}^{(\ell)opt}, \ldots, d_K^{(\ell)opt})$$

defined in (7.52)–(7.56) satisfies

$$E\{Y^*(\overline{a}_{\ell-1}, d^{(\ell)})|\overline{X}_\ell^{(p)} = \overline{x}_\ell, \overline{A}_{\ell-1}^{(p)} = \overline{a}_{\ell-1}\}$$
$$\leq E\{Y^*(\overline{a}_{\ell-1}, d^{(\ell)opt})|\overline{X}_\ell^{(p)} = \overline{x}_\ell, \overline{A}_{\ell-1}^{(p)} = \overline{a}_{\ell-1}\}$$

for all $d^{(\ell)} \in \mathcal{D}^{(\ell)}$, and thus in this sense $d^{(\ell)opt}$ is an optimal midstream regime.

Comparison of (7.52)–(7.57) to (7.14)–(7.20) shows that the ℓth to Kth decision rules of an optimal regime $d^{(1)opt}$ that would be followed by a patient presenting at Decision 1 may not be the same as those of an optimal midstream regime $d^{(\ell)opt}$ that would be followed by a patient presenting at Decision ℓ who was treated according to routine clinical practice up to that point. In particular, noting that the conditioning sets in (7.14)–(7.18) are $\mathcal{W}_{1,K}$ and $\mathcal{W}_{1,k}$, the rules in $d^{(\ell)opt}$ are ℓ-dependent through the dependence of the conditioning sets $\mathcal{W}_{\ell,k}$, $\ell = 1, \ldots, k$, $k = \ell, \ldots, K$ on ℓ.

Under certain conditions, however, the rules in $d^{(\ell)opt}$ can be shown to coincide with the ℓth to Kth decision rules in $d^{(1)opt}$. If a midstream patient presents at Decision ℓ with realized history $h_\ell = (\overline{x}_\ell, \overline{a}_{\ell-1}) \in \Gamma_\ell^{(\ell)}$ that is consistent with having followed some Ψ-specific regime $d^{(1)}$ from Decision 1 through Decision $\ell - 1$, then $h_\ell \in \Gamma_\ell$. Assume henceforth that $h_\ell \in \Gamma_\ell$, and furthermore make the sequential randomization assumption

$$W^* \perp\!\!\!\perp A_k^{(p)} | \overline{X}_k^{(p)}, \overline{A}_{k-1}^{(p)}, \quad k = 1, \ldots, \ell - 1, \tag{7.58}$$

where (7.58) implies that treatment assignment in routine practice at Decisions $1, \ldots, \ell - 1$ is based only on a patient's past history and not additionally on potential outcomes. Then, with $h_\ell \in \Gamma_\ell$, the consistency assumption (7.48), and (7.58), it is possible to show by an argument similar to that used in demonstrating (6.26) via repeated application of Lemma 6.2.1 that, letting $X_{K+1}^*(\overline{a}_K) = Y^*(\overline{a})$,

$$P\{X_k^*(\overline{a}_{k-1}) = x_k \mid \mathcal{W}_{\ell,k-1}\} \tag{7.59}$$
$$= P\{X_k^*(\overline{a}_{k-1}) = x_k \mid \overline{X}_{k-1}^*(\overline{a}_{k-2}) = \overline{x}_{k-1}\}, \quad k = \ell + 1, \ldots, K + 1.$$

Then, from (7.2)–(7.3) and (7.50)–(7.51), $\Gamma_k^{(\ell)} = \Gamma_k$, $k = \ell+1, \ldots, K+1$.

The equality of the conditional distributions in (7.59) implies that the conditional expectations in the definition of $d^{(\ell)opt}$ in (7.52)–(7.56) coincide with those in the definition of $d^{(1)opt}$ in (7.14)-(7.17) for Decisions $K, \ldots, \ell$. Thus, under these conditions, the rules in an optimal midstream regime $d^{(\ell)opt}$ do not depend on ℓ and are identical to the ℓth to Kth rules in an optimal regime $d^{(1)opt}$. That is, for $\ell = 1, \ldots, K$ and $k = \ell, \ldots, K$,

$$d_k^{(\ell)opt}(h_k) = d_k^{(1)opt}(h_k), \quad h_k \in \Gamma_k.$$

It follows that the single set of rules $d^{(1)opt}$ is relevant regardless of when a patient presents. That is, as long as the above conditions hold, selection of treatment at the ℓth decision point for a patient who presents at Decision 1 and has followed the rules in $d^{(1)opt}$ through Decision $\ell - 1$ and selection of treatment for a patient who presents for the first time at Decision ℓ would be determined by the same rule $d_\ell^{(1)opt}$ evaluated at the patient's history h_ℓ to that point.

In fact, under SUTVA (6.16), the SRA (6.17), and the positivity assumption (7.7), because $d^{(1)opt}$ can be expressed equivalently in terms of the observed data as shown in Section 7.2.4, under these conditions, an optimal midstream regime can be estimated based on observed data.

7.4   Estimation of an Optimal Regime

7.4.1   Q-learning

As in Section 5.7.1, the characterization of a Ψ-specific optimal regime $d^{opt} \in \mathcal{D}$ in (7.34)–(7.41) of Section 7.2.4 in terms of the observed data leads immediately to the method of Q-learning. Here, for completeness, we present this method again in the context of Ψ-specific regimes and note special considerations that arise in this setting. The reader should refer to Section 5.7.1 for additional discussion, particularly of practical considerations.

From (7.35), (7.38), and (7.41), an optimal Ψ-specific regime d^{opt} can be represented in terms of the Q-functions

$$Q_K(h_K, a_K) = Q_K(\overline{x}_K, \overline{a}_K) = E(Y|\overline{X}_K = \overline{x}_K, \overline{A}_K = \overline{a}_K); \quad (7.60)$$

and, for $k = K - 1, \ldots, 1$,

$$Q_k(h_k, a_k) = Q_k(\overline{x}_k, \overline{a}_k) = E\{V_{k+1}(\overline{x}_k, X_{k+1}, \overline{a}_k)|\overline{X}_k = \overline{x}_k, \overline{A}_k = \overline{a}_k\}, \quad (7.61)$$

where, for $k = 1, \ldots, K$,

$$V_k(h_k) = V_k(\overline{x}_k, \overline{a}_{k-1}) = \max_{a_k \in \Psi_k(h_k)} Q_k(h_k, a_k). \quad (7.62)$$

Note that, in contrast to (5.87), maximization in (7.62) is over options in $\Psi_k(h_k)$. Estimation of d^{opt} via Q-learning based on observed data

$$(X_{1i}, A_{1i}, \ldots, X_{Ki}, A_{Ki}, Y_i), \quad i = 1, \ldots, n,$$

is accomplished by positing models for the Q-functions $Q_k(h_k, a_k)$,

$$Q_k(h_k, a_k; \beta_k) = Q_k(\overline{x}_k, \overline{a}_k; \beta_k), \quad k = K, K - 1, \ldots, 1,$$

depending on finite-dimensional parameters β_k, $k = 1, \ldots, K$. As discussed in Section 5.7.1, the models can be linear or nonlinear in β_k and include main effects and interactions among elements of $\overline{x}_k$ and $\overline{a}_k$. Estimators $\widehat{\beta}_k$ are obtained in a backward iterative fashion for $k = K, K - 1, \ldots, 1$ by solving appropriate estimating equations; for example, those corresponding to OLS or WLS.

At Decision K, the estimator $\widehat{\beta}_K$ for β_K is found by solving an estimating equation of the form

$$\sum_{i=1}^n \frac{\partial Q_K(H_{Ki}, A_{Ki}; \beta_K)}{\partial \beta_K} \Sigma_K^{-1}(H_{Ki}, A_{Ki})\{Y_i - Q_K(H_{Ki}, A_{Ki}; \beta_K)\} = 0, \quad (7.63)$$

where $\Sigma_K(\overline{x}_K, \overline{a}_K)$ is a working variance model as in (5.89), taken to be equal to 1 if homoscedasticity is assumed. Substituting the model $Q_K(h_K, a_K; \beta_K)$ in (7.35) leads to the estimator for $d_K^{opt}(h_K)$ given by

$$\widehat{d}_{Q,K}^{opt}(h_K) = \underset{a_K \in \Psi_K(h_K)}{\arg\max} \, Q_K(h_K, a_K; \widehat{\beta}_K), \quad (7.64)$$

where, comparing to (5.90), the maximization in (7.64) is over options in $\Psi_K(h_K)$. We discuss the implications of this for implementation momentarily. Form the pseudo outcomes

$$\widetilde{V}_{Ki} = \max_{a_K \in \Psi_K(H_{Ki})} Q_K(H_{Ki}, a_K; \widehat{\beta}_K).$$

For Decisions $k = K - 1, \ldots, 1$, one then obtains $\widehat{\beta}_k$ for each k by solving an estimating equation of the form

$$\sum_{i=1}^{n} \frac{\partial Q_k(H_{ki}, A_{ki}; \beta_k)}{\partial \beta_k} \Sigma_k^{-1}(H_{ki}, A_{ki})\{\widetilde{V}_{k+1,i} - Q_k(H_{ki}, A_{ki}; \beta_k)\} = 0,$$

$$(7.65)$$

where $\Sigma_k(h_k, a_k)$ is a working variance model. The corresponding estimated rule is

$$\widehat{d}_{Q,k}^{opt}(h_k) = d_k^{opt}(h_k; \widehat{\beta}_k) = \arg\max_{a_k \in \Psi_k(h_k)} Q_k(h_k, a_k; \widehat{\beta}_k), \qquad (7.66)$$

where, again, the maximization in (7.66) is over options in $\Psi_k(h_k)$. Form the pseudo outcomes

$$\widetilde{V}_{ki} = \max_{a_k \in \Psi_k(H_{ki})} Q_k(H_{ki}, a_k; \widehat{\beta}_k).$$

An estimated optimal Ψ-specific regime is then given by

$$\widehat{d}_Q^{opt} = \{\widehat{d}_{Q,1}^{opt}(h_1), \ldots, \widehat{d}_{Q,K}^{opt}(h_K)\}.$$

With

$$\widetilde{V}_{1i} = \max_{a_1 \in \Psi_1(H_{1i})} Q_1(H_{1i}, a_1; \widehat{\beta}_1), \quad i = 1, \ldots, n,$$

from (7.47), an estimator for the value $\mathcal{V}(d^{opt})$ is given by

$$\widehat{\mathcal{V}}_Q(d^{opt}) = n^{-1} \sum_{i=1}^{n} \widetilde{V}_{1i} = n^{-1} \sum_{i=1}^{n} \max_{a_1 \in \Psi_1(H_{1i})} Q_1(H_{1i}, a_1; \widehat{\beta}_1). \quad (7.67)$$

As noted after (5.98) in Section 5.7.1, $\widehat{\mathcal{V}}_Q(d^{opt})$ is a nonregular estimator for $\mathcal{V}(d^{opt})$, so that inference on the true value of an optimal regime d^{opt} is not straightforward; see Chapter 10.

Modeling and Implementation Considerations for Q-learning

The issues related to modeling and practical implementation discussed at the end of Section 5.7.1 persist in this more complex formulation involving feasible sets of treatment options at each decision point.

As in the remark following (5.98), except at Decision K, where standard asymptotic theory applies to deduce an efficient estimating equation for obtaining $\widehat{\beta}_K$ by choice of the leading term in the summand (5.99), derivation of efficient estimating equations for $k = 1, \ldots, K - 1$ is challenging. Moreover, as demonstrated in detail for $K = 2$ in Section 5.7.1 in the example of linear models for the Q-functions at each decision point, misspecification of the Q-function models at all but the final, Kth decision point is almost certain and propagates through the models at Decisions $K - 1, \ldots, 1$. Accordingly, the caveats noted in Sections 5.7.1 and 5.7.4 apply here.

In fact, positing models for the Q-functions is itself more complicated in this setting, analogous to the considerations discussed in Remark (iii) of Section 6.4.2 for the backward induction approach to estimation of the value of a fixed regime. As noted there, if for Decision k $\Psi_k(h_k)$ comprises the same treatment options in $\mathcal{A}_k$ for all h_k, then a single model $Q_k(h_k, a_k; \beta_k)$ can be postulated. However, as reviewed in Section 7.2.1, it is likely, particularly for $k > 1$, that there are ℓ_k distinct subsets of $\mathcal{A}_k$ that are feasible sets determined by a few key components or functions of components of h_k; e.g., response status at Decision 2 in the acute leukemia setting. As before, denote for each $k = 1, \ldots, K$ the lth distinct subset by $\mathcal{A}_{k,l} \subseteq \mathcal{A}_k$, $l = 1, \ldots, \ell_k$. As in Remark (iii), it is often the case that the subsets $\mathcal{A}_{k,l}$ are nonoverlapping. If each $\mathcal{A}_{k,l}$ involves at least two treatment options in $\mathcal{A}_k$, with $s_k(h_k)$ defined as in Section 7.2.1 to be the indicator of to which of these ℓ_k distinct subsets $\Psi_k(h_k)$ corresponds, then ℓ_k separate models $Q_{k,l}(h_k, a_k; \beta_{kl})$, $l = 1, \ldots, \ell_k$, can be posited, and, analogous to (6.71),

$$Q_k(h_k, a_k; \beta_k) \tag{7.68}$$

$$= \sum_{l=1}^{\ell_k} \mathrm{I}\{s_k(h_k) = l\} Q_{k,l}(h_k, a_k; \beta_{kl}), \quad \beta_k = (\beta_{k1}^T, \ldots, \beta_{k\ell_k}^T)^T.$$

In (7.68), it is understood that a_k takes values in the feasible set $\Psi_k(h_k)$ for which $s_k(h_k) = l$; i.e., $\mathcal{A}_{k,l}$.

From (7.68), the estimating equations (7.63) can then be written as

$$\sum_{i=1}^{n} \left[\sum_{l=1}^{\ell_K} \mathrm{I}\{s_K(H_{Ki}) = l\} \frac{\partial Q_{K,l}(H_{Ki}, A_{Ki}; \beta_{Kl})}{\partial \beta_{Kl}} \Sigma_{K,l}^{-1}(H_{Ki}, A_{Ki}) \right.$$

$$\left. \times \{Y_i - Q_{K,l}(H_{Ki}, A_{Ki}; \beta_{Kl})\} \right] = 0; \tag{7.69}$$

in (7.69) and (7.70) below, we allow the possibility of a different working variance model for each distinct subset. If the β_{Kl} do not contain common components, so are variationally independent, then (7.69) reduces to ℓ_K separate equations that can be solved individually in each of $\beta_{K1}, \ldots, \beta_{K\ell_K}$, respectively. Clearly, for each l, the equation is based on data from only individuals i whose realized histories make them eligible for the lth distinct subset of feasible treatment options. The estimated rule for h_K such that $s_K(h_K) = l$ is then

$$\widehat{d}^{opt}_{Q,K,l}(h_K) = \arg\max_{a_K \in \mathcal{A}_{K,l}} Q_{K,l}(h_K, a_K; \widehat{\beta}_{Kl}),$$

so that, from (7.4),

$$\widehat{d}^{opt}_{Q,K}(h_K) = \sum_{l=1}^{\ell_K} I\{s_K(h_K) = l\} \widehat{d}^{opt}_{Q,K,l}(h_K);$$

and the pseudo outcome for individual i for whom $s_K(H_{Ki}) = l$ is found as

$$\widetilde{V}_{Ki} = \max_{a_K \in \mathcal{A}_{K,l}} Q_{K,l}(H_{Ki}, a_K; \widehat{\beta}_{Kl}).$$

Similarly, for $k = K - 1, \ldots, 1$, (7.65) becomes

$$\sum_{i=1}^{n} \left[\sum_{l=1}^{\ell_K} I\{s_k(H_{ki}) = l\} \frac{\partial Q_{k,l}(H_{ki}, A_{ki}; \beta_{kl})}{\partial \beta_{kl}} \Sigma^{-1}_{k,l}(H_{ki}, A_{ki}) \right.$$

$$\left. \times \{\widetilde{V}_{k+1,i} - Q_{k,l}(H_{ki}, A_{ki}; \beta_{kl})\} \right] = 0, \tag{7.70}$$

yielding ℓ_k separate equations for $\beta_{k1}, \ldots, \beta_{k\ell_k}$ when these parameters are nonoverlapping; and

$$\widehat{d}^{opt}_{Q,k,l}(h_k) = \arg\max_{a_k \in \mathcal{A}_{k,l}} Q_{k,l}(h_k, a_k; \widehat{\beta}_{kl}),$$

$$\widehat{d}^{opt}_{Q,k}(h_k) = \sum_{l=1}^{\ell_k} I\{s_k(h_k) = l\} \widehat{d}^{opt}_{Q,k,l}(h_k).$$

The pseudo outcome for individual i with $s_k(H_{ki}) = l$ is

$$\widetilde{V}_{ki} = \max_{a_k \in \mathcal{A}_{k,l}} Q_{k,l}(H_{ki}, a_k; \widehat{\beta}_{kl}).$$

If the distinct subsets contain common options, so are overlapping at Decision k, in principle, problem-specific modeling and estimation approaches that incorporate the overlap can be developed to posit and fit the Q-function $Q_k(h_k, a_k; \beta_k)$. Of course, it is possible to posit and fit separate Q-function models for each subset, downplaying the overlap, which may be a more practically feasible approach.

As discussed in Remark (iv) of Section 6.4.2, it may be that only one treatment option in $\mathcal{A}_k$ is feasible for some patients at Decision k depending on their histories h_k; e.g., if the only option for a responder is to continue the current intervention, as at Decision 2 in the ADHD example in Section 1.2.2. In this situation, any Decision k rule must select this single, feasible option; accordingly, if the lth distinct subset $\mathcal{A}_{k,l}$ contains a single option, $\widehat{d}_{Q,k,l}^{opt}(h_k)$, and thus $\widehat{d}_{Q,k}^{opt}(h_k)$, must return this option when h_k is such that $s_k(h_k) = l$. Here, then, no corresponding Q-function model is required, and the estimating equation for β_k in the overall model $Q_k(h_k, a_k; \beta_k)$ can be restricted to involve only individuals whose histories dictate other feasible sets with more than one option. For example, with $M_k(h_k)$ denoting the number of options in $\Psi_k(h_k)$ as in Remark (iv), (7.65) becomes

$$\sum_{i:M_k(H_{ki})>1} \left[\frac{\partial Q_k(H_{ki}, A_{ki}; \beta_k)}{\partial \beta_k} \Sigma_k^{-1}(H_{ki}, A_{ki}) \right.$$
$$\left. \times \{\widetilde{V}_{k+1,i} - Q_k(H_{ki}, A_{ki}; \beta_k)\} \right] = 0,$$

which can be recast as in (7.70), where the sum over l is now over only those distinct subsets with more than one option.

Moreover, for individuals i for whom $M_k(H_{ki}) = 1$, so having only one feasible option, by an argument almost identical to that in Remark (iv) of Section 6.4.2, we can take $\widetilde{V}_{ki} = \widetilde{V}_{k+1,i}$ and thus "carry backward" the pseudo outcome from the previous step of the algorithm.

7.4.2 A-learning

As in Sections 3.5.2 and 3.5.5 in the case of a single decision, it is possible to deduce a strategy for estimation of an optimal Ψ-specific regime based on modeling of so-called contrast functions rather than of the full Q-functions at each decision point. The class of techniques referred to as advantage or A-learning that we now discuss in the multiple decision setting is thus an alternative to Q-learning that involves making fewer assumptions on the Q-functions and can yield results that are more robust to model misspecification.

For simplicity, we describe this approach and the A-learning method known as g-estimation for fitting the models in the situation where the feasible sets $\Psi_k(h_k) = \mathcal{A}_k$ for all h_k, $k = 1, \ldots, K$, and discuss considerations arising when this is not the case later in this section. As in Section 3.5.5, we take $\mathcal{A}_k$ to comprise m_k options, coded so that

$$\mathcal{A}_k = \{0, 1, \ldots, m_k - 1\},$$

where the option coded as 0 is a control or reference treatment. Of course, the options so coded need not be the same for each k.

From (7.60) and (7.61), the Q-functions are

$$Q_K(h_K, a_K) = Q_K(\overline{x}_K, \overline{a}_K) = E(Y|\overline{X}_K = \overline{x}_K, \overline{A}_K = \overline{a}_K);$$

and, for $k = K - 1, \ldots, 1,$

$$Q_k(h_k, a_k) = Q_k(\overline{x}_k, \overline{a}_k) = E\{V_{k+1}(\overline{x}_k, X_{k+1}, \overline{a}_k)|\overline{X}_k = \overline{x}_k, \overline{A}_k = \overline{a}_k\},$$

where, from (7.62),

$$V_k(h_k) = \max_{a_k \in \Psi_k(h_k)} Q_k(h_k, a_k), \quad k = 1, \ldots, K,$$

so that the value functions under these conditions are given by

$$V_k(h_k) = \max_{j \in \{0,1,\ldots,m_k-1\}} Q_k(h_k, j), \quad k = 1, \ldots, K. \tag{7.71}$$

Then an optimal regime comprises rules of the form

$$d_k^{opt}(h_k) = d_k^{opt}(\overline{x}_k, \overline{a}_{k-1}) = \underset{j \in \{0,1,\ldots,m_k-1\}}{\arg\max} Q_k(h_k, j), \quad k = 1, \ldots, K. \tag{7.72}$$

In fact, using (7.72), (7.71) can be expressed equivalently as

$$V_k(h_k) = Q_k\{h_k, d_k^{opt}(h_k)\}, \quad k = 1, \ldots, K, \tag{7.73}$$

which proves useful momentarily.

From (7.72), because $\Psi_k(h_k) = \mathcal{A}_k = \{0, 1, \ldots, m_k - 1\}$ for all h_k for each $k = 1, \ldots, K$, it suffices to know the contrast functions

$$C_{kj}(h_k) = Q_k(h_k, j) - Q_k(h_k, 0), \quad j = 0, \ldots, m_k - 1, \tag{7.74}$$

where $C_{k0}(h_k) \equiv 0$, to deduce $d_k^{opt}(h_k)$, as it is immediate using (7.74) that

$$d_k^{opt}(h_k) = \underset{j \in \{0,1,\ldots,m_k-1\}}{\arg\max} C_{kj}(h_k), \quad k = 1, \ldots, K. \tag{7.75}$$

Analogous to the single decision case, (7.75) shows that, rather than knowing or modeling entire Q-functions for each k, one need only know or model the contrast functions to characterize or estimate an optimal regime. Before we discuss the A-learning approach that exploits this premise, we note a particular interpretation of the contrast functions defined in (7.74).

The functions $C_{kj}(h_k)$, $k = 1, \ldots, K$, can be regarded as *optimal blip to zero functions* in the sense discussed by Robins (2004) and Moodie et al. (2007) for multiple decisions. We illustrate this concept in the case of $K = 2$ decision points. At Decision 2, by the definition (7.74),

$$
\begin{aligned}
C_{2j}(h_2) &= E(Y \mid H_2 = h_2, A_2 = j) - E(Y \mid H_2 = h_2, A_2 = 0) \\
&= E\{Y^*(a_1, j) \mid H_2 = h_2, A_2 = j\} - E\{Y^*(a_1, 0) \mid H_2 = h_2, A_2 = 0\} \\
&= E\{Y^*(a_1, j) \mid H_2 = h_2\} - E\{Y^*(a_1, 0) \mid H_2 = h_2\}, \qquad (7.76)
\end{aligned}
$$

where the first equality follows by SUTVA (6.16), and (7.76) follows by the SRA (6.17). From (7.76), $C_{2j}(h_2)$ can be interpreted as the difference in expected outcome an individual with realized history h_2 would have if she were to receive the option coded as j relative to the control option 0 at Decision 2; that is, if she were to receive a "blip" of treatment (via option j) versus control at Decision 2. By definition and using (7.73),

$$
\begin{aligned}
Q_1(h_1, a_1) &= E\left[E\{Y \mid H_2, A_2 = d_2^{opt}(H_2)\} \mid H_1 = h_1, A_1 = a_1 \right] \\
&= E\Bigg\{ E\left(Y^*[a_1, d_2^{opt}\{h_1, X_2^*(a_1), a_1\}] \mid H_1 = h_1, X_2^*(a_1), A_1 = a_1, \right. \\
&\qquad\qquad \left. A_2 = d_2^{opt}\{h_1, X_2^*(a_1), a_1\} \right) \Bigg| H_1 = h_1, A_1 = a_1 \Bigg\} \\
&= E\left(Y^*[a_1, d_2^{opt}\{h_1, X_2^*(a_1), a_1\}] \mid H_1 = h_1 \right)
\end{aligned}
$$

using SUTVA and the SRA. It follows that

$$
\begin{aligned}
C_{1j}(h_1) &= E\left(Y^*[j, d_2^{opt}\{h_1, X_2^*(j), j\}] \mid H_1 = h_1 \right) \\
&\quad - E\left(Y^*[0, d_2^{opt}\{h_1, X_2^*(0), 0\}] \mid H_1 = h_1 \right). \qquad (7.77)
\end{aligned}
$$

The representation (7.77) shows that $C_{1j}(h_1)$ can be interpreted as the difference in expected outcome an individual with realized history h_1 would have if he were to receive option j versus option 0 at Decision 1, so receive a blip of treatment relative to control at Decision 1, and then follow an optimal regime at the final decision point. It should be clear that this backward argument can be extended to general K to show that the contrast functions $C_{kj}(h_k)$, $k = K - 1, \ldots, 1$, can be interpreted as the difference in expected outcome an individual with realized history h_k would have if she were to receive a blip of treatment versus control at Decision k and then follow an optimal regime at Decisions $k + 1, \ldots, K$ thereafter.

As in the single decision case, because an arbitrary function $Q_k(h_k, a_k)$ can be written as

$$
Q_k(h_k, a_k) = \nu_k(h_k) + \sum_{j=1}^{m_k - 1} I(a_k = j) C_{kj}(h_k),
$$

where $\nu_k(h_k) = Q_k(h_k, 0)$, the representation of $d_k(h_k)$ in (7.75) holds; and, from (7.71), the value functions can be expressed as

$$V_k(h_k) = \nu_k(h_k) + \max_{j \in \{0, 1, \ldots, m_k - 1\}} C_{kj}(h_k), \quad k = 1, \ldots, K.$$

The A-learning method for estimation of an optimal regime we now discuss is based on positing models for the contrast/optimal blip to zero functions $C_{kj}(h_k)$. In the discussion here, we take these models to depend on parameters ψ_{kj}; namely,

$$C_{kj}(h_k; \psi_{kj}), \quad j = 1, \ldots, m_k - 1, \ k = 1, \ldots, K. \tag{7.78}$$

They in turn imply models for the Q-functions of the form

$$\nu_k(h_k) + \sum_{j=1}^{m_k-1} \mathrm{I}(a_k = j) C_{kj}(h_k; \psi_{kj}), \quad k = 1, \ldots, K, \tag{7.79}$$

$$\psi_k = (\psi_{k1}^T, \ldots, \psi_{k,m_k-1}^T)^T.$$

The models (7.78) are a type of *structural nested mean model* for estimation of an optimal regime proposed by Robins (2004). If there are values of the parameters ψ_{kj} such that $C_{kj}(h_k; \psi_{kj}) = 0$ for all $k = 1, \ldots, K$ and $j = 1, \ldots, m_k - 1$, then, from (7.79), the model includes the causal null hypothesis that all regimes in $\mathcal{D}$ achieve the same value; see Robins (2004). Vansteelandt and Joffe (2014) present an overview of structural nested models in the context of inference on causal effects of treatment sequences.

As in Section 5.5.2, for $a_k = 0, 1, \ldots, m_k - 1$, let

$$\omega_k(h_k, a_k) = P(A_k = a_k | H_k = h_k), \quad k = 1, \ldots, K,$$

$$\omega_k(h_k, m_k - 1) = 1 - \sum_{a_k=0}^{m_k-2} \omega_k(h_k, a_k); \tag{7.80}$$

note that (7.80) differs from (5.65) and (5.66) in that the m_k treatment options are coded as $\{0, 1, \ldots, m_k - 1\}$ rather than $\{1, \ldots, m_k\}$. Models $\omega_k(h_k, a_k; \gamma_k)$, $k = 1, \ldots, K$, e.g., multinomial (polytomous) logistic regression models such as that in (3.97), can be posited and fitted via maximum likelihood.

The A-learning procedure follows a backward recursive scheme similar to that for Q-learning. Consider the Kth decision point. Robins (1997, 2004) showed using semiparametric theory that all consistent, asymptotically normal estimators for ψ_K are solutions to estimating equations of the form

$$
\sum_{i=1}^{n} \left(\left[\sum_{j=1}^{m_K-1} \lambda_{Kj}(H_{Ki}) \left\{ \mathrm{I}(A_{Ki} = j) - \omega_K(H_{Ki}, j) \right\} \right] \right. \tag{7.81}
$$
$$
\left. \times \left\{ Y_i - \sum_{j=1}^{m_K-1} \mathrm{I}(A_{Ki} = j) C_{Kj}(H_{Ki}; \psi_K) + \theta_K(H_{Ki}) \right\} \right) = 0
$$

for arbitrary vector-valued functions $\lambda_{Kj}(h_k)$, $j = 1, \ldots, m_K - 1$, of the same dimension as ψ_K; and arbitrary real-valued function $\theta_K(h_K)$. If the components ψ_{Kj}, $j = 1, \ldots, m_K - 1$, are nonoverlapping and thus variationally independent, (7.81) reduces to $m_K - 1$ separate equations

$$
\sum_{i=1}^{n} \left[\lambda_{Kj}(H_{Ki}) \left\{ \mathrm{I}(A_{Ki} = j) - \omega_K(H_{Ki}, j) \right\} \right. \tag{7.82}
$$
$$
\left. \times \left\{ Y_i - \sum_{j'=1}^{m_K-1} \mathrm{I}(A_{Ki} = j') C_{Kj'}(H_{Ki}; \psi_{Kj'}) + \theta_K(H_{Ki}) \right\} \right] = 0,
$$

$j = 1, \ldots, m_K - 1$, where $\lambda_{Kj}(h_K)$, $j = 1, \ldots, m_K - 1$, are now arbitrary vector-valued functions of the same dimension as ψ_{Kj}. As in the single decision case in Sections 3.5.2 and 3.5.5, if the contrast function models $C_{Kj}(h_K; \psi_{Kj})$, $j = 1, \ldots, m_K - 1$, are correctly specified, then the optimal choice of $\theta_K(h_K)$ on efficiency grounds is $\theta_K(h_K) = -\nu_K(h_K)$, and if moreover $\mathrm{var}(Y \mid H_K = h_K, A_K = a_K)$ is constant, then the optimal choices of $\lambda_{Kj}(h_K)$ in (7.81) and (7.82) are

$$
\frac{\partial C_{Kj}(h_K; \psi_K)}{\partial \psi_K} \quad \text{and} \quad \frac{\partial C_{Kj}(h_K; \psi_{Kj})}{\partial \psi_{Kj}}, \tag{7.83}
$$

respectively. If the variance is nonconstant, the optimal $\lambda_{Kj}(h_K)$ are complicated, and the specifications in (7.83) are reasonable for practical use.

As in the single decision case, to exploit these developments in practice, a model $\nu_K(h_K; \phi_K)$ can be posited. Then, focusing on (7.82) as an example, the parameters ψ_{Kj}, $j = 1, \ldots, m_K - 1$; ϕ_K; and γ_K can be estimated jointly by solving the stacked estimating equations

$$
\sum_{i=1}^{n} \left[\frac{\partial C_{Kj}(H_{Ki}; \psi_{Kj})}{\partial \psi_{Kj}} \left\{ \mathrm{I}(A_{Ki} = j) - \omega_K(H_{Ki}, j; \gamma_K) \right\} \right.
$$
$$
\left. \times \left\{ Y_i - \sum_{j'=1}^{m_K-1} \mathrm{I}(A_{Ki} = j') C_{Kj'}(H_{Ki}; \psi_{Kj'}) - \nu_K(H_{Ki}; \phi_K) \right\} \right] = 0,
$$
$$
j = 1, \ldots, m_K - 1, \tag{7.84}
$$

$$\sum_{i=1}^{n} \left[\frac{\partial \nu_K(H_{Ki}; \phi_K)}{\partial \phi_K} \right.$$

$$\left. \times \left\{ Y_i - \sum_{j'=1}^{m_K-1} \mathrm{I}(A_{Ki} = j') C_{Kj'}(H_{Ki}; \psi_{Kj'}) - \nu_K(H_{Ki}; \phi_K) \right\} \right] = 0,$$

along with the maximum likelihood score equations for γ_K. Analogous to the case $K = 1$ in Section 3.5.2, under SUTVA (6.16), the SRA (6.17), and the positivity assumption (7.7), if the models for the contrast functions are correctly specified, the resulting estimator $\widehat{\psi}_K$ for ψ_K will be consistent and asymptotically normal if either or both of the models $\omega_K(h_K, a_K; \gamma_K)$ or $\nu_K(h_K; \phi_K)$ are correctly specified; the argument when $\omega_K(h_K, a_K; \gamma_K)$ is correctly specified is similar to that given in (3.65)–(3.69) of Section 3.5.2. That is, the estimator $\widehat{\psi}_K$ is doubly robust.

It follows from (7.75) with $k = K$ that an optimal rule at Decision K can be estimated by

$$\widehat{d}_{A,K}^{opt}(h_K) = \underset{j \in \{0,1,\ldots,m_K-1\}}{\arg\max} \, C_{Kj}(h_K; \widehat{\psi}_{Kj}).$$

By manipulations similar to those at the end of Section 3.5.2, for $k = K - 1, \ldots, 1$,

$$E \left\{ V_{k+1}(H_{k+1}) + \underset{j \in \{0,1,\ldots,m_k-1\}}{\max} C_{kj}(H_k) - \sum_{j=1}^{m_k-1} \mathrm{I}(A_k = j) C_{kj}(H_k) \middle| H_k \right\}$$

$$= E \left[E\{V_{k+1}(H_{k+1}) \mid H_k, A_k\} + \underset{j \in \{0,1,\ldots,m_k-1\}}{\max} C_{kj}(H_k) - \right.$$

$$\left. - \sum_{j=1}^{m_k-1} \mathrm{I}(A_k = j) C_{kj}(H_k) \middle| H_k \right] \qquad (7.85)$$

$$= E \left\{ Q_k(H_k, A_k) + \underset{j \in \{0,1,\ldots,m_k-1\}}{\max} C_{kj}(H_k) \right.$$

$$\left. - \sum_{j=1}^{m_k-1} \mathrm{I}(A_k = j) C_{kj}(H_k) \middle| H_k \right\}$$

$$= E \left\{ \nu_k(H_k) + \underset{j \in \{0,1,\ldots,m_k-1\}}{\max} C_{kj}(H_k) \middle| H_k \right\} = V_k(H_k)$$

almost surely. Taking $k = K$ and replacing $V_{k+1}(H_{k+1})$ by Y in (7.85), these same steps lead to

$$E\left\{Y + \max_{j\in\{0,1,\ldots,m_K-1\}} C_{Kj}(H_K) - \sum_{j=1}^{m_K-1} C_{Kj}(H_K)\mathrm{I}(A_K = j)\,\middle|\, H_K\right\}$$

$$= V_K(H_K) \qquad (7.86)$$

almost surely. Then (7.85)–(7.86) suggest defining recursively the pseudo outcomes

$$\widetilde{V}_{ki} = \widetilde{V}_{k+1,i} + \max_{j\in\{0,1,\ldots,m_k-1\}} C_{kj}(H_{ki};\widehat{\psi}_{kj}) \qquad (7.87)$$

$$- \sum_{j=1}^{m_k-1} \mathrm{I}(A_{ki} = j)C_{kj}(H_{ki};\widehat{\psi}_{kj}), \quad k = K, K-1,\ldots,1,$$

where $\widetilde{V}_{K+1,i} = Y_i$, and forming estimating equations analogous to (7.84).

Accordingly, as with Q-learning, the A-learning algorithm proceeds in a backward, iterative fashion, yielding $\widehat{\psi}_k$, $k = K-1,\ldots,1$. At the kth decision point, given models $C_{kj}(h_k;\psi_{kj})$, $j = 1,\ldots,m_k-1$, for the contrast functions and models $\nu_k(h_k;\phi_k)$ and $\omega_k(h_k, a_k;\gamma_k)$; and taking ψ_{kj} to be variationally independent, solve jointly in $(\psi_k^T, \phi_k^T, \gamma_k^T)^T$ the stacked estimating equations

$$\sum_{i=1}^{n}\left[\frac{\partial C_{kj}(H_{ki};\psi_{kj})}{\partial \psi_{kj}}\{\mathrm{I}(A_{ki} = j) - \omega_k(H_{ki}, j;\gamma_k)\}\right.$$

$$\times\left.\left\{\widetilde{V}_{k+1,i} - \sum_{j'=1}^{m_k-1}\mathrm{I}(A_{ki} = j')C_{kj'}(H_{ki};\psi_{kj'}) - \nu_k(H_{ki};\phi_k)\right\}\right] = 0$$

$$j = 1,\ldots,m_k-1, \qquad (7.88)$$

$$\sum_{i=1}^{n}\left[\frac{\partial \nu_k(H_{ki};\phi_k)}{\partial \phi_k}\right.$$

$$\times\left.\left\{\widetilde{V}_{k+1,i} - \sum_{j'=1}^{m_k-1}\mathrm{I}(A_{ki} = j')C_{kj'}(H_{ki};\psi_{kj'}) - \nu_k(H_{ki};\phi_k)\right\}\right] = 0,$$

with the maximum likelihood score equation for γ_k. As for K, the optimal choice of $\lambda_k(h_k;\psi_k)$ is complex; taking

$$\lambda_k(h_k;\psi_k) = \frac{\partial C_k(h_k;\psi_k)}{\partial \psi_k}$$

as in (7.88) is reasonable in practice. If the ψ_{kj} are overlapping, the obvious version of (7.81) can be substituted in (7.88).

The A-learning estimator for the rule $d_k^{opt}(h_k)$, $k = K - 1, \ldots, 1$, is then

$$\widehat{d}_{A,k}^{opt}(h_k) = \underset{j \in \{0,1,\ldots,m_k-1\}}{\arg \max} C_{kj}(h_k; \widehat{\psi}_{kj}),$$

and, continuing in this fashion, the A-learning estimator for an optimal regime is

$$\widehat{d}_A^{opt} = \{\widehat{d}_{A,1}^{opt}(h_1), \ldots, \widehat{d}_{A,K}^{opt}(h_K)\}.$$

How well $\widehat{d}_A^{opt}$ estimates d^{opt} depends on how close the posited models $C_{kj}(h_k; \psi_k)$, $k = 1, \ldots, K$, $j = 1, \ldots, m_k - 1$, for the contrast functions are to the true contrast functions, as well as correct specification of at least one of the models for $\nu_k(h_k)$ or $\omega_k(h_k, a_k)$ for each $k = 1, \ldots, K$.

Murphy (2003) proposes an A-learning approach based instead on direct modeling of the advantage or regret function. Analogous to (3.72) in the single decision case, in the formulation here, the advantage or regret function at Decision k can be written as

$$\underset{j \in \{0,1,\ldots,m_k-1\}}{\max} C_{kj}(H_k) - \sum_{j=1}^{m_k-1} \mathrm{I}(A_k = j)C_{kj}(H_k),$$

and can be interpreted as the advantage in expected outcome gained by administering an optimal option at Decision k relative to that actually received, or, equivalently, the regret associated with not receiving an optimal option. Given models for these functions, Murphy (2003) proposes an alternative fitting strategy referred to by Moodie et al. (2007) as iterative minimization for optimal regimes; see this reference for details of this approach.

Modeling and Implementation Considerations for A-learning

The foregoing developments introduce A-learning in the simplest situation in which $\Psi_k(h_k) = \mathcal{A}_k$, $k = 1, \ldots, K$. As we have discussed, this is not the case for many multiple decision problems, where there are two or more distinct subsets of $\mathcal{A}_k$ that are feasible sets. The A-learning approach can be adapted readily to estimation of a Ψ-specific optimal regime for a general specification of feasible sets Ψ, as we now outline.

As in Section 7.2.1 and the discussion of modeling considerations for Q-learning in the previous section, at Decision k, suppose that there are ℓ_k distinct subsets of $\mathcal{A}_k$ that are feasible sets at Decision k, $\mathcal{A}_{k,l} \subseteq \mathcal{A}_k$, $l = 1, \ldots, \ell_k$; let $s_k(h_k) = 1, \ldots, \ell_k$ indicate which of these distinct subsets corresponds to $\Psi_k(h_k)$, and let $M_k(h_k)$ denote the number of options in $\Psi_k(h_k)$, $k = 1, \ldots, K$. As in (7.4),

$$d_k(h_k) = \sum_{l=1}^{\ell_k} \mathrm{I}\{s_k(h_k) = l\}\, d_{k,l}(h_k), \tag{7.89}$$

where $d_{k,l}(h_k)$ is the rule for the lth distinct subset at Decision k.

Assume first that these subsets are all nonoverlapping and that $M_k(h_k) > 1$ for all h_k. Let m_{kl} denote the number of options in $\mathcal{A}_{k,l}$, where one of these is a control or reference option, coded as 0, and the remaining options are coded as $1, \ldots, m_{kl} - 1$, so that $\mathcal{A}_{k,l} = \{0, 1, \ldots, m_{kl} - 1\}$. Then, at Decision k, the contrast functions (7.74) are of necessity different for each of the distinct feasible sets, which involve different treatment options. Thus, by analogy to (7.68) for Q-learning, separate contrast function models

$$C_{kj,l}(h_k; \psi_{kj,l}), \quad j = 1, \ldots, m_{kl} - 1,$$

must be posited for h_k such that $s_k(h_k) = l$ for each $l = 1, \ldots, \ell_k$. Consistent with this, to achieve a representation of the Q-function $Q_{k,l}(h_k, a_k)$ for the lth subset as in (7.68), one must posit models

$$\nu_{k,l}(h_k; \phi_{kl}), l = 1, \ldots, \ell_k,$$

depending on parameters ϕ_{kl}. These parameters would ordinarily be taken as nonoverlapping across l. Finally, as discussed at the end of Section 6.4.3, one must also posit propensity models

$$\omega_{k,l}(h_k, a_k; \gamma_{kl}), \quad l = 1, \ldots, \ell_k,$$

where here a_k takes values in $\{0, 1, \ldots, m_{kl} - 1\}$, which can be fitted by maximum likelihood based on the data from individuals for whom $s_k(h_k) = l$ to yield estimators $\widehat{\gamma}_{kl}$, $l = 1, \ldots, \ell_k$.

With these specifications, it is possible to carry out arguments similar to those earlier in this section, which, by analogy to (7.87), lead to defining the pseudo outcomes recursively as

$$\widetilde{V}_{ki} = \widetilde{V}_{k+1,i} + \sum_{l=1}^{\ell_k} \mathrm{I}\{s_k(H_{ki}) = l\} \left[\max_{j \in \{0,1,\ldots,m_{kl}-1\}} C_{kj,l}(H_{ki}; \widehat{\psi}_{kj,l}) \right.$$
$$\left. - \sum_{j=1}^{m_{kl}-1} \mathrm{I}(A_{ki} = j) C_{kj,l}(H_{ki}; \widehat{\psi}_{kj,l}) \right], \quad k = K, K-1, \ldots, 1,$$

where $\widetilde{V}_{K+1,i} = Y_i$. Taking all of the parameters $\psi_{kj,l}$ and ϕ_{kl} to be variationally independent across j and l, the stacked A-learning estimating equations (7.88) at the kth decision point are now

$$
\sum_{i=1}^{n} \left[\sum_{l=1}^{\ell_k} \mathrm{I}\{s_k(H_{ki}) = l\} \frac{\partial C_{kj,l}(H_{ki}; \psi_{kj,l})}{\partial \psi_{kj,l}} \left\{ \mathrm{I}(A_{ki} = j) - \omega_{k,l}(H_{ki}, j; \gamma_{kl}) \right\} \right.
$$
$$
\left. \times \left\{ \widetilde{V}_{k+1,i} - \sum_{j'=1}^{m_{kl}-1} \mathrm{I}(A_{ki} = j') C_{kj',l}(H_{ki}; \psi_{kj',l}) - \nu_{k,l}(H_{ki}; \phi_{kl}) \right\} \right] = 0
$$

$$
j = 1, \ldots, m_{kl} - 1,
$$

$$
\sum_{i=1}^{n} \left[\sum_{l=1}^{\ell_k} \mathrm{I}\{s_k(H_{ki}) = l\} \frac{\partial \nu_{k,l}(H_{ki}; \phi_{kl})}{\partial \phi_{kl}} \right.
$$
$$
\left. \times \left\{ \widetilde{V}_{k+1,i} - \sum_{j'=1}^{m_{kl}-1} \mathrm{I}(A_{ki} = j') C_{kj',l}(H_{ki}; \psi_{kj',l}) - \nu_{k,l}(H_{ki}; \phi_{kl}) \right\} \right] = 0,
$$

with the maximum likelihood score equations for γ_{kl}, $l = 1, \ldots, \ell_k$.

The A-learning estimator for the rule $d_{k,l}^{opt}(h_k)$ for h_k corresponding to the lth distinct subset $\mathcal{A}_{k,l}$ is then

$$
\widehat{d}_{A,k,l}^{opt}(h_k) = \underset{j \in \{0,1,\ldots,m_{kl}-1\}}{\arg \max} \; C_{kj,l}(h_k; \widehat{\psi}_{kj,l}),
$$

so that, from (7.89),

$$
\widehat{d}_{A,k}^{opt}(h_k) = \sum_{l=1}^{\ell_k} \mathrm{I}\{s_k(h_k) = l\} \, \widehat{d}_{A,k,l}^{opt}(h_k).
$$

As for Q-learning, if the distinct subsets are overlapping at Decision k, it may be possible to deduce a problem-specific strategy for modeling the contrast functions that incorporates this structure. However, adopting separate contrast function models for each $l = 1, \ldots, \ell_k$ may be more practically appealing from the point of view of ease of implementation.

Likewise, if for some h_k the relevant feasible set contains a single treatment option, so that $M_k(h_k) = 1$, then if this is the lth distinct subset $\mathcal{A}_{k,l}$, the estimated corresponding rule $\widehat{d}_{A,k,l}^{opt}(h_k)$ must return this option for h_k with $s_k(h_k) = l$. In this case, no contrast function model is necessary, and there is no corresponding estimating equation. For individuals i for whom $M_k(H_{ki}) = 1$, as for Q-learning, the pseudo outcome $\widetilde{V}_{k+1,i}$ can be "carried backward" to the next step of the algorithm; i.e., for Decision $k - 1$, take $\widetilde{V}_{k,i} = \widetilde{V}_{k+1,i}$.

Although the A-learning approach does not require modeling of the full Q-functions and offers robustness of estimation of contrast function parameters to mismodeling of the propensities or of $\nu_k(h_k)$, just as the validity of Q-learning is predicated on correct specification of the Q-functions, the method requires correct specification of the contrast function models to achieve faithful estimation of d^{opt}. The contrast functions at Decision K represent differences in expected observed outcome, so that familiar modeling techniques can be exploited. However, as for Q-learning, modeling of the contrast functions at Decisions $k < K$ is a nonstandard statistical problem, raising the strong possibility of misspecification, analogous to the demonstration for Q-learning in the case $K = 2$ in Section 5.7.1.

7.4.3 Value Search Estimation

From the discussion at the beginning of Section 5.7.2, the posited parametric Q-function or contrast function models involved in Q- and A-learning, respectively, can be viewed as inducing indirectly a class of multiple decision Ψ-specific regimes whose rules have a form determined by these functions and are indexed by the K sets of parameters in the models. Thus, these methods restrict the search for an optimal regime d^{opt} in the class $\mathcal{D}$ of all Ψ-specific regimes to this induced class. Moreover, if these models are misspecified, as is likely for $k < K$ for either method, the resulting estimators for d^{opt} may be suspect.

As in Sections 3.5.3 and 5.7.2, an alternative approach is to specify directly a restricted class $\mathcal{D}_\eta$ of K-decision Ψ-specific regimes, indexed by a parameter η, which is deliberately chosen on the basis of interpretability, cost, or ease and/or context of implementation. As in Section 5.7.2, a regime $d_\eta \in \mathcal{D}_\eta$ comprises K rules; i.e.,

$$d_\eta = \{d_1(h_1; \eta_1), \ldots, d_K(h_K; \eta_K)\}, \quad \eta = (\eta_1^T, \ldots, \eta_K^T)^T,$$

where the rule at each decision point k is indexed by a parameter η_k; and, as in Section 5.7.2, we often write for brevity

$$d_{\eta,k}(h_k) = d_k(h_k; \eta_k), \quad k = 1, \ldots, K.$$

Of necessity, specification of the rules $d_k(h_k; \eta_k)$, $k = 1, \ldots, K$, should be consistent with the nature of the feasible sets. At Decision k, if there are ℓ_k distinct subsets of $\mathcal{A}_k$ that are feasible sets, suppose that the lth subset $\mathcal{A}_{k,l} \subseteq \mathcal{A}_k$, $l = 1, \ldots, \ell_k$, comprises m_{kl} options coded as $\{1, \ldots, m_{kl}\}$. Then rules should be of the form

$$d_k(h_k; \eta_k) = \sum_{l=1}^{\ell_k} I\{s_k(h_k) = l\} d_{k,l}(h_k; \eta_{kl}), \quad \eta_k = (\eta_{k1}^T, \ldots, \eta_{k\ell_k}^T)^T,$$

$$(7.90)$$

$k = 1, \ldots, K$, where $d_{k,l}(h_k; \eta_{kl})$ is the rule relevant for histories h_k for which the feasible treatment options at Decision k are in the lth distinct subset $\mathcal{A}_{k,l}$, indexed by a parameter η_{kl}. As above, letting $d_{\eta,k,l}(h_k) = d_{k,l}(h_k; \eta_{kl})$, (7.90) can be written briefly as

$$d_{\eta,k}(h_k) = \sum_{l=1}^{\ell_k} \mathrm{I}\{s_k(h_k) = l\} \, d_{\eta,k,l}(h_k), \quad k = 1, \ldots, K.$$

With these definitions, as in (5.105), an optimal regime d_η^{opt} in $\mathcal{D}_\eta$ is given by

$$d_\eta^{opt} = \{d_1(h_1; \eta_1^{opt}), \ldots, d_K(h_K; \eta_K^{opt})\},$$
$$\eta^{opt} = (\eta_1^{opt\,T}, \ldots, \eta_K^{opt\,T})^T = \arg\max_\eta \mathcal{V}(d_\eta). \qquad (7.91)$$

Given an estimator $\widehat{\mathcal{V}}(d)$ for the value of a fixed regime d, (7.91) suggests obtaining

$$\widehat{\eta}^{opt} = (\widehat{\eta}_1^{opt\,T}, \ldots, \widehat{\eta}_K^{opt\,T})^T = \arg\max_\eta \widehat{\mathcal{V}}(d_\eta)$$

and estimating an optimal restricted regime d_η^{opt} by the value search (or direct or policy search) estimator

$$\widehat{d}_\eta^{opt} = \{d_1(h_1, \widehat{\eta}_1^{opt}), \ldots, d_K(h_K, \widehat{\eta}_K^{opt})\}. \qquad (7.92)$$

Value search estimation based on the simple inverse probability weighted estimator for the value is introduced in Section 5.7.2; we briefly review this approach in the context of Ψ-specific regimes and $\mathcal{A}_k$ that may contain more than two options and then discuss estimation of an optimal regime based on an augmented inverse probability weighted estimator.

As in Section 6.4.3, at Decision k, $k = 1, \ldots, K$, for the lth distinct subset $\mathcal{A}_{k,l} \subseteq \mathcal{A}_k$ comprising m_{kl} options coded as $1, \ldots, m_{kl}$, $l = 1, \ldots, \ell_k$, and $a_k \in \mathcal{A}_{k,l}$,

$$\omega_{k,l}(h_k, a_k) = P(A_k = a_k | H_k = h_k),$$
$$\omega_{k,l}(h_k, m_{kl}) = 1 - \sum_{a_k=1}^{m_{kl}-1} \omega_{k,l}(h_k, a_k) \qquad (7.93)$$

as in (6.104). Here, $\omega_{k,l}(h_k, 1) \equiv 1$ if the lth subset has a single element ($m_{kl} = 1$). Assume that models

$$\omega_{k,l}(h_k, a_k; \gamma_{kl}), \quad l = 1, \ldots, \ell_k, \qquad (7.94)$$

are posited for $k = 1, \ldots, K$ when $m_{kl} \geq 2$. As in Section 5.5.2, with

$d_{\eta,1}(h_1) = d_{\eta,1}(x_1)$, recall the recursive representation of the treatment options selected by d_η through Decision k, given here for $k = 2, \ldots, K$ as

$$\overline{d}_{\eta,k}(\overline{x}_k) = [d_{\eta,1}(x_1), d_{\eta,2}\{\overline{x}_2, d_{\eta,1}(x_1)\}, \ldots, d_{\eta,k}\{\overline{x}_k, \overline{d}_{\eta,k-1}(\overline{x}_{k-1})\}],$$

with $\overline{d}_\eta(\overline{x}) = \overline{d}_{\eta,K}(\overline{x}_K)$; and define

$$\mathcal{C}_{d_\eta} = \mathrm{I}\{\overline{A} = \overline{d}_\eta(\overline{X})\}.$$

From (6.86), with $\overline{\eta}_k = (\eta_1^T, \ldots, \eta_k)^T$, $k = 2, \ldots, K$, define

$$\pi_{d_\eta,1}(X_1; \eta_1) = p_{A_1|X_1}\{d_{\eta,1}(X_1)|X_1\},$$
$$\pi_{d_\eta,k}(\overline{X}_k; \overline{\eta}_k) = p_{A_k|\overline{X}_k, \overline{A}_{k-1}}[d_{\eta,k}\{\overline{X}_k, \overline{d}_{\eta,k-1}(\overline{X}_{k-1})\} \qquad (7.95)$$
$$|\overline{X}_k, \overline{d}_{\eta,k-1}(\overline{X}_{k-1})], \quad k = 2, \ldots, K.$$

The considerations in Section 6.4.3 can be exploited to obtain models for the quantities in (7.95). Namely, representing (7.95) as in (6.107), given propensity models (7.94),

$$\pi_{d_\eta,1}(X_1; \eta_1, \gamma_1) = \sum_{l=1}^{\ell_1} \mathrm{I}\{s_1(h_1) = l\} \prod_{a_1=1}^{m_{1l}} \omega_{1,l}(X_1, a_1; \gamma_{1l})^{\mathrm{I}\{d_{\eta,1}(X_1)=a_1\}}$$

$$\pi_{d_\eta,k}(\overline{X}_k; \overline{\eta}_k, \gamma_k) = \sum_{l=1}^{\ell_k} \mathrm{I}\{s_k(h_k) = l\} \qquad (7.96)$$

$$\times \prod_{a_k=1}^{m_{kl}} \omega_{k,l}\{\overline{X}_k, \overline{d}_{\eta,k-1}(\overline{X}_{k-1}), a_k; \gamma_{kl}\}^{\mathrm{I}[d_{\eta,k}\{\overline{X}_k, \overline{d}_{\eta,k-1}(\overline{X}_{k-1})\}=a_k]},$$

$$k = 2, \ldots, K,$$

analogous to (6.108).

As discussed in Section 6.4.3 and the previous section, for each $l = 1, \ldots, \ell_k$, $k = 1, \ldots, K$, the models (7.94) can be fitted by maximum likelihood using the data from individuals i for whom $s_k(H_{ki}) = l$, yielding estimators $\widehat{\gamma}_k = (\widehat{\gamma}_{k1}^T, \ldots, \widehat{\gamma}_{k\ell_k}^T)^T$. Substituting these estimators in (7.96), the inverse probability weighted estimator for $\mathcal{V}(d_\eta)$ for fixed η, and thus fixed d_η, is given by

$$\widehat{\mathcal{V}}_{IPW}(d_\eta) = n^{-1} \sum_{i=1}^n \frac{\mathcal{C}_{d_\eta,i} Y_i}{\left\{\prod_{k=2}^K \pi_{d_\eta,k}(\overline{X}_{ki}; \overline{\eta}_k, \widehat{\gamma}_k)\right\} \pi_{d_\eta,1}(X_{1i}; \eta_1, \widehat{\gamma}_1)}. \qquad (7.97)$$

As in Section 5.7.2, under SUTVA (6.16), the SRA (6.17), and the positivity assumption (7.7), if the models $\omega_{k,l}(h_k, a_k; \gamma_{kl})$ in (7.94) are all correctly specified, $l = 1, \ldots, \ell_k$, $k = 1, \ldots, K$, so that the implied models in (7.96) are also correctly specified, then $\widehat{V}_{IPW}(d_\eta)$ in (7.97) is a consistent estimator for $\mathcal{V}(d_\eta)$. An alternative estimator that shares this property but is more efficient in practice follows from (5.108) with the definitions above; see Section 5.7.2.

Maximizing (7.97) in η leads to the estimator

$$\widehat{\eta}_{IPW}^{opt} = (\widehat{\eta}_{1,IPW}^{opt\,T}, \ldots, \widehat{\eta}_{K,IPW}^{opt\,T})^T.$$

Then, from (7.92), the value search estimator for d_η^{opt} based on simple inverse probability weighting is given by

$$\widehat{d}_{\eta,IPW}^{opt} = \{d_1(h_1; \widehat{\eta}_{1,IPW}^{opt}), \ldots, d_K(h_K; \widehat{\eta}_{K,IPW}^{opt})\},$$

and the corresponding estimator $\widehat{V}_{IPW}(d_\eta^{opt})$ for $\mathcal{V}(d_\eta^{opt})$ is obtained by substituting $\widehat{\eta}_{IPW}^{opt}$ in $\widehat{V}_{IPW}(d_\eta)$ (7.97).

Unfortunately, from the discussion in Section 5.7.4, this estimator can exhibit poor performance in finite samples. The value estimator $\widehat{V}_{IPW}(d_\eta)$ involves data only from individuals for whom $\mathcal{C}_{d_\eta} = 1$, so for whom the treatment options actually received at all K decision points are consistent with following regime d_η. For larger and larger K, the number of individuals for whom this is true can be a smaller and smaller proportion of the entire sample, leading to instability and inefficiency for K larger than 2 or 3. Moreover, consistency of $\widehat{V}_{IPW}(d_\eta)$ as an estimator for $\mathcal{V}(d_\eta)$ is predicated on correct specification of the propensity models (7.94). The propensities are known when the data are from a SMART, in which case $\widehat{V}_{IPW}(d_\eta)$ is consistent, but are subject to possible misspecification when the data are from an observational study. These features can have deleterious effects on the resulting estimator $\widehat{d}_{\eta,IPW}^{opt}$.

Citing these drawbacks, Zhang et al. (2013) propose value search estimation based on augmented inverse probability weighted estimators for $\mathcal{V}(d_\eta)$; for a fixed regime, these estimators are discussed in Section 6.4.4. For $d_\eta \in \mathcal{D}_\eta$, let $\widehat{\overline{\gamma}}_k = (\widehat{\gamma}_1^T, \ldots, \widehat{\gamma}_k^T)^T$, $k = 1, \ldots, K$; and, as in (6.110), define for brevity

$$\overline{\pi}_{d_\eta,1}(X_1; \widehat{\gamma}_1) = \pi_{d_\eta,1}(X_1; \eta_1, \widehat{\gamma}_1)$$

$$\overline{\pi}_{d_\eta,k}(\overline{X}_k; \widehat{\overline{\gamma}}_k) = \left\{ \prod_{j=2}^{k} \pi_{d_\eta,j}(\overline{X}_j; \overline{\eta}_j, \widehat{\gamma}_j) \right\} \pi_{d_\eta,1}(X_1; \eta_1, \widehat{\gamma}_1), \quad k = 2, \ldots, K,$$

with $\overline{\pi}_{d_\eta,0} \equiv 1$. As in (6.83), let

$$\mathcal{C}_{\overline{d}_\eta,k} = \mathrm{I}\{\overline{A}_k = \overline{d}_{\eta,k}(\overline{X}_k)\}, \quad k = 1, \ldots, K, \tag{7.98}$$

be the indicator that the treatment options received through Decision k

are consistent with those dictated by the first k rules in d_η, where, clearly, $\mathcal{C}_{\overline{d}_{\eta,K}} = \mathcal{C}_{d_\eta}$; and define $\mathcal{C}_{\overline{d}_{\eta,0}} \equiv 1$. Then, from (6.112), an augmented inverse probability weighted estimator for $\mathcal{V}(d_\eta)$ for fixed $d_\eta \in \mathcal{D}_\eta$ is

$$\widehat{\mathcal{V}}_{AIPW}(d_\eta) = n^{-1} \sum_{i=1}^{n} \left[\frac{\mathcal{C}_{d_\eta,i} Y_i}{\left\{ \prod_{k=2}^{K} \pi_{d_\eta,k}(\overline{X}_{ki}; \overline{\eta}_k, \widehat{\gamma}_k) \right\} \pi_{d_\eta,1}(X_{1i}; \eta_1, \widehat{\gamma}_1)} \right.$$

$$\left. + \sum_{k=1}^{K} \left\{ \frac{\mathcal{C}_{\overline{d}_{\eta,k-1},i}}{\pi_{d_\eta,k-1}(\overline{X}_{k-1,i}; \widehat{\overline{\gamma}}_{k-1})} - \frac{\mathcal{C}_{\overline{d}_{\eta,k},i}}{\pi_{d_\eta,k}(\overline{X}_{ki}, \widehat{\overline{\gamma}}_k)} \right\} L_k(\overline{X}_{ki}) \right], \tag{7.99}$$

where $L_k(\overline{x}_k)$ are arbitrary functions of $\overline{x}_k$, $k = 1, \ldots, K$.

As noted following (6.112) in Section 6.4.4, with $L_k(\overline{x}_k) \equiv 0$, $\widehat{\mathcal{V}}_{AIPW}(d_\eta)$ reduces to the inverse probability weighted estimator (7.97); and, when $K = 1$, (7.99) is the estimator (3.27) introduced in the single decision setting, evaluated at the fixed regime d_η. Under SUTVA (6.16), the SRA (6.17), and the positivity assumption (7.7), as long as the propensity models (7.94) are correctly specified, it can be shown that (7.99) is a consistent estimator for the true value $\mathcal{V}(d_\eta)$. The optimal choice of $L_k(\overline{x}_k)$ yielding the smallest asymptotic variance among estimators of the form (7.99) follows from semiparametric theory (Tsiatis, 2006) and is given by, from (6.113),

$$L_k(\overline{x}_k) = E\{Y^*(d_\eta) \mid \overline{X}_k^*(\overline{d}_{\eta,k-1}) = \overline{x}_k\}, \quad k = 1, \ldots, K. \tag{7.100}$$

The result (7.100) suggests positing models for the conditional expectations $E\{Y^*(d_\eta) | \overline{X}_k^*(\overline{d}_{\eta,k-1}) = \overline{x}_k\}$, $k = 1, \ldots, K$, in terms of parameters β_k and substituting the fitted models for $L_k(\overline{x}_k)$, $k = 1, \ldots, K$, in (7.99). As we discuss shortly, the approaches reviewed in Section 6.4.4 for developing and fitting these models can be used for this purpose. Analogous to (6.119), let

$$\mathcal{Q}_{d_\eta,k}(\overline{x}_k; \beta_k), \quad k = 1, \ldots, K, \tag{7.101}$$

denote these models, which, as (7.100) and (7.101) imply, depend on d_η and thus η; and let $\widehat{\beta}_k$ be the corresponding estimators for β_k. The augmented inverse probability weighted estimator for $\mathcal{V}(d_\eta)$ is then

$$\widehat{\mathcal{V}}_{AIPW}(d_\eta) = n^{-1} \sum_{i=1}^{n} \left[\frac{\mathcal{C}_{d_\eta,i} Y_i}{\left\{ \prod_{k=2}^{K} \pi_{d_\eta,k}(\overline{X}_{ki}; \overline{\eta}_k, \widehat{\gamma}_k) \right\} \pi_{d_\eta,1}(X_{1i}; \eta_1, \widehat{\gamma}_1)} \right.$$

$$\left. + \sum_{k=1}^{K} \left\{ \frac{\mathcal{C}_{\overline{d}_{\eta,k-1},i}}{\pi_{d_\eta,k-1}(\overline{X}_{k-1,i}; \widehat{\overline{\gamma}}_{k-1})} - \frac{\mathcal{C}_{\overline{d}_{\eta,k},i}}{\pi_{d_\eta,k}(\overline{X}_{ki}, \widehat{\overline{\gamma}}_k)} \right\} \mathcal{Q}_{d_\eta,k}(\overline{X}_{ki}; \widehat{\beta}_k) \right]. \tag{7.102}$$

The estimator (7.102) is a consistent estimator for the true value $\mathcal{V}(d_\eta)$ if either the models for the propensities (7.94) or the models (7.101) for $E\{Y^*(d) \mid \overline{X}_k^*(\overline{d}_k) = \overline{x}_k\}$, $k = 1, \ldots, K$, are correctly specified and thus is doubly robust; see Section 6.4.4 for discussion.

As for the simple inverse probability weighted estimator (7.97), one maximizes the augmented estimator $\widehat{\mathcal{V}}_{AIPW}(d_\eta)$ in (7.102) in η to obtain

$$\widehat{\eta}_{AIPW}^{opt} = (\widehat{\eta}_{1,AIPW}^{opt\,T}, \ldots, \widehat{\eta}_{K,AIPW}^{opt\,T})^T.$$

The value search estimator for d_η^{opt} based on the augmented inverse probability weighted estimator is then given by

$$\widehat{d}_{\eta,AIPW}^{opt} = \{d_1(h_1; \widehat{\eta}_{1,AIPW}^{opt}), \ldots, d_K(h_K, \widehat{\eta}_{K;AIPW}^{opt})\},$$

and substituting $\widehat{\eta}_{AIPW}^{opt}$ in (7.102) for η leads to the estimator $\widehat{\mathcal{V}}_{AIPW}(d_\eta^{opt})$ for $\mathcal{V}(d_\eta^{opt})$.

Modeling and Implementation Considerations for Value Search Estimation

Throughout this discussion, we continue to assume that, at Decision k, $k = 1, \ldots, K$, there are ℓ_k distinct subsets of $\mathcal{A}_k$ that are feasible sets, the lth of which, $\mathcal{A}_{k,l} \subseteq \mathcal{A}_k$, comprises m_{kl} treatment options coded as $\{1, \ldots, m_{kl}\}$. Clearly, for both $\widehat{\mathcal{V}}_{IPW}(d_\eta)$ and $\widehat{\mathcal{V}}_{AIPW}(d_\eta)$, propensity models (7.94) relevant to each distinct subset must be developed, as discussed in Section 6.4.3. Formulation of the models (7.101) for $L_k(\overline{x}_k)$, $k = 1, \ldots, K$, used in construction of the augmented inverse probability weighted estimator $\widehat{\mathcal{V}}_{AIPW}(d_\eta)$ in (7.102) must also respect the nature of the feasible sets, in the spirit of Remark (iii) in Section 6.4.2; these models are discussed below.

Although maximizing (7.97) or (7.102) in η to obtain $\widehat{\eta}_{IPW}^{opt}$ or $\widehat{\eta}_{AIPW}^{opt}$ and thus estimators $\widehat{d}_{\eta,IPW}^{opt}$ or $\widehat{d}_{\eta,AIPW}^{opt}$ for $d_\eta^{opt} \in \mathcal{D}_\eta$ is conceptually straightforward, as noted in Sections 5.7.3 and 5.7.4, implementation is challenging on several fronts. Maximization of both value estimators in η is a nonsmooth optimization problem, so standard techniques cannot be used. Moreover, and more ominously, two additional issues arise that can render this optimization problem practically infeasible.

The first challenge, discussed briefly in Section 5.7.3 and on which we now expand, is that the dimension of η can be large enough in a multiple decision setting to make the optimization of either $\widehat{\mathcal{V}}_{IPW}(d_\eta)$ or $\widehat{\mathcal{V}}_{AIPW}(d_\eta)$ itself computationally intractable. From (7.90), at Decision k, a rule $d_k(h_k; \eta_k)$ for a regime $d_\eta \in \mathcal{D}_\eta$ is a collection of rules; namely,

$$d_k(h_k; \eta_k) = \sum_{l=1}^{\ell_k} \mathrm{I}\{s_k(h_k) = l\} d_{k,l}(h_k; \eta_{kl}), \quad \eta_k = (\eta_{k1}^T, \ldots, \eta_{k\ell_k}^T)^T,$$

where $d_{k,l}(h_k; \eta_{kl})$ is the rule corresponding to realized histories h_k that render an individual eligible for the options in $\mathcal{A}_{k,l}$. If, as would ordinarily be the case, the rules $d_{k,l}(h_k; \eta_{kl})$, $l = 1, \ldots, \ell_k$, involve nonoverlapping parameters η_{kl}, the dimension of η_k is equal to the sum of the dimensions of $\eta_{k1}, \ldots, \eta_{k\ell_k}$. Then, even if the rules $d_{k,l}(h_k; \eta_{kl})$ have relatively simple forms, for general K and ℓ_k, $k = 1, \ldots, K$, the overall dimension of η can be considerable. As an illustration, suppose that, for each of Decisions $k = 1, \ldots, K$, $x_k = (x_{k1}, x_{k2})^T$; $\ell_k = 2$, so that there are two distinct subsets of $\mathcal{A}_k$ that are feasible sets at each decision point; each distinct subset $\mathcal{A}_{k,l}$, $l = 1, 2$, comprises $m_{kl} = 2$ options coded as 0 and 1; and the subset-specific rules are of the form

$$d_{k,l}(h_k; \eta_{kl}) = \mathrm{I}(x_{k1} < \eta_{kl,1}, x_{k2} < \eta_{kl,2}), \quad \eta_{kl} = (\eta_{kl,1}, \eta_{kl,2})^T, \quad l = 1, 2.$$

Then $\eta_k = (\eta_{k1}^T, \eta_{k2}^T)^T$ is four dimensional, so that, with $K = 3$, say, $\dim(\eta) = 12$. Maximization of the nonsmooth functions $\widehat{\mathcal{V}}_{IPW}(d_\eta)$ or $\widehat{\mathcal{V}}_{AIPW}(d_\eta)$ of η in 12 dimensions using, for example, a genetic algorithm (Goldberg, 1989) as discussed in Section 5.7.4, can be a significant computational challenge. Clearly, for general K; ℓ_k, $k = 1, \ldots, K$; and numbers of options m_{kl}, $l = 1, \ldots, \ell_k$ in the distinct subsets $\mathcal{A}_{k,l}$, the dimension of η can be substantially larger. Implementation of value search estimation via a backward iterative algorithm, as reviewed for $\widehat{\mathcal{V}}_{IPW}(d_\eta)$ in Section 5.7.3, is an approach to addressing this challenge; we present a detailed account in the next section.

The second issue is relevant to the augmented inverse probability weighted estimator $\widehat{\mathcal{V}}_{AIPW}(d_\eta)$ and has to do with positing and fitting the models $\mathcal{Q}_{d_\eta,k}(\overline{x}_k; \beta_k)$ in (7.101) for $L_k(\overline{x}_k)$, $k = 1, \ldots, K$, in the context of obtaining and maximizing (7.102). We demonstrate by considering the three approaches to this task reviewed in Section 6.4.4.

One strategy is to use the g-computation algorithm, as outlined in Section 6.4.4, to obtain estimators for $L_k(\overline{X}_{ki})$ for each individual i via Monte Carlo integration based on models for the relevant conditional densities $p_{Y|\overline{X},\overline{A}}(y|\overline{x}, \overline{a}; \beta_{K+1})$, $p_{X_k|\overline{X}_{k-1},\overline{A}_{k-1}}(x_k|\overline{x}_{k-1}, \overline{a}_{k-1}; \beta_k)$, $k = 2, \ldots, K$, and $p_{X_1}(x_1; \beta_1)$ as in (6.117) in terms of parameters $\beta_1, \ldots, \beta_{K+1}$. These models must obviously take into account the nature of the feasible sets, and β_k can be estimated by $\widehat{\beta}_k$, $k = 1, \ldots, K+1$, maximizing an appropriate partial likelihood. Then, for each individual i and each $k = 1, \ldots, K$, the analyst would carry out steps 1–3 of the Monte Carlo simulation algorithm given in Section 6.4.4 M times using these fitted models to obtain the estimators for $L_k(\overline{X}_{ki})$ empirically, which can then be substituted for $\mathcal{Q}_{d_\eta,k}(\overline{X}_{ki}; \widehat{\beta}_k)$, $k = 1, \ldots, K$, in (7.102). Inspection of this algorithm shows that generation of the required simulated values from the fitted densities at each step is based on d_η; e.g., in the first step, one generates $x_{k+1,r}$, $r = 1, \ldots, M$, from

$$p_{X_{k+1}|\overline{X}_k, \overline{A}_k}\{x_{k+1} \mid \overline{x}_k, \overline{d}_{\eta,k}(\overline{x}_k); \widehat{\beta}_k\}.$$

Thus, although the models for the conditional densities do not depend on d_η and need be posited and fitted only once, obtaining the estimate of $L_k(\overline{X}_{ki})$ for each i depends on d_η and thus η. Accordingly, in each internal iteration of an optimization algorithm used to maximize $\widehat{\mathcal{V}}_{AIPW}(d_\eta)$ in η, evaluation of $\widehat{\mathcal{V}}_{AIPW}(d_\eta)$ at the current iterate of η requires that the estimates of $L_k(\overline{X}_{ki})$ for $k = 1, \ldots, K$ for each individual $i = 1, \ldots, n$ be recalculated using this current iterate. Clearly, this could be quite computationally intensive.

From (6.74), with

$$\mu_k^{d_\eta}(\overline{x}_k) = E\{Y^*(d_\eta) \mid \overline{X}_k^*(\overline{d}_{\eta,k-1}) = \overline{x}_k\},$$

another strategy involves positing models $\mu_k^{d_\eta}(\overline{x}_k; \beta_k)$ for these conditional expectations directly; obtaining estimators $\widehat{\beta}_k$, $k = 1, \ldots, K$, via the monotone coarsening approach in Section 6.4.2; and taking

$$\mathcal{Q}_{d_\eta,k}(\overline{X}_{ki}; \widehat{\beta}_k) = \mu_k^{d_\eta}(\overline{X}_{ki}; \widehat{\beta}_k), \quad k = 1, \ldots, K, \tag{7.103}$$

for each $i = 1, \ldots, n$ in (7.102). As noted in the remark at the end of Section 6.4.2, not only must these models take into account the nature of the feasible sets, positing and backward iterative fitting of these models depends on the regime d_η and thus on η. In particular, in the backward fitting algorithm outlined in (6.82) and (6.84), the indicators $\mathcal{C}_{\overline{d}_{\eta,k,i}}$ for each i, $k = K, \ldots, 1$, determining the set of individuals whose data is included in in each fit, depend on d_η and thus η. Consequently, as for estimation of $L_k(\overline{X}_{ki})$ via the g-computation algorithm, the models $\mu_k^{d_\eta}(\overline{x}_k; \beta_k)$ must be refitted, and thus the backward fitting scheme carried out anew, for the value of η at each internal iteration of the optimization algorithm used to maximize $\widehat{\mathcal{V}}_{AIPW}(d_\eta)$ in η. Although for fixed η this method for estimation of the $L_k(\overline{X}_{ki})$ is not as intensive as the simulation-based approach used in g-computation, repeated implementation of the backward fitting algorithm in the context of maximization of $\widehat{\mathcal{V}}_{AIPW}(d_\eta)$ in η renders this approach computationally demanding.

A third method is based on the result in (6.115). Namely, as in Section 6.4.4, with $Q_K^{d_\eta}(h_K, a_K) = E(Y|H_K = h_K, A_K = a_K)$ and, for $k = K - 1, \ldots, 1$,

$$Q_k^{d_\eta}(h_k, a_k) = E\{V_{k+1}^{d_\eta}(H_{k+1}) \mid H_k = h_k, A_k = a_k\},$$
$$V_k^{d_\eta}(h_k) = Q_k^{d_\eta}\{h_k, d_{\eta,k}(h_k)\}, \quad k = 1, \ldots, K, \tag{7.104}$$

from (6.115),

$$V_k^{d_\eta}\{\overline{x}_k, \overline{d}_{\eta,k-1}(\overline{x}_{k-1})\} = E\{Y^*(d_\eta) \mid \overline{X}_k^*(\overline{d}_{\eta,k-1}) = \overline{x}_k\}.$$

Remark. As in the remark at the beginning of Section 6.4.2, with the exception that $Q_K^{d_\eta}(h_K, a_K) = Q_K(h_K, a_K) = E(Y|H_K = h_K, A_K = a_K)$, $Q_k^{d_\eta}(h_k, a_k)$ and $V_k^{d_\eta}(h_k)$ in (7.104) are different from the Q-functions $Q_k(h_k, a_k)$ and value functions $V_k(h_k)$ in (7.61) and (7.62), and the superscript in the former emphasizes dependence on d_η.

This suggests developing models $Q_k^{d_\eta}(h_k, a_k; \beta_k)$, $k = 1, \ldots, K$; obtaining estimators $\widehat{\beta}_k$, $k = K, K-1, \ldots, 1$, using the backward induction algorithm in Section 6.4.2; and, letting

$$V_k^{d_\eta}\{\overline{x}_k, \overline{d}_{\eta,k-1}(\overline{x}_{k-1}); \beta_k\} = Q_k^{d_\eta}\{\overline{x}_k, \overline{d}_{\eta,k}(\overline{x}_k); \beta_k\},$$

taking

$$\begin{aligned} \mathcal{Q}_{d_\eta,k}(\overline{X}_{ki}; \widehat{\beta}_k) &= V_k^{d_\eta}\{\overline{X}_{ki}, \overline{d}_{\eta,k-1}(\overline{X}_{k-1,i}); \widehat{\beta}_k\}, \\ &= Q_k^{d_\eta}\{\overline{X}_{ki}, \overline{d}_{\eta,k}(\overline{X}_{ki}); \widehat{\beta}_k\}, \quad k = 1, \ldots, K, \end{aligned} \tag{7.105}$$

for $i = 1, \ldots, n$ in (7.102). Inspection of the backward induction algorithm shows that, with the exception of development and fitting of the model $Q_K^{d_\eta}(h_K, a_K; \beta_K)$ for $E(Y|H_K = h_K, A_K = a_K)$, the models and pseudo outcomes at steps $K - 1, \ldots, 1$ depend on d_η and thus η. Thus, as with the previous two approaches, the backward induction algorithm for fitting the models $Q_k^{d_\eta}(h_k, a_k; \beta_k)$, $k = 1, \ldots, K$, must be repeated at each internal iteration of the optimization scheme used to maximize $\widehat{\mathcal{V}}_{AIPW}(d_\eta)$ in η.

The foregoing developments indicate that implementation of value search estimation can involve formidable computational obstacles. When the dimension of η is not large, the data analyst might be tempted to avoid the need for repeated fitting of the models (7.101) in the augmentation term of $\widehat{\mathcal{V}}_{AIPW}(d_\eta)$ in (7.102) at each internal iteration of the optimization by basing estimation of d_η^{opt} on $\widehat{\mathcal{V}}_{IPW}(d_\eta)$ instead. However, as discussed in Section 7.4.9, this is at the expense of substantial loss of efficiency and likely instability of estimation of $\mathcal{V}(d_\eta^{opt})$ and thus of d_η^{opt}. Accordingly, Zhang et al. (2013) propose two practical, ad hoc strategies for implementation of value search estimation based on $\widehat{\mathcal{V}}_{AIPW}(d_\eta)$ that circumvent this difficulty.

The strategy advocated in (7) of Zhang et al. (2013) involves first carrying out Q-learning as described in Section 7.4.1. That is, posit models $Q_k(h_k, a_k; \beta_k)$ for the Q-functions $Q_k(h_k, a_k)$, $k = 1, \ldots, K$, in

(7.60) and (7.61). These models and the backward scheme to fit them do not depend on d_η or η, so can be fitted by a single, preliminary invocation of the Q-learning algorithm given in Section 7.4.1, yielding

$$Q_k(h_k, a_k; \widehat{\beta}_k) = Q_k(\overline{x}_k, \overline{a}_k; \widehat{\beta}_k), \quad k = 1, \ldots, K.$$

Then take in (7.102)

$$\mathcal{Q}_{d_\eta, k}(\overline{X}_{ki}; \widehat{\beta}_k) = Q_k\{\overline{X}_{ki}, \overline{d}_{\eta, k}(\overline{X}_{ki}); \widehat{\beta}_k\}, \quad k = 1, \ldots, K. \tag{7.106}$$

Note that the quantities in (7.106) are functions of η only through substitution of $\overline{d}_{\eta, k}(\overline{X}_{ki})$ in the second argument and do not need to be refitted at each internal iteration of the optimization algorithm. Using (7.106) in the augmentation term thus eliminates this computational challenge. Of course, strictly speaking, (7.106) do not represent fitted models for the conditional expectations $E\{Y^*(d_\eta) | \overline{X}_k^*(\overline{d}_{\eta, k-1}) = \overline{x}_k\}$; nonetheless, the hope is that they will be "close enough." Zhang et al. (2013) advocate this approach primarily for the situation in which the functional forms of the rules $d_k(h_k; \eta_k)$ are the same as those for an optimal regime induced by the Q-function models. As a simple example, if $\Psi_k(h_k) = \mathcal{A}_k = \{0, 1\}$, $k = 1, \ldots, K$; the class $\mathcal{D}_\eta$ is taken to comprise regimes with rules $d_k(h_k; \eta_k) = \text{I}(\widetilde{h}_k^T \eta_k > 0)$, $\widetilde{h}_k = (1, h_k^T)^T$, $k = 1, \ldots, K$; and the Q-functions are of the form

$$Q_k(h_k, a_k; \beta_k) = \widetilde{h}_k^T \beta_{k1} + a_k(\widetilde{h}_k^T \beta_{k2}), \quad k = 1, \ldots, K,$$

as in (5.100) and (5.102), then the optimal rules induced by these Q-functions have the same form as $d_k(h_k; \eta_k)$. The authors present empirical evidence that using (7.106) leads to performance of the resulting estimators for $\mathcal{V}(d_\eta^{opt})$ and d_η^{opt} close to that of the estimators for these quantities based on the full, computationally intensive monotone coarsening approach discussed above.

The second method, proposed in Section 6 of the supplemental material to Zhang et al. (2013), involves an iterative three step strategy, as follows: (i) Obtain a preliminary estimator $\widehat{\eta}_{(0)}^{opt}$, say, by maximizing $\widehat{\mathcal{V}}_{IPW}(d_\eta)$ or $\widehat{\mathcal{V}}_{AIPW}(d_\eta)$ with (7.106), and let $r = 0$. (ii) Posit models $\mu_k^{d_\eta}(\overline{X}_{ki}; \beta_k)$, $k = 1, \ldots, K$, and estimate β_k using the monotone coarsening algorithm with η fixed at $\widehat{\eta}_{(r)}^{opt}$, to obtain $\widehat{\beta}_k^{(r)}$, $k = 1, \ldots, K$. (iii) Take

$$\mathcal{Q}_{d_\eta, k}(\overline{X}_{ki}; \widehat{\beta}_k^{(r)}) = \mu_k^{d_\eta}(\overline{X}_{ki}; \widehat{\beta}_k^{(r)}), \quad k = 1, \ldots, K,$$

as in (7.103), with η fixed at $\widehat{\eta}_{(r)}^{opt}$, and maximize $\widehat{\mathcal{V}}_{AIPW}(d_\eta)$ in η where it appears elsewhere to obtain $\widehat{\eta}_{(r+1)}^{opt}$. One can stop and declare $\widehat{\eta}_{AIPW}^{opt} = \widehat{\eta}_{(r+1)}^{opt}$, or let $r = r + 1$ and return to (ii) and iterate between steps

(ii) and (iii) one or more times. This strategy could also be implemented based on models $Q_k^{d_\eta}(h_k, a_k; \beta_k)$, $k = 1, \ldots, K$, in the obvious way.

These ad hoc approaches can be used to implement value search estimation based on $\widehat{\mathcal{V}}_{AIPW}(d_\eta)$ when the dimension of η is not too large, with the understanding that their performance may be problem specific. However, when η is of sufficiently high dimension, global maximization of both $\widehat{\mathcal{V}}_{IPW}(d_\eta)$ and $\widehat{\mathcal{V}}_{AIPW}(d_\eta)$ in η may be computationally prohibitive, making even these simplified approaches problematic.

7.4.4 Backward Iterative Estimation

In this section, we continue to assume that interest focuses on a restricted class of regimes $\mathcal{D}_\eta$ with elements of the form $d_\eta = \{d_1(h_1; \eta_1), \ldots, d_K(h_K; \eta_K)\} = \{d_{\eta,1}(h_1), \ldots, d_{\eta,K}(h_K)\}$. The challenge of global maximization of value estimators in η is one motivation for the alternative strategies we now discuss. These strategies exploit a backward iterative approach first used by Zhao et al. (2015a) with simple inverse weighted estimators and sketched in Section 5.7.3 and by Zhang and Zhang (2018a) with a doubly robust augmented inverse probability weighted estimator, both from a classification perspective discussed in the next section. We first discuss how this approach can be used to reduce the global optimization of $\widehat{\mathcal{V}}_{IPW}(d_\eta)$ or $\widehat{\mathcal{V}}_{AIPW}(d_\eta)$ in η to a recursive series of lower-dimensional maximizations in η_k, $k = K, \ldots, 1$. The reader may wish to review Section 5.7.3 before proceeding with the more formal and detailed account based on augmented inverse probability weighted estimators given here.

Backward Iterative Implementation of Value Search Estimation

Consider $\widehat{\mathcal{V}}_{AIPW}(d_\eta)$ with $\mathcal{Q}_{d_\eta,k}(\overline{X}_{ki}; \widehat{\beta}_k)$ as in (7.105), so that, for $k = 1, \ldots, K$,

$$
\begin{aligned}
\mathcal{Q}_{d_\eta,k}(\overline{X}_{ki}; \widehat{\beta}_k) &= V_k^{d_\eta}\{\overline{X}_{ki}, \overline{d}_{\eta,k-1}(\overline{X}_{k-1,i}); \widehat{\beta}_k\} \\
&= Q_k^{d_\eta}\{\overline{X}_{ki}, \overline{d}_{\eta,k}(\overline{X}_{ki}); \widehat{\beta}_k\} \qquad (7.107) \\
&= Q_k^{d_\eta}\left[\overline{X}_{ki}, \overline{d}_{\eta,k-1}(\overline{X}_{k-1,i}), d_{\eta,k}\{\overline{X}_{ki}, \overline{d}_{\eta,k-1}(\overline{X}_{k-1,i})\}; \widehat{\beta}_k\right].
\end{aligned}
$$

We begin by presenting an equivalent expression for $\widehat{\mathcal{V}}_{AIPW}(d_\eta)$ in (7.102), which proves convenient here and in an analogous formulation for censored time-to-event outcome in Chapter 8.

In (7.102), it is straightforward to observe that the kth summand in the augmentation term is equal to zero unless

$$
\overline{A}_{k-1,i} = \overline{d}_{\eta,k-1}(\overline{X}_{k-1,i}),
$$

because, from (7.98), $\mathcal{C}_{\overline{d}_{\eta,k-1},i} = \mathcal{C}_{\overline{d}_{\eta,k},i} = 0$ if this does not hold. From (7.107), this suggests that $\mathcal{Q}_{d_\eta,k}(\overline{X}_{ki}; \widehat{\beta}_k)$ can be replaced by

$$V_k^{d_\eta}(\overline{X}_{ki}, \overline{A}_{k-1,i}; \widehat{\beta}_k) = Q_k^{d_\eta}\{\overline{X}_{ki}, \overline{A}_{k-1,i}, d_{\eta,k}(\overline{X}_{ki}, \overline{A}_{k-1,i}); \widehat{\beta}_k\}$$
$$= Q_k^{d_\eta}\{H_{ki}, d_{\eta,k}(H_{ki}); \widehat{\beta}_k\} = Q_k^{d_\eta}\{H_{ki}, d_k(H_{ki}; \eta_k); \widehat{\beta}_k\}, \quad (7.108)$$

$k = 1, \ldots, K$, where the last expression in (7.108) emphasizes that the dependence on η is only through η_k dictating the kth rule in d_η. In what follows, we use mostly the streamlined notation $d_{\eta,k}(h_k)$ rather than $d_k(h_k; \eta_k)$ for brevity.

From (7.93), with the propensities

$$\omega_k(h_k, a_k) = \sum_{l=1}^{\ell_k} \mathrm{I}\{s_k(h_k) = l\}\, \omega_{k,l}(h_k, a_k), \quad k = 1, \ldots, K,$$

where the argument a_k takes values in the relevant distinct subset $\mathcal{A}_{k,l}$, define

$$\varpi_k(h_k, a_k) = \prod_{j=1}^{k} \omega_j(h_j, a_j), \quad k = 1, \ldots, K, \qquad (7.109)$$

the probability of receiving treatment options $\overline{a}_k$ through Decision k; and define $\varpi_0 \equiv 1$. As in (6.106), with $\gamma_k = (\gamma_{k1}^T, \ldots, \gamma_{k\ell_k}^T)^T$, let models for the propensities $\omega_k(h_k, a_k)$ be given by, for $k = 1, \ldots, K$,

$$\omega_k(h_k, a_k; \gamma_k) = \sum_{l=1}^{\ell_k} \mathrm{I}\{s_k(h_k) = l\}\, \omega_{k,l}(h_k, a_k; \gamma_{kl}),$$

inducing models for (7.109)

$$\varpi_k(h_k, a_k; \overline{\gamma}_k) = \prod_{j=1}^{k} \omega_j(h_j, a_j; \gamma_j),$$

where $\overline{\gamma}_k = (\gamma_1^T, \ldots, \gamma_k^T)^T$. As previously, let $\widehat{\gamma}_k$ denote the maximum likelihood estimator for γ_k, and write $\widehat{\overline{\gamma}}_k = (\widehat{\gamma}_1^T, \ldots, \widehat{\gamma}_k^T)^T$, $k = 1, \ldots, K$.

Because $\mathcal{C}_{d_\eta} = 1$ only if the treatment options actually received through all K decisions are consistent with those selected by d_η, it is then straightforward to deduce that the leading term in the summand of (7.102) can be written equivalently as

$$\frac{\mathcal{C}_{d_\eta,i} Y_i}{\left\{\prod_{k=2}^{K} \pi_{d_\eta,k}(\overline{X}_{ki}; \overline{\eta}_k, \widehat{\gamma}_k)\right\} \pi_{d_\eta,1}(X_{1i}; \eta_1, \widehat{\gamma}_1)} = \frac{\mathcal{C}_{d_\eta,i} Y_i}{\varpi_K(H_{Ki}, A_{Ki}; \widehat{\overline{\gamma}}_K)},$$

analogous to (5.110). By similar reasoning and some rearrangement, and using (7.107) and (7.108), it is straightforward to show that the ith summand in the augmentation term in (7.102),

$$\sum_{k=1}^{K} \left\{ \frac{\mathcal{C}_{\overline{d}_{\eta,k-1},i}}{\overline{\pi}_{d_{\eta},k-1}(\overline{X}_{k-1,i}; \widehat{\overline{\gamma}}_{k-1})} - \frac{\mathcal{C}_{\overline{d}_{\eta,k},i}}{\overline{\pi}_{d_{\eta},k}(\overline{X}_{ki}; \widehat{\overline{\gamma}}_{k})} \right\} \mathcal{Q}_{d_{\eta},k}(\overline{X}_{ki}; \widehat{\beta}_{k}),$$

can be reexpressed as

$$-\sum_{k=1}^{K} \left(\frac{\mathcal{C}_{\overline{d}_{\eta,k-1},i}}{\varpi_{k-1}(H_{k-1,i}, A_{k-1,i}; \widehat{\overline{\gamma}}_{k-1})} \right.$$
$$\times \left[\frac{I\{A_{ki} = d_{\eta,k}(H_{ki})\} - \omega_{k}\{H_{ki}, d_{\eta,k}(H_{ki}); \widehat{\gamma}_{k}\}}{\omega_{k}\{H_{ki}, d_{\eta,k}(H_{ki}); \widehat{\gamma}_{k}\}} \right]$$
$$\left. \times Q_{k}^{d_{\eta}}\{H_{ki}, d_{\eta,k}(H_{ki}); \widehat{\beta}_{k}\} \right).$$

In fact, by reasoning similar to that in the remark following (3.30) in Section 3.3.3, this can be further rewritten as

$$-\sum_{k=1}^{K} \left(\frac{\mathcal{C}_{\overline{d}_{\eta,k-1},i}}{\varpi_{k-1}(H_{k-1,i}, A_{k-1,i}; \widehat{\overline{\gamma}}_{k-1})} \right.$$
$$\left. \times \left[\frac{I\{A_{ki} = d_{\eta,k}(H_{ki})\} - \omega_{k}(H_{ki}, A_{ki}; \widehat{\gamma}_{k})}{\omega_{k}(H_{ki}, A_{ki}; \widehat{\gamma}_{k})} \right] Q_{k}^{d_{\eta}}\{H_{ki}, d_{\eta,k}(H_{ki}); \widehat{\beta}_{k}\} \right).$$

Then (7.102) can be written, using $\varpi_{0} \equiv 1$ and $\mathcal{C}_{d_{\eta,0}} \equiv 0$, as

$$\widehat{\mathcal{V}}_{AIPW}(d_{\eta}) = n^{-1} \sum_{i=1}^{n} \left\{ \frac{\mathcal{C}_{d_{\eta},i} Y_{i}}{\varpi_{K}(H_{Ki}, A_{Ki}; \widehat{\overline{\gamma}}_{K})} \right.$$
$$- \left[\frac{I\{A_{1i} = d_{\eta,1}(H_{1i})\} - \omega_{k}(H_{1i}, A_{1i}; \widehat{\gamma}_{1})}{\omega_{k}(H_{1i}, A_{1i}; \widehat{\gamma}_{1})} \right] Q_{1}^{d_{\eta}}\{H_{1i}, d_{\eta,1}(H_{1i}); \widehat{\beta}_{1}\}$$
$$- \sum_{k=2}^{K} \left(\frac{\mathcal{C}_{\overline{d}_{\eta,k-1},i}}{\varpi_{k-1}(H_{k-1,i}, A_{k-1,i}; \widehat{\overline{\gamma}}_{k-1})} \right. \tag{7.110}$$
$$\left. \left. \times \left[\frac{I\{A_{ki} = d_{\eta,k}(H_{ki})\} - \omega_{k}(H_{ki}, A_{ki}; \widehat{\gamma}_{k})}{\omega_{k}(H_{ki}, A_{ki}; \widehat{\gamma}_{k})} \right] Q_{k}^{d_{\eta}}\{H_{ki}, d_{\eta,k}(H_{ki}); \widehat{\beta}_{k}\} \right) \right\}.$$

For $k = 1, \ldots, K$, as in (5.111), let

$$\underline{d}_{\eta,k} = (d_{\eta,k}, d_{\eta,k+1}, \ldots, d_{\eta,K}),$$

so $\underline{d}_{\eta,1} = d_{\eta}$, define $\underline{\gamma}_{k} = (\gamma_{k}^{T}, \ldots, \gamma_{K}^{T})^{T}$ and $\underline{\beta}_{k} = (\beta_{k}^{T}, \ldots, \beta_{K}^{T})^{T}$, and define $\widehat{\underline{\gamma}}_k$ and $\widehat{\underline{\beta}}_k$ similarly. For $r \geq \ell = 1, \ldots, K$, define $\underline{\gamma}_{\ell,r} = (\gamma_\ell^T, \ldots, \gamma_r^T)^T$, so that $\underline{\gamma}_{k,K} = \underline{\gamma}_k$; and, generalizing (5.109), let

$$\underline{\omega}_{\ell,r}(h_r, a_r; \underline{\gamma}_{\ell,r}) = \prod_{j=\ell}^{r} \omega_j(h_j, a_j; \gamma_j), \quad r \geq \ell = 1, \ldots, K, \qquad (7.111)$$

so that $\underline{\omega}_{1,k}(h_k, a_k; \underline{\gamma}_{1,k}) = \varpi_k(h_k, a_k; \overline{\gamma}_k)$. Define

$$\mathfrak{C}_{d_\eta,\ell,r} = \mathrm{I}\{A_\ell = d_{\eta,\ell}(H_\ell), \ldots, A_r = d_{\eta,r}(H_r)\}, \quad r \geq \ell = 1, \ldots, K, \qquad (7.112)$$

the indicator of treatment options consistent with those dictated by the ℓth through rth rules in d_η, generalizing (5.112); clearly, from (7.112), $\mathfrak{C}_{d_\eta,1,k} = \mathcal{C}_{\overline{d}_{\eta,k}}$ and $\mathfrak{C}_{d_\eta,1,K} = \mathcal{C}_{d_\eta}$.

With these definitions, for $k = 1, \ldots, K$, analogous to (5.113) in the case of the simple inverse weighted estimator, let

$$\mathcal{G}_{AIPW,k}(\underline{d}_{\eta,k}; \underline{\gamma}_k, \underline{\beta}_k) = \frac{\mathfrak{C}_{d_\eta,k,K} Y}{\underline{\omega}_{k,K}(H_K, A_K; \underline{\gamma}_{k,K})}$$

$$- \left[\frac{\mathrm{I}\{A_k = d_{\eta,k}(H_k)\} - \omega_k(H_k, A_k; \gamma_k)}{\omega_k(H_k, A_k; \gamma_k)} \right] Q_k^{d_\eta}\{H_k, d_{\eta,k}(H_k); \beta_k\}$$

$$\qquad (7.113)$$

$$- \mathrm{I}(k < K) \sum_{r=k+1}^{K} \left(\frac{\mathfrak{C}_{d_\eta,k,r-1}}{\underline{\omega}_{k,r-1}(H_{r-1}, A_{r-1}; \underline{\gamma}_{k,r-1})} \right.$$

$$\left. \times \left[\frac{\mathrm{I}\{A_r = d_{\eta,r}(H_r)\} - \omega_r(H_r, A_r; \gamma_r)}{\omega_r(H_r, A_r; \gamma_r)} \right] Q_r^{d_\eta}\{H_r, d_{\eta,r}(H_r); \beta_r\} \right),$$

where dependence on the observed data $(\overline{X}, \overline{A}, Y) = (H_K, A_K, Y)$ is suppressed for brevity, the third term on the right-hand side of (7.113) is equal to zero when $k = K$, and $\mathcal{G}_{AIPW,ki}(\underline{d}_{\eta,k}; \underline{\gamma}_k, \underline{\beta}_k)$ denotes evaluation at (H_{Ki}, A_{Ki}, Y_i). Then, using (7.113), with the choice of models (7.107) and (7.108), (7.110) and thus (7.102) can be written equivalently as

$$\widehat{\mathcal{V}}_{AIPW}(d_\eta) = n^{-1} \sum_{i=1}^{n} \mathcal{G}_{AIPW,1i}(\underline{d}_{\eta,1}; \widehat{\underline{\gamma}}_1, \widehat{\underline{\beta}}_1)$$

$$\qquad (7.114)$$

$$= n^{-1} \sum_{i=1}^{n} \mathcal{G}_{AIPW,1i}(d_\eta; \widehat{\overline{\gamma}}_K, \widehat{\overline{\beta}}_K),$$

where $\widehat{\overline{\beta}}_k = (\widehat{\beta}_1^T, \ldots, \widehat{\beta}_k^T)^T$.

Note that, because $\widehat{\mathcal{V}}_{IPW}(d_\eta)$ is found by replacing $\mathcal{Q}_{d_\eta,k}(\overline{X}_{ki};\widehat{\beta}_k)$ by zero, $k = 1,\ldots,K$, in (7.102), defining

$$\mathcal{G}_{IPW,k}(\underline{d}_{\eta,k};\underline{\gamma}_k) = \frac{\mathfrak{C}_{d_\eta,k,K}Y}{\underline{\omega}_{k,K}(H_K,A_K;\underline{\gamma}_{k,K})}, \qquad (7.115)$$

$$\widehat{\mathcal{V}}_{IPW}(d_\eta) = n^{-1}\sum_{i=1}^{n}\mathcal{G}_{IPW,1i}(\underline{d}_{\eta,1};\widehat{\underline{\gamma}}_1) = n^{-1}\sum_{i=1}^{n}\mathcal{G}_{IPW,1i}(d_\eta;\widehat{\overline{\gamma}}_K)$$

as in (5.113) and (5.114). We continue to focus on the augmented inverse probability weighted estimator, but the same developments apply to (7.115).

The alternative representation (7.114) is advantageous in the formulation of the backward iterative algorithm for estimation of d_η^{opt}, which is based on the principle of backward induction and involves successive maximization of certain value estimators in $\eta_K, \eta_{K-1}, \ldots, \eta_1$. The following algorithm generalizes that given in Section 5.7.3 based on the simple inverse probability weighted estimator (7.97).

At Decision K, an individual has already achieved history H_K, so, as noted in Section 5.6, selection of a Decision K treatment option is analogous to a single decision problem in which an individual presents with "baseline" information H_K. With $Q_K^{d_\eta}(h_K, a_K;\beta_K)$ a model for $E(Y|H_K = h_K, A_K = a_K)$, using (7.113) and the facts that $\underline{\omega}_{K,K}(h_K,a_K;\underline{\gamma}_{K,K}) = \omega_K(h_K,a_K;\gamma_K)$ and $\mathfrak{C}_{d_\eta,K,K} = I\{A_K = d_{\eta,K}(H_K)\}$ from (7.111) and (7.112), let

$$\widehat{\mathcal{V}}^{(K)}_{AIPW}(d_{\eta,K}) = n^{-1}\sum_{i=1}^{n}\mathcal{G}_{AIPW,Ki}(d_{\eta,K};\widehat{\gamma}_K,\widehat{\beta}_K)$$

$$= n^{-1}\sum_{i=1}^{n}\left(\frac{I\{A_{Ki} = d_{\eta,K}(H_{Ki})\}Y_i}{\omega_K(H_{Ki},A_{Ki};\widehat{\gamma}_K)}\right. \qquad (7.116)$$

$$\left. - \left[\frac{I\{A_{Ki} = d_{\eta,K}(H_{Ki})\} - \omega_K(H_{Ki},A_{Ki};\widehat{\gamma}_{Ki})}{\omega_K(H_{Ki},A_{Ki};\widehat{\gamma}_{Ki})}\right]\right.$$

$$\left. \times Q_K^{d_\eta}\{H_{Ki},d_{\eta,K}(H_{Ki});\widehat{\beta}_K\}\right),$$

where $\widehat{\beta}_K$ is obtained as in Section 6.4.2 by solving the estimating equation (6.64). It is straightforward to deduce that (7.116) is of the same form as the augmented estimator (3.99) in the single decision case, with Decision K playing the role of the single decision; H_{Ki}, A_{Ki}, and $d_{\eta,K}$ corresponding to H_{1i}, A_{1i}, and $d_{\eta,1}$, respectively; and, from above, $Q_K^{d_\eta}\{h_K,d_{\eta,K}(h_K);\beta_K\}$ playing the role of (3.98).

As in Sections 5.7.3, 6.4.2, and 7.2.3, let

$$Y^*(\overline{a}_{k-1}, d_{\eta,k}, \ldots, d_{\eta,K}) = Y^*(\overline{a}_{k-1}, \underline{d}_{\eta,k}), \quad k = 1, \ldots, K,$$

be the potential outcome if an individual were to receive options $a_1, \ldots, a_{k-1}$ at Decisions 1 to $k-1$ and then be treated according to the rules $d_{\eta,k}, \ldots, d_{\eta,K}$ at Decisions k to K. Let γ_K^* and β_K^* be the limits in probability of $\widehat{\gamma}_K$ and $\widehat{\beta}_K$. Then, if at least one of either of the models $\omega_K(h_K, a_K; \gamma_K)$ or $Q_K^{d_\eta}(h_K, a_K; \beta_K)$ is correctly specified, so that at least one of γ_K^* or β_K^* is equal to the true value $\gamma_{K,0}$ or $\beta_{K,0}$ of these parameters, respectively, it can be shown, by virtue of the double robustness property of (7.116), that

$$E\{\mathcal{G}_{AIPW,K}(d_{\eta,K}; \gamma_K^*, \beta_K^*) \mid H_K\} = E\{Y^*(\overline{A}_{K-1}, d_{\eta,K}) \mid H_K\}, \tag{7.117}$$

so that

$$E\{\mathcal{G}_{AIPW,K}(d_{\eta,K}; \gamma_K^*, \beta_K^*)\} = E\{Y^*(\overline{A}_{K-1}, d_{\eta,K})\}. \tag{7.118}$$

It follows that, for fixed $d_{\eta,K}$, $\widehat{\mathcal{V}}_{AIPW}^{(K)}(d_{\eta,K})$ is a consistent estimator for $E\{\mathcal{G}_{AIPW,K}(d_{\eta,K}; \gamma_K^*, \beta_K^*)\}$, and thus, from (7.118), for $E\{Y^*(\overline{A}_{K-1}, d_{\eta,K})\}$. Accordingly, $E\{Y^*(\overline{A}_{K-1}, d_{\eta,K})\}$ plays the role of the value of the "single decision regime" $d_{\eta,K}$ in the analogy to a single decision problem, where, of course, $\overline{A}_{K-1}$ is part of the "baseline" information; and $E\{Y^*(\overline{A}_{K-1}, d_{\eta,K})\}$ depends on η_K.

Under this analogy, let

$$d_{\eta,K,B}^{opt}(h_K) = d_K(h_K; \eta_{K,B}^{opt}), \qquad \eta_{K,B}^{opt} = \arg\max_{\eta_K} E\{Y^*(\overline{A}_{K-1}, d_{\eta,K})\}. \tag{7.119}$$

Note that $\eta_{K,B}^{opt}$ defined in (7.119) need not necessarily be the same as the component η_K^{opt} of η^{opt} globally maximizing $\mathcal{V}(d_\eta)$ defined in (7.91); we discuss conditions under which $\eta_{K,B}^{opt} = \eta_K^{opt}$ below.

Based on these developments, the first step of the algorithm, at Decision K, is thus to maximize $\widehat{\mathcal{V}}_{AIPW}^{(K)}(d_{\eta,K})$ in (7.116) in η_K to obtain $\widehat{\eta}_{K,B,AIPW}^{opt}$, an estimator for $\eta_{K,B}^{opt}$, and the estimator

$$\widehat{d}_{\eta,K,B}^{opt}(h_K) = d_K(h_K; \widehat{\eta}_{K,B,AIPW}^{opt}). \tag{7.120}$$

for (7.119). In this maximization, $Q_K^{d_\eta}\{H_{Ki}, d_{\eta,K}(H_{Ki}); \widehat{\beta}_K\}$ depends on η_K only through substitution of $d_{\eta,K}(h_K)$, so that the model $Q_K^{d_\eta}(h_K, a_k; \beta_K)$ need not be refitted at each internal iteration.

Now consider Decision $K - 1$. Using (7.113), define

$$\widehat{\mathcal{V}}_{AIPW}^{(K-1)}(\underline{d}_{\eta,K-1}) = n^{-1} \sum_{i=1}^{n} \mathcal{G}_{AIPW,K-1,i}(\underline{d}_{\eta,K-1}; \widehat{\underline{\gamma}}_{K-1}, \widehat{\underline{\beta}}_{K-1})$$

$$= n^{-1} \sum_{i=1}^{n} \mathcal{G}_{AIPW,K-1,i}(d_{\eta,K-1}, d_{\eta,K}; \widehat{\underline{\gamma}}_{K-1}, \widehat{\underline{\beta}}_{K-1}),$$

(7.121)

where now

$$\mathcal{G}_{AIPW,K-1}(\underline{d}_{\eta,K-1}; \underline{\gamma}_{K-1}, \underline{\beta}_{K-1}) = \frac{\mathfrak{C}_{d_\eta,K-1,K} Y}{\underline{\omega}_{K-1,K}(H_K, A_k; \underline{\gamma}_{K-1,K})}$$

$$- \left[\frac{I\{A_{K-1} = d_{\eta,K-1}(H_{K-1})\} - \omega_{K-1}(H_{K-1}, A_{K-1}; \gamma_{K-1})}{\omega_{K-1}(H_{K-1}, A_{K-1}; \gamma_{K-1})} \right]$$

$$\times Q_{K-1}^{d_\eta}\{H_{K-1}, d_{\eta,K-1}(H_{K-1}); \beta_{K-1}\}$$

(7.122)

$$- \frac{\mathfrak{C}_{d_\eta,K-1,K}}{\underline{\omega}_{K-1,K}(H_K, A_K; \underline{\gamma}_{K-1,K})} \left[\frac{I\{A_K = d_{\eta,K}(H_K)\} - \omega_K(H_K, A_K; \gamma_K)}{\omega_K(H_K, A_K; \gamma_K)} \right]$$

$$\times Q_K^{d_\eta}\{H_K, d_{\eta,K}(H_K); \beta_K\},$$

and $Q_{K-1}^{d_\eta}(h_{K-1}, a_{K-1}; \beta_{K-1})$ is a model for which positing and fitting is discussed below. By analogy to a two-decision problem, with Decisions $K - 1$ and K playing the roles of Decisions 1 and 2 and "baseline" information H_{K-1}, and by reasoning similar to that above, $\widehat{\mathcal{V}}_{AIPW}^{(K-1)}(\underline{d}_{\eta,K-1})$ in (7.121) is a doubly robust estimator for

$$E\{Y^*(\overline{A}_{K-2}, d_{\eta,K-1}, d_{\eta,K})\}.$$

(7.123)

Similar to (7.119), define

$$d_{\eta,K-1,B}^{opt}(h_{K-1}) = d_{K-1}(h_{K-1}; \eta_{K-1,B}^{opt}),$$

$$\eta_{K-1,B}^{opt} = \arg\max_{\eta_{K-1}} E\{Y^*(\overline{A}_{K-2}, d_{\eta,K-1}, d_{\eta,K,B}^{opt})\}.$$

(7.124)

In (7.124), $d_{\eta,K}$ is fixed at $d_{\eta,K,B}^{opt}$, so that $\eta_{K-1,B}^{opt}$ is not necessarily the global maximizer of (7.123) in $(\eta_{K-1}^T, \eta_K^T)^T$, nor is $\eta_{K-1,B}^{opt}$ necessarily equal to η_{K-1}^{opt} globally maximizing $\mathcal{V}(d_\eta)$ as defined in (7.91); this is discussed below.

Given these developments, $\widehat{\mathcal{V}}_{AIPW}^{(K-1)}(d_{\eta,K-1}, d_{\eta,K,B}^{opt})$ is a doubly robust estimator for $E\{Y^*(\overline{A}_{K-1}, d_{\eta,K-1}, d_{\eta,K,B}^{opt})\}$, so that the obvious estimator for $\eta_{K-1,B}^{opt}$ in (7.124) is found by substituting $\widehat{d}_{\eta,K,B}^{opt}$ in (7.120) for $d_{\eta,K}$ in (7.121), obtaining

$$\widehat{\mathcal{V}}_{AIPW}^{(K-1)}(d_{\eta,K-1}, \widehat{d}_{\eta,K,B}^{opt}),$$

(7.125)

and maximizing this estimator in η_{K-1} to obtain $\widehat{\eta}^{opt}_{K-1,B,AIPW}$ and

$$\widehat{d}^{opt}_{\eta,K-1,B}(h_{K-1}) = d_{K-1}(h_{K-1}; \widehat{\eta}^{opt}_{K-1,B,AIPW}). \tag{7.126}$$

From (7.122), $Q^{d_\eta}_K\{H_{Ki}, \widehat{d}^{opt}_{\eta,K,B}(H_{Ki}); \widehat{\beta}_K\}$ in the third term is fixed for each i. The fitted model $Q^{d_\eta}_{K-1}(h_{K-1}, a_{K-1}; \widehat{\beta}_{K-1})$ in the second term must respect evaluation of (7.121) at $\widehat{d}^{opt}_{\eta,K,B}$; accordingly, the posited model $Q^{d_\eta}_{K-1}(h_{K-1}, a_{K-1}; \beta_{K-1})$ should be a model for

$$E\{V^{d^{opt}_\eta}_K(H_K) \mid H_{K-1} = h_{K-1}, A_{K-1} = a_{K-1}\},$$

say, where

$$V^{d^{opt}_\eta}_K(h_K) = Q^{d_\eta}_K\{h_K, d^{opt}_{\eta,K,B}(h_K)\}.$$

This suggests in the backward induction algorithm in Section 6.4.2 forming pseudo outcomes

$$\widetilde{V}^{d_\eta}_{Ki} = Q^{d_\eta}_K\{H_{Ki}, \widehat{d}^{opt}_{\eta,K,B}(H_{Ki}); \widehat{\beta}_K\}, \quad i = 1, \ldots, n, \tag{7.127}$$

by substituting the estimator (7.120); as in (6.65), positing the model $Q^{d_\eta}_{K-1}(h_{K-1}, a_{K-1}; \beta_{K-1})$ based on the considerations discussed in Remarks (i)–(iv) in Section 6.4.2; and obtaining $\widehat{\beta}_{K-1}$ by solving the estimating equation (6.66) for β_{K-1} using the pseudo outcomes $\widetilde{V}^{d_\eta}_{Ki}$ in (7.127). The pseudo outcomes $\widetilde{V}^{d_\eta}_{Ki}$ are fixed with respect to η_{K-1}, and $Q^{d_\eta}_{K-1}\{H_{K-1,i}, d_{\eta,K-1}(H_{K-1,i}); \widehat{\beta}_{K-1})\}$ depends for each i on η_{K-1} only through substitution of $d_{\eta,K-1}(H_{K-1})$ so that the model $Q^{d_\eta}_{K-1}(h_{K-1}, a_{K-1}; \beta_{K-1})$ need not be refitted at every internal iteration of the optimization algorithm used to maximize (7.125) in η_{K-1}.

Continuing in this fashion for $k = K-2, \ldots, 1$, at Decision k, define

$$\begin{aligned}\widehat{\mathcal{V}}^{(k)}_{AIPW}(\underline{d}_{\eta,k}) &= n^{-1}\sum_{i=1}^{n}\mathcal{G}_{AIPW,ki}(\underline{d}_{\eta,k}; \widehat{\underline{\gamma}}_k, \widehat{\underline{\beta}}_k) \\ &= n^{-1}\sum_{i=1}^{n}\mathcal{G}_{AIPW,ki}(d_{\eta,k}, \underline{d}_{\eta,k+1}; \widehat{\underline{\gamma}}_k, \widehat{\underline{\beta}}_k),\end{aligned} \tag{7.128}$$

which can be viewed as a doubly robust estimator for

$$E\{Y^*(\overline{A}_{k-1}, \underline{d}_{\eta,k})\} = E\{Y^*(\overline{A}_{k-1}, d_{\eta,k}, \underline{d}_{\eta,k+1})\}. \tag{7.129}$$

As above, define

$$\begin{aligned}d^{opt}_{\eta,k,B}(h_k) &= d_k(h_k; \eta^{opt}_{k,B}), \\ \eta^{opt}_{k,B} &= \arg\max_{\eta_k} E\{Y^*(\overline{A}_{k-1}, d_{\eta,k}, \underline{d}^{opt}_{\eta,k+1,B})\},\end{aligned} \tag{7.130}$$

where
$$\underline{d}_{\eta,k+1,B}^{opt} = (d_{\eta,k+1,B}^{opt}, \dots, d_{\eta,K,B}^{opt});$$

and, with $\underline{d}_{\eta,k+1}^{opt}$ fixed at $\underline{d}_{\eta,k+1,B}^{opt}$, $\eta_{k,B}^{opt}$ is not necessarily the global maximizer of (7.129) nor equal to η_k^{opt} globally maximizing $\mathcal{V}(d_\eta)$ in (7.91). Substitute

$$\widehat{\underline{d}}_{\eta,k+1,B}^{opt} = (\widehat{d}_{\eta,k+1,B}^{opt}, \dots, \widehat{d}_{\eta,K,B}^{opt})$$

from the previous steps for $\underline{d}_{\eta,k+1}$ in (7.128) to obtain

$$\widehat{\mathcal{V}}_{AIPW}^{(k)}(d_{\eta,k}^{opt}, \widehat{\underline{d}}_{\eta,k+1,B}^{opt}), \tag{7.131}$$

and maximize in η_k to obtain $\widehat{\eta}_{k,B,AIPW}^{opt}$ and

$$\widehat{d}_{\eta,k,B}^{opt}(h_k) = d_k(h_k; \widehat{\eta}_{k,B,AIPW}^{opt}). \tag{7.132}$$

As for $k = K - 1$, the fitted model $Q_k^{d_\eta}(h_k, a_k; \widehat{\beta}_k)$ must respect substitution of $\widehat{\underline{d}}_{\eta,k+1,B}^{opt}$ in (7.128), so that $Q_k^{d_\eta}(h_k, a_k; \beta_k)$ is a model for $E\{V_{k+1}^{d_\eta}(H_{k+1}) \mid H_k = h_k, A_k = a_k\}$, where $V_{k+1}^{d_\eta^{opt}}(h_k) = Q_{k+1}^{d_\eta}\{h_{k+1}, d_{\eta,k+1,B}^{opt}(h_{k+1})\}$. This is accomplished by forming the pseudo outcomes

$$\widetilde{V}_{k+1,i}^{d_\eta} = Q_{k+1}^{d_\eta}\{H_{k+1,i}, \widehat{d}_{\eta,k+1,B}^{opt}(H_{k+1,i}); \widehat{\beta}_{k+1}\}, \quad i = 1, \dots, n;$$

in the backward induction algorithm, positing the model $Q_k^{d_\eta}(h_k, a_k; \beta_k)$ based on the considerations in Remarks (i)–(iv) in Section 6.4.2, and solving the estimating equation (6.68) for β_k using the pseudo outcomes $\widetilde{V}_{k+1,i}^{d_\eta}$. Here, as above, fitting of the model $Q_k^{d_\eta}(h_k, a_k; \beta_k)$ does not depend on η_k so does not need to be repeated at every internal iteration of the optimization algorithm.

At the conclusion of this scheme at Decision 1, the estimator for

$$d_{\eta,B}^{opt} = \{d_{\eta,1,B}^{opt}(h_1), \dots, d_{\eta,K,B}^{opt}(h_K)\}, \tag{7.133}$$

where $d_{\eta,k,B}^{opt}(h_k)$, $k = 1, \dots, K$, are defined in (7.119), (7.124), and (7.130), is given by

$$\widehat{d}_{\eta,B,AIPW}^{opt} = \{d_1(h_1; \widehat{\eta}_{1,B,AIPW}^{opt}), \dots, d_K(h_K; \widehat{\eta}_{K,B,AIPW}^{opt})\}. \tag{7.134}$$

Substituting $\widehat{d}_{\eta,B,AIPW}^{opt}$ in (7.102), or, equivalently, in (7.114), yields the estimator $\widehat{\mathcal{V}}_{B,AIPW}(d_{\eta,B}^{opt})$, say, for the value $\mathcal{V}(d_{\eta,B}^{opt})$.

Analogous to (7.134), as presented in Section 5.7.3, an estimator

$\widehat{d}^{opt}_{\eta,B,IPW}$ for $d^{opt}_{\eta,B}$ in (7.133) is obtained by a similar backward algorithm, where the value estimators at each step are defined in terms of (7.115). The value estimators so defined, $\widehat{\mathcal{V}}^{(K)}_{IPW}(d_{\eta,K})$ and $\widehat{\mathcal{V}}^{(k)}_{IPW}(\underline{d}_{\eta,k})$, $k = K-1,\ldots,1$, are consistent estimators for the corresponding conditional expectations (7.118) and (7.129), respectively, for fixed d_η only if the propensity models $\omega_k(h_k, a_k; \gamma_k)$ are correctly specified, $k = 1,\ldots,K$. Thus, this approach is predicated on these models being correct.

Remark. As emphasized in the formulation of the backward algorithm, $\eta^{opt}_{k,B}$ defined at each step $k = K,\ldots,1$ does not necessarily maximize $E\{Y^*(\overline{A}_{k-1}, \underline{d}_{\eta,k})\}$ in $(\eta^T_k, \ldots, \eta^T_K)^T$, $k = 1,\ldots,K$, so does not maximize $\mathcal{V}(d_\eta) = E\{Y^*(d_\eta)\}$ globally in η. Accordingly, it is not necessarily the case that $\widehat{d}^{opt}_{\eta,B,AIPW}$ in (7.134) is an estimator for an optimal restricted Ψ-specific regime $d^{opt}_\eta \in \mathcal{D}_\eta$ defined in (7.91). It is natural to ask if, and under what conditions, the resulting estimator $\widehat{d}^{opt}_{\eta,B,AIPW}$ is a valid estimator for d^{opt}_η.

Consider regimes $d = (d_1, \ldots, d_K) \in \mathcal{D}$, the class of all possible Ψ-specific regimes, where $d^{opt}_k = d^{(1)opt}_k, \ldots, d^{opt}_K = d^{(1)opt}_K$ as in (7.46) are the kth to Kth rules characterizing an optimal regime $d^{opt} \in \mathcal{D}$. Under SUTVA (6.16), the SRA (6.17), and the positivity assumption (7.7), it can be shown by arguments in a similar spirit to those in Sections 7.2 and 7.3 that, for each $k = 1,\ldots,K$, $d^{opt}_k, \ldots, d^{opt}_K$ maximize

$$E\{Y^*(\overline{A}_{k-1}, d_k, \ldots, d_K) \mid H_k\},$$

so that

$$\underline{d}^{opt}_k = (d^{opt}_k, \ldots, d^{opt}_K) = \arg\max_{d_k,\ldots,d_K} E\{Y^*(\overline{A}_{k-1}, d_k, \ldots, d_K)\}, \; k = 1,\ldots,K.$$

$$(7.135)$$

Thus, if the restricted class $\mathcal{D}_\eta$ of interest is such that

$$d^{opt} \in \mathcal{D}_\eta,$$

so that the form of regimes in $\mathcal{D}_\eta$ includes that of an optimal $d^{opt} \in \mathcal{D}$, then $\mathcal{V}(d^{opt}_\eta) = \mathcal{V}(d^{opt})$, and in this sense d^{opt}_η and d^{opt} are equivalent. It follows in this case from (7.135) and the definitions of $d^{opt}_{\eta,B,k}$, $k = 1,\ldots,K$, in (7.119), (7.124), and (7.130) that in fact $\mathcal{V}(d^{opt}_{\eta,B}) = \mathcal{V}(d^{opt}_\eta) = \mathcal{V}(d^{opt})$, so that $d^{opt}_{\eta,B}$ in (7.133) is equivalent to an optimal regime d^{opt} and thus d^{opt}_η. Moreover,

$$\widehat{\eta}^{opt}_{B,AIPW} = (\widehat{\eta}^{opt\,T}_{1,B,AIPW}, \ldots, \widehat{\eta}^{opt\,T}_{K,B,AIPW})^T$$

resulting from the backward iterative algorithm globally maximizes

$\widehat{\mathcal{V}}_{AIPW}(d_\eta)$ in η, so is a valid estimator for η^{opt}, and $\widehat{d}_{\eta,B,AIPW}^{opt}$ in (7.134) is indeed the desired value search estimator for d_η^{opt}. Further, $\widehat{\mathcal{V}}_{B,AIPW}(d_\eta^{opt})$ found by substituting $\widehat{\eta}_{B,AIPW}^{opt}$ in $\widehat{\mathcal{V}}_{AIPW}(d_\eta)$ is a valid estimator for $\mathcal{V}(d_\eta^{opt})$. These results apply equally to the estimators $\widehat{\eta}_{B,IPW}^{opt}$, $\widehat{\mathcal{V}}_{IPW}(d_\eta)$, and $\widehat{d}_{\eta,B,IPW}^{opt}$, say, that result from basing the algorithm on (7.115) instead.

When the restricted class $\mathcal{D}_\eta$ does not contain $d^{opt} \in \mathcal{D}$, this argument does not apply. Then it is no longer necessarily the case that $\mathcal{V}(d_{\eta,B}^{opt}) = \mathcal{V}(d_\eta^{opt})$, so that $d_{\eta,B}^{opt}$ is not necessarily equivalent to d_η^{opt} in this sense. Thus, $\widehat{\eta}_{B,AIPW}^{opt}$ in (7.134) need not maximize $\widehat{\mathcal{V}}_{AIPW}(d_\eta)$ in η, and the resulting estimator $\widehat{d}_{\eta,B,AIPW}^{opt}$ in (7.134) need not estimate an optimal restricted regime $d_\eta^{opt} \in \mathcal{D}_\eta$, and similarly for $\widehat{\eta}_{B,IPW}^{opt}$ and $\widehat{d}_{\eta,B,IPW}^{opt}$. Nonetheless, simulation evidence presented by Zhao et al. (2015a) and Hager et al. (2018) suggests that estimators obtained via the backward iterative strategy can perform well as estimators for d_η^{opt} and $\mathcal{V}(d_\eta^{opt})$ in practice.

As noted at the outset of this discussion, the backward iterative approach outlined here replaces direct, global maximization of the value estimators $\widehat{\mathcal{V}}_{IPW}(d_\eta)$ or $\widehat{\mathcal{V}}_{AIPW}(d_\eta)$, which is likely to be of insurmountably high dimension, with a series of lower-dimensional maximizations in each of $\eta_K, \ldots, \eta_1$. However, from an implementation perspective, the successive maximizations of $\widehat{\mathcal{V}}_{AIPW}^{(K)}(d_{\eta,K})$ or $\widehat{\mathcal{V}}_{IPW}^{(K)}(d_{\eta,K})$ in η_K and each of $\widehat{\mathcal{V}}_{AIPW}^{(k)}(d_{\eta,k}^{opt}, \underline{\widehat{d}}_{k+1,B}^{opt})$ or $\widehat{\mathcal{V}}_{IPW}^{(k)}(d_{\eta,k}^{opt}, \underline{\widehat{d}}_{k+1,B}^{opt})$ in η_k, $k = K - 1, \ldots, 1$, although of lower dimension, are still challenging optimization tasks, owing to the nonsmooth nature of these objective functions, analogous to the discussion at the end of Section 4.2. As in that section, this suggests representing value search estimation for multiple decisions as a series of weighted classification problems. This is discussed in Section 7.4.5.

Backward Iterative Estimation via Regression Modeling

In the context of estimation of an optimal regime in the restricted class of regimes whose rules are in the form of decision lists, reviewed in Section 7.4.6 later in this chapter, Zhang et al. (2018) propose an alternative backward iterative strategy for estimation of an optimal restricted multiple decision regime. This method is motivated by an approach advocated by Taylor et al. (2015) in the single decision case, discussed in Section 4.5, a generalization of which we first review.

With $K = 1$, $\mathcal{D}_\eta$ consists of regimes of the form $d_\eta = \{d_1(h_1; \eta_1)\}$. For comparison with developments in Section 4.5, suppose that $\mathcal{A}_1$ com-

prises $m_1 \geq 2$ treatment options that are feasible for all individuals; this
condition can be relaxed to involve a specification of feasible sets with
additional notation. Then, with $Q_1^{d_\eta}(h_1, a_1) = E(Y \mid H_1 = h_1, A_1 = a_1)$,
under SUTVA, the SRA, and the positivity assumption, from (3.12) and
generalizing (4.12),

$$
\mathcal{V}(d_\eta) = E\{Y^*(d_\eta)\} = \sum_{a_1 \in \mathcal{A}_1} E[Q_1^{d_\eta}(H_1, a_1) \, \mathrm{I}\{d_1(H_1; \eta_1) = a_1\}]
$$

$$
= E[Q_1^{d_\eta}\{H_1, d_1(H_1; \eta_1)\}], \tag{7.136}
$$

for fixed $d_\eta \in \mathcal{D}_\eta$, using

$$
Q_1^{d_\eta}\{h_1, d_1(h_1; \eta_1)\} = \sum_{a_1 \in \mathcal{A}_1} Q_1^{d_\eta}(h_1, a_1) \, \mathrm{I}\{d_1(h_1; \eta_1) = a_1\}.
$$

In fact, as in (7.104) with $K = 1$,

$$
V_1^{d_\eta}(h_1) = Q_1^{d_\eta}\{h_1, d_1(h_1; \eta_1)\} = E\{Y^*(d_\eta) \mid H_1 = h_1\}, \tag{7.137}
$$

where the second equality in (7.137) is a special case of the result (6.54)
proved in Section 6.4.2, and (7.136) can be derived as

$$
E\{V_1^{d_\eta}(H_1)\} = E[Q_1^{d_\eta}\{H_1, d_1(H_1; \eta_1)\}] = E\{Y^*(d_\eta)\} = \mathcal{V}(d_\eta). \tag{7.138}
$$

Let $\widehat{Q}_1^{d_\eta}(h_1, a_1)$ be a nonparametric regression estimator for
$Q_1^{d_\eta}(h_1, a_1)$; for example, obtained using random forests, kernel regression, or other flexible method. Then, from the foregoing results, analogous to (4.54),

$$
n^{-1} \sum_{i=1}^{n} \widehat{Q}_1^{d_\eta}\{H_{1i}, d_1(H_{1i}; \eta_1)\} \tag{7.139}
$$

is an estimator for the value $\mathcal{V}(d_\eta)$. This suggests estimating

$$
\eta_1^{opt} = \arg\max_{\eta_1} \mathcal{V}(d_\eta)
$$

defining an optimal restricted regime $d_\eta^{opt} = \{d_1(h_1; \eta_1^{opt})\}$ in $\mathcal{D}_\eta$ by $\widehat{\eta}_{1,Q}^{opt}$
maximizing (7.139) in η_1 and thus d_η^{opt} by

$$
\widehat{d}_\eta^{opt} = \{d_1(h_1; \widehat{\eta}_{1,Q}^{opt})\}.
$$

Evidently, this is a form of value search estimation that uses a value
estimator based on direct regression modeling rather than on inverse

weighting. As noted after (4.54) in Section 4.5, flexible modeling and estimation of $Q_1^{d_\eta}(h_1, a_1)$ via nonparametric regression methods is meant to mitigate the effect of model misspecification that might be of concern if a parametric model were used in (7.139) so that a faithful representation of $\mathcal{V}(d_\eta)$ is achieved.

Zhang et al. (2018) propose generalization of this idea to estimation of an optimal restricted multiple decision regime via a backward algorithm similar to that above but replaces maximization of augmented or simple inverse weighted estimators for $E\{Y^*(\overline{A}_{K-1}, d_{\eta,K})\}$ and

$$E\{Y^*(\overline{A}_{k-1}, \underline{d}_{\eta,k})\} = E\{Y^*(\overline{A}_{k-1}, d_{\eta,k}, \underline{d}_{\eta,k+1})\}, \quad k = K-1, \ldots, 1,$$

in (7.129) at each step by a maximization of estimators based on direct regression modeling analogous to (7.139). The algorithm proceeds as follows.

At Decision K, with $Q_K^{d_\eta}(h_K, a_K) = E(Y \mid H_K = h_K, A_K = a_K)$, as in (7.104) and analogous to (7.137), for fixed $d_\eta \in \mathcal{D}_\eta$, let

$$V_K^{d_\eta}(h_K) = Q_K^{d_\eta}\{h_K, d_K(h_K; \eta_K)\} = E\{Y^*(\overline{a}_{K-1}, d_{\eta,K}) \mid H_K = h_K\},$$
$$(7.140)$$

where the second equality in (7.140) is immediate from (6.54) proved in Section 6.4.2 under SUTVA (6.16) and the SRA (6.17). Analogous to (7.138), it follows that

$$E\{V_K^{d_\eta}(H_K)\} = E[Q_K^{d_\eta}\{H_K, d_K(H_K; \eta_K)\}] = E\{Y^*(\overline{A}_{K-1}, d_{\eta,K})\}.$$
$$(7.141)$$

As in (7.119), define

$$d_{\eta,K,B}^{opt}(h_K) = d_K(h_K; \eta_{K,B}^{opt}), \quad \eta_{K,B}^{opt} = \arg\max_{\eta_K} E\{Y^*(\overline{A}_{K-1}, d_{\eta,K})\},$$
$$(7.142)$$

where, as above, $\eta_{K,B}^{opt}$ need not be the same as the component η_K^{opt} of η^{opt} globally maximizing $\mathcal{V}(d_\eta)$. Based on (7.141), obtain the estimator $\widehat{\eta}_{K,B,Q}^{opt}$ for $\eta_{K,B}^{opt}$ by maximizing in η_K the estimator for $E\{Y^*(\overline{A}_{K-1}, d_{\eta,K})\}$ given by

$$n^{-1} \sum_{i=1}^n \widehat{Q}_K^{d_\eta}\{H_{Ki}, d_K(H_{Ki}; \eta_K)\}, \quad (7.143)$$

where $\widehat{Q}_K^{d_\eta}(h_K, a_K)$ is a nonparametric estimator for $Q_K^{d_\eta}(h_K, a_K)$ obtained by regressing the observed Y on (H_K, A_K). Note that (7.143) depends on η_K only through substitution of $d_K(H_K; \eta_K)$ for A_K in the nonparametric regression representation. From (7.142), estimate $d_{\eta,K,B}^{opt}(h_K)$ by

$$\widehat{d}_{\eta,K,B}^{opt}(h_K) = d_K(h_K; \widehat{\eta}_{K,B,Q}^{opt}).$$

At Decision $K - 1$, from (7.104),

$$Q_{K-1}^{d_\eta}(h_{K-1}, a_{K-1}) = E\{V_K^{d_\eta}(H_K) \mid H_{K-1} = h_{K-1}, A_{K-1} = a_{K-1}\}. \tag{7.144}$$

Using (6.54) under SUTVA and the SRA,

$$
\begin{aligned}
V_{K-1}^{d_\eta}(h_{K-1}) &= Q_{K-1}^{d_\eta}\{h_{K-1}, d_{K-1}(h_{K-1}; \eta_{K-1})\} \\
&= E\{Y^*(\bar{a}_{K-2}, d_{\eta,K-1}, d_{\eta,K}) \mid H_{K-1} = h_{K-1}\},
\end{aligned}
$$

so that

$$
\begin{aligned}
E\{V_{K-1}^{d_\eta}(H_{K-1})\} &= E[Q_{K-1}^{d_\eta}\{H_{K-1}, d_{K-1}(H_{K-1}; \eta_{K-1})\}] \\
&= E\{Y^*(\bar{A}_{K-2}, d_{\eta,K-1}, d_{\eta,K})\}. \tag{7.145}
\end{aligned}
$$

As in (7.124), define

$$
\begin{aligned}
d_{\eta,K-1,B}^{opt}(h_{K-1}) &= d_{K-1}(h_{K-1}; \eta_{K-1,B}^{opt}), \\
\eta_{K-1,B}^{opt} &= \arg\max_{\eta_{K-1}} E\{Y^*(\bar{A}_{K-1}, d_{\eta,K-1}, d_{\eta,K,B}^{opt})\}. \tag{7.146}
\end{aligned}
$$

As noted previously, because $d_{\eta,K}$ is fixed at $d_{\eta,K,B}^{opt}$, $\eta_{K-1,B}^{opt}$ is not necessarily the global maximizer of (7.145) in $(\eta_{K-1}^T, \eta_K^T)^T$, nor is $\eta_{K-1,B}^{opt}$ necessarily equal to η_{K-1}^{opt} globally maximizing $\mathcal{V}(d_\eta)$.

As in the previous backward algorithm, from (7.146), we thus wish to maximize in η_{K-1} an estimator for $E\{Y^*(\bar{A}_{K-1}, d_{\eta,K-1}, d_{\eta,K,B}^{opt})\}$, which, from (7.145) and as in (7.143), can be obtained as the sample average across individuals of predicted values from a fitted model for $Q_{K-1}^{d_\eta}(h_{K-1}, a_{K-1})$ that respects evaluation of $E\{Y^*(\bar{A}_{K-2}, d_{\eta,K-1}, d_{\eta,K})\}$ at $d_{\eta,K,B}^{opt}$. An appropriate such model thus should be a model for

$$E\{V_K^{d_\eta^{opt}}(H_K) \mid H_{K-1} = h_{K-1}, A_{K-1} = a_{K-1}\},$$

$$V_K^{d_\eta^{opt}}(h_K) = Q_K^{d_\eta}\{h_K, d_{\eta,K,B}^{opt}(h_K)\}.$$

This suggests forming the pseudo outcomes

$$\widetilde{V}_{Ki}^{d_\eta} = \widehat{Q}_K^{d_\eta}\{H_{Ki}, \widehat{d}_{\eta,K,B}^{opt}(H_{Ki})\}, \quad i = 1, \ldots, n,$$

and estimating $Q_{K-1}^{d_\eta}(h_{K-1}, a_{K-1})$ in (7.144) by a nonparametric estimator $\widehat{Q}_{K-1}^{d_\eta}(h_{K-1}, a_{K-1})$ obtained by regressing these pseudo outcomes on the observed (H_{K-1}, A_{K-1}). Then, from (7.145), form the estimator

$$n^{-1} \sum_{i=1}^n \widehat{Q}_{K-1}^{d_\eta}\{H_{K-1,i}, d_{K-1}(H_{K-1,i}; \eta_{K-1})\} \tag{7.147}$$

for $E\{Y^*(\overline{A}_{K-1}, d_{\eta,K-1}, d_{\eta,K,B}^{opt})\}$, estimate $\eta_{K-1,B}^{opt}$ in (7.146) by $\widehat{\eta}_{K-1,B,Q}^{opt}$ maximizing (7.147) in η_{K-1}, and estimate $d_{\eta,K-1,B}^{opt}(h_{K-1})$ by

$$\widehat{d}_{\eta,K-1,B}^{opt}(h_{K-1}) = d_{K-1}(h_{K-1}; \widehat{\eta}_{K-1,B,Q}^{opt}).$$

As in the previous backward algorithm, the pseudo outcomes $\widetilde{V}_{Ki}^{d_\eta}$ are fixed with respect to η_K by substitution of $\widehat{\eta}_{K,B,Q}^{opt}$, and the fitted model depends on η_{K-1} only through substitution of $d_{\eta,K-1}(H_{K-1,i})$, so that the model need not be refitted at each internal iteration of the algorithm used to maximize (7.147).

Continuing, at Decision $k = K - 2, \ldots, 1$,

$$Q_k^{d_\eta}(h_k, a_k) = E\{V_{k+1}^{d_\eta}(H_{k+1}) \mid H_k = h_k, A_k = a_k\} \qquad (7.148)$$

from (7.104); and, by (6.54) under SUTVA and the SRA,

$$V_k^{d_\eta}(h_k) = Q_k^{d_\eta}\{h_k, d_k(h_k; \eta_k)\} = E\{Y^*(\overline{A}_{k-1}, d_{\eta,k}, \underline{d}_{\eta,k+1}) \mid H_k = h_k\}$$

from (7.129), and thus

$$E\{V_k^{d_\eta}(H_k)\} = E[Q_k^{d_\eta}\{H_k, d_k(H_k; \eta_k)\}] = E\{Y^*(\overline{A}_{k-1}, d_{\eta,k}, \underline{d}_{\eta,k+1})\}.$$

$$(7.149)$$

Let

$$d_{\eta,k,B}^{opt}(h_k) = d_k(h_k; \eta_{k,B}^{opt}),$$
$$\eta_{k,B}^{opt} = \arg\max_{\eta_k} E\{Y^*(\overline{A}_{k-1}, d_{\eta,k}, \underline{d}_{\eta,k+1,B}^{opt})\}, \qquad (7.150)$$

where $\underline{d}_{\eta,k+1,B}^{opt} = (d_{\eta,k+1,B}^{opt}, \ldots, d_{\eta,K,B}^{opt})$, and again $\eta_{k,B}^{opt}$ is not necessarily the global maximizer of (7.149) nor equal to η_k^{opt} globally maximizing $\mathcal{V}(d_\eta)$. Then, by the same reasoning as above, form the estimator for $E\{Y^*(\overline{A}_{k-1}, d_{\eta,k}, \underline{d}_{\eta,k+1,B}^{opt})\}$ given by

$$n^{-1} \sum_{i=1}^{n} \widehat{Q}_k^{d_\eta}\{H_{ki}, d_k(H_{ki}; \eta_k)\}, \qquad (7.151)$$

where the nonparametric estimator $\widehat{Q}_k^{d_\eta}(h_k, a_k)$ for $Q_k^{d_\eta}(h_k, a_k)$ in (7.148) respecting evaluation of (7.149) at $\underline{d}_{\eta,k+1,B}^{opt}$ is found by regressing the pseudo outcomes

$$\widetilde{V}_{k+1,i}^{d_\eta} = \widehat{Q}_{k+1}^{d_\eta}\{H_{k+1,i}, \widehat{d}_{\eta,k+1,B}^{opt}(H_{k+1,i})\}, \quad i = 1, \ldots, n,$$

on the observed (H_{ki}, A_{ki}). The estimator $\widehat{\eta}_{k,B,Q}^{opt}$ for $\eta_{k,B}^{opt}$ in (7.150) is then obtained by maximizing (7.151) in η_k, and the estimator for $d^{opt}_{\eta,k,B}(h_k)$ is

$$\widehat{d}^{opt}_{\eta,k,B}(h_k) = d_k(h_k; \widehat{\eta}^{opt}_{k,B,Q}).$$

At the completion of this process, the estimator for $d^{opt}_{\eta,B} = \{d^{opt}_{\eta,1,B}(h_1), \ldots, d^{opt}_{\eta,K,B}(h_K)\}$ is given by

$$\widehat{d}^{opt}_{\eta,B,Q} = \{d_1(h_1; \widehat{\eta}^{opt}_{1,B,Q}), \ldots, d_K(h_K; \widehat{\eta}^{opt}_{K,B,Q})\}. \tag{7.152}$$

Similar to (6.53), from (7.149) with $k = 1$, for fixed d_η,

$$E\{V^{d_\eta}_1(H_1)\} = E[Q^{d_\eta}_1\{H_1, d_1(H_1; \eta_1)\}] = E\{Y^*(d_{\eta 1})\} = \mathcal{V}(d_\eta),$$

which suggests estimating $\mathcal{V}(d^{opt}_{\eta,B})$ by

$$\widehat{\mathcal{V}}_{B,Q}(d^{opt}_{\eta,B}) = n^{-1} \sum_{i=1}^{n} \widehat{Q}^{d_\eta}_1\{H_{1i}, d_1(H_{1i}; \widehat{\eta}^{opt}_{1,B,Q})\}.$$

As in the remark following the presentation of the backward algorithm based on augmented and simple inverse weighted estimators above, $\eta^{opt}_{k,B}$ defined at each step $k = K, \ldots, 1$ do not necessarily maximize $E\{Y^*(\overline{A}_{k-1}, \underline{d}_{\eta,k})\}$ in $(\eta^T_k, \ldots, \eta^T_K)^T$, $k = 1, \ldots, K$, so do not maximize $\mathcal{V}(d_\eta) = E\{Y^*(d_\eta)\}$ globally in η. Thus, analogous to $\widehat{d}^{opt}_{\eta,B,AIPW}$ in (7.134), $\widehat{d}^{opt}_{\eta,B,Q}$ in (7.152) is not necessarily an estimator for an optimal restricted Ψ-specific regime $d^{opt}_\eta \in \mathcal{D}_\eta$ defined in (7.91). The same considerations discussed in the remark regarding if and under what conditions $\widehat{d}^{opt}_{\eta,B,AIPW}$ is a valid estimator for d^{opt}_η apply to $\widehat{d}^{opt}_{\eta,B,Q}$.

7.4.5 Classification Perspective

In Section 4.2, following the general formulation in Zhang et al. (2012a), we demonstrate how, in the single decision case, when $\mathcal{A}_1$ comprises exactly two options that are feasible for all individuals, value search estimation of the single decision rule $d^{opt}_1(h_1; \eta_1)$ characterizing an optimal restricted regime d^{opt}_η can be cast as a weighted classification problem. Under this analogy, the rule $d_1(h_1; \eta_1)$ plays the role of a classifier, and the form of the restricted class $\mathcal{D}_\eta$ is dictated by the choice of a particular family of classifiers. This idea is the foundation for the method of outcome weighted learning (OWL, Zhao et al., 2012) based on an inverse probability weighted value estimator discussed in Section 4.3. The correspondence to a weighted classification problem allows well-known approaches in the classification literature for optimization of non-smooth, nonconvex objective functions to be exploited in implementation of value search estimation based on inverse weighted and augmented inverse weighted value estimators for the single decision case.

As noted at the end of Section 5.7.3, for multiple decision problems in which $\mathcal{A}_k$ comprises two options that are feasible for all h_k, $k = 1, \ldots, K$, Zhao et al. (2015a) propose an extension of OWL, which they refer to as *backward outcome weighted learning* (BOWL). BOWL is based on a backward iterative scheme as in Section 7.4.4 using simple inverse weighted value estimators in which each step is represented as minimization of a weighted classification error. Here, we discuss how a classification perspective akin to that in Section 4.2 can be taken at each of the K steps of the general backward iterative algorithm, allowing techniques for optimization of nonsmooth, nonconvex objective functions favored in the classification literature to be used to maximize $\widehat{\mathcal{V}}^{(K)}_{AIPW}(d_{\eta,K})$ in η_K and each of $\widehat{\mathcal{V}}^{(k)}_{AIPW}(d_{\eta,k}, \widehat{d}^{opt}_{k+1,B})$ in η_k, $k = K - 1, \ldots, 1$ (or, similarly, the analogous simple inverse weighted estimators). The approach of Zhang and Zhang (2018a) using augmented inverse probability weighted estimators is similar in spirit to the general formulation here.

In what follows, we assume for simplicity that, at each Decision k, $\mathcal{A}_k$ comprises two options coded as 0 and 1; i.e., $\mathcal{A}_k = \{0, 1\}$, $k = 1, \ldots, K$, which are feasible for all individuals, where of course the two options need not be the same at each decision point. The developments can be extended to the case of general $\mathcal{A}_k$, where there are ℓ_k distinct subsets of $\mathcal{A}_k$, $\mathcal{A}_{k,l}$, $l = 1, \ldots, \ell_k$, that are feasible sets, $k = 1, \ldots, K$, where each subset $\mathcal{A}_{k,l}$ comprises one or two options, at the expense of more complicated notation.

The reader may wish to review the argument in Section 4.2 for the single decision case before proceeding, as the following development is based on entirely similar manipulations.

General Classification Analogy

As in the description of the backward iterative algorithm in Section 7.4.4, consider $\widehat{\mathcal{V}}_{AIPW}(d_\eta)$ with $\mathcal{Q}_{d_\eta,k}(\overline{X}_{ki}; \widehat{\beta}_k)$ replaced by $Q^{d_\eta}_k\{H_{ki}, d_k(H_{ki}; \eta_k); \widehat{\beta}_k\}$ in (7.108), which, using the definition of

$$\mathcal{G}_{AIPW,k}(\underline{d}_{\eta,k}, \underline{\gamma}_k, \underline{\beta}_k), \quad k = 1, \ldots, K,$$

in (7.113), can be written equivalently as

$$\widehat{\mathcal{V}}_{AIPW}(d_\eta) = n^{-1} \sum_{i=1}^{n} \mathcal{G}_{AIPW,1i}(d_\eta; \underline{\widehat{\gamma}}_k, \underline{\widehat{\beta}}_k)$$

as in (7.114). An entirely similar argument applies to $\widehat{\mathcal{V}}_{IPW}(d_\eta)$ defined in terms of $\mathcal{G}_{IPW,k}(\underline{d}_{\eta,k}; \underline{\gamma}_k)$ in (7.115).

From Section 7.4.4, the first step of the algorithm, at Decision K, is to maximize (7.116); namely,

$$\widehat{\mathcal{V}}^{(K)}_{AIPW}(d_{\eta,K}) = n^{-1} \sum_{i=1}^{n} \mathcal{G}_{AIPW,Ki}(d_{\eta,K}; \widehat{\gamma}_K, \widehat{\beta}_K), \qquad (7.153)$$

in η_K to obtain $\widehat{\eta}^{opt}_{K,B,AIPW}$ and thus the estimated rule $\widehat{d}^{opt}_{\eta,K,B}(h_K) = d_K(h_K; \widehat{\eta}^{opt}_{K,B,AIPW})$ in (7.120). Analogous to (4.10) in the single decision case, it is straightforward to deduce that (7.153) can be expressed
equivalently as

$$\widehat{\mathcal{V}}^{(K)}_{AIPW}(d_{\eta,K}) = n^{-1} \sum_{i=1}^{n} \Big[\mathcal{G}_{AIPW,Ki}(1; \widehat{\gamma}_K, \widehat{\beta}_K) \mathrm{I}\{d_{\eta,K}(H_{Ki}) = 1\}$$
$$+ \mathcal{G}_{AIPW,Ki}(0; \widehat{\gamma}_K, \widehat{\beta}_K) \mathrm{I}\{d_{\eta,K}(H_{Ki}) = 0\} \Big], \quad (7.154)$$

where $\mathcal{G}_{AIPW,Ki}(a; \widehat{\gamma}_K, \widehat{\beta}_K)$ replaces $d_{\eta,K}(H_{Ki})$ wherever it appears by
option a, $a = 0, 1$. Define

$$\widehat{C}_{Ki} = \mathcal{G}_{AIPW,Ki}(1; \widehat{\gamma}_K, \widehat{\beta}_K) - \mathcal{G}_{AIPW,Ki}(0; \widehat{\gamma}_K, \widehat{\beta}_K), \qquad (7.155)$$

where dependence on (H_{Ki}, A_{Ki}, Y_i) is suppressed for brevity and which
does not depend on η_K. It follows by algebra analogous to that leading
to (4.14) and (4.17) that (7.154) and thus (7.153) can be written as

$$\widehat{\mathcal{V}}^{(K)}_{AIPW}(d_{\eta,K}) = n^{-1} \sum_{i=1}^{n} \Big\{ d_K(H_{Ki}; \eta_K) \widehat{C}_{Ki} + \mathcal{G}_{AIPW,Ki}(0; \widehat{\gamma}_K, \widehat{\beta}_K) \Big\}.$$

As the second term in the summand does not involve η_K, maximizing
(7.153) in η_K is equivalent to maximizing

$$n^{-1} \sum_{i=1}^{n} d_K(H_{Ki}; \eta_K) \widehat{C}_{Ki}. \qquad (7.156)$$

By manipulations identical to those in (4.18), it follows that maximiz-
ing (7.156), and thus $\widehat{\mathcal{V}}^{(K)}_{AIPW}(d_{\eta,K})$ in (7.153), in η_K is equivalent to
minimizing in η_K the weighted classification error

$$n^{-1} \sum_{i=1}^{n} |\widehat{C}_{Ki}| \left\{ \mathrm{I}(\widehat{C}_{Ki} > 0) - d_K(H_{Ki}; \eta_K) \right\}^2$$
$$= n^{-1} \sum_{i=1}^{n} |\widehat{C}_{Ki}| \mathrm{I}\left\{ \mathrm{I}(\widehat{C}_{Ki} > 0) \neq d_K(H_{Ki}; \eta_K) \right\}. \qquad (7.157)$$

Thus, as discussed in Section 4.2, if the restricted class $\mathcal{D}_\eta$ is taken to comprise regimes having rules $d_{\eta,k}(h_k)$, $k = 1, \ldots, K$, induced by a particular choice of classifier, such as support vector machines (Cortes and Vapnik, 1995) or classification and regression trees (Breiman et al., 1984), standard algorithms and software for minimizing a weighted classification error can be applied to (7.157) to maximize $\widehat{\mathcal{V}}^{(K)}_{AIPW}(d_{\eta,K})$ in η_K and obtain $\widehat{\eta}^{opt}_{K,B,AIPW}$ and $\widehat{d}^{opt}_{\eta,K,B}(h_K) = d_K(h_K; \widehat{\eta}^{opt}_{K,B,AIPW})$ in (7.120).

Analogous to (4.24), writing

$$d_K(h_K; \eta_K) = \text{I}\{f_K(h_K; \eta_K) > 0\}$$

for some decision function $f_K(h_K; \eta_K)$, as for the single decision case in (4.27), the objective function (7.157) can be written in terms of the nonconvex 0-1 loss function $\ell_{0\text{-}1}(x) = I(x \le 0)$ in (4.26) as

$$n^{-1} \sum_{i=1}^{n} |\widehat{C}_{Ki}| \, \ell_{0\text{-}1}\left[\left\{2\text{I}(\widehat{C}_{Ki} > 0) - 1\right\} f_K(H_{Ki}; \eta_K)\right]. \qquad (7.158)$$

which, as in the discussion at the end of Section 4.2, makes explicit why this optimization problem is so challenging.

For Decisions $K - 1, \ldots, 1$, this same argument can be applied. At Decision k, $k = K - 1, \ldots, 1$, from (7.128) and (7.131), we wish to maximize in η_k

$$\widehat{\mathcal{V}}^{(k)}_{AIPW}(d_{\eta,k}, \widehat{\underline{d}}^{opt}_{\eta,k+1,B}) = n^{-1} \sum_{i=1}^{n} \mathcal{G}_{AIPW,ki}(d_{\eta,k}, \widehat{\underline{d}}^{opt}_{\eta,k+1,B}; \widehat{\gamma}_k, \widehat{\underline{\beta}}_k).$$
$$(7.159)$$

Analogous to (7.154), reexpress (7.159) as

$$\widehat{\mathcal{V}}^{(k)}_{AIPW}(d_{\eta,k}, \widehat{\underline{d}}^{opt}_{\eta,k+1,B})$$
$$= n^{-1} \sum_{i=1}^{n} \left[\mathcal{G}_{AIPW,ki}(1, \widehat{\underline{d}}^{opt}_{\eta,k+1,B}; \widehat{\gamma}_k, \widehat{\underline{\beta}}_k)\text{I}\{d_{\eta,k}(H_{ki}) = 1\} \right.$$
$$\left. + \mathcal{G}_{AIPW,ki}(0, \widehat{\underline{d}}^{opt}_{\eta,k+1,B}; \widehat{\gamma}_k, \widehat{\underline{\beta}}_k)\text{I}\{d_{\eta,k}(H_{ki}) = 0\} \right],$$

where $\mathcal{G}_{AIPW,ki}(a, \widehat{\underline{d}}^{opt}_{\eta,k+1,B})$ replaces $d_{\eta,k}(H_{ki})$ wherever it appears by option a, $a = 0, 1$; and define

$$\widehat{C}_{ki}(\underline{d}_{\eta,k+1}) \qquad\qquad (7.160)$$
$$= \mathcal{G}_{AIPW,ki}(1, \underline{d}_{\eta,k+1}; \widehat{\gamma}_k, \widehat{\underline{\beta}}_k) - \mathcal{G}_{AIPW,ki}(0, \underline{d}_{\eta,k+1}; \widehat{\gamma}_k, \widehat{\underline{\beta}}_k),$$

which does not depend on η_k. It then follows by the same manipulations as above that maximizing $\widehat{\mathcal{V}}^{(k)}_{AIPW}(d_{\eta,k}, \widehat{\underline{d}}^{opt}_{\eta,k+1,B})$ in (7.159) in η_k is the same as maximizing in η_k

$$n^{-1} \sum_{i=1}^{n} d_k(H_{ki}; \eta_k) \widehat{C}_{ki}(\widehat{\underline{d}}^{opt}_{\eta,k+1,B}). \tag{7.161}$$

Moreover, maximizing (7.161) in η_k is equivalent to minimizing in η_k the weighted classification error

$$n^{-1} \sum_{i=1}^{n} |\widehat{C}_{ki}(\widehat{\underline{d}}^{opt}_{\eta,k+1,B})| \left[\mathrm{I}\{\widehat{C}_{ki}(\widehat{\underline{d}}^{opt}_{\eta,k+1,B}) > 0\} - d_k(H_{ki}; \eta_k) \right]^2$$

$$= n^{-1} \sum_{i=1}^{n} |\widehat{C}_{ki}(\widehat{\underline{d}}^{opt}_{\eta,k+1,B})| \, \mathrm{I}\left[\mathrm{I}\{\widehat{C}_{ki}(\widehat{\underline{d}}^{opt}_{\eta,k+1,B}) > 0\} \neq d_k(H_{ki}; \eta_k) \right]. \tag{7.162}$$

Then, as with (7.157) for Decision K, if the restricted class $\mathcal{D}_\eta$ is induced by a particular choice of classifier, standard algorithms and software for minimizing a weighted classification error can be applied to (7.162) to maximize $\widehat{\mathcal{V}}^{(k)}_{AIPW}(d_{\eta,k}, \widehat{\underline{d}}^{opt}_{\eta,k+1,B})$ in η_k to obtain $\widehat{\eta}^{opt}_{k,B,AIPW}$ and $\widehat{d}^{opt}_{\eta,k,B}(h_K) = d_k(h_K; \widehat{\eta}^{opt}_{k,B,AIPW})$. As above, (7.162) can be expressed in a form analogous to (7.158), demonstrating the nonsmooth, nonconvex nature of this objective function.

At Decision K, from (7.117), analogous to (4.15) and (4.16) in the single decision case, let

$$C_K(H_K) = E\{Y^*(\overline{A}_{K-1}, 1) - Y^*(\overline{A}_{K-1}, 0) \mid H_K\}$$

denote the "contrast function" corresponding to the difference in expected outcome for an individual with history H_K were he to receive option 1 versus option 0 at Decision K. Then

$$\widehat{C}_{Ki} = \mathcal{G}_{AIPW,Ki}(1; \widehat{\gamma}_K, \widehat{\beta}_K) - \mathcal{G}_{AIPW,Ki}(0; \widehat{\gamma}_K, \widehat{\beta}_K)$$

in (7.155) can be viewed as a predictor of $C_K(H_{Ki})$ for individual i. Similarly, for $k = K - 1, \ldots, 1$, let

$$C_k(H_k, \underline{d}_{\eta,k+1}) = E\{Y^*(\overline{A}_{k-1}, 1, \underline{d}_{\eta,k+1}) - Y^*(\overline{A}_{k-1}, 0, \underline{d}_{\eta,k+1}) \mid H_k\}$$

be the "contrast function" corresponding to the difference in expected outcomes for an individual with history H_k were he to receive option 1 versus option 0 at Decision k and then follow the rules $(d_{\eta,k+1}, \ldots, d_{\eta,K})$ at Decisions $k + 1, \ldots, K$ thereafter. Then, from (7.160), $\widehat{C}_{ki}(\widehat{\underline{d}}^{opt}_{\eta,k+1,B})$ can be interpreted as a predictor of $C_k(H_{ki}, \underline{d}^{opt}_{\eta,k+1,B})$, where, as in Section 7.4.4, the rules $(d^{opt}_{\eta,k+1,B}, \ldots, d^{opt}_{\eta,K,B})$ are defined in (7.120), (7.126), and (7.132).

The foregoing developments demonstrate that, when there are two feasible treatment options at each decision point for all individuals, taking $\mathcal{D}_\eta$ to comprise regimes whose rules $d_{\eta,k}(h_k)$, $k = 1, \ldots, K$, are induced by a particular choice of classifier, each step of the backward iterative algorithm in Section 7.4.4 can be cast as a separate weighted classification problem reminiscent of that in the single decision case in Section 4.2. That is, at step $k = K, K-1, \ldots, 1$, a weighted classification error is minimized in η_k, just as (4.22) is minimized in η_1.

As noted above, a backward formulation of this type was first proposed in the particular context of maximizing a simple inverse probability weighted estimator for the value $\mathcal{V}(d_\eta)$ of a multiple decision restricted regime by Zhao et al. (2015a), who sought to generalize OWL to this case. We now discuss this approach.

Backward Outcome Weighted Learning

For comparison with BOWL as proposed by Zhao et al. (2015a) and with Section 4.3, code the two options in $\mathcal{A}_k$, $k = 1, \ldots, K$, as 1 and -1, so that $\omega_k(h_k, a_k) = P(A_k = a_k \mid H_k = h_k)$ is defined for $a_k = 1, -1$. Zhao et al. (2015a) did not consider positing and fitting appropriate models $\omega_k(h_k, a_k; \gamma_k)$, but this extension is immediate. Then, from (7.115), the goal is to maximize

$$\widehat{\mathcal{V}}_{IPW}(d_\eta) = n^{-1} \sum_{i=1}^{n} \mathcal{G}_{IPW,1i}(d_\eta; \widehat{\underline{\gamma}}_1)$$

$$= n^{-1} \sum_{i=1}^{n} \left[\prod_{j=1}^{K} \frac{Y_i \mathrm{I}\{A_{ji} = d_j(H_{ji}; \eta_j)\}}{\omega_j(H_{ji}, A_{ji}; \widehat{\gamma}_j)} \right].$$

The BOWL algorithm for this purpose is as follows. As for OWL in (4.33) in the single decision case, in what follows, represent the rule at Decision k in terms of a decision function $f_k(h_k; \eta_k)$ as

$$d_k(h_k; \eta_k) = \mathrm{sign}\{f_k(h_k; \eta_k)\}, \quad k = 1, \ldots, K.$$

From (7.115), at Decision K, analogous to (7.153), we wish to maximize in η_K

$$\widehat{\mathcal{V}}_{IPW}^{(K)}(d_{\eta,K}) = n^{-1} \sum_{i=1}^{n} \mathcal{G}_{IPW,Ki}(d_{\eta,K}; \widehat{\gamma}_K)$$

$$= n^{-1} \sum_{i=1}^{n} \frac{\mathrm{I}\{A_{Ki} = d_{\eta,K}(H_{Ki})\} Y_i}{\omega_K(H_{Ki}, A_{Ki}; \widehat{\gamma}_K)},$$

which is equivalent to minimizing in η_K

$$n^{-1} \sum_{i=1}^{n} \frac{Y_i \mathrm{I}\{A_{Ki} \neq d_{\eta,K}(H_{Ki})\}}{\omega_K(H_{Ki}, A_{Ki}; \widehat{\gamma}_K)}$$

$$= n^{-1} \sum_{i=1}^{n} \frac{Y_i \mathrm{I}[A_{Ki} \neq \mathrm{sign}\{f_K(H_{Ki}; \eta_K)\}]}{\omega_K(H_{Ki}, A_{Ki}; \widehat{\gamma}_K)}. \tag{7.163}$$

Analogous to the single decision case,

$$\mathrm{I}[A_{Ki} \neq \mathrm{sign}\{f_K(H_{Ki}; \eta_K)\}] = \mathrm{I}\{A_{Ki} f_K(H_{Ki}; \eta_K) \leq 0\}$$
$$= \ell_{0\text{-}1}\{A_{Ki} f_K(H_{Ki}; \eta_K)\},$$

where as before $\ell_{0\text{-}1}(x) = I(x \leq 0)$ is the 0-1 loss function in (4.26), showing that (7.163) is a nonconvex objective function. As for OWL, Zhao et al. (2015a) propose replacing the 0-1 loss function by the convex surrogate hinge loss function

$$\ell_{hinge}(x) = (1-x)_+, \quad x_+ = \max(0, x)$$

in (4.35) and instead minimizing

$$n^{-1} \sum_{i=1}^{n} \frac{Y_i}{\omega_K(H_{Ki}, A_{Ki}; \widehat{\gamma}_K)} \{1 - A_{Ki} f_1(H_{Ki}; \eta_K)\}_+ + \lambda_{K,n} \|f_K\|^2,$$
$$\tag{7.164}$$

which is (2.4) of Zhao et al. (2015a). In (7.164), as in (4.36) in OWL in the single decision case, $\| \cdot \|$ is a suitable norm for f_K, $\lambda_{K,n}$ is a scalar tuning parameter, and the second term in (7.164) is a penalty controlling the complexity of f_K in η_K. As in the general case, let $\widehat{\eta}_{K,B,BOWL}^{opt}$ be the minimizer of (7.164) and

$$\widehat{d}_{\eta,K,B}^{opt}(h_K) = d_K(h_K; \widehat{\eta}_{K,B,BOWL}^{opt}) = \mathrm{sign}\{f_K(h_K; \widehat{\eta}_{K,B,BOWL}^{opt})\}$$

be the estimated Decision K rule.

Continuing in this fashion, at Decision $k = K-1, \ldots, 1$, from (7.115) and analogous to (7.159), we wish to maximize in η_k

$$\widehat{\mathcal{V}}_{IPW}^{(k)}(d_{\eta,k}, \widehat{\underline{d}}_{\eta,k+1,B}^{opt}) = n^{-1} \sum_{i=1}^{n} \mathcal{G}_{IPW,ki}(d_{\eta,k}, \widehat{\underline{d}}_{\eta,k+1,B}^{opt}; \widehat{\underline{\gamma}}_k)$$

$$= n^{-1} \sum_{i=1}^{n} \frac{\prod_{j=k+1}^{K} \mathrm{I}\{A_{ji} = d_j(H_{ji}; \widehat{\eta}_{j,B,BOWL}^{opt})\} Y_i}{\prod_{j=k}^{K} \omega_j(H_{ji}, A_{ji}; \widehat{\gamma}_j)} \mathrm{I}\{A_{ki} = d_k(H_{ki}; \eta_k)\},$$

which, as above, is equivalent to minimizing in η_k

$$n^{-1} \sum_{i=1}^{n} \left(\frac{\prod_{j=k+1}^{K} Y_i \mathrm{I}\{A_{ji} = d_j(H_{ji}; \widehat{\eta}_{j,B,BOWL}^{opt})\}}{\prod_{j=k}^{K} \omega_j(H_{ji}, A_{ji}; \widehat{\gamma}_j)} \right. \tag{7.165}$$
$$\left. \times \mathrm{I}[A_{ki} \neq \mathrm{sign}\{f_k(H_{ki}; \eta_k)\}] \right).$$

Replacing the 0-1 loss function by the convex surrogate hinge loss function in (7.165) as above, Zhao et al. (2015a) propose minimizing in η_k

$$n^{-1} \sum_{i=1}^{n} \frac{\prod_{j=k+1}^{K} Y_i \mathrm{I}\{A_{ji} = d_j(H_{ji}; \widehat{\eta}_{j,B,BOWL}^{opt})\}}{\prod_{j=k}^{K} \omega_j(H_{ji}, A_{ji}; \widehat{\gamma}_j)} \{1 - A_{ki} f_k(H_{ki}; \eta_k)\}_+$$
$$+ \lambda_{k,n} \|f_k\|^2, \tag{7.166}$$

which is their (2.5), where, as in (7.164), $\lambda_{k,n}$ is a scalar tuning parameter, and the second term in (7.166) is a penalty controlling the complexity of f_k in η_k. Letting $\widehat{\eta}_{k,B,BOWL}^{opt}$ be the minimizer of (7.166), the estimated rule at Decision k, $k = K - 1, \ldots, 1$, is

$$\widehat{d}_{\eta,k,B}^{opt}(h_k) = d_k(h_k; \widehat{\eta}_{k,B,BOWL}^{opt}) = \mathrm{sign}\{f_k(h_k; \widehat{\eta}_{k,B,BOWL}^{opt})\}.$$

As for OWL in the single decision case in Section 4.3, the objective functions (7.164) and (7.166), in which the 0-1 loss function is replaced by the hinge loss, are different from (7.163) and (7.165). Thus, analogous to the comment after (4.36) in that section, it is not necessarily the case that the resulting estimators $d_k(h_k; \widehat{\eta}_{k,B,BOWL}^{opt})$ at each step are equivalent to those minimizing the original objective functions.

Zhao et al. (2015a) propose using a very flexible class of decision functions, and thus classification method, for each $k = 1, \ldots, K$ to represent potentially complex relationships between high-dimensional h_k and treatment options. This choice corresponds to a restricted class of regimes $\mathcal{D}_\eta$ whose rules are richly parameterized in terms of high-dimensional η_k, $k = 1, \ldots, K$. The hope is that such a flexible class $\mathcal{D}_\eta$ contains the global d^{opt}, as discussed in the remark at the end of the description of the backward iterative implementation of value search estimation. Of course, as in Section 4.3, the decision functions also can be taken to belong to a much simpler class corresponding to simpler classification methods such as linear support vector machines.

Because BOWL is based on simple inverse probability weighting, the number of individuals whose actual treatments received are consistent with the first k rules of a regime decreases as k increases, so that, for K not small, the objective function is based on data from a limited number of individuals and can be unstable. Zhao et al. (2015a) propose an iterative version of BOWL meant to increase the stability of the procedure. The authors also describe an approximation to direct maximization of $\widehat{\mathcal{V}}_{IPW}(d_\eta)$ in which the indicator functions are replaced by continuous and concave surrogate functions. See Zhao et al. (2015a) for details on these methods.

As discussed in Section 4.3 in the single decision problem, the approach of Zhao et al. (2015a) is applicable to the general case of the backward iterative algorithm based on maximizing $\widehat{\mathcal{V}}_{AIPW}(d_\eta)$ or $\widehat{\mathcal{V}}_{IPW}(d_\eta)$ in η. Expressing the weighted classification errors (7.157) and (7.162) at each step $k = K, K-1, \ldots, 1$ in terms of decision functions $f_k(h_k; \eta_k)$ and the 0-1 loss function as in (7.158), replacing the 0-1 loss function by the surrogate hinge loss function, and adopting a very flexible representation of the decision functions as in Zhao et al. (2015a), one can minimize penalized versions of the resulting objective functions analogous to (7.164) and (7.166) at each step. The resulting estimators are subject to the same caveat noted above regarding the equivalence to those obtained by minimizing the original objective functions at each step.

7.4.6 Interpretable Regimes via Decision Lists

Taking the classification perspective as in the previous section, and adopting a very flexible classifier and thus representation of decision functions as in BOWL, likely induces a restricted class of regimes $\mathcal{D}_\eta$ whose decision rules are complex and depend on high-dimensional η. The advantage of such flexibility in the representation of decision rules is that the threat of model misspecification is mitigated, and the resulting estimated regime may come close to achieving the performance of an optimal regime in $\mathcal{D}$, the class of all possible regimes. However, this may be at the expense of interpretability. In particular, the rules may be unintelligible to clinicians and patients, and new scientific insights and hypotheses may be impossible to achieve on their basis.

To address the need to restrict attention to parsimonious, interpretable regimes when the primary goal is to advance scientific knowledge or provide clinicians and patients with understandable decision support, Zhang et al. (2015) focus in the single decision case on the restricted class of regimes whose rules are in the form of decision lists. The authors propose a strategy for estimation of an optimal regime within this class. The salient features of this approach, including examples of rules in the form of a decision list, are presented in Section 4.4.

For the multiple decision case, Zhang et al. (2018) propose a method for estimation of an optimal regime in the class of regimes with rules in the form of decision lists. We provide here a brief sketch of the approach and refer the reader to Zhang et al. (2018) for details of implementation and theoretical results. The reader may wish to review Section 4.4 before proceeding, as the concept of decision rules that are expressible as decision lists is covered in some detail there and is not repeated here.

As in Zhang et al. (2018), consider the setting in which all $m_k \geq 2$ options in $\mathcal{A}_k$, $k = 1, \ldots, K$, are feasible for all individuals; extension to the case of a specification Ψ of feasible sets is possible although not presented explicitly by the authors. Analogous to (4.42), Zhang et al. (2018) consider rules for each decision point k, $k = 1, \ldots, K$, in the form of a decision list of length L_k given by

$$
\begin{aligned}
&\text{If } c_{k1} \text{ then } \mathsf{a}_{k1}; \\
&\text{else if } c_{k2} \text{ then } \mathsf{a}_{k2}; \\
&\qquad\qquad \vdots \\
&\text{else if } c_{kL_k} \text{ then } \mathsf{a}_{kL_k},
\end{aligned}
\tag{7.167}
$$

which can be summarized as $\{(c_{k1}, \mathsf{a}_{k1}), \ldots, (c_{kL_k}, \mathsf{a}_{kL_k})\}$. In (7.167), $c_{k1}, \ldots, c_{kL_k}$ are logical conditions that are true or false for each h_k; and $\mathsf{a}_{k\ell}$, $\ell = 0, 1, \ldots, L_k$, are the corresponding recommended treatment options in $\mathcal{A}_k$. The formulation in (7.167) is slightly different from (4.42) in that the list does not have a final "else" condition; this is for computational reasons discussed below. Examples of logical conditions in the context of the acute leukemia example in Section 1.2.1 are given in (4.40) and (4.41). As in Section 4.4, for $k = 1, \ldots, K$, let

$$
\mathcal{T}_k(c_{k\ell}) = \{h_k : c_{k\ell} \text{ is true }\}, \quad \ell = 1, \ldots, L_k,
$$

be subsets of $\mathcal{H}_k$, in which case (7.167) can be expressed equivalently as

$$
\begin{aligned}
&\text{If } h_k \in \mathcal{T}_k(c_{k1}) \text{ then } \mathsf{a}_{k1}; \\
&\text{else if } h_k \in \mathcal{T}_k(c_{k2}) \text{ then } \mathsf{a}_{k2}; \\
&\qquad\qquad \vdots \\
&\text{else if } h_k \in \mathcal{T}_k(c_{kL_k}) \text{ then } \mathsf{a}_{kL_k}
\end{aligned}
\tag{7.168}
$$

as in (1) of Zhang et al. (2018). Henceforth, for consistency with Zhang et al. (2018), we express decision lists in the equivalent form (7.168).

As in Zhang et al. (2015) for the single decision case in Section 4.4, because arbitrary logical conditions $c_{k\ell}$, $\ell = 1, \ldots, L_k$, can involve h_k in complicated ways, to maintain parsimony and interpretability, as in (4.44), Zhang et al. (2018) restrict attention to logical conditions $c_{k\ell}$ and thus sets $\mathcal{T}_k(c_{k\ell})$, $\ell = 1, \ldots, L_k$, $k = 1, \ldots, K$, involving at most two components of h_k. Letting p_k be the number of components in h_k and

$j_1 < j_2 \in \{1, \ldots, p_k\}$ be the indices of two arbitrary components, the sets $\mathcal{T}_k(c_{k\ell})$ can be of any of the forms

$$
\begin{aligned}
\{h_k : h_{kj_1} \leq \tau_{k1}\}, &\qquad \{h_k : h_{kj_1} > \tau_{k1}\} \\
\{h_k : h_{kj_1} \leq \tau_{k1} \text{ and } h_{kj_2} \leq \tau_{k2}\} & \\
\{h_k : h_{kj_1} \leq \tau_{k1} \text{ and } h_{kj_2} > \tau_{k2}\} &\qquad (7.169) \\
\{h_k : h_{kj_1} > \tau_{k1} \text{ and } h_{kj_2} \leq \tau_{k2}\} & \\
\{h_k : h_{kj_1} > \tau_{k1} \text{ and } h_{kj_2} > \tau_{k2}\}, &
\end{aligned}
$$

where τ_{k1} and τ_{k2} are scalar threshold values. In contrast to (4.44), sets involving an "or" condition analogous to those in the right column of (4.44) are omitted because a list involving such sets can be reexpressed in terms of clauses involving sets in (7.169), as a decision list need not be unique, as discussed in Section 4.4. For example, the clause "if $h_k \in \{h_k : h_{kj_1} \leq \tau_{k1} \text{ or } h_{kj_2} \leq \tau_{k2}\}$ then a_{k1}" can be written equivalently as "if $h_k \in \{h_k : h_{kj_1} \leq \tau_{k1}\}$ then a_{k1}; else if $h_k \in \{h_k : h_{kj_2} \leq \tau_{k2}\}$ then a_{k1}." This version allows ascertainment of h_{kj_2} to be "short circuited" for individuals for whom $h_{kj_1} \leq \tau_{k1}$, thereby reducing the potential cost of implementation, as discussed in Section 4.4. See Zhang et al. (2018) for additional considerations regarding (7.169).

For brevity, write $\mathcal{T}_{k\ell}$ to denote a subset of $\mathcal{H}_k$ of any of the forms in (7.169), so defined by corresponding logical conditions $c_{k\ell}$. Analogous to Section 4.4, the restricted class of regimes $\mathcal{D}_\eta$ of interest is then defined as follows. Under (7.169), for each $k = 1, \ldots, K$, let

$$
\eta_k = \{(\mathcal{T}_{k\ell}, \mathsf{a}_{k\ell})\}_{\ell=1}^{L_k} = \{(\mathcal{T}_{k1}, \mathsf{a}_{k1}), \ldots, (\mathcal{T}_{kL_k}, \mathsf{a}_{kL_k})\}
$$

be a collection of L_k subsets $\mathcal{T}_{k\ell}$ of $\mathcal{H}_k$, each of which is the form of one of those in (7.169); and a set of corresponding treatment options. Zhang et al. (2018) impose an upper bound L_{max} on list length for all K decision points; i.e., $L_k \leq L_{max}$, $k = 1, \ldots, K$. A rule at the kth decision point, $k = 1, \ldots, K$, can then be characterized in terms of η_k and written as $d_k(h_k; \eta_k)$. Letting $\eta = \{\eta_1, \ldots, \eta_K\}$ comprise all K collections of subsets and treatment options, the restricted class of regimes $\mathcal{D}_\eta$ of interest consists of all possible regimes $d_\eta = \{d_1(h_1; \eta_1), \ldots, d_K(h_K; \eta_K)\}$ indexed by η for which

$$
\eta_k \in \left\{ \{(\mathcal{T}_{k\ell}, \mathsf{a}_{k\ell})\}_{\ell=1}^{L_k} : \mathcal{T}_{k\ell} \in \mathcal{T}_k, \mathsf{a}_{k\ell} \in \mathcal{A}_k, \ell = 1, \ldots, L_k; L_k \leq L_{max} \right\},
$$

$k = 1, \ldots, K$, where, as in (2) of Zhang et al. (2018), $\mathcal{T}_k$ denotes the collection of all subsets of $\mathcal{H}_k$ of the forms in (7.169).

Clearly, estimation of an optimal regime d_η^{opt} in the class $\mathcal{D}_\eta$ by direct maximization in η of an augmented or simple inverse probability weighted estimator for $\mathcal{V}(d_\eta)$, as in Zhang et al. (2015) and described in Section 4.4, is an insurmountable challenge. Accordingly,

Zhang et al. (2018) propose exploiting the backward iterative strategy using regression modeling introduced in Section 7.4.4 to estimate each rule successively. To obtain the nonparametric estimators $\widehat{Q}_k^{d_\eta}(h_k, a_k)$ for $Q_k^{d_\eta}(h_k, a_k)$, $k = 1, \ldots, K$, the authors use kernel ridge regression, in which $Q_k^{d_\eta}(h_k, a_k)$ is estimated by regressing the pseudo outcomes $\widetilde{V}_{k+1,i}^{d_\eta}$ on the observed (H_k, A_k) via penalized least squares.

We outline the basic premise of the approach, which at each decision point $k = K, \ldots, 1$ constructs an estimator for $d_{\eta,k,B}^{opt}(h_k)$ defined in (7.142), (7.146) and (7.150) using a greedy optimization algorithm one clause at a time.

At Decision K, as in Section 7.4.4, obtain the nonparametric estimator $\widehat{Q}_K^{d_\eta}(h_K, a_K)$ for $Q_K^{d_\eta}(h_K, a_K) = E(Y \mid H_K = h_K, A_K = a_K)$ by regressing Y on the observed (H_K, A_K) as above. Note that, if we consider all possible Decision K rules for regimes $d \in \mathcal{D}$, the class of all possible regimes, so not restricting to rules of the form $d_{\eta,K}(h_K)$, as in Q-learning in Sections 5.7.1 and 7.4.1, an estimator for an optimal unrestricted rule $d_K^{opt}(h_K)$ at Decision K is

$$\widehat{d}_K^{opt}(h_K) = \underset{a_K \in \mathcal{A}_K}{\arg\max} \, \widehat{Q}_K^{d_\eta}(h_K, a_K).$$

Presumably, if the nonparametric regression method used to estimate $Q_K^{d_\eta}(h_K, a_K)$ is sufficiently flexible, $\widehat{d}_K^{opt}(h_K)$ is a good estimator for $d_K^{opt}(h_K)$ in that it closely resembles $d_K^{opt}(h_K)$. The rule $d_K^{opt}(h_K)$, and thus $\widehat{d}_K^{opt}(h_K)$, may be complex, depending on h_K in a complicated way, but it is optimal if no restrictions are imposed.

To estimate $(\mathcal{T}_{K1}^{opt}, a_{K1}^{opt})$, say, characterizing the first clause in $d_{\eta,K,B}^{opt}(h_K)$, consider the rule in the form of a decision list

$$
\begin{aligned}
&\text{If } h_K \in \mathcal{T} \text{ then a;} \\
&\text{else if } h_K \in \mathcal{H}_K \text{ then } d_K^{opt}(h_K).
\end{aligned}
\tag{7.170}
$$

By the same reasoning used to develop the backward iterative strategy, an estimator for $E\{Y^*(\overline{A}_{K-1}, d_{\eta,K})\}$, where $d_{\eta,K}$ is given in (7.170), is

$$n^{-1} \sum_{i=1}^n \left[\mathrm{I}(H_{Ki} \in \mathcal{T}) \, \widehat{Q}_K^{d_\eta}(H_{Ki}, \mathrm{a}) + \mathrm{I}(H_{Ki} \notin \mathcal{T}) \, \widehat{Q}_K^{d_\eta}\{H_{Ki}, \widehat{d}_K^{opt}(H_{Ki})\} \right].$$

$$\tag{7.171}$$

Zhang et al. (2018) propose estimating $(\mathcal{T}_{K1}^{opt}, a_{K1}^{opt})$ by maximizing (7.171) in $(\mathcal{T}, \mathrm{a})$. The difference between an estimator for $E\{Y^*(\overline{A}_{K-1}, d_K^{opt})\}$ and (7.171) is

$$\sum_{i=1}^n \mathrm{I}(H_{Ki} \in \mathcal{T}) \left[\widehat{Q}_K^{d_\eta}\{H_{Ki}, \widehat{d}_K^{opt}(H_{Ki})\} - \widehat{Q}_K^{d_\eta}(H_{Ki}, \mathrm{a}) \right],$$

which can be interpreted as reflecting the decrease in expected outcome when some part of $d_K^{opt}(h_K)$ is replaced by an if-then clause and thus the price paid for interpretability. This price is minimized by maximizing (7.171). Zhang et al. (2018) actually maximize a penalized version of (7.171) that favors subsets $\mathcal{T}$ of $\mathcal{H}_K$ that are large and involve checking fewer components of h_K.

Having obtained $(\widehat{\mathcal{T}}_{K1}^{opt}, \widehat{\mathsf{a}}_{K1}^{opt})$ via this maximization, to estimate the second clause characterized by $(\mathcal{T}_{K2}^{opt}, \mathsf{a}_{K2}^{opt})$, consider the rule in the form of a decision list

$$\text{If } h_K \in \widehat{\mathcal{T}}_{K1}^{opt} \text{ then } \widehat{\mathsf{a}}_{K1}^{opt};$$

$$\text{else if } h_K \in \mathcal{T} \text{ then } \mathsf{a}; \qquad (7.172)$$

$$\text{else if } h_K \in \mathcal{H}_K \text{ then } d_K^{opt}(h_K).$$

As above, an estimator for $E\{Y^*(\overline{A}_{K-1}, d_{\eta,K})\}$, where $d_{\eta,K}$ is given in (7.172), is

$$n^{-1} \sum_{i=1}^{n} \Big[\text{I}(H_{Ki} \in \widehat{\mathcal{T}}_{K1}^{opt}) \, \widehat{Q}_K^{d_\eta}(H_{Ki}, \widehat{\mathsf{a}}_{K1})$$

$$+ \text{I}(H_{Ki} \notin \widehat{\mathcal{T}}_{K1}^{opt}, H_{Ki} \in \mathcal{T}) \, \widehat{Q}_K^{d_\eta}(H_{Ki}, \mathsf{a})$$

$$+ \text{I}(H_{Ki} \notin \widehat{\mathcal{T}}_{K1}^{opt}), H_{Ki} \notin \mathcal{T}) \, \widehat{Q}_K^{d_\eta}\{H_{Ki}, \widehat{d}_K^{opt}(H_{Ki})\} \Big]. \quad (7.173)$$

The first term in the summand of (7.173) does not depend on $(\mathcal{T}, \mathsf{a})$; thus, maximize (7.173) with this term eliminated to obtain $(\widehat{\mathcal{T}}_{K2}^{opt}, \widehat{\mathsf{a}}_{K2}^{opt})$. As for (7.171), Zhang et al. (2018) propose maximizing a penalized version of this objective function.

This scheme continues until either every individual receives a recommended treatment option, so $\mathcal{T}_{K\ell} = \mathcal{H}_K$ for some ℓ or the maximum list length L_{max} is reached, in which case $\mathcal{T}_{KL_{max}}$ is set equal to $\mathcal{H}_K$ to ensure an option is selected by the estimated rule for every $h_K \in \mathcal{H}_k$, with $\widehat{\mathsf{a}}_{KL_{max}}^{opt}$ the estimated option for all remaining h_K. With the number of steps required equal to L_K, letting

$$\widehat{\eta}_{K,B,DL}^{opt} = \{(\widehat{\mathcal{T}}_{K\ell}^{opt}, \widehat{\mathsf{a}}_{K\ell}^{opt})\}_{\ell=1}^{L_K},$$

the estimated optimal restricted rule maximizing $E\{Y^*(\overline{A}_{K-1}, d_{\eta,K})\}$ is taken to be $d_K(h_K; \widehat{\eta}_{K,B,DL}^{opt})$.

At Decisions $k = K-1, \ldots, 1$, estimation of $d_{\eta,k,B}^{opt}(h_k)$ follows the same principle. Form the pseudo outcomes

$$\widetilde{V}_{k+1,i}^{d_\eta} = \widehat{Q}_{k+1}^{d_\eta}\{H_{k+1,i}, \widehat{d}_{\eta,k+1,B}^{opt}(H_{k+1,i})\}, \quad i = 1, \ldots, n,$$

and regress these on the observed (H_k, A_k) as described above to obtain the nonparametric estimator $\widehat{Q}_k^{d_\eta}(h_k, a_k)$ for $Q_k^{d_\eta}(h_k, a_k)$ in (7.148). As for Decision K, an estimator for an unrestricted optimal rule $d_k^{opt}(h_k)$ at Decision k that maximizes in d_k $E\{Y^*(\overline{A}_{k-1}, d_k, \underline{d}_{\eta,k+1,B}^{opt})\}$ and thus assumes that the restricted rules $\underline{d}_{\eta,k+1,B}^{opt}$ are followed in the future, is

$$\widehat{d}_k^{opt}(h_k) = \underset{a_k \in \mathcal{A}_k}{\arg\max} \, \widehat{Q}_k^{d_\eta}(h_k, a_k).$$

Then, by analogy to the procedure for Decision K, to estimate $d_{\eta,k,B}^{opt}(h_k)$, Zhang et al. (2018) propose estimating $(\mathcal{T}_{k1}^{opt}, \mathsf{a}_{k1}^{opt})$ characterizing the first clause in $d_{\eta,k,B}^{opt}(h_K)$ by considering the rule $d_{\eta,k}$:

$$\text{If } h_k \in \mathcal{T} \text{ then } \mathsf{a};$$
$$\text{else if } h_k \in \mathcal{H}_k \text{ then } d_k^{opt}(h_k) \tag{7.174}$$

and maximizing in $(\mathcal{T}, \mathsf{a})$ a penalized version of the estimator for $E\{Y^*(\overline{A}_{k-1}, d_{\eta,k}, \underline{d}_{\eta,k+1,B}^{opt})\}$ given by

$$n^{-1} \sum_{i=1}^{n} \left[\mathrm{I}(H_{ki} \in \mathcal{T}) \, \widehat{Q}_k^{d_\eta}(H_{ki}, \mathsf{a}) + \mathrm{I}(H_{ki} \notin \mathcal{T}) \, \widehat{Q}_k^{d_\eta}\{H_{ki}, \widehat{d}_k^{opt}(H_{ki})\} \right],$$
$$\tag{7.175}$$

where $d_{\eta,k}$ is given in (7.174). Then, given the resulting $(\widehat{\mathcal{T}}_{k1}^{opt}, \widehat{\mathsf{a}}_{k1}^{opt})$, as in (7.172), consider the rule $d_{\eta,k}$:

$$\text{If } h_k \in \widehat{\mathcal{T}}_{k1}^{opt} \text{ then } \widehat{\mathsf{a}}_{k1}^{opt};$$
$$\text{else if } h_k \in \mathcal{T} \text{ then } \mathsf{a}; \tag{7.176}$$
$$\text{else if } h_k \in \mathcal{H}_k \text{ then } d_k^{opt}(h_k)$$

and estimate the second clause characterized by $(\mathcal{T}_{k2}^{opt}, \mathsf{a}_{k2}^{opt})$ by maximizing in $(\mathcal{T}, \mathsf{a})$ a penalized version of the estimator for $E\{Y^*(\overline{A}_{k-1}, d_{\eta,k}, \underline{d}_{\eta,k+1,B}^{opt})\}$ given by

$$n^{-1} \sum_{i=1}^{n} \left[\mathrm{I}(H_{ki} \in \widehat{\mathcal{T}}_{k1}^{opt}) \, \widehat{Q}_k^{d_\eta}(H_{ki}, \widehat{\mathsf{a}}_{k1}) \right.$$
$$+ \mathrm{I}(H_{ki} \notin \widehat{\mathcal{T}}_{k1}^{opt}, H_{ki} \in \mathcal{T}) \, \widehat{Q}_k^{d_\eta}(H_{ki}, \mathsf{a})$$
$$\left. + \mathrm{I}(H_{ki} \notin \widehat{\mathcal{T}}_{k1}^{opt}, H_{ki} \notin \mathcal{T}) \, \widehat{Q}_k^{d_\eta}\{H_{ki}, \widehat{d}_k^{opt}(H_{ki})\} \right], \tag{7.177}$$

analogous to (7.173). As for Decision K, continue until either every individual receives a recommended treatment option or the maximum list length L_{max} is reached as described above, and denote the resulting estimator for the kth optimal restricted rule as $d_k(h_k; \hat{\eta}^{opt}_{k,B,DL})$, where

$$\hat{\eta}^{opt}_{k,B,DL} = \{(\hat{\mathcal{T}}^{opt}_{k\ell}, \mathfrak{a}^{opt}_{k\ell})\}^{L_k}_{\ell=1}.$$

The estimator for $d^{opt}_{\eta,B} = \{d^{opt}_{\eta,1,B}(h_1), \ldots, d^{opt}_{\eta,K,B}(h_K)\}$ is obtained after Decision 1 and is given by

$$\hat{d}^{opt}_{\eta,B,DL} = \{d_1(h_1; \hat{\eta}^{opt}_{1,B,DL}), \ldots, d_K(h_K; \hat{\eta}^{opt}_{K,B,DL})\}. \qquad (7.178)$$

As with the objective functions maximized at each decision point k in the general backward iterative strategies in Section 7.4.4, maximization of (7.171), (7.173), (7.175), (7.177), and similar estimators in the foregoing scheme is a nonstandard optimization problem, as these objective functions are nonsmooth and nonconvex. Moreover, a brute force search over all possible η_k to achieve the maximum involves considerable computational burden and is not suitable for practical use. Zhang et al. (2018) propose a strategy that reduces the computational complexity and supports feasible implementation in practice.

It is not readily apparent that the proposed approach should yield valid estimators for rules $d_{\eta,k,B}(h_k)$, $k = 1, \ldots, K$, in (7.142), (7.146) and (7.150). Zhang et al. (2018) present theoretical results demonstrating that $\hat{d}^{opt}_{\eta,B,DL}$ in (7.178) does represent a valid estimator for $d^{opt}_{\eta,B}$ in a certain sense.

7.4.7 Estimation via Marginal Structural Models

In Section 6.4.5, we present a strategy for estimation of the value of a fixed regime in a restricted class of regimes $\mathcal{D}_\eta \subset \mathcal{D}$ whose rules can be represented in terms of a low-dimensional parameter η using a posited marginal structural model, based on work of Orellana et al. (2010a,b). We now discuss how estimation of an optimal regime in a restricted class can be based on this approach. The reader may wish to review Section 6.4.5 before proceeding, as the developments here build on that section.

As defined in Section 6.4.5, for $d_\eta \in \mathcal{D}_\eta$ of the form

$$d_\eta = \{d_1(h_1; \eta_1), \ldots, d_K(h_K; \eta_K)\}, \quad \eta = (\eta^T_1, \ldots, \eta^T_K)^T,$$

if $\mathcal{V}(d_\eta) = E\{Y^*(d_\eta)\} = \mu(\eta)$ for some real-valued function $\mu(\cdot)$, as in (6.125), a marginal structural model is a parametric model for $\mu(\eta)$ of the form

$$\mu(\eta; \alpha), \qquad (7.179)$$

depending on a finite-dimensional parameter α. The use of marginal structural models is particularly attractive when the class $\mathcal{D}_\eta$ is simple, as demonstrated in the example of treatment of HIV-infected patients in Section 6.4.5, where the outcome of interest is negative viral load ($-$viral RNA copies/ml) measured after K monthly clinic visits, so that larger values are preferred. In this situation, $\eta = \eta_1 = \cdots = \eta_K$ is a scalar threshold such that, at each of the K monthly decision points, a regime $d_\eta \in \mathcal{D}_\eta$ has decision rule of the form in (6.124),

$$d_k(h_k; \eta) = \mathrm{I}(\mathsf{CD4}_k \leq \eta), \quad k = 1, \ldots, K, \tag{7.180}$$

where $\mathsf{CD4}_k$ is the patient's CD4 T cell count (cells/mm^3) immediately prior to Decision k; and the two treatment options at any decision point are take (do not take) antiretroviral therapy for the next month, coded as 1 (0), which are feasible for all individuals. The rules (7.180), and thus regimes in $\mathcal{D}_\eta$, are of a very simple form, involving comparison of current CD4 count to a common threshold η at all K decision points.

With $Y^*(d_\eta)$ an HIV-infected patient's negative viral load at a final clinic visit if he were to be administered antiretroviral therapy according to regime d_η with K rules of the form (7.180), in Section 6.4.5, we discuss estimation of the value $\mathcal{V}(d_{\eta^*}) = E\{Y^*(d_{\eta^*})\}$ for a particular threshold η^*, and thus particular fixed regime d_{η^*}, based on a marginal structural model of the form (7.179). As noted in that section, η plays the role of a "covariate," and, given suitable data comprising information on CD4 count at each decision point k and final negative viral load value, we present methods for estimation of the parameter α. See Section 6.4.5 for details, which are not repeated here. Denoting the resulting estimator by $\widehat{\alpha}$, an estimator for $\mathcal{V}(d_{\eta^*})$ is then given by $\widehat{\mathcal{V}}_{MSM}(d_{\eta^*}) = \mu(\eta^*; \widehat{\alpha})$. More generally, for any fixed η,

$$\widehat{\mathcal{V}}_{MSM}(d_\eta) = \mu(\eta; \widehat{\alpha}) \tag{7.181}$$

is an estimator for the value $\mathcal{V}(d_\eta)$. As discussed in Section 6.4.5, if the structural model is a correct specification of the true relationship between value $\mathcal{V}(d_\eta)$ and η within a range of η values of interest, intuitively, (7.181) is a consistent estimator for the true value for any fixed η.

By analogy to value search estimation in Section 7.4.3, an optimal regime d_η^{opt} in $\mathcal{D}_\eta$ is such that its rules satisfy (7.91), which here becomes

$$d_\eta^{opt} = \{d_1(h_1; \eta^{opt}), \ldots, d_K(h_K; \eta^{opt})\},$$
$$\eta^{opt} = \arg\max_\eta \mathcal{V}(d_\eta).$$

Then an obvious strategy for estimation of an optimal regime d_η^{opt} in $\mathcal{D}_\eta$

is to maximize (7.181) in η to obtain $\widehat{\eta}^{opt}$ and estimate the rules in d_η^{opt} by

$$\widehat{d_\eta^{opt}} = \{d_1(h_1, \widehat{\eta}^{opt}), \ldots, d_K(h_K, \widehat{\eta}^{opt})\},$$

so that in this example the estimator for an optimal rule of the form (7.180) at Decision k is given by

$$d_k(h_k; \widehat{\eta}^{opt}) = \mathrm{I}(\mathsf{CD4}_k \leq \widehat{\eta}^{opt}), \quad k = 1, \ldots, K.$$

Because η is a scalar, maximization of (7.181) in η is entirely computationally feasible. Indeed, in the example of a quadratic marginal structural model in (6.126); namely,

$$\mu(\eta; \alpha) = \alpha_1 + \alpha_2\eta + \alpha_3\eta^2, \quad \alpha = (\alpha_1, \alpha_2, \alpha_3)^T,$$

the maximum is found directly by straightforward differentiation.

In general, the foregoing approach to estimation of an optimal regime in a restricted class based on marginal structural models is appealing in settings where the regimes in the class of interest have rules characterized by a low-dimensional parameter η. Clearly, the quality of the resulting estimator for an optimal regime in the class is predicated on how well the marginal structural model represents the relationship between $\mathcal{V}(d_\eta)$ and η. We have sketched the basic premise of this approach here. See Orellana et al. (2010a,b) for more extensive discussion. Related references include Hernán et al. (2006), Bembom and van der Laan (2007), van der Laan and Petersen (2007b,a), Robins et al. (2008), and Moodie (2009).

7.4.8 Additional Approaches

As noted in Section 4.5, there is a burgeoning literature on estimation of optimal treatment regimes in both the single and multiple decision cases. Here and in Chapters 3, 4, and 5 we do not attempt to present a comprehensive survey of this vast and expanding catalog of approaches. Rather, we have discussed in some detail a few fundamental methods and the ideas that underlie them with the goal of providing the reader with a solid foundation for tackling the broader literature and latest advances. We highlight here some additional approaches for estimation of optimal multiple decision regimes not covered in this chapter and refer the reader to the cited articles for details; this is by no means an exhaustive account.

As discussed in Section 4.5 in the single decision case and in Section 7.4.1, Q-learning is ordinarily implemented using parametric models for the Q-functions. However, the true relationships these models are meant to represent can be complex; and, as the demonstration for $K = 2$ in Section 5.7.1 emphasizes, conventional parametric linear modeling leads to almost certain misspecification at all but the final, Kth decision point. Concern over the consequences of model misspecification has inspired proposals for adoption of flexible, nonparametric representations of the Q-functions. For example, Moodie et al. (2014) study Q-learning using generalized additive models to represent the Q-functions, so accommodating both continuous and discrete outcomes.

Other authors focus on frameworks that embed some robustness to model misspecification. Henderson et al. (2010) propose an approach they call regret-regression based on direct parametric modeling of the regret or advantage functions that is closely related to both Q- and A-learning (g-estimation). Wallace and Moodie (2015) introduce an approach to estimation of an optimal regime that shares features of Q- and A-learning and enjoys a double robustness property. Using a form of A-learning (g-estimation) as an example, Wallace et al. (2015) argue that the double robustness of methods such as A-learning and value search estimation based on an augmented inverse probability weighted estimator can be exploited to assess whether or not the required models have been misspecified.

A common theme of many approaches is the incorporation of machine learning techniques in various ways to provide flexible representations of relevant quantities and circumvent the potentially deleterious effects of model misspecification. Methods for estimation of an optimal multiple decision regime and its value based on targeted maximum likelihood estimation (e.g., van der Laan and Rubin, 2006; van der Laan, 2010; Schuler and Rose, 2017), in which machine learning algorithms have been integrated into a semiparametric causal model framework, have been proposed; see Chaffee and van der Laan (2012), van der Laan and Luedtke (2015) Luedtke and van der Laan (2016b), and Part VII of van der Laan and Rose (2018).

Laber et al. (2014a) propose an alternative strategy for estimation of an optimal treatment regime in the case $K = 2$, referred to as interactive Q-learning (IQ-learning), owing to the feature that standard, interactive model building techniques can be used at both decision points. In this approach, the nonstandard regression problem of modeling pseudo outcomes is replaced by an ordinary mean-variance function modeling problem; this is discussed further in Sections 10.3 and 10.4.

As is evident throughout this book and in the cited literature, approaches to estimation of optimal treatment regimes are overwhelmingly frequentist. There is work placing this problem in a parametric Bayesian framework; e.g., see Saarela et al. (2015) and the references cited therein. Xu et al. (2016) propose a nonparametric Bayesian approach to estimation of the value of a fixed regime; see also Zajonc (2012).

The standard criterion for optimality of a treatment regime is maximization of the value; that is, for an unrestricted or restricted class of regimes $\mathcal{D}$, maximization of $\mathcal{V}(d) = E\{Y^*(d)\}$ over all $d \in \mathcal{D}$. This criterion forms the basis for fundamental methods for estimating an optimal regime, and, accordingly, we focus in this book mainly on approaches predicated on this definition. In some contexts, an alternative criterion may be more meaningful. For example, when the distribution of the potential outcome of interest is significantly skewed or when interest focuses on benefiting individuals with the poorest potential outcomes, a more appropriate criterion may be maximization of the median or other quantile. Wang et al. (2018) propose estimation of an optimal regime defined by such criteria via maximizing appropriate simple inverse probability weighted estimators in the cases $K = 1$ and 2. Linn et al. (2017) propose an approach analogous to IQ-learning when $K = 2$, where the optimality criterion involves maximization of the cumulative distribution function of the outcome at a fixed outcome value or of a prespecified quantile.

As noted in Section 4.5, the standard classification problem involves two classes or labels, so that the methods discussed in Section 7.4.5, which are based on an explicit analogy to binary classification, are limited to at most two treatment options feasible for all individuals at each decision point. When there are possibly more than two treatments at some or all decision points that are feasible for all individuals, Tao and Wang (2017) propose a backward iterative strategy that can be viewed as a generalization and variant of that in Section 7.4.5 based on an augmented inverse probability weighted estimator. At each decision point, objective functions akin to (7.156) and (7.161) are adopted, which are predictors for the contrast functions, referred to as adaptive contrasts by the authors, comparing treatment options based on an estimated ordering of their associated values for each individual; for example, the options yielding the largest and smallest estimated value. This formulation allows standard approaches for minimizing a weighted classification error in the case of binary treatment to be used to optimize the objective function.

See Chapter 11 for additional discussion and references.

7.4.9   Implementation and Practical Performance

The approaches to estimation of an optimal multiple decision treatment regime presented in Sections 7.4.1–7.4.8 provide the analyst with a spectrum of options for use in substantive applications. We conclude our review of methods with a brief discussion of considerations for implementation in practice.

Implementation

Clearly, implementation of any of the methods presented in this chapter is challenging, even if specialized software is available (and particularly so without such software). A key task is positing and fitting of the required models, and we have already discussed specific issues associated with this for Q-learning, A-learning, and value search estimation. Considerations for the latter carry over to the backward iterative estimation strategies in Section 7.4.4 and to methods based on the classification perspective. Although dedicated software implementing these methods may be available, the user is still faced with many issues. One is the need to specify and critique unconventional models; for example, for the conditional expectations of the value functions given past history in Q-learning and for analogous quantities in value search estimation based on an augmented inverse probability weighted estimator. With methods deduced from a classification perspective, the user must select the classifier inducing the restricted class of regimes to be considered, and implementation can involve selection of tuning parameters to which results can be sensitive. Similarly, when highly flexible representations are employed, as for the decision functions at each decision point in BOWL and for $Q_k^{d_\eta}(h_k, a_k)$, $k = 1, \ldots, K$, in the method based on decision lists, not only is modeling of nonstandard quantities involved, but appropriate penalties to avoid overfitting must be chosen. When there are different feasible sets of treatment options for different individuals based on their past histories, as demonstrated in Sections 7.4.1–7.4.3, yet another complication is introduced.

From a purely operational point of view, Q-learning is attractive to users because off the shelf regression software can be used to fit the models for the Q-functions. As in Section 3.5.4 in the single decision case, each step of the backward A-learning algorithm involves solution of a stacked set of M-estimating equations and in principle can also often be solved using regression software. Propensity models can be posited and fitted using standard methods for binary or polytomous regression. Likewise, for the user implementing the methods from scratch, value search estimation via the backward iterative strategy with two feasible options at each decision point can be cast as a weighted classification problem and implemented using existing software for a particular choice of classifier, such as for classification and regression trees (CART). Of course, in general, maximization of the nonsmooth, nonconvex objective functions that arise in value search estimation, both global maximization of a value estimator in η indexing the restricted class of regimes $\mathcal{D}_\eta$ of interest or of a series of value estimators in one of the backward strategies, is a significant challenge because of both the nature of these objective functions and the potentially high dimension of η.

Practical Performance

As for methods in the single decision case, there is no consensus on a universally preferred approach for practical use, and evidence favoring any one method over others is inconclusive.

Analogous to that in the single decision case in Section 3.5.4, a standard measure of performance of an estimator for an optimal multiple decision regime is the extent to which its value approaches the value of a true optimal regime. In particular, if $\widehat{d}^{opt}$ is an estimated optimal multiple decision regime and were followed by the entire patient population, the average outcome achieved, $\mathcal{V}(\widehat{d}^{opt})$, can be compared to the value of a true optimal regime d^{opt}, $\mathcal{V}(d^{opt})$. As emphasized in Section 3.5.4, $\mathcal{V}(\widehat{d}^{opt})$ is different from $\widehat{\mathcal{V}}(d^{opt})$, the latter being an estimator for $\mathcal{V}(d^{opt})$. The considerations discussed for evaluation of $\mathcal{V}(\widehat{d}^{opt})$ in Section 3.5.4 carry over to this setting. In simulation studies, for which the generative data distribution is known, $\mathcal{V}(\widehat{d}^{opt})$ can be approximated numerically for each simulated data set as described in that section. Likewise, $\mathcal{V}(d^{opt})$ is often not available in a closed form and must be calculated via simulation. Simulation studies involving competing methods for estimation of optimal multiple decision regimes in the literature typically are based on calculation and inspection of these measures.

In fact, it is not difficult to appreciate by considering the underlying potential outcomes framework that development of generative data scenarios under which to evaluate competing methods is considerably more complicated than in the single decision case. Ordinarily, it is difficult to derive directly an optimal regime and its value for a given generative data model. When a particular restricted class of regimes is studied, the forms of the rules at each decision point are known, in which case one can deduce optimal rules numerically; see Hager et al. (2018) for an example.

Reports of simulation studies comparing subsets of the methods reviewed in this chapter and others are scattered across the literature. Most studies embed SUTVA, the SRA, and the positivity assumption; and involve $K = 2$ or at most 3 decision points, relatively simple generative models, and various forms of model misspecification. Very few simulations involve situations in which not all treatment options in $\mathcal{A}_k$ are feasible for all individuals. Because the multiple decision problem is more complex than that of a single decision, it can be difficult to deduce the features of a simulation scenario implicated in the relative performance of methods, so that it is not possible to glean general insights.

Accordingly, we do not present a detailed account of simulation experiments reported in the literature. Instead, we highlight a few recurring themes in empirical work by Zhang et al. (2013), Schulte et al. (2014),

Zhao et al. (2015a), Zhang et al. (2018), Tao and Wang (2017), and others comparing subsets of the methods presented in Sections 7.4.1–7.4.6. Overall, Q- and A-learning based on parametric modeling perform similarly over a range of conditions; comparisons between them under different types of model misspecification are qualitatively similar to those reported for $K = 1$ by Schulte et al. (2014), reviewed in Section 3.5.4. Comparisons of these methods to various value search approaches are more striking: in many studies, estimated regimes based on forms of augmented inverse probability weighted estimators can achieve performance similar to Q- and A-learning when the latter are based on correctly specified models for contrast functions but can vastly outperform Q- and A-learning when these models are misspecified. Not unexpectedly, methods based on simple inverse probability weighted value estimators, can suffer serious degradation of performance under misspecification of propensity models and exhibit substantially greater variability relative to methods based on augmented inverse probability weighted estimators or Q- and A-learning based on correctly specified models. Methods based on augmented estimators can perform well under model misspecification owing to the double robustness property. Under complex, highly nonlinear and high-dimensional generative data scenarios, methods that incorporate very flexible representations, such as BOWL, can outperform methods using lower-dimensional, parametric modeling. Simulations reported by Zhang et al. (2018) suggest that restricting attention to regimes with rules in the form of decision lists implemented using flexible models as discussed in Section 7.4.6 can yield competitive performance even under complex generative models and for K as large as 10.

Obviously, relative performance of methods is strongly tied to the true distribution of the data and a complex combination of other factors, so is likely highly problem specific. As advocated in Section 3.5.4, we recommend implementing more than one approach suitable to the practical context under modeling assumptions and choices that induce the same form of decision rules characterizing the class of regimes of interest. The extent of qualitative agreement of results in concert with domain science expertise can guide insights and inform further analyses.

7.5   Application

Implementations of several of the estimators for an optimal multiple decision regime introduced in this chapter are demonstrated on the book's companion website given in the Preface. All codes used to generate simulated data and to implement each method are available on the website.

Chapter 8

Regimes Based on Time-to-Event Outcomes

8.1 Introduction

In much of cancer and other chronic disease research, the outcome of primary interest is a time to an event; for example, overall survival time (time to death or failure) or disease-free or progression-free survival time. Clinical trials or observational studies in this context are of limited duration, so that for some participants the time-to-event outcome is not observed by the end of the study and thus is censored. This type of censoring, which arises because the event of interest may not have occurred by the time of study termination, is referred to as administrative censoring. Censoring of the outcome also results because an individual drops out of the study and is lost to follow up before the event is ascertained.

As discussed briefly in Section 5.2, when the outcome of interest is a time to an event, challenges arise that necessitate a specialized statistical framework for the study of dynamic treatment regimes. Moreover, because the available data from a randomized or observational study are almost certain to involve censoring of the outcome, methodology for estimation of the value of a fixed regime and for estimation of an optimal regime from such data must take censoring into appropriate account. In this chapter, we develop the required statistical framework and present methods for estimating the value of a fixed dynamic treatment regime and for estimation of an optimal regime and its value when the outcome of interest is a possibly censored time to an event in both the single decision and multiple decision cases.

For the single decision problem, where all individuals receive treatment at the sole decision point and the time-to-event outcome is to be ascertained subsequently, the main challenge is to develop techniques based on outcome regression modeling or inverse probability weighted estimators for the value as in Chapters 3 and 4 that incorporate the possibility of censoring of the outcome in the available data. A survey of such methods for the single decision case is presented in Section 8.2.

In the multiple decision setting, the available data also are almost certain to involve censoring of the outcome. Development of methods is further complicated by the fact that the outcome can occur at any time following the first decision point, so that, for some individuals, the outcome may occur before all K decision points have been reached. For example, in the acute leukemia setting of Section 1.2.1, with $K = 2$, if the outcome of interest is overall or progression-free survival time, after receiving an induction chemotherapeutic option at Decision 1, a patient could experience the outcome prior to reaching Decision 2. Such a patient would be observed only to have received treatment at the first of the two possible decision points, while others not experiencing the outcome before Decision 2 would be observed to have received treatment at both decision points. Moreover, the times at which the latter patients are ascertained to have achieved response or not might be different for different patients. Accordingly, both the number of decision points and the times at which decision points are observed to be reached should be regarded as random. In Section 8.3, we introduce an appropriate statistical framework in terms of potential outcomes that incorporates these features and is the foundation for development of methods for estimation of the value of a fixed regime and of an optimal regime from corresponding observed data subject to possible censoring. This framework is rather involved, so that this section is a bit more technical.

We assume that the reader has some familiarity with the fundamentals of survival analysis. Readers seeking an introduction to key considerations for regimes based on time-to-event outcomes and approaches for taking account of censoring of the outcome in observed data should review the account for the single decision case in Section 8.2 and the material on the multiple decision case in Sections 8.3.1 and 8.3.2 and the discussion of the g-computation algorithm in Section 8.3.3. Readers wishing more in-depth coverage should also read the remainder of Section 8.3. Technical arguments are collected in Section 8.5.

8.2 Single Decision Treatment Regimes

The developments in this section draw heavily on those in Chapters 2 and 3, so the reader may wish to review this material before proceeding.

8.2.1 Statistical Framework

Potential Outcomes

As in previous chapters, let X_1 be the vector of baseline information for a randomly chosen individual in the population, so that the individual has history $H_1 = X_1$ at the time of the decision. For simplicity, we consider the case of two treatment options, $\mathcal{A}_1 = \{0, 1\}$, paralleling the formulation in Chapter 3, but the developments can be generalized to the case where $\mathcal{A}_1$ contains a finite number of values as in Section 3.5.5.

Analogous to the definition of potential outcomes in Chapter 2, let $T^*(a_1)$ be the potential time-to-event for such a randomly chosen individual if he were to receive treatment $a_1 \in \mathcal{A}_1$, so that

$$W^* = \{T^*(0), T^*(1)\}$$

is the set of all potential outcomes. Interest focuses on treatment regimes $d = \{d_1(h_1)\}$ in $\mathcal{D}$, the class of all possible treatment regimes d. For any $d \in \mathcal{D}$, analogous to (3.3), define the potential outcome

Need to be expanded

$$T^*(d) = T^*(1)\mathrm{I}\{d_1(H_1) = 1\} + T^*(0)\mathrm{I}\{d_1(H_1) = 0\}. \qquad (8.1)$$

As in previous chapters, $T^*(d)$ is interpreted as the time-to-event that a randomly chosen individual in the population would achieve if he were to receive treatment according to regime d.

Certain functions of the time-to-event outcome are often of interest. Define the primary (potential) outcome of interest as

$$f\{T^*(d)\},$$

where $f(\cdot)$ is a known, monotone nondecreasing function. This encompasses many common situations. If $f(t) = t$, then the outcome itself is the focus. If $f(t) = \mathrm{I}(t \geq r)$ for some fixed time r, then $f\{T^*(d)\}$ is the indicator of whether or not an individual would survive to time r if he were to receive treatment according to regime d. Likewise, if $f(t) = \min(t, L)$ for some fixed time L, then $f\{T^*(d)\}$ is the truncated time-to-event through time L under regime d, often referred to as the restricted lifetime. Restricted lifetime may be considered when survival to some prespecified time is of clinical interest, for example, survival to $L = 1$ year when the effect of treatment is expected to manifest within the first year following administration. Often, investigators are limited to considering restricted lifetime because participants in a study are followed only for a finite amount of time, as discussed further below, in which case L should be chosen to be smaller than the maximum follow-up time.

For given $f(\cdot)$, of interest are then

$$\mathcal{V}(d) = E[f\{T^*(d)\}], \qquad (8.2)$$

the value of any fixed regime $d \in \mathcal{D}$, and identifying an optimal regime $d^{opt} \in \mathcal{D}$ satisfying $\mathcal{V}(d^{opt}) \geq \mathcal{V}(d)$ for all $d \in \mathcal{D}$. Note that if $f(t) = \mathrm{I}(t \geq r)$, then $E[f\{T^*(d)\}] = P\{T^*(d) \geq r\}$, the survival probability at time r; and, if $f(t) = \min(t, L)$, $E[f(T^*(d)\}]$ is the mean restricted lifetime, respectively, for the population if all individuals were to receive treatment according to d. Thus, depending on the choice of

$f(\cdot)$, the value of a regime d corresponds to a quantity typically of interest in the time-to-event setting.

Data

Observed data suitable for these tasks would arise from a point exposure study in which each subject received one of the treatment options in $\mathcal{A}_1$ at baseline. For any subject, let A_1 be the treatment actually received, taking values $a_1 \in \mathcal{A}_1$. Ideally, there would be no censoring, and thus the time-to-event outcome T under the treatment received would be observed for each subject, in which case the observed data would be (H_1, A_1, T), and the methods in Chapters 3 and 4 could be adapted straightforwardly.

As noted in Section 8.1, in practice, the outcome is typically censored for some subjects. In this case, U, the time to the event or censoring, whichever comes first, is observed, along with an indicator Δ taking on the value 1 if U is the event time and 0 if U is the time of censoring. Because T may be censored and thus not observed, it is conventional in the survival analysis literature to view T as a potential survival time, to define C to be the potential time to censoring, and to represent $U = \min(T, C)$ and $\Delta = I(T \leq C)$. The observable data are thus (H_1, A_1, U, Δ), and the data from a study involving n participants can be summarized as

$$(H_{1i}, A_{1i}, U_i, \Delta_i), \quad i = 1, \ldots, n. \tag{8.3}$$

The major objectives are to estimate $\mathcal{V}(d) = E[f\{T^*(d)\}]$ in (8.2) for any fixed regime $d \in \mathcal{D}$ and to estimate an optimal regime $d^{opt} \in \mathcal{D}$ and its value $\mathcal{V}(d^{opt})$ based on the observed data in (8.3).

Identifiability Assumptions

As in Chapters 3–4, estimation of $\mathcal{V}(d)$ and of an optimal regime in $\mathcal{D}$ requires that the distribution of $f\{T^*(d)\}$, and more generally that of $[H_1, f\{T^*(d)\}]$, which depends on that of (H_1, W^*), be identifiable from the distribution of (H_1, A_1, U, Δ). As in those chapters, this is possible under appropriate versions of SUTVA and the no unmeasured confounders and positivity assumptions as in Chapters 2–4.

Here, SUTVA is written, analogous to (3.6), as

$$T_i = T_i^*(1)A_{1i} + T_i^*(0)(1 - A_{1i}), \quad i = 1, \ldots, n, \tag{8.4}$$

so that the survival time, whether observed or not, is equal to the survival time that would be achieved under the treatment actually received.

The no unmeasured confounders assumption, analogous to (3.7), becomes

$$\{T^*(1), T^*(0)\} \perp\!\!\!\perp A_1 | H_1; \quad \text{equivalently,} \quad W^* \perp\!\!\!\perp A_1 | H_1. \tag{8.5}$$

We also make the assumption of noninformative censoring, stated as

$$\{T^*(1), T^*(0)\} \perp\!\!\!\perp C | H_1, A_1; \quad \text{equivalently,} \quad W^* \perp\!\!\!\perp C | H_1, A_1. \tag{8.6}$$

Under SUTVA in (8.4), (8.6) implies that

$$T \perp\!\!\!\perp C | H_1, A_1. \tag{8.7}$$

The noninformative censoring assumption in (8.6) and (8.7) is standard and underlies many popular conventional survival analysis methods.

The positivity assumption here is more involved than (3.8) owing to the possibility of censoring of the outcome. First, we require that

$$P(A_1 = a_1 | H_1 = h_1) > 0, \quad a_1 = 0, 1, \tag{8.8}$$

for all $h_1 \in \mathcal{H}_1$ such that $P(H_1 = h_1) > 0$ as in (3.8). There also should be a positive probability that the event time is not censored; namely,

$$P(C \geq T \mid T = u, H_1 = h_1, A_1 = a_1)$$
$$= P(C \geq u \mid T = u, H_1 = h_1, A_1 = a_1) > 0 \tag{8.9}$$

for all $u \geq 0$, h_1, and a_1 such that

$$P(T = u, H_1 = h_1, A_1 = a_1) > 0. \tag{8.10}$$

Under the assumption of noninformative censoring in (8.6) and (8.7), (8.9) can be simplified to

$$P(C \geq u \mid H_1 = h_1, A_1 = a_1) > 0 \tag{8.11}$$

for all u, h_1, and a_1 satisfying (8.10).

As noted above, it is often the case that the data arise from a study of finite length. Thus, data on event or censoring time are available only through the maximum follow-up time. Clearly, it is not possible to estimate $E[f\{T^*(d)\}]$ for $f(t) = t$ from these data unless the support of T is contained in the interval from 0 to the maximum follow-up time or by making a strong, unverifiable distributional assumption on $T^*(d)$. In this situation, investigators instead consider restricted lifetime, $f(t) = \min(t, L)$, where L is some time less than the maximum follow-up time. Likewise, if interest focuses on $f(t) = I(t \geq r)$, estimation of $E[f\{T^*(d)\}]$ is possible only if r is less than or equal to the maximum follow-up time.

Accordingly, estimation of the value of a fixed regime and of an optimal regime using the methods introduced later in this section must be possible under these conditions. For general $f(t)$, it is necessary to restrict attention to a truncated version of $f(t)$ such that $f(t)$ is redefined to satisfy $f(t) = f(L)$ for $t \geq L$, which of course is already the case for restricted lifetime. Under these conditions, the positivity assumption in (8.9) is modified to

$$P\{C \geq \min(u, L) \mid T = u, H_1 = h_1, A_1 = a_1)\} > 0$$

and similarly for (8.11). In the sequel, we note explicitly considerations for estimation when interest focuses on a general truncated version of $f(t)$ as defined above, which include those for restricted lifetime $f(t) = \min(t, L)$ as a special case.

Remark. In conventional survival analyses in practice, interest usually focuses on estimation of a hazard ratio or of survival distributions under competing treatments, often via the assumption of a proportional hazards model. These inferential tasks are straightforward from data involving a restricted time L, and no special considerations are required. However, when the objective is estimation of the expectation of a function of survival time, as in the present context, inference is limited to functions that involve truncation at L, as above.

In the next three sections, under SUTVA, the no unmeasured confounders, noninformative censoring, and positivity assumptions in (8.4)–(8.11), we describe several approaches to estimation of $\mathcal{V}(d)$ for fixed $d \in \mathcal{D}$ and of an optimal regime in $\mathcal{D}$ and its value. We take these assumptions to hold without comment throughout.

8.2.2 Outcome Regression Estimators

It follows from arguments identical to those in Section 3.3.1 that, for any regime $d \in \mathcal{D}$,

$$\mathcal{V}(d) = E[Q_1(H_1, 1)I\{d_1(H_1) = 1\} + Q_1(H_1, 0)I\{d_1(H_1) = 0\}],$$

as in (3.14), where now

$$Q_1(h_1, a_1) = E\{f(T)|H_1 = h_1, A_1 = a_1\}. \tag{8.12}$$

Moreover, analogous to (3.40), an optimal regime d^{opt} thus can be expressed in terms of the observed data as

$$d^{opt}(h_1) = I\{Q_1(h_1, 1) > Q_1(h_1, 0)\}.$$

This suggests that we consider estimation of $\mathcal{V}(d)$ and d^{opt} by positing a model $Q_1(h_1, a_1; \beta_1)$ for $Q_1(h_1, a_1)$ in terms of a parameter β_1, fitting the model to the observed data (8.3), and substituting the fitted model in the above expressions.

Many approaches to modeling the distribution of a time-to-event outcome have been proposed in the survival analysis literature. Thus, an appealing strategy for specifying a model for $Q_1(h_1, a_1)$ is to exploit the fact that such a model can be deduced from a model for the distribution of T or $f(T)$ given H_1 and A_1. Among the most popular is the proportional hazards regression model. Letting $\lambda_{T1}(u|H_1, A_1)$ denote the hazard function of an event at time u given H_1 and A_1, namely,

$$\lambda_{T1}(u|h_1, a_1) = \lim_{du \to 0} du^{-1} P(u \leq T < u + du \mid T \geq u, H_1 = h_1, A_1 = a_1),$$

the proportional hazards model has the form

$$\lambda_{T1}(u|h_1, a_1; \beta_1) = \lambda_{T10}(u) \exp\{g_{T1}(h_1, a_1; \xi_1)\}, \qquad (8.13)$$

where $\lambda_{T10}(u)$ is an arbitrary baseline hazard function, and $g_{T1}(h_1, a_1; \xi_1)$ is a function of h_1 and a_1 in terms of a finite-dimensional parameter ξ_1. For example, we might take

$$g_{T1}(h_1, a_1; \xi_1) = \xi_{11}^T \tilde{h}_1 + \xi_{12} a_1 + \xi_{13}^T \tilde{h}_1 a_1,$$

where $\tilde{h}_1$ is a vector of known functions of elements of h_1; and $\xi_1 = (\xi_{11}^T, \xi_{12}, \xi_{13}^T)^T$, in which case $\beta_1 = \{\lambda_{T01}(\cdot), \xi_1^T\}^T$. The proportional hazards model (8.13) is a semiparametric model n that it involves both a finite-dimensional parametric component ξ_1 and an infinite-dimensional component $\lambda_{T01}(\cdot)$; here, we use β_1 to denote the collection of both components. Under the assumption of noninformative censoring (8.6), ξ_1 can be estimated from the observed data (8.3) by $\widehat{\xi}_1$ maximizing the usual partial likelihood (Cox, 1972, 1975), and $\lambda_{T01}(\cdot)$ can be estimated using the Breslow estimator $\widehat{\lambda}_{T01}(\cdot)$ (Breslow, 1972). Both of these estimators are available in standard survival analysis software.

Remark. As noted above, if interest focuses on a version of $f(t)$ truncated at L, such as restricted lifetime, $f(t) = \min(t, L)$, fitting of the model for $\lambda_{T1}(u|H_1, A_1)$ can be carried out directly based on the observed data.

A model for the survival function $\mathcal{S}_{T1}(u|h_1, a_1) = P(T \geq u|H_1 = h_1, A_1 = a_1)$ follows from (8.13) by the relationship between the hazard and survival functions given by

$$\mathcal{S}_{T1}(u|h_1, a_1) = \exp\left\{-\int_0^u \lambda_{T1}(w|h_1, a_1)\, dw\right\}. \qquad (8.14)$$

Denote the resulting model by $\mathcal{S}_{T1}(u|h_1, a_1; \beta_1)$. The implied model for $Q_1(h_1, a_1)$ is then given by

$$Q_1(h_1, a_1; \beta_1) = \int_0^\infty f(u)\{-d\mathcal{S}_{T1}(u|h_1, a_1; \beta_1)\}, \qquad (8.15)$$

in which case we can estimate $Q_1(h_1, a_1)$ in (8.12) by $Q_1(h_1, a_1; \widehat{\beta}_1)$, where $\widehat{\beta}_1 = \{\widehat{\lambda}_{01}(\cdot), \widehat{\xi}_1^T\}^T$.

Remark. In the case of restricted time L, with $f(t)$ redefined to be truncated at L, following from the discussion below (8.11), it is straightforward that the integral in (8.15) becomes

$$\int_0^L f(u)\{-d\mathcal{S}_{T1}(u|h_1, a_1; \beta_1)\} + f(L)\mathcal{S}_{T1}(L|h_1, a_1; \beta_1).$$

If interest focuses on restricted lifetime, so that $f(t) = \min(t, L)$, then, (8.15) becomes

$$\int_0^L u\{-d\mathcal{S}_{T1}(u|h_1, a_1; \beta_1)\} + L\mathcal{S}_{T1}(L|h_1, a_1; \beta_1).$$

By analogy to the methods developed in Sections 3.3.1 and 3.5.1, the outcome regression estimator for $\mathcal{V}(d)$ is given by

$$\widehat{\mathcal{V}}_Q(d) = n^{-1} \sum_{i=1}^n \Big[Q_1(H_{1i}, 1; \widehat{\beta}_1) I\{d_1(H_{1i}) = 1\} \qquad (8.16)$$
$$+ Q_1(H_{1i}, 0; \widehat{\beta}_1) I\{d_1(H_{1i}) = 0\}\Big],$$

and the estimator for the rule $d_1^{opt}(h_1)$ characterizing d^{opt} is

$$\widehat{d}_{Q,1}^{opt}(h_1) = I\{Q_1(h_1, 1; \widehat{\beta}_1) > Q_1(h_1, 0; \widehat{\beta}_1)\}. \qquad (8.17)$$

An estimator for $\mathcal{V}(d^{opt})$ is then

$$\widehat{\mathcal{V}}_Q(d^{opt}) = n^{-1} \sum_{i=1}^n \Big[Q_1(H_{1i}, 1; \widehat{\beta}_1) I\{\widehat{d}_{Q,1}^{opt}(H_{1i}) = 1\} \qquad (8.18)$$
$$+ Q_1(H_{1i}, 0; \widehat{\beta}_1) I\{\widehat{d}_{Q,1}^{opt}(H_{1i}) = 0\}\Big].$$

In the foregoing development, we focus on use of the semiparametric proportional hazards model to deduce a model for $Q_1(h_1, a_1)$. However, any other approach to modeling the conditional distribution of T given given H_1 and A_1 could be substituted. For example, one could posit a semiparametric transformation model or a fully parametric regression model based on an exponential, Weibull, or other suitable distribution.

8.2.3 Inverse Probability of Censoring Regression Estimators

In the previous section, a model for $Q_1(h_1, a_1) = E\{f(T)|H_1 = h_1, A_1 = a_1\}$ was obtained indirectly from a model for the hazard function of T. One of the advantages when considering models for the hazard function, such as the proportional hazards regression model, is that, under the assumption of noninformative censoring (8.7), consistent estimators for the parameters characterizing the hazard function model can be obtained without making any assumptions on the distribution of censoring. That is, the conditional distribution of C given H_1 and A_1 need not be specified. Thus, in the previous section, the resulting estimators for the value of a regime $d \in \mathcal{D}$ and an optimal regime can be obtained without having to specify this distribution.

An alternative class of estimators for $\mathcal{V}(d)$ and d^{opt} is based instead on positing a model for $Q_1(h_1, a_1)$ directly in terms of a finite number of parameters β_1 rather than indirectly, fitting the model using an appropriate technique, and substituting the fitted model in appropriate expressions for $\mathcal{V}(d)$ and d^{opt}, in the same spirit as the approach in Sections 3.3 and 3.5.1 when there is no censoring of the outcome. For example, if interest focuses on restricted lifetime, so that $f(t) = \min(t, L)$, we can specify a model directly for the mean restricted lifetime $Q_1(h_1, a_1) = E\{\min(T, L)|H_1 = h_1, A_1 = a_1\}$, e.g.,

$$Q_1(h_1, a_1; \beta_1) = \exp(\beta_{11} + \beta_{12}^T h_1 + \beta_{13} a_1 + \beta_{14}^T h_1 a_1),$$

where $\beta_1 = (\beta_{11}, \beta_{12}^T, \beta_{13}, \beta_{14}^T)^T$ is a finite-dimensional parameter.

With no censoring, so that T_i is observed for all $i = 1, \ldots, n$, β_1 can be estimated straightforwardly using standard regression methods such as least squares; i.e., the estimator $\widehat{\beta}_1$ is the solution to the estimating equation

$$\sum_{i=1}^{n} \frac{\partial Q_1(H_{1i}, A_{1i}; \beta_1)}{\partial \beta_1} \{f(T_i) - Q_1(H_{1i}, A_{1i}; \beta_1)\} = 0. \qquad (8.19)$$

If the model $Q_1(h_1, a_1; \beta_1)$ is correctly specified, then by the argument in Section 2.5, the estimator $\widehat{\beta}_1$ solving (8.19) is a consistent and asymptotically normal estimator for the true value of β_1.

With censoring, T_i is not observed for all $i = 1, \ldots, n$, so estimation of β_1 by solving (8.19) is not possible. When $\Delta_i = 1$, T_i is observed; otherwise, it is censored and thus "missing." From this point of view, appealing to the same rationale underlying the inverse probability weighted estimators in Chapters 2 and 3 to the estimating equation (8.19) leads to the class of estimators for β_1 known as *inverse probability of censoring estimators.* Specifically, let

$$\mathcal{K}(u|h_1, a_1) = P(C \geq u \mid H_1 = h_1, A_1 = a_1)$$
$$= \exp\left\{ -\int_0^u \lambda_C(w|h_1, a_1)\, dw \right\} \tag{8.20}$$

be the "survival function" for censoring conditional on H_1 and A_1, where, with

$$\lambda_C(u|h_1, a_1) = \lim_{du \to 0} du^{-1} P(u \leq C < u + du \mid C \geq u, H_1 = h_1, A_1 = a_1) \tag{8.21}$$

denoting the hazard function of being censored at time u given H_1 and A_1, the second equality in (8.20) follows analogous to (8.14).

We now show that the solution $\widehat{\beta}_1$ to the estimating equation

$$\sum_{i=1}^n \frac{\Delta_i}{\mathcal{K}(U_i|H_{1i}, A_{1i})} \frac{\partial Q_1(H_{1i}, A_{1i}; \beta_1)}{\partial \beta_1} \{f(U_i) - Q_1(H_{1i}, A_{1i}; \beta_1)\} = 0. \tag{8.22}$$

is a consistent, asymptotically normal estimator for the true value of β_1 when the model $Q_1(h_1, a_1; \beta_1)$ is correctly specified. Note that, by the noninformative censoring and positivity assumptions (8.7) and (8.11), $\mathcal{K}(u|h_1, a_1) > 0$ for all u, h_1, and a_1 occurring with positive probability, so that the estimating equation (8.22) is well defined.

Remark. When interest focuses on a truncated version of $f(t)$, with truncation at L, in (8.22), define $T^L = \min(T, L)$. Then, it follows from the discussion after (8.11) that the positivity assumption (8.11) can be expressed equivalently as

$$P(C \geq u \mid T^L = u, H_1 = h_1, A_1 = a_1) > 0$$

for all u, h_1, and a_1 such that

$$P(T^L = u, H_1 = h_1, A_1 = a_1) > 0,$$

where it follows that $u \leq L$. Define $U^L = \min(T^L, C) = \min(T, L, C)$ and $\Delta^L = I(T^L \leq C) = I\{\min(T, L) \leq C\}$, so that $\Delta^L = 1$ if $U \geq L$, because $T^L = \min(T, L) = L$ regardless of whether the event time is ultimately censored or not. Then replace U_i and Δ_i in (8.22) by U_i^L and Δ_i^L, respectively.

To demonstrate that the solution to (8.22) is consistent and asymptotically normal, appealing to the developments for M-estimation in Section 2.5, we show that the estimating function in (8.22) is unbiased. That is, we demonstrate that

$$E_\beta \left[\frac{\Delta}{\mathcal{K}(U|H_1, A_1)} \frac{\partial Q_1(H_1, A_1; \beta_1)}{\partial \beta_1} \{f(U) - Q_1(H_1, A_1; \beta_1)\} \right] = 0,$$

(8.23)

where, as in (2.31), this notation implies that the expectation is taken with respect to the distribution of (H_1, A_1, U, Δ) evaluated at β_1. To show this, note that, when $\Delta = I(C \geq T) = 1, U = T$, and the left-hand side of (8.23) can be written as

$$E_\beta \left[\frac{I(C \geq T)}{\mathcal{K}(T|H_1, A_1)} \frac{\partial Q_1(H_1, A_1; \beta_1)}{\partial \beta_1} \{f(T) - Q_1(H_1, A_1; \beta_1)\} \right]. \quad (8.24)$$

By conditioning first on T, H_1, and A_1, it follows that (8.24) can be expressed equivalently as

$$E_\beta \left[\frac{E\{I(C \geq T)|T, H_1, A_1\}}{\mathcal{K}(T|H_1, A_1)} \frac{\partial Q_1(H_1, A_1; \beta_1)}{\partial \beta_1} \{f(T) - Q_1(H_1, A_1; \beta_1)\} \right].$$

(8.25)

Under the assumption (8.7) that censoring is noninformative, it follows from (8.9)–(8.11) and the definition of $\mathcal{K}(u|h_1, a_1)$ in (8.20) that

$$E\{I(C \geq T) \mid T, H_1, A_1\} = \mathcal{K}(T|H_1, A_1)$$

almost surely, in which case (8.25) becomes

$$E_\beta \left[\frac{\partial Q_1(H_1, A_1; \beta_1)}{\partial \beta_1} \{f(T) - Q_1(H_1, A_1; \beta_1)\} \right]. \quad (8.26)$$

The expectation in (8.26) involves the "complete case" estimating function in (8.19), which is unbiased as noted above, so that (8.26) is equal to zero when the model $Q_1(h_1, a_1; \beta_1)$ is correctly specified, demonstrating the result. In the case of $f(t)$ truncated at restricted time L, an entirely analogous development holds with T, U, and Δ replaced by T^L, U^L, and Δ^L.

The estimating equation (8.22) depends on the conditional distribution of censoring through $\mathcal{K}(u|h_1, a_1) = P(C \geq u \mid H_1 = h_1, A_1 = a_1)$ in (8.20), which is not known. An obvious approach is to posit a model for $\mathcal{K}(u|h_1, a_1)$, fit the model, and substitute the fitted model in (8.22). By reversing the roles of the time-to-event outcome T and the censoring variable C and considering the "data"

$$(H_{1i}, A_{1i}, U_i, 1 - \Delta_i), \quad i = 1, \ldots, n, \quad (8.27)$$

this can be accomplished using standard survival analysis regression methods as in the previous section.

We demonstrate using a proportional hazards regression model for this purpose. With $\lambda_C(u|h_1, a_1)$ the hazard function for censoring as in (8.20), a proportional hazards model for $\lambda_C(u|h_1, a_1)$ has the form

$$\lambda_C(u|h_1, a_1; \beta_C) = \lambda_{0C}(u) \exp\{g_C(h_1, a_1; \xi_C)\}, \qquad (8.28)$$

where $\lambda_{0C}(u)$ is an unspecified baseline hazard function, $g_C(h_1, a_1; \xi_C)$ is a function of h_1 and a_1 in terms of a finite-dimensional parameter ξ_C, and $\beta_C = \{\lambda_{0C}(\cdot), \xi_C^T\}^T$. A model $\mathcal{K}(u|h_1, a_1; \beta_C)$ then follows from (8.20) and (8.28). As in the previous section, ξ_C and $\lambda_{0C}(u)$ can be estimated by standard methods for this model using the data (8.27). Letting the resulting estimator be $\widehat{\beta}_C$, and denoting the corresponding estimator for $\mathcal{K}(u|h_1, a_1)$ by

$$\widehat{\mathcal{K}}(u|h_1, a_1) = \mathcal{K}(u|h_1, a_1; \widehat{\beta}_C),$$

the estimator $\widehat{\beta}_1$ for β_1 is then the solution to

$$\sum_{i=1}^n \frac{\Delta_i}{\widehat{\mathcal{K}}(U_i|H_{1i}, A_{1i})} \frac{\partial Q_1(H_{1i}, A_{1i}; \beta_1)}{\partial \beta_1} \{f(U_i) - Q_1(H_{1i}, A_{1i}; \beta_1)\} = 0,$$
$$(8.29)$$

where, for $f(t)$ truncated at L, U_i and Δ_i are replaced by U_i^L and Δ_i^L, respectively. The estimating equation (8.29) can be solved using standard software implementing nonlinear weighted least squares regression.

Once the estimator $\widehat{\beta}_1$ solving (8.29) is in hand, $\mathcal{V}(d)$, d^{opt}, and $\mathcal{V}(d^{opt})$ can be estimated by substituting the fitted model $Q_1(h_1, a_1; \widehat{\beta}_1)$ as in (8.16), (8.17), and (8.18) to yield estimators $\widehat{\mathcal{V}}_{IPCW}(d)$, $\widehat{d}_{IPCW}^{opt}$, and $\widehat{\mathcal{V}}_{IPCW}(d^{opt})$. This strategy is that proposed by Goldberg and Kosorok (2012) in the special case of a single decision. These authors adapted the method of Q-learning discussed in Sections 5.7.1 and 7.4.1 for estimating an optimal treatment regime in the case of multiple decisions to the setting of a censored time-to-event outcome using similar ideas of inverse probability of censoring estimators. A generalization of this approach is outlined later in this chapter when we discuss the multiple decision setting.

8.2.4 Inverse Probability Weighted and Value Search Estimators

Analogous to the developments in Sections 3.3.2 and 3.3.3, an alternative approach to estimation of the value $\mathcal{V}(d) = E[f\{T^*(d)\}]$ for given $f(\cdot)$ and fixed $d \in \mathcal{D}$ is to derive a suitable inverse probability weighted estimator $\widehat{\mathcal{V}}(d)$. Moreover, as discussed in Section 3.5.3, a drawback of methods for estimation of an optimal regime based on outcome regression modeling, as in the previous two sections, is that the estimated optimal regime can be far from a true optimal regime $d^{opt} \in \mathcal{D}$ if the model $Q_1(h_1, a_1; \beta_1)$ is misspecified. This concern carries over naturally to this setting.

This suggests, as argued in Section 3.5.3, restricting attention to a class of regimes $\mathcal{D}_\eta \subset \mathcal{D}$ indexed by parameter $\eta = \eta_1$, with elements $d_\eta = \{d_1(h_1; \eta_1)\}$, and focusing on estimation of

$$d_\eta^{opt} = \{d_1(h_1; \eta_1^{opt})\}, \quad \eta_1^{opt} = \arg\max_{\eta_1} \mathcal{V}(d_\eta).$$

The class $\mathcal{D}_\eta$ can be chosen based on considerations of feasibility, interpretability, or cost; e.g., with $h_1 = x_1 = (x_{11}, x_{12})^T$, where x_{11} and x_{12} are scalar baseline covariates, $\mathcal{D}_\eta$ might be taken to comprise regimes d_η characterized by rules involving rectangular regions involving x_{11} and x_{12}, for example,

$$d(h_1; \eta_1) = I(x_{11} < \eta_{11}, x_{12} < \eta_{12}), \quad \eta_1 = (\eta_{11}, \eta_{12})^T,$$

as in (3.83). Further examples are given in Section 3.5.3. As in that section, η_1^{opt} can then be estimated by $\hat{\eta}^{opt}$ maximizing an inverse probability weighted estimator $\widehat{\mathcal{V}}(d_\eta)$ in η, leading to the value search estimator

$$\widehat{d}_\eta^{opt} = \{d_1(h_1; \hat{\eta}^{opt})\}, \quad \hat{\eta}^{opt} = \arg\max_{\eta_1} \widehat{\mathcal{V}}(d_\eta)$$

for an optimal restricted regime d_η^{opt}.

We now discuss derivation of inverse probability weighted estimators for $\mathcal{V}(d)$ for a specified function $f(\cdot)$ of the event time and fixed regime $d = \{d_1(h_1)\}$ based on censored, time-to-event data (8.3). We focus mainly on augmented estimators, which, as noted in Chapters 2 and 3, are expected to be more efficient and stable in practice than their simple inverse weighted counterparts.

If there were no censoring, the augmented inverse probability weighted estimator (3.30) adapted to this setting would be

$$\widehat{\mathcal{V}}_{AIPW}(d) = n^{-1} \sum_{i=1}^n \left\{ \frac{\mathcal{C}_{d,i} f(T_i)}{\pi_{d,1}(H_{1i}; \hat{\gamma}_1)} - \frac{\mathcal{C}_{d,i} - \pi_{d,1}(H_{1i}; \hat{\gamma}_1)}{\pi_{d,1}(H_{1i}; \hat{\gamma}_1)} \mathcal{Q}_{d,1}(H_{1i}; \hat{\beta}_1) \right\};$$

(8.30)

the corresponding simple inverse probability weighted estimator involves the leading term on the right-hand side of (8.30) only. In (8.30), as in Section 3.3.3,

$$\mathcal{C}_d = I\{A_1 = d_1(H_1)\} = A_1 I\{d_1(H_1) = 1\} + (1 - A_1) I\{d_1(H_1) = 0\}$$

is the indicator of consistency of treatment received with that dictated by d; $\pi_{d,1}(H_1, \widehat{\gamma})$ is the estimator for $\pi_{d,1}(H_1) = P(\mathcal{C}_d = 1|H_1)$ as in (3.21) given by

$$\pi_{d,1}(H_1; \widehat{\gamma}_1) = \pi_1(H_1; \widehat{\gamma}_1)\mathrm{I}\{d_1(H_1) = 1\}+\{1-\pi_1(H_1; \widehat{\gamma}_1)\}\mathrm{I}\{d_1(H_1) = 0\},$$

depending on a posited model $\pi_1(h_1; \gamma_1)$ for the propensity score $\pi_1(h_1) = P(A_1 = 1|H_1 = h_1)$ with γ_1 estimated by $\widehat{\gamma}_1$; and $\mathcal{Q}_{d,1}(H_1; \beta_1)$ is a model for $E[f\{T^*(d)\}|H_1]$, which, from (3.29), can be estimated by

$$\mathcal{Q}_{d,1}(H_1; \widehat{\beta}_1) = Q_1(H_1, 1; \widehat{\beta}_1)\mathrm{I}\{d_1(H_1) = 1\}+Q_1(H_1, 0; \widehat{\beta}_1)\mathrm{I}\{d_1(H_1) = 0\}$$
$$= Q_1\{H_1, d_1(H_1); \widehat{\beta}_1\},$$

where $Q_1(h_1, a_1; \beta_1)$ is a posited model for $E\{f(T)|H_1 = h_1, A_1 = a_1\}$ with β_1 estimated by $\widehat{\beta}_1$.

As in Sections 3.3.2 and 3.3.3, the estimator (8.30) is well defined if $\pi_{d,1}(H_1) > 0$ for all $d \in \mathcal{D}$; this holds under the positivity assumption (8.8), which implies $0 < \pi_1(H_1) < 1$ almost surely.

When the observed data involve censoring of the event time for some individuals, an estimator for $\mathcal{V}(d)$ in the same spirit as (8.30) can be derived as follows. Now, because of censoring, T is observed only when $\Delta = 1$, and, analogous to the discussion in Section 3.3.2, $T^*(d)$ is thus observed for individuals with $\mathcal{C}_d = 1$ and $\Delta = 1$. This suggests that the leading inverse probability weighted term in the augmented estimator (8.30) should be modified to depend only on such individuals.

To this end, we first derive an expression for the probability that $T^*(d)$ is observed, conditional on $T^*(1)$, $T^*(0)$, and H_1. We have

$$P\{\mathcal{C}_d = 1, \Delta = 1|T^*(1), T^*(0), H_1\} \qquad (8.31)$$
$$= P\{\mathcal{C}_d = 1|T^*(1), T^*(0), H_1\}P\{\Delta = 1|\mathcal{C}_d = 1, T^*(1), T^*(0), H_1\}.$$

Because $\mathcal{C}_d$ depends on H_1 and A_1, by the no unmeasured confounders assumption (8.5), the first term on the right-hand side of (8.31) satisfies

$$P\{\mathcal{C}_d = 1|T^*(1), T^*(0), H_1\} = P\{\mathcal{C}_d = 1|H_1\} = \pi_{d,1}(H_1).$$

The second term on the right-hand side of (8.31) can be written, using the definition of Δ, as

$$P\{C \geq T|\mathcal{C}_d = 1, T^*(1), T^*(0), H_1\}$$
$$= P\{C \geq T^*(d)|\mathcal{C}_d = 1, T^*(1), T^*(0), H_1\} \qquad (8.32)$$
$$= P\{C \geq T^*(1)|\mathcal{C}_d = 1, T^*(1), T^*(0), H_1\}\mathrm{I}\{d_1(H_1) = 1\}$$
$$\quad + P\{C \geq T^*(0)|\mathcal{C}_d = 1, T^*(1), T^*(0), H_1\}\mathrm{I}\{d_1(H_1) = 0\} \qquad (8.33)$$
$$= P\{C \geq T^*(1)|T^*(1), T^*(0), A_1 = 1, d_1(H_1) = 1, H_1\}\mathrm{I}\{d_1(H_1) = 1\}$$

$$+ P\{C \geq T^*(0)|T^*(1), T^*(0), A_1 = 0, d_1(H_1) = 0, H_1\}I\{d_1(H_1) = 0\} \tag{8.34}$$

$$= P\{C \geq T^*(d)|T^*(1), T^*(0), A_1 = 1, H_1\}I\{d_1(H_1) = 1\}$$
$$+ P\{C \geq T^*(d)|T^*(1), T^*(0), A_1 = 0, H_1\}I\{d_1(H_1) = 0\}$$
$$= \mathcal{K}\{T^*(d)|H_1, 1\}I\{d_1(H_1) = 1\} + \mathcal{K}\{T^*(d)|H_1, 0\}I\{d_1(H_1) = 0\}, \tag{8.35}$$

where (8.32) follows because of SUTVA (8.4) and the definition of $T^*(d)$ in (8.1), the equality (8.33) holds almost surely because $I\{d_1(H_1) = 1\} + I\{d_1(H_1) = 0\} = 1$, (8.34) follows because of the definition of $\mathcal{C}_d$, and (8.35) follows by the assumption of noninformative censoring (8.6). Thus, combining the above and defining

$$\mathcal{K}_d(u|H_1) = \mathcal{K}(u|H_1, 1)I\{d_1(H_1) = 1\} + \mathcal{K}(u|H_1, 0)I\{d_1(H_1) = 0\}$$
$$= \mathcal{K}\{u|H_1, d_1(H_1)\},$$

it follows from (8.31) that

$$P\{\mathcal{C}_d = 1, \Delta = 1|T^*(1), T^*(0), H_1\} = \pi_{d,1}(H_1)\mathcal{K}_d\{T^*(d)|H_1\}. \tag{8.36}$$

Using these developments and an argument similar to that in Section 3.3.2, it is straightforward that

$$E\left\{\frac{\mathcal{C}_d\Delta f(U)}{\pi_{d,1}(H_1)\mathcal{K}_d(U|H_1)}\right\} = E\left\{\frac{\mathcal{C}_d\Delta f(T)}{\pi_{d,1}(H_1)\mathcal{K}_d(T|H_1)}\right\}$$
$$= E\left[\frac{\mathcal{C}_d\Delta f\{T^*(d)\}}{\pi_{d,1}(H_1)\mathcal{K}_d\{T^*(d)|H_1\}}\right]$$
$$= E\left(E\left[\frac{\mathcal{C}_d\Delta f\{T^*(d)\}}{\pi_{d,1}(H_1)\mathcal{K}_d\{T^*(d)|H_1\}}\middle| T^*(1), T^*(0), H_1\right]\right)$$
$$= E\left[\frac{f\{T^*(d)\}E\{\mathcal{C}_d\Delta|T^*(1), T^*(0), H_1\}}{\pi_{d,1}(H_1)\mathcal{K}_d\{T^*(d)|H_1\}}\right]$$
$$= E[f\{T^*(d)\}] = \mathcal{V}(d), \tag{8.37}$$

where (8.37) follows from the fact that

$$E\{\mathcal{C}_d\Delta|T^*(1), T^*(0), H_1\} = P\{\mathcal{C}_d = 1, \Delta = 1|T^*(1), T^*(0), H_1\}$$

and (8.36). This suggests immediately the inverse probability weighted estimator

$$\widehat{\mathcal{V}}_{IPW}(d) = n^{-1}\sum_{i=1}^{n} \frac{\mathcal{C}_{d,i}\Delta_i f(U_i)}{\pi_{d,1}(H_{1i}; \widehat{\gamma}_1)\widehat{\mathcal{K}}_d(U_i|H_{1i})}, \tag{8.38}$$

where

$$\widehat{\mathcal{K}}_d(u|H_1) = \widehat{\mathcal{K}}(u|H_1,1)\mathrm{I}\{d_1(H_1) = 1\} + \widehat{\mathcal{K}}(u|H_1,0)\mathrm{I}\{d_1(H_1) = 0\}$$
$$= \widehat{\mathcal{K}}\{u|H_1, d_1(H_1)\}, \tag{8.39}$$

$\widehat{\mathcal{K}}(u|h_1, a_1)$ is a fitted model for $\mathcal{K}(u|h_1, a_1)$ as in the previous section, and $\pi_{d,1}(H_{1i}; \widehat{\gamma}_1)$ is based on a fitted model for the propensity score as above.

Remark. If $f(t)$ is truncated at restricted time L, with $T^L = \min(T, L)$, as in the previous section, replace U_i and Δ_i in (8.38) by $U_i^L = \min(T_i^L, C_i)$ and $\Delta_i^L = \mathrm{I}(T_i^L \leq C_i)$, respectively.

Analogous to (3.24), the estimator (8.38) is a consistent estimator for the true value $\mathcal{V}(d)$ of the fixed regime $d \in \mathcal{D}$ as long as both the propensity score model $\pi_1(h_1; \gamma)$ and that for the censoring distribution, $\mathcal{K}(u|h_1, a_1; \beta_C)$, are correctly specified.

As in Section 3.3.3, it is possible to improve on the simple inverse weighted estimator $\widehat{\mathcal{V}}_{IPW}(d)$. A model $Q_1(h_1, a_1; \beta_1)$ for $E\{f(T)|H_1 = h_1, A_1 = a_1\}$ can be specified indirectly or directly, and β_1 can be estimated based on the (censored) data (8.3) using one of the methods in the previous two sections. Then with $Q_{d,1}(H_1; \widehat{\beta}_1) = Q_1\{H_1, d_1(H_1); \widehat{\beta}_1\}$ defined as above, an augmented inverse probability weighted estimator for $\mathcal{V}(d)$ is given by

$$\widehat{\mathcal{V}}_{AIPW}(d) = n^{-1} \sum_{i=1}^{n} \left\{ \frac{\mathcal{C}_{d,i} \Delta_i f(U_i)}{\pi_{d,1}(H_{1i}; \widehat{\gamma}_1) \widehat{\mathcal{K}}_d(U_i|H_{1i})} \right. \tag{8.40}$$
$$\left. - \frac{\mathcal{C}_{d,i} - \pi_{d,1}(H_{1i}; \widehat{\gamma}_1)}{\pi_{d,1}(H_{1i}; \widehat{\gamma}_1)} Q_{d,1}(H_{1i}; \widehat{\beta}_1) \right\}.$$

As above, if interest focuses on $f(t)$ truncated at L, then U_i and Δ_i in the first term in the summand of (8.40) should be replaced by U_i^L and Δ_i^L, respectively.

The second term in the summand of (8.40) is the "augmentation term," which, as remarked in Section 3.3.3, can be viewed as an attempt to recapture some of the "missing information" from the individuals in the data set for whom $\mathcal{C}_d = 0$, who actually received treatment that was not consistent with that dictated by the regime d and are thus not included in the leading inverse probability weighted term. With censored data, there is yet another type of missing information. Specifically, there are also individuals for whom $\mathcal{C}_d = 1$, who did receive treatment consistent with d, but whose time-to-event outcome is "missing" due to censoring and thus have $\Delta = 0$; these individuals also are not included in the leading term.

Bai et al. (2017) show that it is possible to modify the estimator $\widehat{V}_{AIPW}(d)$ in (8.40) to recover information from these individuals through an additional augmentation term and, by doing so, obtain the locally efficient estimator for $\mathcal{V}(d)$ (Tsiatis, 2006, Chapter 11). Define the martingale increment for censoring at time u, conditional on H_1 and A_1, as

$$dM_{C,1}(u|h_1, a_1) = dN_C(u) - \lambda_C(u|h_1, a_1)Y(u)\, du, \qquad (8.41)$$

with $N_C(u) = \mathrm{I}(U \leq u, \Delta = 0)$, $Y(u) = \mathrm{I}(U \geq u)$, and the hazard function for censoring $\lambda_C(u|h_1, a_1)$ as in (8.21). Then this augmentation term has the form

$$\frac{\mathcal{C}_d}{\pi_{d,1}(H_1)} \int_0^\infty \frac{dM_{C,d}(u|H_1)}{\mathcal{K}_d(u|H_1)} m_{d,1}(u|H_1), \qquad (8.42)$$

where

$$\begin{aligned}
dM_{C,d}(u|h_1) &= dM_{C,1}(u|h_1, 1)\mathrm{I}\{d_1(h_1) = 1\} \\
&\quad + dM_{C,1}(u|h_1, 0)\mathrm{I}\{d_1(h_1) = 0\} \\
&= dM_{C,1}\{u|h_1, d_1(h_1)\},
\end{aligned}$$

$$\begin{aligned}
m_{d,1}(u|h_1) &= m_1(u|h_1, 1)\mathrm{I}\{d_1(h_1) = 1\} + m_1(u|h_1, 0)\mathrm{I}\{d_1(h_1) = 0\} \\
&= m_1\{u|h_1, d_1(h_1)\},
\end{aligned}$$

$$m_1(u|h_1, a_1) = E\{f(T)|T \geq u, H_1 = h_1, A_1 = a_1\}. \qquad (8.43)$$

To implement the locally efficient estimator that incorporates this term, it is necessary to estimate the quantities in (8.42). As discussed in the previous section, a model for the censoring hazard function $\lambda_C(u|h_1, a_1)$, $\lambda_C(u|h_1, a_1; \beta_C)$, e.g., a proportional hazards regression model as in (8.28), can be posited and fitted based on the data (8.3), from which a model for the censoring survival function $\mathcal{K}(u|h_1, a_1)$, $\mathcal{K}(u|h_1, a_1; \beta_C)$, is implied. An estimator for $dM_{C,d}(u|h_1)$ then can be constructed as

$$d\widehat{M}_{C,d}(u|h_1) = d\widehat{M}_{C,1}\{u|h_1, d_1(h_1)\},$$

where

$$d\widehat{M}_{C,1}(u|h_1, a_1) = dN_C(u) - \lambda_C(u|h_1, a_1; \widehat{\beta}_C)Y(u)\, du;$$

and an estimator for $\mathcal{K}_d(u|H_1)$ is as in (8.39). Given a model $\mathcal{S}_{T1}(u|h_1, a_1; \beta_1)$ for $\mathcal{S}_{T1}(u|h_1, a_1)$, posited and fitted as discussed in Section 8.2.2, an estimator for $m_1(u|h_1, a_1)$ can be deduced as

$$m_1(u|h_1, a_1; \widehat{\beta}_1) = \int_u^\infty f(w)\frac{\{-d\mathcal{S}_{T1}(w|h_1, a_1; \widehat{\beta}_1)\}}{\mathcal{S}_{T1}(u|h_1, a_1; \widehat{\beta}_1)},$$

and thus an estimator for $m_{d,1}(u|h_1)$ is

$$m_{d,1}(u|h_1; \widehat{\beta}_1) = m_1\{u|h_1, d_1(h_1); \widehat{\beta}_1\}.$$

The resulting locally efficient estimator for $\mathcal{V}(d)$ is given by

$$
\begin{aligned}
\widehat{\mathcal{V}}_{LE}(d) = n^{-1} \sum_{i=1}^{n} & \left\{ \frac{\mathcal{C}_{d,i}\Delta_i f(U_i)}{\pi_{d,1}(H_{1i}; \widehat{\gamma}_1)\widehat{\mathcal{K}}_d(U_i|H_{1i})} \right. \\
& - \frac{\mathcal{C}_{d,i} - \pi_{d,1}(H_{1i}; \widehat{\gamma}_1)}{\pi_{d,1}(H_{1i}; \widehat{\gamma}_1)} \mathcal{Q}_{d,1}(H_{1i}; \widehat{\beta}_1) \\
& \left. + \frac{\mathcal{C}_{d,i}}{\pi_{d,1}(H_{1i}, \widehat{\gamma}_1)} \int_0^\infty \frac{d\widehat{M}_{C,d}(u|H_{1i})}{\widehat{\mathcal{K}}_d(u|H_{1i})} m_{d,1}(u|H_{1i}; \widehat{\beta}_1) \right\}.
\end{aligned}
\tag{8.44}
$$

Remarks. (i) When $f(t)$ is truncated at L, the foregoing developments are modified as follows. The additional augmentation term (8.42) becomes

$$\frac{\mathcal{C}_d}{\pi_{d,1}(H_1)} \int_0^L \frac{dM_{C,d}(u|H_1)}{\mathcal{K}_d(u|H_1)} m_{d,1}(u|H_1),$$

$m_1(u|H_1, a_1)$ in (8.43) is defined for $u \leq L$, and the estimator $m_1(u|h_1, a_1; \widehat{\beta}_1)$ is thus given by

$$m_1(u|h_1, a_1; \widehat{\beta}_1) = \int_u^L f(w) \frac{\{-d\mathcal{S}_{T1}(w|h_1, a_1; \widehat{\beta}_1)\}}{\mathcal{S}_{T1}(u|h_1, a_1; \widehat{\beta}_1)} + f(L) \frac{\mathcal{S}_{T1}(L|h_1, a_1)}{\mathcal{S}_{T1}(u|h_1, a_1)}.$$
$$\tag{8.45}$$

The locally efficient estimator is then given by (8.44) with U_i and Δ_i replaced by U_i^L and Δ_i^L in the first term in the summand and the third term in the summand modified by substitution of $m_1(u|h_1, a_1; \widehat{\beta}_1)$ in (8.45) and changing the upper limit of integration from ∞ to L.

(ii) Analogous to the remarks in Sections 3.3.2 and 3.3.3, it is possible to express the locally efficient estimator (8.44) in an alternative form; these same substitutions apply also to the simple and augmented inverse probability weighted estimators (8.38) and (8.40). Because when $\mathcal{C}_d = 1$, $A_1 = d_1(H_1)$, the estimator is unchanged if $\pi_{d,1}(H_{1i}; \widehat{\gamma}_1)$ is replaced by

$$
\begin{aligned}
\pi_1(H_{1i}; \widehat{\gamma}_1)\mathrm{I}(A_{1i} = 1) &+ \{1 - \pi_1(H_{1i}; \widehat{\gamma}_1)\}\mathrm{I}(A_{1i} = 0) \\
&= \pi_1(H_{1i}; \widehat{\gamma}_1)A_{1i} + \{1 - \pi_1(H_{1i}; \widehat{\gamma}_1)\}(1 - A_{1i})
\end{aligned}
$$

as in (3.26). Similarly, $\widehat{\mathcal{K}}_d(u|H_{1i})$ can be replaced by $\widehat{\mathcal{K}}(u|H_{1i}, A_{1i})$, $d\widehat{M}_{C,d}(u|H_{1i})$ can be replaced by $d\widehat{M}_{C,1}(u|H_{1i}, A_{1i})$, and $m_{d,1}(u|H_{1i}; \widehat{\beta}_1)$

can be replaced by $m_1(u|H_{1i}, A_{1i}; \widehat{\beta}_1)$ in the leading and third terms of (8.44) without altering the value of the estimator. These modifications simplify evaluation of the estimator somewhat in practice. In the extension of these developments to the multiple decision case in Section 8.3.3, we adopt a similar formulation to simplify the presentation.

As demonstrated in Bai et al. (2017), the locally efficient estimator (8.44) enjoys a double robustness property in that $\widehat{\mathcal{V}}_{LE}(d)$ is a consistent estimator for $\mathcal{V}(d)$ if either both the propensity score model $\pi_1(h_1; \gamma_1)$ and the censoring distribution model $\mathcal{K}(u|H_1, A_1; \beta_C)$ are correctly specified or if the model for the failure time distribution $\mathcal{S}_{T1}(u|h_1, a_1; \beta_1)$ is correctly specified.

Any of the estimators $\widehat{\mathcal{V}}_{IPW}(d)$, $\widehat{\mathcal{V}}_{AIPW}(d)$, or $\widehat{\mathcal{V}}_{LE}(d)$ in (8.38), (8.40), or (8.44) can be used to estimate the value $\mathcal{V}(d)$ of a fixed regime d. The locally efficient estimator $\widehat{\mathcal{V}}_{LE}(d)$ has the advantage of being the most precise asymptotically if the models for the propensity score, censoring distribution, and failure time distribution are correctly specified, and furthermore is doubly robust, so offering some protection against mismodeling. However, implementation of this estimator is somewhat more complex.

Remark. If the data (8.3) are from a randomized study, the propensity score $\pi_1(H_1) = P(A_1 = 1|H_1)$ is known and likely not dependent on H_1. If in addition there was no loss to follow-up in the study, so that all censoring of time-to-event outcomes is due to study termination (i.e., all censoring is administrative), then it is reasonable to assume that $\mathcal{K}(u|H_1, A_1) = P(C \geq u|H_1, A_1) = \mathcal{K}(u)$ and thus does not depend on H_1, A_1. Then the model (8.28) is correctly specified as long as $g_C(H_1, A_1; \xi_C) = 0$ for some ξ_C. Alternatively, one can estimate $\mathcal{K}(u)$ by the Kaplan-Meier estimator for the "survival function" for censoring based on the "data" $\{U_i, 1 - \Delta_i\}$, $i = 1, \ldots, n$. Under these conditions, all of these estimators are consistent for the true $\mathcal{V}(d)$, including (8.38), and $\widehat{\mathcal{V}}_{AIPW}(d)$ and $\widehat{\mathcal{V}}_{LE}(d)$ are generally more efficient than $\widehat{\mathcal{V}}_{IPW}$, as they attempt to recover information from individuals who did not receive treatment consistent with d or who were censored.

As in Section 3.5.3, estimation of an optimal regime d_η^{opt} within a specified restricted class $\mathcal{D}_\eta$ comprising regimes of the form $d_\eta = \{d_1(h_1; \eta_1)\}$ can be accomplished by maximizing any of $\widehat{\mathcal{V}}_{IPW}(d_\eta)$, $\widehat{\mathcal{V}}_{AIPW}(d_\eta)$, or $\widehat{\mathcal{V}}_{LE}(d_\eta)$ in η_1 to obtain $\widehat{\eta}_{1,IPW}^{opt}$, $\widehat{\eta}_{1,AIPW}^{opt}$, or $\widehat{\eta}_{1,LE}^{opt}$, respectively, and substituting these in $d_1(h_1; \eta_1)$ to obtain the value search estimators for d_η^{opt} given by

$$\widehat{d}_{\eta,IPW}^{opt} = \{d_1(h_1, \widehat{\eta}_{1,IPW}^{opt})\}, \quad \widehat{d}_{\eta,AIPW}^{opt} = \{d_1(h_1, \widehat{\eta}_{1,AIPW}^{opt})\},$$

$$\text{or} \quad \widehat{d}_{\eta,LE}^{opt} = \{d_1(h_1, \widehat{\eta}_{1,LE}^{opt})\}.$$

The value achieved by $d_\eta^{opt} \in \mathcal{D}_\eta$ likewise can be estimated in the obvious way by substitution of $\widehat{d}_{\eta,IPW}^{opt}$, $\widehat{d}_{\eta,AIPW}^{opt}$, or $\widehat{d}_{\eta,LE}^{opt}$ in (8.38), (8.40), or (8.44) to yield corresponding estimators $\widehat{\mathcal{V}}_{IPW}(d_\eta^{opt})$, $\widehat{\mathcal{V}}_{AIPW}(d_\eta^{opt})$, and $\widehat{\mathcal{V}}_{LE}(d_\eta^{opt})$. As discussed in Section 3.5.3, intuitively, the estimators for d_η^{opt} and $\mathcal{V}(d_\eta^{opt})$ based on the locally efficient estimator $\widehat{\mathcal{V}}_{LE}(d)$ are expected to be of higher quality.

8.2.5 Discussion

We conclude with remarks on special considerations involved in assessment of uncertainty, additional approaches, and the perspective on censoring we adopt in the rest of this chapter.

Approximate Distribution for Estimators for the Value of a Fixed Regime

In principle, measures of uncertainty such as standard errors and confidence intervals for the estimators for $\mathcal{V}(d)$ for fixed $d \in \mathcal{D}$, $\widehat{\mathcal{V}}_Q(d)$ given in (8.16); $\widehat{\mathcal{V}}_{IPCW}(d)$ discussed in Section 8.2.3; and $\widehat{\mathcal{V}}_{IPW}(d)$, $\widehat{\mathcal{V}}_{AIPW}(d)$, and $\widehat{\mathcal{V}}_{LE}(d)$ in (8.38), (8.40), and (8.44) can be derived by appealing to the theory of M-estimation as in Section 2.5.

In the case of the regression estimator $\widehat{\mathcal{V}}_Q(d)$, if the model $\mathcal{S}_{T1}(u|h_1, a_1; \beta_1)$ for the survival function $\mathcal{S}_{T1}(u|h_1, a_1)$ for the outcome T, and thus the implied model $Q_1(h_1, a_1; \beta_1)$, is based on a fully parametric specification as discussed at the end of Section 8.2.2, then an approximate large sample distribution for $\widehat{\mathcal{V}}_Q(d)$ can be derived by viewing $\widehat{\mathcal{V}}_Q(d)$ and $\widehat{\beta}_1$ as solving a set of stacked estimating equations and appealing to the general M-estimation theory in Section 2.5. Likewise, if the censoring distribution $\mathcal{K}(u|h_1, a_1)$ is represented by a fully parametric model, an approximate large sample distribution for $\widehat{\mathcal{V}}_{IPCW}(d)$ can be deduced analogously. If the models for all of $\mathcal{S}_{T1}(u|h_1, a_1)$, $\mathcal{K}(u|h_1, a_1)$, and the propensity score $\pi_1(h_1)$ are fully parametric, approximate large sample distributions for the inverse weighted estimators $\widehat{\mathcal{V}}_{IPW}(d)$, $\widehat{\mathcal{V}}_{AIPW}(d)$, and $\widehat{\mathcal{V}}_{LE}(d)$ follow similarly.

If the models for $\mathcal{S}_{T1}(u|h_1, a_1)$ and $\mathcal{K}(u|h_1, a_1)$ are derived from semiparametric proportional hazards models as proposed in (8.13) and (8.28), respectively, or are instead based on semiparametric transformation models, then the models involve infinite-dimensional components, and derivation of approximate large sample distributions for all of these estimators for $\mathcal{V}(d)$ is more involved. One can show that these estimators are regular and asymptotically linear, derive their associated influence functions, and appeal to the theory of semiparametrics to deduce a large sample distribution as outlined in general in Tsiatis (2006, Chapters 7–9). See Chen and Tsiatis (2001), Anstrom and Tsiatis (2001), Bai et al. (2013), and Bai et al. (2017) for related derivations that demonstrate the considerations involved.

Because $\widehat{\mathcal{V}}_Q(d)$, $\widehat{\mathcal{V}}_{IPCW}(d)$, $\widehat{\mathcal{V}}_{IPW}(d)$, $\widehat{\mathcal{V}}_{AIPW}(d)$, and $\widehat{\mathcal{V}}_{LE}(d)$ can be shown to be regular and asymptotically linear, a more feasible alternative for practical use, which we recommend, is to implement a standard nonparametric bootstrap to obtain approximate standard errors.

Nonregularity of Estimators for an Optimal Regime

Analogous to the developments in Sections 3.5.1, 3.5.2, and 3.5.3, the estimators $\widehat{\mathcal{V}}_Q(d^{opt})$ and $\widehat{\mathcal{V}}_{IPCW}(d^{opt})$ for the value of $d^{opt} \in \mathcal{D}$ and $\widehat{\mathcal{V}}_{IPW}(d_\eta^{opt})$, $\widehat{\mathcal{V}}_{AIPW}(d_\eta^{opt})$, and $\widehat{\mathcal{V}}_{LE}(d_\eta^{opt})$ for d_η^{opt} in a specified restricted class of regimes $\mathcal{D}_\eta$ are nonregular. Accordingly, inference on the true value of an optimal regime or restricted optimal regime is problematic. In the case of the inverse probability weighted locally efficient estimator $\widehat{\mathcal{V}}_{LE}(d_\eta^{opt})$ for the value $\mathcal{V}(d_\eta^{opt})$ of an optimal restricted regime, Bai et al. (2017) show that a result similar to that of Zhang et al. (2012b) in the uncensored case discussed at the end of Section 3.5.3 holds. Specifically, these authors argue that, when $\mathcal{V}(d_\eta)$ is a smooth function in η_1 with a unique maximum and when all of the models $\mathcal{S}_{T1}(u|h_1, a_1; \beta_1)$, $\mathcal{K}(u|h_1, a_1; \beta_C)$, and $\pi_1(h_1; \gamma)$ are all correctly specified in constructing $\widehat{\mathcal{V}}_{LE}(d_\eta^{opt})$, standard asymptotic theory can be used to derive an approximate normal sampling distribution for $\widehat{\mathcal{V}}_{LE}(d_\eta^{opt})$ with variance that can be estimated by the sandwich technique. Bai et al. (2017) present simulation evidence suggesting that, under these conditions, appealing to this result leads to reliable standard errors for $\widehat{\mathcal{V}}_{LE}(d_\eta^{opt})$ and associated confidence intervals that achieve nominal coverage. However, as noted at the end of Section 3.5.3, this approximation can fail under certain configurations of the true distribution of the data.

Other Approaches

Other methods are available for estimation of an optimal regime from censored data in the single decision case. We briefly note several approaches; this is not a comprehensive account of additional methods.

Jiang et al. (2017a) focus on estimation of an optimal regime within a restricted class $\mathcal{D}_\eta$, where $f(t) = I(t \geq r)$ for fixed r, so that $E[f\{T^*(d)\}]$

is the r year survival probability. Under the assumptions here, they propose simple and augmented inverse probability weighted Kaplan-Meier estimators for $\mathcal{V}(d_\eta) = P\{T^*(d_\eta) \geq r\}$ for fixed $\eta = \eta_1$ and maximize these estimators in η_1 to obtain estimators for an optimal restricted regime in $\mathcal{D}_\eta$. Because these value estimators are highly nonsmooth in η_1, they propose smoothing them via kernel smoothing and maximizing the smoothed versions in η_1. Geng et al. (2015) propose an approach in the spirit of A-learning as in Section 3.5.2 in the case of independent censoring that incorporates a penalty for overfitting.

Zhao et al. (2015b) focus on $f(t) = \min(t, L)$ for fixed L and propose a modification of outcome weighted learning (OWL, Section 4.3) in which censoring is handled similarly to the approach in Section 8.2.4 by including additional inverse weighting by an estimator of the censoring distribution. They propose both simple and augmented estimators for the value of a fixed regime, the latter of which can be shown to be doubly robust, although they do not consider a locally efficient estimator. As with OWL in the uncensored case, they cast maximization of these estimators as a weighted classification problem, restrict attention to regimes that can be represented in terms of linear combinations of elements of h_1 and a_1, and use support vector machines via the convex surrogate hinge loss function for implementation as in Section 4.3.

Similarly, by manipulations analogous to those in Section 4.2.2, Bai et al. (2017) demonstrate that maximization in η of the locally efficient estimator $\widehat{\mathcal{V}}_{LE}(d_\eta)$ for the value of a fixed restricted regime $d_\eta \in \mathcal{D}_\eta$ can be accomplished by minimization of a weighted classification error. They describe implementation when the class $\mathcal{D}_\eta$ is induced by linear support vector machines using a convex surrogate loss function, which can be accomplished via linear programming. Díaz et al. (2018) propose an efficient approach that is particularly suited to high-dimensional patient information.

Remarks on Censoring

In Section 8.2.1, we adopt the conventional formulation in the survival analysis literature that the observed time to the event of interest or censoring, whichever comes first, can be represented as $U = \min(T, C)$. Here, T is the event time (which would be observed if there were no censoring) and can be written in terms of the potential event times $T^*(0)$ and $T^*(1)$ in W^* under SUTVA in (8.4), C is a potential time to censoring, and $\Delta = I(T \leq C)$. The assumption of noninformative censoring in (8.6) states that C is independent of W^* given H_1, A_1, or, equivalently under SUTVA, that C is independent of T given H_1, A_1 as in (8.7). A slightly weaker noninformative censoring assumption is expressed in terms of the cause-specific hazard as

$$\lambda_C(u|H_1, A_1, W^*)$$
$$= \lim_{du \to 0} du^{-1}P(u \leq U < u + du, \Delta = 0 \,|\, U \geq u, H_1, A_1, W^*)$$
$$= \lim_{du \to 0} du^{-1}P(u \leq U < u + du, \Delta = 0 \,|\, U \geq u, H_1, A_1)$$
$$= \lambda_C(u|H_1, A_1), \tag{8.46}$$

similar in spirit to specifications in Robins and Rotnitzky (1992), Robins (1993), and Hernán et al. (2000). Of course, (8.6) implies (8.46), but the converse need not be true. In the multiple decision case in the next section, we formulate the assumption of noninformative censoring in terms of the cause-specific hazard, analogous to (8.46).

Although in the conventional setup in the last paragraph C is referred to as a "potential" censoring time, we do not introduce potential outcomes $C^*(a_1)$, say, for $a_1 \in \mathcal{A}_1$, analogous to $T^*(a_1)$. We view censoring as an external process, similar in spirit to treatment assignment. That is, censoring is a mechanism that occurs when individuals are observed in practice. For example, if censoring is for administrative reasons, because an individual is a participant in a study of known, finite length, a given individual's censoring time is determined at study entry (baseline) and is equal to the time from baseline to the end of the study. Here, the censoring time is known for all individuals and is unrelated to treatment received, although the event time may precede it for some individuals. When censoring is due to dropout, an individual may be lost to follow up, and thus have censored event time. Here, in line with the noninformative censoring assumption, dropout is viewed as depending only on the observed past history and not on potential outcomes. We continue to take this perspective in the multiple decision case in Section 8.3.

Remarks on Competing Risks

In the survival analysis literature, censoring of the outcome is sometimes attributed to the fact that competing risks prevent observation of the time-to-event outcome of interest. For example, if the event is "death due to cancer," death due to some other cause is a competing risk. There is an extensive literature on approaches to inference on and interpretation of competing risks. In this chapter, we do not consider issues associated with competing risks, and, as above, we view censoring as an external process. As discussed in Section 2 of Tsiatis (2014), we take the point of view that, because of the well-known challenges of evaluating a single risk in isolation, which involves making assumptions that are not verifiable from the observed data, the focus should be on quantities that can be identified from the observed data. From this perspective, the time-to-event outcome of interest in the above example would be taken to be "death from any cause." See Tsiatis (2014) and the references therein for further discussion.

8.3 Multiple Decision Treatment Regimes

We now consider the case of multiple decision points, which of necessity is considerably more complex. The reader may wish to review Chapter 5 as background before proceeding. The developments also make use of material in Chapters 6 and 7; these are noted in the text. In most of what follows, for the sake of continuity for readers interested mainly in the key ideas and considerations for implementation, we defer longer proofs of results to Section 8.5.

8.3.1 Multiple Decision Regimes

Consider the situation where there is a maximum of K decision points that individuals could experience, where K is a prespecified, finite positive integer, and focus on $K \geq 2$. As in Section 5.2, for each $k = 1, \ldots, K$, let $\mathcal{A}_k$ denote the set of treatment options available at Decision k, where a_k is an option in $\mathcal{A}_k$, and write $\overline{\mathcal{A}}_k = \mathcal{A}_1 \times \cdots \times \mathcal{A}_k$, $k = 1, \ldots, K$, and $\overline{\mathcal{A}} = \overline{\mathcal{A}}_K$. Although all individuals present at Decision 1 and are eligible to receive a treatment option in $\mathcal{A}_1$, not all individuals would reach all K decisions. In the context here, this is because the time-to-event outcome of interest can occur at any time following Decision 1, and, once the event time has been achieved, no further treatment decisions are required. Moreover, as noted in Section 8.1, the timing of decision points can be different for different individuals.

We now describe the form of a regime d in the class $\mathcal{D}$ of all possible regimes under these conditions. As in Section 5.2, an individual presents at baseline, so at time $\tau_1 = 0$, with information $x_1 \in \mathcal{X}_1$. Let $h_1 = (\tau_1, x_1)$ denote the individual's history at baseline, where we include $\tau_1 = 0$ for completeness. Let $a_1 \in \mathcal{A}_1$ be the treatment option administered at Decision 1. For $k = 2, \ldots, K$, if an individual does not experience the event between Decisions $k - 1$ and k, let the time Decision k is reached, measured from baseline, be τ_k; let $x_k \in \mathcal{X}_k$ denote additional information that arises between these decision points; and let $a_{k-1} \in \mathcal{A}_{k-1}$ denote the treatment option selected at Decision $k - 1$. Then, for $k = 2, \ldots, K$, the history h_k of accrued information on an individual who reaches Decision k without yet having experienced the event, similar to (5.1), is

$$h_k = (\tau_1, x_1, a_1, \tau_2, x_2, a_2, \ldots, \tau_{k-1}, x_{k-1}, a_{k-1}, \tau_k, x_k) = (\overline{\tau}_k, \overline{x}_k, \overline{a}_{k-1}),$$

where $\overline{\tau}_k = (\tau_1, \ldots, \tau_k)$, $k = 1, \ldots, K$. An individual who achieves the time-to-event outcome between Decisions $k-1$ and k has history h_j for each $j = k, \ldots, K$ given by $h_j = (\tau_1, x_1, a_1, \ldots, \tau_{k-1}, x_{k-1}, a_{k-1}, t) = (\overline{\tau}_{k-1}, \overline{x}_{k-1}, \overline{a}_{k-1}, t)$, where t is the time the event was achieved, measured from baseline. We define potential and observable histories more precisely in Section 8.3.2.

A treatment regime d is then a collection of decision rules, i.e., $d = \{d_1(h_1), \ldots, d_K(h_K)\}$, where each rule $d_k(h_k)$ maps an individual's history to a treatment option in $\mathcal{A}_k$ as long as h_k indicates that the event of interest has not yet occurred. As in Section 6.2.2, the feasible options for a given such history h_k may comprise a subset $\Psi_k(h_k) \subseteq \mathcal{A}_k$ depending on h_k, $k = 1, \ldots, K$. For example, in the acute leukemia setting, at Decision 2, with $\mathcal{A}_2 = \{\mathsf{M}_1, \mathsf{M}_2, \mathsf{S}_1, \mathsf{S}_2\}$, $\Psi_2(h_2)$ comprises the two maintenance options, $\Psi_2(h_2) = \{\mathsf{M}_1, \mathsf{M}_2\} \subset \mathcal{A}_2$ for all h_2 indicating that an individual has not yet achieved the time-to-event outcome and has responded to Decision 1 chemotherapy; and $\Psi_2(h_2) = \{\mathsf{S}_1, \mathsf{S}_2\} \subset \mathcal{A}_2$, the two salvage options, for all h_2 indicating the time to event has not yet been achieved and nonresponse to Decision 1 chemotherapy. As formalized in (6.8) in Section 6.2.2, the rule $d_k(h_k)$ is then a collection of rules, each corresponding to a distinct feasible subset of $\mathcal{A}_k$.

If, for $k = 2, \ldots, K$, h_k indicates that the time-to-event outcome was achieved prior to Decision k, then $d_k(h_k)$ is understood to make no selection of a treatment option from $\mathcal{A}_k$. That is, the set of feasible treatment options $\Psi_k(h_k)$ is the empty set, so that $d_k(h_k)$ can be considered as null if h_k indicates that the event has occurred prior to Decision k. Thus, this construction dictates that, effectively, for an individual who experiences the time-to-event outcome between Decisions $k-1$ and k, there are no decisions to be made at decision points $k, \ldots, K$. The class $\mathcal{D}$ comprises all possible regimes d that satisfy these conditions.

Recursive Representation of a Regime $d \in \mathcal{D}$

At the end of Section 5.2, a recursive representation of the rules in a regime if they are followed by an individual is presented, which depends only on the evolving information on the individual. In the discussion of methods for estimation of the value of a fixed regime and of an optimal regime in upcoming sections, a similar recursive representation of the rules in a regime $d = (d_1, \ldots, d_K)$ if they are followed by an individual is required, which we now present. As defined formally later, let $\varkappa \leq K$ denote the number of decision points ultimately reached by an individual following d; although $\varkappa$ is not known as the individual progresses, at any Decision k, whether or not $\varkappa \geq k$ is known.

If an individual presents at baseline with information $h_1 = (\tau_1, x_1)$ as above, the option selected at Decision 1 is $d_1(h_1) = d_1(\tau_1, x_1)$. If the individual then reaches Decision 2 without experiencing the event, so that $\varkappa \geq 2$, $h_2 = (\tau_1, x_1, a_1, \tau_2, x_2) = (\overline{\tau}_2, \overline{x}_2, a_1)$, as in Section 5.2, the option selected depends on that selected at Decision 1 and is given by

$$d_2\{\overline{\tau}_2, \overline{x}_2, d_1(\tau_1, x_1)\}.$$

If instead the individual does not reach Decision 2, as above, d_2 and all subsequent rules can be considered as null. If $\varkappa \geq 3$, so that the individual reaches Decision 3, $h_3 = (\overline{\tau}_3, \overline{x}_3, \overline{a}_2)$, and the option selected at Decision 3 is then

$$d_3[\overline{\tau}_3, \overline{x}_3, d_1(\tau_1, x_1), d_2\{\overline{\tau}_2, \overline{x}_2, d_1(\tau_1, x_1)\}].$$

If instead the individual reaches Decision 2 but does not reach Decision 3, d_3 and all subsequent rules can be considered as null.

In general, analogous to (5.6), for $k \leq \varkappa$, define recursively

$$\overline{d}_2(\overline{\tau}_2, \overline{x}_2) = [d_1(\tau_1, x_1), d_2\{\overline{\tau}_2, \overline{x}_2, d_1(\tau_1, x_1)\}]$$
$$\overline{d}_3(\overline{\tau}_3, \overline{x}_3) = [d_1(\tau_1, x_1), d_2\{\overline{\tau}_2, \overline{x}_2, d_1(\tau_1, x_1)\}, d_3\{\overline{\tau}_3, \overline{x}_3, \overline{d}_2(\overline{\tau}_2, \overline{x}_2)\}]$$

$$\vdots \tag{8.47}$$

$$\overline{d}_k(\overline{\tau}_k, \overline{x}_k) = [d_1(\tau_1 x_1), d_2\{\overline{\tau}_2, \overline{x}_2, d_1(\tau_1, x_1)\}, \ldots,$$
$$d_k\{\overline{\tau}_k, \overline{x}_k, \overline{d}_{k-1}(\overline{\tau}_{k-1}, \overline{x}_{k-1})\}],$$

so that, if an individual reaches all K decision points, $\varkappa = K$,

$$\overline{d}_K(\overline{\tau}_K, \overline{x}_K) = [d_1(\tau_1, x_1), d_2\{\overline{\tau}_2, \overline{x}_2, d_1(\tau_1, x_1)\}, \ldots,$$
$$d_K\{\overline{\tau}_K, \overline{x}_K, \overline{d}_{K-1}(\overline{\tau}_{K-1}, \overline{x}_{K-1})\}].$$

8.3.2 Statistical Framework

Potential Outcomes

We now present a potential outcomes framework for this setting, where there is a maximum number of decision points K. Because an individual can experience the time-to-event outcome before reaching the final, Kth decision point, and, as noted in Section 8.1, different individuals may reach decision points at different times, a relevant framework must accommodate these features. In particular, both the number of decision points reached and the timing of these should be random variables, as in the following formulation.

Consider a randomly chosen individual in the population who presents with baseline information X_1 at Decision 1 and a given treatment sequence $\overline{a} = (a_1, \ldots, a_K) \in \overline{\mathcal{A}}$. For $k = 2, \ldots, K$, let

$$\varkappa_k^*(\overline{a}_{k-1}) = 1 \quad \text{if the individual would reach Decision } k$$
$$= 0 \quad \text{otherwise}, \tag{8.48}$$

and define $\varkappa_1 = 1$, reflecting that all individuals reach Decision 1. In (8.48), if $\varkappa_k^*(\bar{a}_{k-1}) = 1$, then it must be that $\varkappa_j^*(\bar{a}_{j-1}) = 1$ for $j = 2, \ldots, k - 1$; likewise, if $\varkappa_k^*(\bar{a}_{k-1}) = 0$, then $\varkappa_j^*(\bar{a}_{j-1}) = 0$ for $j = k + 1, \ldots, K$. Let

$$\varkappa^*(\bar{a}) = \max_j \{j : \varkappa_j^*(\bar{a}_{j-1}) = 1\}$$

be the largest decision point k for which $\varkappa_k^*(\bar{a}_{k-1}) = 1$. Thus, if $\varkappa_k^*(\bar{a}_{k-1}) = 1$ and $\varkappa_{k+1}^*(\bar{a}_k) = 0$, it must be that $\varkappa^*(\bar{a}) = k$.

For $k = 2, \ldots, \varkappa^*(\bar{a})$, define $T_k^*(\bar{a}_{k-1})$ to be the time of Decision k, measured from baseline, and $T_1 = 0$, the time of Decision 1; and let $X_k^*(\bar{a}_{k-1})$ be the intervening information arising between Decisions $k-1$ and k following administration of options $\bar{a}_{k-1}$ at Decisions $1, \ldots, k - 1$. From the definition of $\varkappa^*(\bar{a})$, the time-to-event outcome is achieved following Decision $\varkappa^*(\bar{a})$; thus, let $T^*(\bar{a}_{\varkappa^*(\bar{a})})$ be the potential event time. Then the potential information available on an individual under a given treatment sequence $\bar{a}$ is

$$\left[\varkappa_1, \varkappa_2^*(a_1), \varkappa_3^*(\bar{a}_2), \ldots, \varkappa_K^*(\bar{a}_{K-1}), \varkappa^*(\bar{a}) = \max_j \{j : \varkappa_j^*(\bar{a}_{j-1}) = 1\}, \right.$$

$$T_1, X_1, T_2^*(a_1), X_2^*(a_1), T_3^*(\bar{a}_2), X_3^*(\bar{a}_2), \ldots, \qquad (8.49)$$

$$\left. T_{\varkappa^*(\bar{a})}^*(\bar{a}_{\varkappa^*(\bar{a})-1}), X_{\varkappa^*(\bar{a})}^*(\bar{a}_{\varkappa^*(\bar{a})-1}), T^*(\bar{a}_{\varkappa^*(\bar{a})}) \right].$$

As in Section 5.3.1, $\varkappa_1$, T_1, and X_1 are not potential outcomes, strictly speaking, but are included for completeness; and (8.49) embeds the assumption that the potential timing of the decision points, the potential intervening information arising between decision points, and the potential event time depend only on the treatment options previously administered.

As there is a set of potential outcomes of the form (8.49) for every $\bar{a} = (a_1, \ldots, a_K) \in \bar{\mathcal{A}}$, we define the set of all possible potential outcomes, disregarding κ_1, T_1, and X_1, as

$$W^* = \left[\varkappa_2^*(a_1), \varkappa_3^*(\bar{a}_2), \ldots, \varkappa_K^*(\bar{a}_{K-1}), \varkappa^*(\bar{a}) = \max_j \{j : \varkappa_j^*(\bar{a}_{j-1}) = 1\}, \right.$$

$$T_2^*(a_1), X_2^*(a_1), T_3^*(\bar{a}_2), X_3^*(\bar{a}_2), \ldots, T_{\varkappa^*(\bar{a})}^*(\bar{a}_{\varkappa^*(\bar{a})-1}), X_{\varkappa^*(\bar{a})}^*(\bar{a}_{\varkappa^*(\bar{a})-1}),$$

$$\left. T^*(\bar{a}_{\varkappa^*(\bar{a})}), \quad \text{for all } \bar{a} \in \bar{\mathcal{A}} \right]. \qquad (8.50)$$

It proves convenient in the sequel to define in terms of (8.49) for a given treatment sequence $\bar{a}$ the potential time to reaching the kth decision point or achieving the event, whichever comes first, given that the $(k-1)$th decision point would be reached under $\bar{a}$, and an associated indicator. Let

$$S_2^*(a_1) = I\{\varkappa_1 = 1, \varkappa_2^*(a_1) = 0\} T^*(a_1) + I\{\varkappa_2^*(a_1) = 1\} T_2^*(a_1),$$

$$\Upsilon_2^*(a_1) = 1 \quad \text{if } \varkappa_1 = 1, \varkappa_2^*(a_1) = 0,$$
$$= -1 \quad \text{if } \varkappa_2^*(a_1) = 1,$$

where we include $\varkappa_1 = 1$ in these expressions for consistency with what follows, and we have used the fact that $\varkappa^*(\bar{a}) = 1$ if $\varkappa_1 = 1$ and $\varkappa_2^*(a_1) = 0$. Thus, $S_2^*(a_1)$ is the potential event time if the individual would not reach the second decision point and is the time of the second decision point otherwise. Likewise, define

$$S_3^*(\bar{a}_2) = I\{\varkappa_2^*(a_1) = 1, \varkappa_3^*(\bar{a}_2) = 0\}\, T^*(\bar{a}_2) + I\{\varkappa_3^*(\bar{a}_2) = 1\} T_3^*(\bar{a}_2),$$
$$\Upsilon_3^*(\bar{a}_2) = 1 \quad \text{if } \varkappa_2^*(a_1) = 1, \varkappa_3^*(\bar{a}_2) = 0,$$
$$= -1 \quad \text{if } \varkappa_3^*(\bar{a}_2) = 1,$$

where, as above, we have used the fact that $\varkappa^*(\bar{a}) = 2$ if $\varkappa_2^*(a_1) = 1$ and $\varkappa_3^*(\bar{a}_2) = 0$. Here, $S_3^*(\bar{a}_2)$ is the potential event time if the individual would reach the second decision point but then achieve the event before the third decision point and is the time of the third decision point otherwise. In general, for $k = 2, \ldots, K$,

$$\begin{aligned}
S_k^*(\bar{a}_{k-1}) &= I\{\varkappa_{k-1}^*(\bar{a}_{k-2}) = 1, \varkappa_k^*(\bar{a}_{k-1}) = 0\}\, T^*(\bar{a}_{k-1}) \\
&\quad + I\{\varkappa_k^*(\bar{a}_{k-1}) = 1\} T_k^*(\bar{a}_{k-1}), \\
\Upsilon_k^*(\bar{a}_{k-1}) &= 1 \quad \text{if } \varkappa_{k-1}^*(\bar{a}_{k-2}) = 1, \varkappa_k^*(\bar{a}_{k-1}) = 0, \\
&= -1 \quad \text{if } \varkappa_k^*(\bar{a}_{k-1}) = 1,
\end{aligned} \tag{8.51}$$

where $\varkappa_1^*(a_0) = \varkappa_1$, and we have used the fact that $\varkappa^*(\bar{a}) = k$ if $\varkappa_k^*(\bar{a}_{k-1}) = 1$ and $\varkappa_{k+1}^*(\bar{a}_k) = 0$. If all K decision points would be reached, so that $\varkappa_K^*(\bar{a}_{K-1}) = 1$ and thus $\varkappa^*(\bar{a}) = K$, let

$$S_{K+1}^*(\bar{a}) = I\{\varkappa^*(\bar{a}) = K\}\, T^*(\bar{a}), \quad \Upsilon_{K+1}^*(\bar{a}) = 1.$$

As in Section 5.3.1 and more formally as in Section 6.2.3, we can define in terms of W^* in (8.50) potential outcomes associated with a regime $d \in \mathcal{D}$ that would be achieved if a randomly chosen individual in the population were to follow d. Defining as in Chapters 5–7 $\bar{d}_k = (d_1, \ldots, d_k)$ to denote the first k rules in d, analogous to (8.48), let $\varkappa_k^*(\bar{d}_{k-1})$ be the indicator of whether or not an individual would reach Decision k if the first $k-1$ rules in d were used to determine treatment at Decisions 1 to $k-1$, and let $\varkappa^*(d) = \max_j\{j : \varkappa_j^*(\bar{d}_{j-1}) = 1\}$ be the largest decision point for which $\varkappa_k^*(\bar{d}_{k-1}) = 1$. Then, for $k = 2, \ldots, \varkappa^*(d)$, write $T_k^*(\bar{d}_{k-1})$ to denote the time of Decision k and $X_k^*(\bar{d}_{k-1})$ to denote the intervening information arising between Decisions $k-1$ and k under the first $k-1$ rules in d. Let $T^*(d) = T^*(\bar{d}_{\varkappa^*(d)})$ be the event time under regime d, which is understood to depend on d only through the rules in d that are not null; that is, corresponding to the first $\varkappa^*(d)$ decision points where decisions have been made. We write the potential outcomes that would be achieved under a given regime $d \in \mathcal{D}$ as

$$\Big[\varkappa_1, \varkappa_2^*(d_1), \varkappa_3^*(\bar{d}_2), \ldots, \varkappa_K^*(\bar{d}_{K-1}), \varkappa^*(d) = \max_j \{ j : \varkappa_j^*(\bar{d}_{j-1}) = 1 \},$$

$$\mathcal{T}_1, X_1, \mathcal{T}_2^*(d_1), X_2^*(d_1), \mathcal{T}_3^*(\bar{d}_2), X_3^*(\bar{d}_2), \ldots,$$

$$\mathcal{T}_{\varkappa^*(d)}^*(\bar{d}_{\varkappa^*(d)-1}), X_{\varkappa^*(d)}^*(\bar{d}_{\varkappa^*(d)-1}), T^*(d) = T^*(\bar{d}_{\varkappa^*(d)}) \Big], \qquad (8.52)$$

where we include $\varkappa_1$, $\mathcal{T}_1$, and X_1 for completeness. It is possible to define the potential outcomes in (8.52) more formally in terms of W^* as in (6.11) in Chapter 6, although we do not present this here.

As in Section 8.2.1 in the case of a single decision, interest is ordinarily in a function of the time-to-event outcome. Within this potential outcomes formulation, the primary (potential) outcome of interest is

$$f\{T^*(d)\},$$

where $f(\cdot)$ is a known, monotone nondecreasing function as in Section 8.2.1. Then, analogous to (5.11) and as in (8.2) in the case of a single decision, for given $f(\cdot)$, we define the value of a fixed regime $d \in \mathcal{D}$ as

$$\mathcal{V}(d) = E[f\{T^*(d)\}]. \qquad (8.53)$$

Based on suitable observed data, discussed next, as in the single decision case, interest focuses on estimation of $\mathcal{V}(d)$ in (8.53) for a given, specified regime d and of an optimal regime $d^{opt} \in \mathcal{D}$ satisfying $\mathcal{V}(d^{opt}) \geq \mathcal{V}(d)$ for all $d \in \mathcal{D}$ and its value $\mathcal{V}(d^{opt})$.

Remark. As discussed in Remark (ii) in Section 6.2.1, the intervening information $\overline{X}_k^*(\bar{a}_{k-1})$ that could be collected between Decisions $k-1$ and k may have certain components that would or would not be collected depending on the treatment options already administered through Decision $k - 1$. For example, if in the acute leukemia setting induction chemotherapy a_1 would lead to nonresponse, it would be unnecessary to measure a variable that would be relevant only to select maintenance therapy for responders. As noted there, we do not make this explicit and take components that would not be collected to be null, where the corresponding components of realized values are also null.

Data, No Censoring

We first describe the data that ideally would be available and then characterize the data that would likely be available, the latter of which involve censoring of the time-to-event outcome for some individuals.

Ideally, as discussed in Section 5.3.2, estimation of $\mathcal{V}(d)$ for given $d \in \mathcal{D}$ and of an optimal regime and its value should be based on data from a longitudinal study in which all subjects are followed from baseline until they experience the time-to-event outcome, through a maximum of K specified decision points. As above, subjects may achieve the outcome prior to the Kth decision, and subjects reach the decision points at possibly different times. In this ideal setting, the event time is thus observed for all study subjects.

Let $\varkappa$ be the observed number of decision points reached by an individual, where, assuming all subjects receive a treatment option in $\mathcal{A}_1$ at Decision 1 at time $\mathcal{T}_1 = 0$, $1 \leq \varkappa \leq K$. Denote the observed times at which the $\varkappa$ decision points are reached by $\mathcal{T}_1, \ldots, \mathcal{T}_\varkappa$; and let A_k, taking values in $\mathcal{A}_k$, be the treatment option actually received at Decision k, $k = 1, \ldots, \varkappa$. With X_1 denoting baseline information, let X_k, $k = 2, \ldots, \varkappa$, denote the information collected on a subject in the intervening period between Decisions $k - 1$ and k. As in the remark above, some components of X_k could be null. Because X_k is used for decision making only if a subject reaches Decision k, we adopt the convention that $\mathcal{T}_k$ precedes X_k in the temporal ordering of the observed data, even if some components of X_k are observed prior to time $\mathcal{T}_k$. This convention is similar in spirit to that in the case of K decisions reached by all individuals in Chapters 5–7 in that observed information arising after the final decision and prior to ascertainment of the outcome is not used for decision making. In this ideal situation, the time-to-event outcome T is observed for all subjects, and the observed data are then realizations of

$$(\varkappa, \mathcal{T}_1, X_1, A_1, \mathcal{T}_2, X_2, A_2, \ldots, \mathcal{T}_\varkappa, X_\varkappa, A_\varkappa, T). \qquad (8.54)$$

We define in terms of the observed data (8.54) the time to reaching the kth decision point or achieving the event, whichever comes first, given that the $(k - 1)$th decision point was reached, and an associated indicator. Let $S_1 = \mathcal{T}_1 = 0$. For $\varkappa \geq 1$, let

$$S_2 = \mathrm{I}(\varkappa = 1)T + \mathrm{I}(\varkappa \geq 2)\mathcal{T}_2,$$
$$\Upsilon_2 = 1 \quad \text{if } \varkappa = 1,$$
$$= -1 \quad \text{if } \varkappa \geq 2,$$

so that S_2 is the event time if the individual did not reach the second decision point and is the time of the second decision point otherwise. Likewise, for $\varkappa \geq 2$, let

$$S_3 = \mathrm{I}(\varkappa = 2)T + \mathrm{I}(\varkappa \geq 3)\mathcal{T}_3,$$

$$\Upsilon_3 = 1 \quad \text{if } \varkappa = 2,$$
$$= -1 \quad \text{if } \varkappa \geq 3,$$

so that S_3 is the event time if the individual did not reach the third decision point and is the time of the third decision otherwise. In general, for $k = 2, \ldots, K$ and $\varkappa \geq k - 1$, let

$$S_k = \mathrm{I}(\varkappa = k - 1)T + \mathrm{I}(\varkappa \geq k)\mathcal{T}_k,$$
$$\Upsilon_k = 1 \quad \text{if } \varkappa = k - 1, \tag{8.55}$$
$$= -1 \quad \text{if } \varkappa \geq k.$$

If all K decision points are reached, so that $\varkappa = K$, let

$$S_{K+1} = \mathrm{I}(\varkappa = K)T, \quad \Upsilon_{K+1} = 1. \tag{8.56}$$

As in (5.14) in Section 5.3.2, define for $k = 1, \ldots, \varkappa$

$$\overline{X}_k = (X_1, \ldots, X_k), \qquad \overline{A}_k = (A_1, \ldots, A_k),$$

and let

$$\overline{\mathcal{T}}_k = (\mathcal{T}_1, \ldots, \mathcal{T}_k).$$

As in Section 8.3.1 and similar to (5.15), the observed history at Decision 1 is

$$H_1 = \{\mathcal{T}_1, X_1\}, \tag{8.57}$$

where we include $\mathcal{T}_1 = 0$ for completeness. As in Section 8.3.1, specification of the observed history at each subsequent decision point reached by a randomly chosen individual is more complex than in (5.15) owing to the fact that the number of decision points $\varkappa$ is random, and $\varkappa \leq K$. It is convenient to define the observed history at all K possible decision points for all individuals, including those for whom $\varkappa < K$. At Decision 2, the observed history for any individual can be represented as

$$H_2 = (\mathcal{T}_1, X_1, A_1, \mathcal{T}_2, X_2) = (\overline{\mathcal{T}}_2, \overline{X}_2, A_1), \quad \varkappa \geq 2,$$
$$= (\mathcal{T}_1, X_1, A_1, T), \qquad \varkappa < 2. \tag{8.58}$$

At Decision k, $k = 3, \ldots, K$, the observed history is

$$H_k = (\mathcal{T}_1, X_1, A_1, \mathcal{T}_2, X_2, A_2, \ldots, \mathcal{T}_k, X_k),$$
$$= (\overline{\mathcal{T}}_k, \overline{X}_k, \overline{A}_{k-1}), \qquad \varkappa \geq k,$$
$$= (\mathcal{T}_1, X_1, A_1, \mathcal{T}_2, X_2, A_2, \ldots, \mathcal{T}_\varkappa, X_\varkappa, A_\varkappa, T), \tag{8.59}$$
$$= (\overline{\mathcal{T}}_\varkappa, \overline{X}_\varkappa, \overline{A}_\varkappa, T) \qquad \varkappa < k.$$

For $k \geq 2$, (8.58)–(8.59) show that, at decisions up to and including the final decision point $\varkappa$, the form of the history is similar to that in Chapters 5–7, with the addition of the timing of the decision points. Once the

$\varkappa$th decision point has been reached, the history available at all future, unrealized decision points is defined to comprise the observed times of all realized decisions, the intervening information and treatments actually received through these decisions, and the time-to-event outcome.

Note that (8.57)–(8.59) can be written succinctly as

$$H_k = \left[\{ \mathrm{I}(\varkappa \geq j), (\mathcal{T}_j, X_j, A_j) \mathrm{I}(\varkappa \geq j), j = 1, \ldots, k-1 \}, \right.$$
$$\left. \mathrm{I}(\varkappa \geq k), (\mathcal{T}_k, X_k) \mathrm{I}(\varkappa \geq k), T \mathrm{I}(\varkappa < k) \right], \quad k = 1, \ldots, K.$$

Remark. Because the time-to-event outcome is achieved after the final decision point reached by an individual, if $\varkappa \geq k$, then $T > \mathcal{T}_k$.

Censored Data

Of course, as noted in Section 8.1, it is likely that the time-to-event outcome is not observed for all subjects in the observed data because it is administratively censored or censored due to loss to follow up. As in Section 8.2.1, under these conditions, U, the time to the event or censoring, whichever comes first, is observed, along with the indicator Δ taking the value 1 if U is the time to the event and 0 if U is the time of censoring of the event time. Following the perspective discussed at the end of Section 8.2.5, we view censoring as an external process. We do not introduce a potential censoring time variable C as in the conventional survival analysis framework; although the developments for the multiple decision problem are considerably more complex than those in the single decision case, such a definition does not simplify the formulation.

Under possible censoring of the event time, the number of decision points observed to be reached by an individual, denoted as κ, is determined by occurrence of either the event or censoring, whichever comes first. The observed data are then given by

$$(\kappa, \mathcal{T}_1, X_1, A_1, \mathcal{T}_2, X_2, A_2, \ldots, \mathcal{T}_\kappa, X_\kappa, A_\kappa, U, \Delta). \qquad (8.60)$$

Remark. Intuitively, κ is always less than or equal to the number of decision points $\varkappa$ that would be reached if there were no censoring.

Under censoring, the definition of the observed history H_k up to Decision k, $k = 2, \ldots, K$, in (8.58)–(8.59) must be modified to take account of censoring as

$$\begin{aligned} H_k &= (\mathcal{T}_1, X_1, A_1, \mathcal{T}_2, X_2, A_2, \ldots, \mathcal{T}_k, X_k), \\ &= (\overline{\mathcal{T}}_k, \overline{X}_k, \overline{A}_{k-1}), & \kappa \geq k, \\ &= (\mathcal{T}_1, X_1, A_1, \mathcal{T}_2, X_2, A_2, \ldots, \mathcal{T}_\kappa, X_\kappa, A_\kappa, U, \Delta), \\ &= (\overline{\mathcal{T}}_\kappa, \overline{X}_\kappa, \overline{A}_\kappa, U, \Delta) & \kappa < k. \end{aligned} \qquad (8.61)$$

As in the ideal case of no censoring, (8.61) is defined for all K possible decision points for all individuals, including those for whom $\kappa < K$. As noted in the remark following (8.60), $\kappa \leq \varkappa$; thus, the observed history at the kth decision point when $\kappa \geq k$ is identical to that in the no censoring case. Analogous to the case of no censoring, the history can be written succinctly as

$$H_k = \big[\{I(\kappa \geq j), (\mathcal{T}_j, X_j, A_j)I(\kappa \geq j), j = 1, \ldots, k-1\},$$
$$I(\kappa \geq k), (\mathcal{T}_k, X_k)I(\kappa \geq k), (U, \Delta)I(\kappa < k)\big], \quad k = 1, \ldots, K.$$

Finally, we define the history of data available on an individual up to time $u > 0$, which will prove convenient momentarily. We make use of this definition only for u such that $U \geq u$, so that neither of the event nor censoring has occurred by time u. For such u, both $\varkappa$ (if there were no censoring) and κ are greater than or equal to u, so we can express this history in terms of either. Note that $I(\kappa \geq k, \mathcal{T}_k \leq u)$ is the indicator that at least k decision points are reached prior to time u. Then the data available up to time u can be represented as

$$H(u) = \{(\mathcal{T}_1, X_1, A_1), I(\kappa \geq 2, \mathcal{T}_2 \leq u),$$
$$I(\kappa \geq 2, \mathcal{T}_2 \leq u)(\mathcal{T}_2, X_2, A_2), \ldots,$$
$$I(\kappa \geq k, \mathcal{T}_k \leq u), I(\kappa \geq k, \mathcal{T}_k \leq u)(\mathcal{T}_k, X_k, A_k), k = 3, \ldots, K, \tag{8.62}$$
$$I(U < u), (U, \Delta)I(U < u)\}.$$

Thus, for example, with $K = 4$, if $\kappa = 2$, for u such that $\mathcal{T}_2 \leq u$ but for which $U \geq u$, (8.62) becomes

$$H(u) = \{(\mathcal{T}_1, X_1, A_1), (\mathcal{T}_2, X_2, A_2)\} = (H_2, A_2).$$

Identifiability Assumptions

As in Chapters 5–7, to deduce the distribution of the potential outcomes and in particular functionals of the distribution of $T^*(d)$ from that of the observed data, we require versions of SUTVA given in (5.17) and (6.16), the sequential randomization assumption (SRA) given in (5.18) and (6.17), and the positivity assumption given in (5.20) and (6.23). We first state these assumptions in the case of no censoring.

SUTVA, also referred to as the consistency assumption, states that the components of the observed data are those that potentially would be achieved under the treatment options actually received. Here, this assumption takes the form

$$\varkappa = \max_j \{j : \varkappa_j^*(\overline{A}_{j-1}) = 1\},$$

$$X_k = X_k^*(\overline{A}_{k-1}), \quad \mathcal{T}_k = \mathcal{T}_k^*(\overline{A}_{k-1}), \quad k = 1, \ldots, \varkappa, \quad T = T^*(\overline{A}_\varkappa). \tag{8.63}$$

Note that, by (8.63), S_k and Υ_k defined in (8.55) satisfy

$$S_k = S_k^*(\overline{A}_{k-1}), \qquad \Upsilon_k = \Upsilon_k^*(\overline{A}_{k-1}).$$

The SRA states that treatment received at each decision point is independent of all potential outcomes, conditional on history. Here, because treatment is administered only through Decision $\varkappa$, the SRA becomes

$$W^* \perp\!\!\!\perp A_k | H_k, \varkappa \geq k, \quad k = 1, \dots, K, \tag{8.64}$$

where (8.64) is relevant only if $\varkappa \geq k$, in which case stage k treatment is observed.

We present the positivity assumption informally, analogous to the development in Section 5.3.3, recognizing that it can be expressed more precisely in terms of feasible sets of treatment options as in Section 6.2.4. As discussed in Section 5.3.3, deducing the distribution of the potential outcomes for any $d \in \mathcal{D}$ defined above in terms of the observed data requires that the feasible treatment options at each decision point be represented in the data. Here, this assumption acknowledges that treatment is administered only through Decision $\varkappa$; namely,

$$P(A_k = a_k \mid H_k = h_k, \varkappa \geq k) > 0, \quad k = 1, \dots, K, \tag{8.65}$$

for all options $a_k \in \mathcal{A}_k$ that are feasible for history h_k and for all possible h_k satisfying

$$P(H_k = h_k, \varkappa \geq k) > 0.$$

When the observed data involve censoring in the multiple decision case, modified versions of (8.63)–(8.65) are required. SUTVA in (8.63) must be revised to recognize that the observed number of decision points reached by an individual is determined by the occurrence of the event or censoring, whichever comes first. Recall that in the potential outcomes framework, there is no censoring, so for given sequence $\overline{a}$, $\varkappa_k^*(\overline{a}_{k-1})$ in (8.48) is equal to 1 if Decision k is reached because the event has not yet taken place, and the time of Decision k is $\mathcal{T}_k^*(\overline{a}_{k-1})$ in this case. Under the perspective that censoring is an external process as discussed at the end of Section 8.2.5, Δ has a similar interpretation to the treatment assignments actually received, taking place when individuals are observed in practice. When $\Delta = 0$, so that censoring of the event time is observed to have occurred, U is the time to censoring and can be viewed similarly as the result of an external process, coming about when individuals are observed. On the other hand, when $\Delta = 1$, U is the event time, which is dictated by underlying potential outcomes under the treatments already received. With these considerations, the addition of censoring then leads to the modification of SUTVA in (8.63) given by

$$\text{If } \Delta = 1, \ \kappa = \max_{j} \ \{j : \ \varkappa_{j}^{*}(\overline{A}_{j-1}) = 1\}, \ \ U = T^{*}(\overline{A}_{\kappa}),$$

$$\text{If } \Delta = 0, \ \kappa = \max_{j} \ \left\{j : \ \varkappa_{j}^{*}(\overline{A}_{j-1}) = 1 \text{ and } U > T_{j}^{*}(\overline{A}_{j-1})\right\},$$

$$X_{k} = X_{k}^{*}(\overline{A}_{k-1}), \quad T_{k} = T_{k}^{*}(\overline{A}_{k-1}), \quad k = 1,\ldots,\kappa. \tag{8.66}$$

From (8.66), when $\Delta = 1$, $\kappa = \varkappa$ and $U = T$, as expected.

With the definition of κ in (8.66), which represents explicitly that κ is determined by the first to occur of the event or censoring, the SRA in (8.64) becomes

$$W^{*} \perp\!\!\!\perp A_{k}|H_{k}, \kappa \geq k, \quad k = 1,\ldots,K, \tag{8.67}$$

which, as with (8.64), is relevant only if $\kappa \geq k$.

As in the single decision case, we make the assumption that censoring is noninformative in the following sense. Analogous to (8.46) in the single decision case, we assume that the cause-specific hazard function for censoring at time u satisfies

$$
\begin{aligned}
\lambda_{C}&\{u|H(u), W^{*}\} \\
&= \lim_{du \to 0} du^{-1} P\{u \leq U < u + du, \Delta = 0 \,|\, U \geq u, H(u), W^{*}\} \\
&= \lim_{du \to 0} du^{-1} P\{u \leq U < u + du, \Delta = 0 \,|\, U \geq u, H(u)\} \\
&= \lambda_{C}\{u|H(u)\},
\end{aligned}
\tag{8.68}
$$

which depends on the history to time u defined in (8.62). As for (8.46), the specification (8.68) indicates that censoring is noninformative in that the hazard at u depends only on information observed through time u and not on unobserved potential outcomes, and it is similar to those in Robins and Rotnitzky (1992), Robins (1993), and Hernán et al. (2000) noted previously.

From (8.62), depending on the range of times u under consideration, in the sequel we often express the cause-specific hazard function $\lambda_{C}\{u|H(u)\}$ explicitly in terms of the components of $H(u)$ relevant to u. Thus, continuing with the example above, if $K = 4$ and $\kappa = 2$, if $T_{2} \leq u \leq U$, so that $H(u) = (H_{2}, A_{2})$, write $\lambda_{C}\{u|H(u)\} = \lambda_{C}(u|H_{2}, A_{2})$. In general, for $k = 1,\ldots,K$, we write, for example,

$$\lambda_{C}\{u|H(u)\} = \lambda_{C}(u|H_{k}, A_{k}) \ \text{ for all } \{u : H(u) = (H_{k}, A_{k})\};$$

and, when referring to a particular realization of $H(u)$, $h(u)$, say, write

$$\lambda_{C}\{u|h(u)\} = \lambda_{C}(u|h_{k}, a_{k}) \ \text{ for all } \{u : h(u) = (h_{k}, a_{k})\}. \tag{8.69}$$

To avoid technical complications, we take $\lambda_C\{u|h(u)\}$ to be continuous in u in what follows.

With censoring, the positivity assumption is more involved than in (8.65) and must be formulated sequentially to take account of possible censoring in the intervening periods between realized decision points. Here, as above, we do not present a formal statement in terms of feasible sets of treatment options and associated histories as in (6.23) in Section 6.2.4, which is of course possible with definition of suitable sets analogous to Γ_k and Λ_k, $k = 1, \ldots, K$, as in that section.

At Decision 1, which is reached by all individuals, so that $\kappa \geq 1$ with certainty, we require that

$$P(A_1 = a_1 \mid H_1 = h_1, \kappa \geq 1) = P(A_1 = a_1 \mid H_1 = h_1) > 0 \qquad (8.70)$$

for all options $a_1 \in \mathcal{A}_1$ that are feasible for history h_1 and for all possible h_1 satisfying

$$P(H_1 = h_1, \kappa \geq 1) = P(H_1 = h_1) > 0.$$

Once treatment has been administered at Decision 1, there must be a positive probability that an individual's event time is not censored before he reaches Decision 2 or achieves the event. This can be expressed as

$$P\{U \geq u \mid S_2^*(a_1) = u, H_1 = h_1, A_1 = a_1, \kappa \geq 1\} > 0 \qquad (8.71)$$

for all feasible a_1, associated histories h_1, and u such that

$$P\{S_2^*(a_1) = u, H_1 = h_1, A_1 = a_1, \kappa \geq 1\} > 0,$$

where we include the certain event $\kappa \geq 1$ in (8.71) for consistency with statements that arise next. From the definition of $S_2^*(a_1)$ in (8.51), the conditioning set in (8.71) implies that either the event or Decision 2 is reached at time u, and thus $U \geq u$ implies that censoring has not occurred by time u.

Under the noninformative censoring assumption in (8.68) and using the definition of $H(u)$ in (8.62), it is possible to write (8.71) equivalently in terms of the cause-specific hazard defined in (8.68), which is useful in the sequel. We demonstrate this heuristically as follows. Using the notion of a product integral as in Andersen et al. (1993), the probability in (8.71) satisfies

$$P\{U \geq u \mid S_2^*(a_1) = u, H_1 = h_1, A_1 = a_1, \kappa \geq 1\}$$
$$= P\{U \geq u \mid S_2^*(a_1) = u, H_1 = h_1, A_1 = a_1\} \qquad (8.72)$$
$$= \prod_{\tau_1 \leq w < u} P\{U \geq w + dw | U \geq w, S_2^*(a_1) = u, H_1 = h_1, A_1 = a_1\}$$

$$= \prod_{\tau_1 \leq w < u} \left[1 - P\{w \leq U < w + dw | U \geq w, S_2^*(a_1) = u, H_1 = h_1, A_1 = a_1\} \right]$$

$$= \prod_{\tau_1 \leq w < u} \left[1 - P\{w \leq U < w + dw, \Delta = 0 | U \geq w, S_2^*(a_1) = u, \right.$$
$$\left. H_1 = h_1, A_1 = a_1\} \right] \tag{8.73}$$

$$= \prod_{\tau_1 \leq w < u} \left[1 - \lambda_C\{w \mid h(w), S_2^*(a_1) = u\} \, dw \right] \tag{8.74}$$

$$= \prod_{\tau_1 \leq w < u} \left[1 - \lambda_C\{w \mid h(w)\} \, dw \right], \tag{8.75}$$

$$= \prod_{\tau_1 \leq w < u} \{ 1 - \lambda_C(w \mid h_1, a_1) \, dw \}, \tag{8.76}$$

$$= \exp \left\{ - \int_0^u \lambda_C(w | h_1, a_1) \, dw \right\}, \tag{8.77}$$

where (8.72) follows because $\kappa \geq 1$ holds with certainty; and because the time to Decision 2 or the event time, whichever comes first, $S_2^*(a_1) = u$ and $u > w$, U can occur between w and $w + dw$ only if $\Delta = 0$, leading to (8.73). Then (8.74) follows because, from (8.62), $H(w) = (\mathcal{T}_1, X_1, A_1) = (H_1, A_1)$, for $\mathcal{T}_1 \leq w < u$; (8.75) follows from the noninformative censoring assumption (8.68); and (8.76) follows from (8.62) and (8.69). This argument, leading to the representation (8.77), is a special case of a more general result for any $k = 2, \ldots, K$, presented in Lemma 8.5.1 in Section 8.5, to which we appeal in what follows.

At Decision 2, we then require that

$$P(A_2 = a_2 \mid H_2 = h_2, \kappa \geq 2) > 0 \tag{8.78}$$

for all options $a_2 \in \mathcal{A}_2$ that are feasible for history h_2, given Decision 2 is reached, and for all possible h_2 satisfying

$$P(H_2 = h_2, \kappa \geq 2) > 0.$$

Following treatment at Decision 2, there must be a positive probability that an individual's event time is not censored before she reaches Decision 3 or achieves the event, namely,

$$P\{U \geq u \mid S_3^*(\bar{a}_2) = u, H_2 = h_2, A_2 = a_2, \kappa \geq 2\} > 0 \tag{8.79}$$

for all feasible a_2, associated histories h_2, and u such that

$$P\{S_3^*(\bar{a}_2) = u, H_2 = h_2, A_2 = a_2, \kappa \geq 2\} > 0.$$

As above, from the definition of $S_3^*(\bar{a}_2)$ in (8.55), the conditioning set in (8.79) implies that censoring did not occur before Decision 2 ($\kappa \geq 2$) and either the event or Decision 3 is reached at time u, so that $U \geq u$ implies that censoring has not yet occurred by u. By Lemma 8.5.1, (8.62), the noninformative censoring assumption (8.68), and (8.69), the probability in (8.79) can be written as

$$P\{U \geq u \mid S_3^*(\bar{a}_2) = u, H_2 = h_2, A_2 = a_2, \kappa \geq 2\}$$
$$= \exp\left\{-\int_{\tau_2}^u \lambda_C(w|h_2, a_2)\, dw\right\}. \tag{8.80}$$

Continuing in this fashion, for $k = 3, \ldots, K - 1$, we require that

$$P(A_k = a_k \mid H_k = h_k, \kappa \geq k) > 0 \tag{8.81}$$

for all options $a_k \in \mathcal{A}_k$ that are feasible for history h_k and for all possible h_k satisfying

$$P(H_k = h_k, \kappa \geq k) > 0;$$

and that, using Lemma 8.5.1, (8.62), and (8.68),

$$P\{U \geq u \mid S_{k+1}^*(\bar{a}_k) = u, H_k = h_k, A_k = a_k, \kappa \geq k\}$$
$$= \exp\left\{-\int_{\tau_k}^u \lambda_C(w|h_k, a_k)\, dw\right\} > 0 \tag{8.82}$$

for all feasible a_k, associated histories h_k, and u such that

$$P\{S_{k+1}^*(\bar{a}_k) = u, H_k = h_k, A_k = a_k, \kappa \geq k\} > 0.$$

Finally, at Decision K, it must be that

$$P(A_K = a_K \mid H_K = h_K, \kappa = K) > 0 \tag{8.83}$$

for all options $a_K \in \mathcal{A}_K$ that are feasible for history h_K and for all possible h_K satisfying

$$P(H_K = h_K, \kappa = K) > 0;$$

and that

$$P\{U \geq u \mid S_{K+1}^*(\bar{a}) = u, H_K = h_K, A_K = a_K, \kappa = K\}$$
$$= \exp\left\{-\int_{\tau_K}^u \lambda_C(w|h_K, a_K)\, dw\right\} > 0 \tag{8.84}$$

for all feasible a_K, associated histories h_K, and u such that

$$P\{S_{K+1}^*(\bar{a}) = u, H_K = h_K, A_K = a_K, \kappa = K\} > 0.$$

Together, (8.70)–(8.84) comprise the positivity assumption, ensuring that there are individuals in the observed data who reach each decision point and receive all feasible options given their observed histories.

Remark. As discussed in the remark following (8.11), when the data arise from a study of finite length, it is necessary to restrict attention to a truncated version of $f(t)$, such as restricted lifetime, $f(t) = \min(t, L)$. Under these conditions, the positivity assumption as presented in (8.70)–(8.84) is modified as follows. Define

$$\kappa^L = \max_k \{k = 1, \ldots, \kappa : \mathcal{T}_k \leq L\}, \tag{8.85}$$

the largest decision point reached before the event time, censoring time, or L, whichever comes first. Then in (8.71), replace $\kappa \geq 1$ by $\kappa^L \geq 1$ and the event $U \geq u$ by $U \geq \min(u, L)$, and replace the upper limit of integration in (8.77) by $\min(u, L)$. Similarly, in (8.79) and (8.80), replace $\kappa \geq 2$ by $\kappa^L \geq 2$ and $U \geq u$ by $U \geq \min(u, L)$, and replace the upper limit of integration in (8.80) by $\min(u, L)$. Likewise, in (8.82), replace $\kappa \geq k$ by $\kappa^L \geq k$, $U \geq u$ by $U \geq \min(u, L)$, and the upper limit of integration by $\min(u, L)$; and, finally, replace $\kappa = K$ by $\kappa^L = K$, $U \geq u$ by $U \geq \min(u, L)$, and the upper limit of integration by $\min(u, L)$ in (8.84).

Because in the foregoing developments H_k, $k = 1, \ldots, K$, is relevant only when $\kappa \geq k$, from the definition of H_k in (8.61), modification of this definition is not necessary.

8.3.3 Estimation of the Value of a Fixed Regime

Estimation via the q-Computation Algorithm

As in Sections 5.4 and 6.3, it is possible to demonstrate that, for any regime $d \in \mathcal{D}$, under SUTVA, the SRA, and the noninformative censoring and positivity assumptions, the joint distribution of the associated potential outcomes

$$W_d^* = \left[\varkappa^*(d), \mathcal{T}_1, X_1, \mathcal{T}_2^*(d_1), X_2^*(d_1), \mathcal{T}_3^*(\bar{d}_2), X_3^*(\bar{d}_2), \ldots, \right. \tag{8.86}$$

$$\left. \mathcal{T}_{\varkappa^*(d)}^*(\bar{d}_{\varkappa^*(d)-1}), X_{\varkappa^*(d)}^*(\bar{d}_{\varkappa^*(d)-1}), T^*(d) = T^*(\bar{d}_{\varkappa^*(d)}) \right]$$

in (8.52) can be expressed in terms of that of the observed data. In (8.86), we include $\mathcal{T}_1 = 0$ for completeness, but $\mathcal{T}_1$ plays no role in the density. We do not prove this result formally; the proof is along the same lines as that in Section 6.3, adapted to account for the fact that the timing and number of decision points are random. Instead, we state the result and provide an intuitive justification.

Consider the case of no censoring, and define the following quantities. As in Sections 5.4 and 6.3, let $p_{X_1}(x_1)$ be the density of X_1. Let

$$\lambda_{T1}(u|\tau_1, x_1, a_1) \tag{8.87}$$
$$= \lim_{du \to 0} du^{-1} P(\tau_1 + u \le S_2 < \tau_1 + u + du, \Upsilon_2 = 1 \,|$$
$$S_2 \ge \tau_1 + u, \mathcal{T}_1 = \tau_1, X_1 = x_1, A_1 = a_1, \varkappa \ge 1),$$

the cause-specific hazard of achieving the event at time u prior to reaching the second decision point, conditional on τ_1, X_1, and A_1; and

$$\lambda_{\tau 1}(u|\tau_1, x_1, a_1) \tag{8.88}$$
$$= \lim_{du \to 0} du^{-1} P(\tau_1 + u \le S_2 < \tau_1 + u + du, \Upsilon_2 = -1 \,|$$
$$S_2 \ge \tau_1 + u, \mathcal{T}_1 = \tau_1, X_1 = x_1, A_1 = a_1, \varkappa \ge 1)$$

the conditional cause-specific hazard of reaching the second decision point at time u prior to experiencing the event. We include $\mathcal{T}_1 = \tau_1 = 0$ in (8.87) and (8.88) for consistency with subsequent definitions below. Let

$$p_{X_2|\mathcal{T}_1, X_1, A_1, \mathcal{T}_2, \varkappa \ge 2}(x_2|\tau_1, x_1, a_1, \tau_2) \tag{8.89}$$

be the density of X_2 given the past through Decision 2, which is relevant only for individuals who reach Decision 2, $\varkappa \ge 2$.

Next, let

$$\lambda_{T2}(u|\overline{\tau}_2, \overline{x}_2, \overline{a}_2) \tag{8.90}$$
$$= \lim_{du \to 0} du^{-1} P(\tau_2 + u \le S_3 < \tau_2 + u + du, \Upsilon_3 = 1 \,|$$
$$S_3 \ge \tau_2 + u, \overline{\mathcal{T}}_2 = \overline{\tau}_2, \overline{X}_2 = \overline{x}_2, \overline{A}_2 = \overline{a}_2, \varkappa \ge 2),$$

the cause-specific hazard of achieving the event u units of time after the second decision point at time τ_2 but prior to reaching the third decision point, conditional on $\overline{\tau}_2$, $\overline{X}_2$, and $\overline{A}_2$; and

$$\lambda_{\tau 2}(u|\overline{\tau}_2, \overline{x}_2, \overline{a}_2) \tag{8.91}$$
$$= \lim_{du \to 0} du^{-1} P(\tau_2 + u \le S_3 < \tau_2 + u + du, \Upsilon_3 = -1 \,|$$
$$S_3 \ge \tau_2 + u, \overline{\mathcal{T}}_2 = \overline{\tau}_2, \overline{X}_2 = \overline{x}_2, \overline{A}_2 = \overline{a}_2, \varkappa \ge 2),$$

the conditional cause-specific hazard of reaching the third decision point u units of time after the second decision time τ_2 prior to experiencing the event. Let

$$p_{X_3|\overline{\mathcal{T}}_2, \overline{X}_2, \overline{A}_2, \mathcal{T}_3, \varkappa \ge 3}(x_3|\overline{\tau}_2, \overline{x}_2, \overline{a}_2, \tau_3) \tag{8.92}$$

be the density of X_3 given the past through Decision 3, which is relevant only for individuals who reach Decision 3, $\varkappa \geq 3$.

Continuing in this fashion, in general, for $k = 1, \ldots, K - 1$, define the conditional cause-specific hazards

$$\lambda_{Tk}(u|\overline{T}_k, \overline{x}_k, \overline{a}_k) \tag{8.93}$$
$$= \lim_{du \to 0} du^{-1} P(\tau_k + u \leq S_{k+1} < \tau_k + u + du, \Upsilon_{k+1} = 1 \mid$$
$$S_{k+1} \geq \tau_k + u, \overline{T}_k = \overline{\tau}_k, \overline{X}_k = \overline{x}_k, \overline{A}_k = \overline{a}_k, \varkappa \geq k),$$

and

$$\lambda_{\tau k}(u|\overline{T}_k, \overline{x}_k, \overline{a}_k) \tag{8.94}$$
$$= \lim_{du \to 0} du^{-1} P(\tau_k + u \leq S_{k+1} < \tau_k + u + du, \Upsilon_{k+1} = -1 \mid$$
$$S_{k+1} \geq \tau_k + u, \overline{T}_k = \overline{\tau}_k, \overline{X}_k = \overline{x}_k, \overline{A}_k = \overline{a}_k, \varkappa \geq k);$$

and the density of X_{k+1} given the past through Decision k, which is relevant only for individuals who reach Decision k, $\varkappa \geq k$,

$$p_{X_{k+1}|\overline{T}_k, \overline{X}_k, \overline{A}_k, T_{k+1}, \varkappa \geq k+1}(x_{k+1}|\overline{T}_k, \overline{x}_k, \overline{a}_k, \tau_{k+1}). \tag{8.95}$$

Finally, let

$$\lambda_{TK}(u|\overline{T}_K, \overline{x}_K, \overline{a}_K) \tag{8.96}$$
$$= \lim_{du \to 0} du^{-1} P(\tau_K + u \leq S_{K+1} < \tau_K + u + du, \Upsilon_{K+1} = 1 \mid$$
$$S_{K+1} \geq \tau_K + u, \overline{T}_K = \overline{\tau}_K, \overline{X}_K = \overline{x}_K, \overline{A}_K = \overline{a}_K, \varkappa = K),$$

where, from (8.56), $S_{K+1} = T$, and $\Upsilon_{K+1} = 1$ is superfluous.

Remark. The cause-specific hazards in (8.93), (8.94), and (8.96) characterize "added life," which is the additional time to reaching the event or the $(k+1)$th decision point given that an individual has reached the kth decision point. This formulation proves convenient for implementation, discussed below.

Define for $k = 1, \ldots, K - 1$

$$S_{\bullet k}(u|\overline{T}_k, \overline{x}_k, \overline{a}_k) \tag{8.97}$$
$$= \exp\left[-\int_0^u \{\lambda_{Tk}(w|\overline{T}_k, \overline{x}_k, \overline{a}_k) + \lambda_{\tau k}(w|\overline{T}_k, \overline{x}_k, \overline{a}_k)\} \, dw\right],$$

and let

$$S_{TK}(u|\overline{T}_K, \overline{x}_K, \overline{a}_K) = \exp\left\{-\int_0^u \lambda_{TK}(w|\overline{T}_K, \overline{x}_K, \overline{a}_K) \, dw\right\}. \tag{8.98}$$

We are now in a position to present the representation of the joint density of the potential outcomes W_d^* in (8.86) for a given regime $d \in \mathcal{D}$,

$$p_{W_d^*}(j, x_1, \tau_2, x_2, \tau_3, x_3, \ldots, \tau_j, x_j, t), \tag{8.99}$$

in terms of that of the observed data under SUTVA (8.4), the SRA (8.64), the noninformative censoring assumption (8.68), and the positivity assumption given in (8.70)–(8.84). As above, although we include $\mathcal{T}_1 = 0$ in W_d^* and in (8.87)–(8.96) for completeness, the density (8.99) really is that of W_d^* excluding $\mathcal{T}_1$, with $\tau_1 = 0$ (a constant).

It can be shown that the density (8.99) can be expressed in terms of the observed data for $j = 1, \ldots, K$ as follows. For $j = 1$, the density is given by

$$p_{X_1}(x_1)\, \mathcal{S}_{\bullet 1}\{t|\tau_1, x_1, d_1(x_1)\}\lambda_{T1}\{t|\tau_1, x_1, d_1(x_1)\}. \tag{8.100}$$

For $j = 2, \ldots, K - 1$, the density is given by, using (8.47),

$$
\begin{aligned}
p_{X_1}(x_1) \prod_{\ell=1}^{j-1} &\Big[\mathcal{S}_{\bullet\ell}\{\tau_{\ell+1} - \tau_\ell | \overline{\tau}_\ell, \overline{x}_\ell, \overline{d}_\ell(\overline{\tau}_\ell, \overline{x}_\ell)\} \\
&\times \lambda_{\tau\ell}\{\tau_{\ell+1} - \tau_\ell | \overline{\tau}_\ell, \overline{x}_\ell, \overline{d}_\ell(\overline{\tau}_\ell, \overline{x}_\ell)\} \\
&\times p_{X_{\ell+1}|\overline{\tau}_\ell, \overline{X}_\ell, \overline{A}_\ell, \tau_{\ell+1}, \varkappa \geq \ell+1}\{x_{\ell+1} | \overline{\tau}_\ell, \overline{x}_\ell, \overline{d}_\ell(\overline{\tau}_\ell, \overline{x}_\ell), \tau_{\ell+1}\} \Big] \\
&\times \mathcal{S}_{\bullet j}\{t - \tau_j | \overline{\tau}_j, \overline{x}_j, \overline{d}_j(\overline{\tau}_j, \overline{x}_j)\}\lambda_{Tj}\{t - \tau_j | \overline{\tau}_j, \overline{x}_j, \overline{d}_j(\overline{\tau}_j, \overline{x}_j)\}.
\end{aligned}
\tag{8.101}
$$

Finally, for $j = K$, the density is

$$
\begin{aligned}
p_{X_1}(x_1) \prod_{\ell=1}^{K-1} &\Big[\mathcal{S}_{\bullet\ell}\{\tau_{\ell+1} - \tau_\ell | \overline{\tau}_\ell, \overline{x}_\ell, \overline{d}_\ell(\overline{\tau}_\ell, \overline{x}_\ell)\} \\
&\times \lambda_{\tau\ell}\{\tau_{\ell+1} - \tau_\ell | \overline{\tau}_\ell, \overline{x}_\ell, \overline{d}_\ell(\overline{\tau}_\ell, \overline{x}_\ell)\} \\
&\times p_{X_{\ell+1}|\overline{\tau}_\ell, \overline{X}_\ell, \overline{A}_\ell, \tau_{\ell+1}, \varkappa \geq \ell+1}\{x_{\ell+1} | \overline{\tau}_\ell, \overline{x}_\ell, \overline{d}_\ell(\overline{\tau}_\ell, \overline{x}_\ell), \tau_{\ell+1}\} \Big] \\
&\times \mathcal{S}_{TK}\{t - \tau_K | \overline{\tau}_K, \overline{x}_K, \overline{d}_K(\overline{\tau}_K, \overline{x}_K)\}\lambda_{TK}\{t - \tau_K | \overline{\tau}_K, \overline{x}_K, \overline{d}_K(\overline{\tau}_K, \overline{x}_K)\}.
\end{aligned}
\tag{8.102}
$$

The fundamental underpinning of the representation of the joint density of the potential outcomes given in (8.99) as in (8.100)–(8.102) is the following set of equalities, which are demonstrated in Section 8.5. It can be shown that the cause-specific hazard functions $\lambda_{Tk}(u|\overline{\tau}_k, \overline{x}_k, \overline{a}_k)$ and $\lambda_{\tau k}(u|\overline{\tau}_k, \overline{x}_k, \overline{a}_k)$, $k = 1, \ldots, K - 1$, and $\lambda_{TK}(u|\overline{\tau}_K, \overline{x}_K, \overline{a}_K)$ defined in (8.93), (8.94), and (8.96), respectively, are equal to corresponding cause-specific hazard functions defined in terms of potential outcomes. Namely, for $k = 1, \ldots, K-1$, $\lambda_{Tk}(u|\overline{\tau}_k, \overline{x}_k, \overline{a}_k)$ in (8.93) can be shown to be equal to

$$\lambda_{Tk}^*(u|\overline{\mathcal{T}}_k, \overline{x}_k, \overline{a}_k) \tag{8.103}$$
$$= \lim_{du \to 0} du^{-1} P\{\tau_k + u \le S_{k+1}^*(\overline{a}_k) < \tau_k + u + du, \Upsilon_{k+1}^*(\overline{a}_k) = 1 \,|$$
$$S_{k+1}^*(\overline{a}_k) \ge \tau_k + u, \overline{\mathcal{T}}_k^*(\overline{a}_{k-1}) = \overline{\tau}_k, \overline{X}_k^*(\overline{a}_{k-1}) = \overline{x}_k, \varkappa^*(\overline{a}_{k-1}) \ge k\},$$

and (8.94) can be shown to be equal to

$$\lambda_{Tk}^*(u|\overline{\mathcal{T}}_k, \overline{x}_k, \overline{a}_k) \tag{8.104}$$
$$= \lim_{du \to 0} du^{-1} P\{\tau_k + u \le S_{k+1}^*(\overline{a}_k) < \tau_k + u + du, \Upsilon_{k+1}^*(\overline{a}_k) = -1 \,|$$
$$S_{k+1}^*(\overline{a}_k) \ge \tau_k + u, \overline{\mathcal{T}}_k^*(\overline{a}_{k-1}) = \overline{\tau}_k, \overline{X}_k^*(\overline{a}_{k-1}) = \overline{x}_k, \varkappa^*(\overline{a}_{k-1}) \ge k\};$$

and (8.96) is equal to

$$\lambda_{TK}^*(u|\overline{\mathcal{T}}_K, \overline{x}_K, \overline{a}_K) \tag{8.105}$$
$$= \lim_{du \to 0} du^{-1} P\{\tau_K + u \le S_{K+1}^*(\overline{a}_K) < \tau_K + u + du, \Upsilon_{K+1}^*(\overline{a}_K) = 1 \,|$$
$$S_{K+1}^*(\overline{a}_K) \ge \tau_K + u, \overline{\mathcal{T}}_K^*(\overline{a}_{K-1}) = \overline{\tau}_K, \overline{X}_K^*(\overline{a}_K) = \overline{x}_K, \varkappa^*(\overline{a}_{K-1}) = K\}.$$

It can also be shown that, for each $k = 1, \ldots, K - 1$, the densities

$$p_{X_{k+1}|\overline{\mathcal{T}}_k, \overline{X}_k, \overline{A}_k, \mathcal{T}_{k+1}, \varkappa \ge k+1}(x_{k+1}|\overline{\tau}_k, \overline{x}_k, \overline{a}_k, \tau_{k+1})$$

given in (8.95) are equal to the densities

$$p_{X_{k+1}^*(\overline{a}_k)|\overline{\mathcal{T}}_k^*(\overline{a}_{k-1}), \overline{X}_k^*(\overline{a}_{k-1}), \mathcal{T}_{k+1}^*(\overline{a}_k), \varkappa_{k+1}^*(\overline{a}_k)=1}(x_{k+1}|\overline{\tau}_k, \overline{x}_k, \tau_{k+1}). \tag{8.106}$$

Intuitively, the equivalence of (8.93), (8.94), and (8.96) to (8.103), (8.104), and (8.105), respectively; and the equivalence of (8.95) and (8.106) can be exploited in a factorization of the joint density of the potential outcomes (8.99) to obtain the representation in terms of the observed data in (8.100)–(8.102).

We now consider how the representation of the joint density of the potential outcomes (8.99) in terms of the observed data given in (8.100)–(8.102) can be used to estimate the value $\mathcal{V}(d) = E[f\{T^*(d)\}]$ in (8.53) for a fixed regime $d \in \mathcal{D}$. As in (5.43) in Section 5.4 and (6.48) in Section 6.3, in principle, it is possible to obtain an expression for $E[f\{T^*(d)\}]$ analytically via integration over the sample space of all possible realizations of numbers and timing of decision points and intervening information, which could form the basis for an estimator by substitution of posited models for $p_{X_1}(x_1)$ and the hazard functions and conditional densities involved in (8.100)–(8.102). However, as discussed in Section 5.5.1, carrying out the required high-dimensional integration is almost certainly infeasible in practice.

An alternative approach is estimation of $\mathcal{V}(d)$ by the g-computation algorithm; that is, approximate the distribution of $T^*(d)$ via Monte Carlo integration in a manner analogous to the strategy outlined in Section 5.5.1. Assume that we posit and fit models for $p_{X_1}(x_1)$ and the hazard functions and conditional densities in (8.87)–(8.96) that characterize (8.100), (8.101), and (8.102). We discuss development and fitting of these models based on both uncensored and censored data shortly. Let $\widehat{p}_{X_1}(x_1)$ be a fitted model for $p_{X_1}(x_1)$, and, from (8.95), for $k = 2, \ldots, K$, let

$$\widehat{p}_{X_k|\overline{T}_{k-1},\overline{X}_{k-1},\overline{A}_{k-1},T_k,\varkappa \geq k}(x_k|\overline{T}_{k-1},\overline{x}_{k-1},\overline{a}_{k-1},\tau_k)$$

be fitted models for

$$p_{X_k|\overline{T}_{k-1},\overline{X}_{k-1},\overline{A}_{k-1},T_k,\varkappa \geq k}(x_k|\overline{T}_{k-1},\overline{x}_{k-1},\overline{a}_{k-1},\tau_k). \tag{8.107}$$

Analogous to (8.98), define for $k = 1, \ldots, K-1$

$$\mathcal{S}_{Tk}(u|\overline{\tau}_k,\overline{x}_k,\overline{a}_k) = \exp\left\{-\int_0^u \lambda_{Tk}(w|\overline{\tau}_k,\overline{x}_k,\overline{a}_k)\,dw\right\}, \tag{8.108}$$

$$\mathcal{S}_{\tau k}(u|\overline{\tau}_k,\overline{x}_k,\overline{a}_k) = \exp\left\{-\int_0^u \lambda_{\tau k}(w|\overline{\tau}_k,\overline{x}_k,\overline{a}_k)\,dw\right\}. \tag{8.109}$$

Let

$$\widehat{\lambda}_{Tk}(u|\overline{\tau}_k,\overline{x}_k,\overline{a}_k), \quad k = 1,\ldots,K, \quad \widehat{\lambda}_{\tau k}(u|\overline{\tau}_k,\overline{x}_k,\overline{a}_k), \quad k = 1,\ldots,K-1,$$

be fitted models for the hazards $\lambda_{Tk}(u|\overline{\tau}_k,\overline{x}_k,\overline{a}_k)$ and $\lambda_{\tau k}(u|\overline{\tau}_k,\overline{x}_k,\overline{a}_k)$; and let

$$\widehat{\mathcal{S}}_{Tk}(u|\overline{\tau}_k,\overline{x}_k,\overline{a}_k), \quad k = 1,\ldots,K, \quad \widehat{\mathcal{S}}_{\tau k}(u|\overline{\tau}_k,\overline{x}_k,\overline{a}_k), \quad k = 1,\ldots,K-1,$$

be obtained by substitution of these fitted hazard models in (8.108) and (8.109).

Then, for $r = 1, \ldots, M$, simulate a realization from the distribution of $T^*(d)$ as follows:

1. Generate random x_{1r} from $\widehat{p}_{X_1}(x_1)$.

2. Generate random $u_{T1,r}$ from

$$\widehat{\mathcal{S}}_{T1}\{u|\tau_1, x_{1r}, d_1(x_{1r})\},$$

and independently generate random $u_{\tau 1,r}$ from

$$\widehat{\mathcal{S}}_{\tau 1}\{u|\tau_1, x_{1r}, d_1(x_{1r})\},$$

where $\tau_1 = 0$. If $u_{T1,r} < u_{\tau 1,r}$, then stop and take $t_r = u_{T1,r}$; otherwise, take $\tau_{2r} = u_{\tau 1,r}$ and continue.

3. Generate x_{2r} from

$$\widehat{p}_{X_2|T_1,X_1,A_1,T_2,\varkappa \geq 2}\{x_2|\tau_1,x_{1r},d_1(x_{1r}),\tau_{2r}\}.$$

4. Generate random $u_{T2,r}$ from

$$\widehat{\mathcal{S}}_{T2}\{u|\overline{\tau}_{2r},\overline{x}_{2r},\overline{d}_2(\overline{\tau}_{2r},\overline{x}_{2r})\},$$

and independently generate random $u_{\tau 2,r}$ from

$$\widehat{\mathcal{S}}_{\tau 2}\{u|\overline{\tau}_{2r},\overline{x}_{2r},\overline{d}_2(\overline{\tau}_{2r},\overline{x}_{2r})\},$$

where $\overline{\tau}_{2r} = (\tau_1,\tau_{2r})$ and $\overline{x}_{2r} = (x_{1r},x_{2r})$. If $u_{T2,r} < u_{\tau 2,r}$, then stop and take $t_r = \tau_{2r} + u_{T2,r}$; otherwise, take $\tau_{3r} = \tau_{2r} + u_{\tau 2,r}$, and continue.

5. Generate x_{3r} from

$$\widehat{p}_{X_3|\overline{T}_2,\overline{X}_2,\overline{A}_2,T_3,\varkappa \geq 3}\{x_3|\overline{\tau}_{2r},\overline{x}_{2r},\overline{d}_2(\overline{\tau}_{2r},\overline{x}_{2r}),\tau_{3r}\}.$$

6. Continue in this fashion for $k = 3,\ldots,K-1$:

   Generate random $u_{Tk,r}$ from

   $$\widehat{\mathcal{S}}_{Tk}\{u|\overline{\tau}_{kr},\overline{x}_{kr},\overline{d}_k(\overline{\tau}_{kr},\overline{x}_{kr})\},$$

   and independently generate random $u_{\tau k,r}$ from

   $$\widehat{\mathcal{S}}_{\tau k}\{u|\overline{\tau}_{kr},\overline{x}_{rk},\overline{d}_k(\overline{\tau}_{kr},\overline{x}_{kr})\},$$

   where $\overline{\tau}_{kr} = (\tau_1,\tau_{2r},\ldots,\tau_{kr})$ and $\overline{x}_{kr} = (x_{1r},x_{2r},\ldots,x_{kr})$. If $u_{Tk,r} < u_{\tau k,r}$, then stop and take $t_r = \tau_{kr} + u_{Tk,r}$; otherwise, take $\tau_{k+1,r} = \tau_{kr} + u_{\tau k,r}$, generate $x_{k+1,r}$ from

   $$\widehat{p}_{X_{k+1}|\overline{T}_k,\overline{X}_k,\overline{A}_k,T_{k+1},\varkappa \geq k+1}\{x_k|\overline{\tau}_{kr},\overline{x}_{kr},\overline{d}_k(\overline{\tau}_{kr},\overline{x}_{kr}),\tau_{k+1,r}\}$$

   and continue.

7. If the previous step continues to $k = K-1$ and Decision K is reached, generate $u_{TK,r}$ from

$$\widehat{\mathcal{S}}_{TK}\{u|\overline{\tau}_{Kr},\overline{x}_{Kr},\overline{d}_K(\overline{\tau}_{Kr},\overline{x}_{Kr})\},$$

and take $t_r = \tau_{Kr} + u_{TK,r}$.

The values $t_1,\ldots,t_M$ are a random sample from the estimated distribution of $T^*(d)$ based on the fitted models. Given this random sample, the value $\mathcal{V}(d) = E[f\{T^*(d)\}]$ for $d \in \mathcal{D}$ is estimated by

$$\widehat{\mathcal{V}}_{GC}(d) = M^{-1}\sum_{r=1}^{M} f(t_r).$$

As in Section 5.5.1, any other functional of the distribution of $T^*(d)$ can be estimated by the analogous sample quantity.

Remark. If interest focuses on a version of $f(t)$ truncated at L, e.g., restricted lifetime $f(t) = \min(t, L)$, at the rth iteration, the foregoing algorithm can be stopped if either of τ_{kr} or t_r exceeds L, in which case take $t_r = L$.

We now discuss development and fitting of the required models for the hazards

$$\lambda_{Tk}(u|\overline{\tau}_k, \overline{x}_k, \overline{a}_k) \text{ and } \lambda_{\tau k}(u|\overline{\tau}_k, \overline{x}_k, \overline{a}_k),$$

$k = 1, \dots, K - 1$, in (8.93) and (8.94);

$$\lambda_{TK}(u|\overline{\tau}_K, \overline{x}_K, \overline{a}_K)$$

in (8.96); and the conditional densities of the covariates

$$p_{X_k|\overline{T}_{k-1}, \overline{X}_{k-1}, \overline{A}_{k-1}, T_k, \varkappa \geq k}(x_k|\overline{\tau}_{k-1}, \overline{x}_{k-1}, \overline{a}_{k-1}, \tau_k), \tag{8.110}$$

$k = 2, \dots, K$, in (8.107). Because this task, based on data without censoring, is a special case of that based on data with possibly censored event times, we discuss only the latter case. Thus, from (8.60), the available data are given by

$$(\kappa_i, \mathcal{T}_{1i}, X_{1i}, A_{1i}, \dots, \mathcal{T}_{\kappa_i i}, X_{\kappa_i i}, A_{\kappa_i i}, U_i, \Delta_i), \quad i = 1, \dots, n, \tag{8.111}$$

i.i.d. across i.

We first discuss modeling of (8.110). For $k = 2, \dots, K$, let

$$p_{X_k|\overline{T}_{k-1}, \overline{X}_{k-1}, \overline{A}_{k-1}, T_k, \kappa \geq k}(x_k|\overline{\tau}_{k-1}, \overline{x}_{k-1}, \overline{a}_{k-1}, \tau_k) \tag{8.112}$$

be the density of X_k given $\overline{X}_{k-1}$, $\overline{A}_{k-1}$, $\overline{T}_k$, and $\kappa \geq k$. This density differs from that in (8.110) through conditioning on $\kappa \geq k$ rather than $\varkappa \geq k$, so that (8.112) is identifiable from the censored data (8.111), as $\overline{X}_{k-1}$, $\overline{A}_{k-1}$, and $\overline{T}_k$ are observed if an individual reaches the kth decision point without experiencing the event or censoring. Under the assumption of noninformative censoring (8.68), it can be shown that (8.110) and (8.112) are in fact equivalent; we defer demonstration of this result to Section 8.5.

Accordingly, models for the densities (8.110) required for implementation of the g-computation algorithm above can be obtained as models for the densities (8.112), which can be fitted based on the observed, censored data (8.111), as can, of course, a model for $p_{X_1}(x_1)$. Development of these models involves the same considerations discussed in Section 5.5.1, which we do not repeat here. As in that section, X_k,

$k = 1, \ldots, K$, may involve both continuous and discrete components and may be high dimensional, in which case the analyst can choose to factorize these densities and develop models for each component of the factorization, analogous to (5.52) and (5.53).

As in Section 5.5.1, denote parametric models for $p_{X_1}(x_1)$ and (8.112) in terms of finite-dimensional parameters ζ_k, $k = 1, \ldots, K$, as

$$p_{X_1}(x_1; \zeta_1), \tag{8.113}$$

$$p_{X_k | \overline{\mathcal{T}}_{k-1}, \overline{X}_{k-1}, \overline{A}_{k-1}, \mathcal{T}_k, \kappa \geq k}(x_k | \overline{\mathcal{T}}_{k-1}, \overline{x}_{k-1}, \overline{a}_{k-1}, \mathcal{T}_k; \zeta_k), \tag{8.114}$$

$$k = 2, \ldots, K.$$

Taking the parameters ζ_k, $k = 1, \ldots, K$, to be nonoverlapping (variationally independent), estimators $\widehat{\zeta}_k$ can be obtained by maximizing appropriate likelihoods for each $k = 1, \ldots, K$. The estimator $\widehat{\zeta}_1$ for ζ_1 in (8.113) can be obtained by maximizing in ζ_1

$$\prod_{i=1}^{n} p_{X_1}(X_{1i}; \zeta_1);$$

and estimators $\widehat{\zeta}_k$ for ζ_k, $k = 2, \ldots, K$, can be obtained by maximizing

$$\prod_{i : \kappa_i \geq k} p_{X_k | \overline{\mathcal{T}}_{k-1}, \overline{X}_{k-1}, \overline{A}_{k-1}, \mathcal{T}_k, \kappa \geq k}(X_{ki} | \overline{\mathcal{T}}_{k-1,i}, \overline{X}_{k-1,i}, \overline{A}_{k-1,i}, \mathcal{T}_{ki}; \zeta_k)$$

in ζ_k, where, of necessity, the product is over only individuals i for whom $\kappa_i \geq k$, so who reached the kth decision point without having experienced the event or being censored. The fitted densities $\widehat{p}_{X_1}(x_1)$ and

$$\widehat{p}_{X_k | \overline{\mathcal{T}}_{k-1}, \overline{X}_{k-1}, \overline{A}_{k-1}, \mathcal{T}_k, \varkappa \geq k}(x_k | \overline{\mathcal{T}}_{k-1}, \overline{x}_{k-1}, \overline{a}_{k-1}, \mathcal{T}_k), \quad k = 2, \ldots, K,$$

in the g-computation algorithm are then given by $p_{X_1}(x_1; \widehat{\zeta}_1)$ and

$$p_{X_k | \overline{\mathcal{T}}_{k-1}, \overline{X}_{k-1}, \overline{A}_{k-1}, \mathcal{T}_k, \kappa \geq k}(x_k | \overline{\mathcal{T}}_{k-1}, \overline{x}_{k-1}, \overline{a}_{k-1}, \mathcal{T}_k; \widehat{\zeta}_k), \quad k = 2, \ldots, K,$$

respectively.

Development and fitting of models for the cause-specific hazard functions in (8.93), (8.94), and (8.96) is facilitated by the following definitions. For $k = 2, \ldots, K$, let

$$S_k^{\dagger} = \mathrm{I}(\kappa = k - 1)U + \mathrm{I}(\kappa \geq k)\mathcal{T}_k,$$

$$\Upsilon_k^{\dagger} = 1 \qquad \text{if } \kappa = k - 1, \Delta = 1$$

$$= 0 \qquad \text{if } \kappa = k - 1, \Delta = 0 \tag{8.115}$$

$$= -1 \quad \text{if } \kappa \geq k.$$

If all K decision points are reached, so that $\kappa = K$, let

$$S_{K+1}^\dagger = I(\kappa = K)U, \quad \Upsilon_{K+1}^\dagger = I(\kappa = K)\Delta. \qquad (8.116)$$

In (8.115) and (8.116), $S_k^\dagger$, $k = 2, \ldots, K$, is the minimum of the time to the event, time to reaching the kth decision point, or time to censoring of the event time, whichever comes first; and $\Upsilon_k^\dagger$ is the associated indicator. These quantities are relevant only to individuals for whom $\kappa \geq k - 1$. For individuals who reach the final, Kth decision point, $S_{K+1}^\dagger = U$ and $\Upsilon_{K+1}^\dagger = \Delta$. Then define the conditional cause-specific hazards in the presence of censoring, analogous to (8.93), (8.94), and (8.96),

$$\lambda_{Tk}^\dagger(u|\overline{\mathcal{T}}_k, \overline{x}_k, \overline{a}_k) \qquad (8.117)$$
$$= \lim_{du \to 0} du^{-1} P(\tau_k + u \leq S_{k+1}^\dagger < \tau_k + u + du, \Upsilon_{k+1}^\dagger = 1 \mid$$
$$S_{k+1}^\dagger \geq \tau_k + u, \overline{\mathcal{T}}_k = \overline{\tau}_k, \overline{X}_k = \overline{x}_k, \overline{A}_k = \overline{a}_k, \kappa \geq k),$$

$$\lambda_{\tau k}^\dagger(u|\overline{\mathcal{T}}_k, \overline{x}_k, \overline{a}_k) \qquad (8.118)$$
$$= \lim_{du \to 0} du^{-1} P(\tau_k + u \leq S_{k+1}^\dagger < \tau_k + u + du, \Upsilon_{k+1}^\dagger = -1 \mid$$
$$S_{k+1}^\dagger \geq \tau_k + u, \overline{\mathcal{T}}_k = \overline{\tau}_k, \overline{X}_k = \overline{x}_k, \overline{A}_k = \overline{a}_k, \kappa \geq k),$$

for $k = 1 \ldots, K - 1$; and

$$\lambda_{TK}^\dagger(u|\overline{\mathcal{T}}_K, \overline{x}_K, \overline{a}_K) \qquad (8.119)$$
$$= \lim_{du \to 0} du^{-1} P(\tau_K + u \leq S_{K+1}^\dagger < \tau_K + u + du, \Upsilon_{K+1}^\dagger = 1 \mid$$
$$S_{K+1}^\dagger \geq \tau_K + u, \overline{\mathcal{T}}_K = \overline{\tau}_K, \overline{X}_K = \overline{x}_K, \overline{A}_K = \overline{a}_K, \kappa = K).$$

As for (8.110) and (8.112) above, it is possible to show that, under the assumption of noninformative censoring, (8.93) and (8.117), (8.94) and (8.118), and (8.96) and (8.119), respectively, are equivalent; see Section 8.5. The cause-specific hazard functions (8.117)–(8.119) are clearly identifiable from the observed, censored data. Consequently, models for the hazards (8.93), (8.94), and (8.96) required for implementation of the g-computation algorithm can be obtained as models for these cause-specific hazards and fitted using the observed data (8.111).

One can posit parametric models

$$\lambda_{Tk}^\dagger(u|\overline{\mathcal{T}}_k, \overline{x}_k, \overline{a}_k; \beta_{Tk}), \quad k = 1, \ldots, K, \qquad (8.120)$$
$$\lambda_{\tau k}^\dagger(u|\overline{\mathcal{T}}_k, \overline{x}_k, \overline{a}_k; \beta_{\tau k}), \quad k = 1, \ldots, K - 1 \qquad (8.121)$$

say, in terms of finite-dimensional parameters β_{Tk} and $\beta_{\tau k}$, respectively.

Because from (8.117)–(8.119) these are models for hazard functions corresponding to possibly censored "added life," which here is the additional time to the event or the $(k+1)$th decision point, whichever comes first, given that an individual reaches Decision k at time $\mathcal{T}_k$, it is possible to use standard survival analysis methods to fit (8.120) and (8.121) for each k based on the following data. For $k = 1, \ldots, K$, for individuals i for whom $\kappa_i \geq k$, define

$$U_{ki}^\dagger = S_{k+1,i}^\dagger - \mathcal{T}_{ki}, \quad \Delta_{Tki}^\dagger = \mathrm{I}(\Upsilon_{k+1,i}^\dagger = 1), \quad \Delta_{\tau ki}^\dagger = \mathrm{I}(\Upsilon_{k+1,i}^\dagger = -1).$$

Here, $U_k^\dagger$ is observed, possibly censored "added life," and $\Delta_{Tki}^\dagger$ and $\Delta_{\tau ki}^\dagger$ indicate whether or not $S_{k+1i}^\dagger$ is the time to event or the time to Decision $k+1$, respectively. Then, for $k = 1, \ldots, K$, β_{Tk} can be estimated by maximizing the likelihood

$$\prod_{i:\kappa_i \geq k} \mathcal{S}_{Tk}^\dagger(U_{ki}^\dagger | \overline{\mathcal{T}}_{ki}, \overline{X}_{ki}, \overline{A}_{ki}; \beta_{Tk}) \left\{ \lambda_{Tk}^\dagger(U_{ki}^\dagger | \overline{\mathcal{T}}_{ki}, \overline{X}_{ki}, \overline{A}_{ki}; \beta_{Tk}) \right\}^{\Delta_{Tki}^\dagger},$$

where, similar to (8.108),

$$\mathcal{S}_{Tk}^\dagger(u | \overline{\mathcal{T}}_k, \overline{x}_k, \overline{a}_k; \beta_{Tk}) = \exp\left\{ -\int_0^u \lambda_{Tk}^\dagger(w | \overline{\mathcal{T}}_k, \overline{x}_k, \overline{a}_k; \beta_{Tk})\, dw \right\}.$$

This can be carried out using standard survival analysis software implementing likelihood methods treating $(\overline{\mathcal{T}}_k, \overline{X}_k, \overline{A}_k)$ as "baseline" covariates. Likewise, for $k = 1, \ldots, K-1$, $\beta_{\tau k}$ can be estimated by maximizing

$$\prod_{i:\kappa_i \geq k} \mathcal{S}_{\tau k}^\dagger(U_{ki}^\dagger | \overline{\mathcal{T}}_{ki}, \overline{X}_{ki}, \overline{A}_{ki}; \beta_{\tau k}) \left\{ \lambda_{\tau k}^\dagger(U_{ki}^\dagger | \overline{\mathcal{T}}_{ki}, \overline{X}_{ki}, \overline{A}_{ki}; \beta_{\tau k}) \right\}^{\Delta_{\tau ki}^\dagger},$$

$$\mathcal{S}_{\tau k}^\dagger(u | \overline{\mathcal{T}}_k, \overline{x}_k, \overline{a}_k; \beta_{\tau k}) = \exp\left\{ -\int_0^u \lambda_{\tau k}^\dagger(w | \overline{\mathcal{T}}_k, \overline{x}_k, \overline{a}_k; \beta_{\tau k})\, dw \right\}$$

as in (8.109).

Alternatively, as in the single decision case in Section 8.2, representing each of (8.120) and (8.121) by semiparametric proportional hazards regression models is a natural choice. Writing $(\overline{\mathcal{T}}_k, \overline{x}_k, \overline{a}_k) = (h_k, a_k)$, these models take the form

$$\lambda_{Tk}^\dagger(u | \overline{\mathcal{T}}_k, \overline{x}_k, \overline{a}_k; \beta_{Tk}) = \lambda_{Tk0}(u) \exp\{g_{Tk}(h_k, a_k; \xi_{Tk})\}, \qquad (8.122)$$

$$\lambda_{\tau k}^\dagger(u | \overline{\mathcal{T}}_k, \overline{x}_k, \overline{a}_k; \beta_{\tau k}) = \lambda_{\tau k0}(u) \exp\{g_{\tau k}(h_k, a_k; \xi_{\tau k})\}, \qquad (8.123)$$

where $\lambda_{Tk0}(u)$ and $\lambda_{\tau k0}(u)$ are arbitrary baseline hazard functions; $g_{Tk}(h_k, a_k; \xi_{Tk})$ and $g_{\tau k}(h_k, a_k; \xi_{\tau k})$ are functions of h_k and a_k depending on finite-dimensional parameters ξ_{Tk} and $\xi_{\tau k}$, respectively; and β_{Tk}

$= \{\lambda_{Tk0}(\cdot), \xi_{Tk}^T\}^T$ and $\beta_{\tau k} = \{\lambda_{\tau k0}(\cdot), \xi_{\tau k}^T\}^T$. For example, with two treatment options $a_k = 0, 1$ feasible for all individuals at Decision k, the analyst might specify

$$g_{Tk}(h_k, a_k; \xi_{Tk}) = \xi_{Tk1}^T h_k + \xi_{Tk2} a_k + \xi_{Tk3}^T h_k a_k,$$

$\xi_{Tk} = (\xi_{Tk1}^T, \xi_{Tk2}, \xi_{Tk3}^T)^T$, and similarly for $g_{\tau k}(h_k, a_k; \xi_{\tau k})$.

Models such as (8.122) and (8.123) for each k can be fitted using standard software implementing proportional hazards regression, treating $(\overline{\mathcal{T}}_k, \overline{X}_k, \overline{A}_k)$ as "baseline" covariates. For each $k = 1, \ldots, K$, ξ_{Tk} can be estimated based on the data $(\overline{\mathcal{T}}_{ki}, \overline{X}_{ki}, \overline{A}_{ki}, U_{ki}^\dagger, \Delta_{Tki}^\dagger)$ for $\{i : \kappa_i \geq k\}$ by $\widehat{\xi}_{Tk}$ maximizing the usual partial likelihood (Cox, 1972, 1975), and $\lambda_{Tk0}(\cdot)$ can be estimated via the Breslow estimator $\widehat{\lambda}_{Tk0}(\cdot)$ (Breslow, 1972). Similarly, for $k = 1, \ldots, K - 1$, $\xi_{\tau k}$ and $\widehat{\lambda}_{\tau k0}(\cdot)$ can be estimated via these methods based on the data $(\overline{\mathcal{T}}_{ki}, \overline{X}_{ki}, \overline{A}_{ki}, U_{ki}^\dagger, \Delta_{\tau ki}^\dagger)$ for $\{i : \kappa_i \geq k\}$, $k = 1, \ldots, K - 1$.

Remark. As noted in Section 8.2.2 for the single decision case, if interest focuses on $f(t)$ truncated at L, fitting of these models is carried out directly based on the observed data as described in the preceding paragraph, with no modification.

Letting $\widehat{\beta}_{Tk}$ and $\widehat{\beta}_{\tau k}$ denote estimators for β_{Tk} and $\beta_{\tau k}$ in the posited parametric or semiparametric models above, the fitted models

$$\widehat{\lambda}_{Tk}(u|\overline{\tau}_k, \overline{x}_k, \overline{a}_k) \text{ and } \widehat{\lambda}_{\tau k}(u|\overline{\tau}_k, \overline{x}_k, \overline{a}_k)$$

and thus

$$\widehat{\mathcal{S}}_{Tk}(u|\overline{\tau}_k, \overline{x}_k, \overline{a}_k) \text{ and } \widehat{\mathcal{S}}_{\tau k}(u|\overline{\tau}_k, \overline{x}_k, \overline{a}_k)$$

required for the g-computation algorithm can be taken to be

$$\lambda_{Tk}^\dagger(u|\overline{\tau}_k, \overline{x}_k, \overline{a}_k; \widehat{\beta}_{Tk}) \text{ and } \lambda_{\tau k}^\dagger(u|\overline{\tau}_k, \overline{x}_k, \overline{a}_k; \widehat{\beta}_{\tau k})$$

and

$$\mathcal{S}_{Tk}^\dagger(u|\overline{\tau}_k, \overline{x}_k, \overline{a}_k; \widehat{\beta}_{Tk}) \text{ and } \mathcal{S}_{\tau k}^\dagger(u|\overline{\tau}_k, \overline{x}_k, \overline{a}_k; \widehat{\beta}_{\tau k}),$$

respectively.

Remark. For the same reasons outlined in Section 5.5.1, although conceptually straightforward, estimation via the g-computation algorithm can be challenging in practice. As discussed there, development of the necessary models (8.113) and (8.114) for the baseline and intervening information when $x_1, \ldots, x_K$ involve complex components and are high dimensional can be daunting and involves the considerations noted above. Simulation of random deviates from these fitted distributions can be complicated in itself. In the current context, models for the cause-specific hazards (8.117)–(8.119) are also required, along with a means to simulate from the implied estimated survival distributions. Finally, obtaining approximate measures of uncertainty for $\widehat{\mathcal{V}}_{GC}(d)$ is not straightforward; use of the bootstrap for this purpose, as discussed in Section 5.5.1, would be computationally demanding.

Accordingly, estimation of the value of a fixed regime $d \in \mathcal{D}$ using this approach is not common in practice. Moreover, as noted in Section 5.5.1, estimation of an optimal regime $d^{opt} \in \mathcal{D}$ via maximization of $\widehat{\mathcal{V}}_{GC}(d)$ is almost certainly computationally prohibitive.

Regression-based Estimation

In Section 6.4.2, we present regression-based methods for estimating the value of a fixed regime $d \in \mathcal{D}$ when an individual treated according to the rules in d would reach all K decision points and would have the outcome of interest observed. We now discuss similar approaches to estimation of $\mathcal{V}(d) = E[f\{T^*(d)\}]$ when the outcome is a possibly censored time to an event, which must take into account that the number and timing of decision points are random.

It is instructive to consider first the case of no censoring. The approach we now describe is analogous to the backward induction strategy outlined in Section 6.4.2 and is based on a similar recursive formulation, adapted to this context. As in the rest of this chapter, we do not highlight feasible sets of treatment options, but the developments of course can be expressed more formally.

For $\varkappa = K$, define for fixed $d \in \mathcal{D}$

$$Q_K^d(h_K, a_K) = E\{f(T)|H_K = h_K, A_K = a_K, \varkappa = K\}, \qquad (8.124)$$

and let

$$V_K^d(h_K) = Q_K^d\{h_K, d_K(h_K)\}, \qquad (8.125)$$

which is (8.124) evaluated at $a_K = d_K(h_K)$. Then for $\varkappa \geq K - 1$, define

$$Q_{K-1}^d(h_{K-1}, a_{K-1}) = E\Big\{I(\varkappa = K - 1)f(T)$$

$$+ I(\varkappa = K)V_K^d(H_K) \mid H_{K-1} = h_{K-1}, A_{K-1} = a_{K-1}, \varkappa \geq K - 1\Big\},$$

$$V_{K-1}^d(h_{K-1}) = Q_{K-1}^d\{h_{K-1}, d_{K-1}(h_{K-1})\}.$$

Continuing in this fashion, for $\varkappa \geq k$, $k = K - 1, \ldots, 1$, let

$$Q_k^d(h_k, a_k) = E\Big\{I(\varkappa = k)f(T) \qquad (8.126)$$

$$+ I(\varkappa \geq k + 1)V_{k+1}^d(H_{k+1}) \mid H_k = h_k, A_k = a_k, \varkappa \geq k\Big\},$$

$$V_k^d(h_k) = Q_k^d\{h_k, d_k(h_k)\}. \tag{8.127}$$

Comparing (8.126) to (6.51) shows that the definition of $Q_k^d(h_k, a_k)$ here accounts for the possibility that the event may be achieved following Decision k, so that Decision $k+1$ and subsequent decision points are not reached.

It is shown in Section 8.5 that

$$\mathcal{V}(d) = E[f\{T^*(d)\}] = E\{V_1^d(H_1)\}. \tag{8.128}$$

The result (8.128) and this formulation suggest a backward recursive algorithm for estimating the value of a given regime $d \in \mathcal{D}$ based on observed data, from (8.54),

$$(\varkappa_i, T_{1i}, X_{1i}, A_{1i}, \dots, T_{\varkappa_i i}, X_{\varkappa_i i}, A_{\varkappa_i i}, T_i,), \quad i = 1, \dots, n, \tag{8.129}$$

i.i.d. across i, by positing models for $Q_k^d(h_k, a_k)$, $k = K, K-1, \dots, 1$, keeping in mind that, for each k, the model is applicable only to individuals i for whom $\varkappa_i \geq k$.

The algorithm is similar to that in Section 6.4.2, starting at Decision K. Note that

$$
\begin{aligned}
Q_K^d(h_K, a_K) &= E\{f(T)|H_K = h_K, A_K = a_K, \varkappa = K\} \\
&= E[f(\tau_K) + \{f(T) - f(\tau_K)\}|H_K = h_K, A_K = a_K, \varkappa = K] \\
&= f(\tau_K) + E[\{f(T) - f(\tau_K)\}|H_K = h_K, A_K = a_K, \varkappa = K],
\end{aligned}
$$

using the fact that, from (8.59), τ_K is a component of h_K when $\varkappa = K$. This suggests that it may be more appropriate to posit a model for

$$Q_K^{R_d}(h_K, a_K) = E[\{f(T) - f(\tau_K)\}|H_K = h_K, A_K = a_K, \varkappa = K], \tag{8.130}$$

as, if $f(\cdot)$ is monotone nondecreasing, then $f(T) \geq f(\tau_K)$, so that models for (8.130) that are strictly nonnegative respect the monotonicity of $f(\cdot)$. Modeling (8.130) is also consistent with the concept of rewards in the reinforcement learning literature, as discussed in Remark (i) in Section 6.2.1, where the overall outcome is given as the sum of variables that accrue in the intervening periods between decision points. Here,

$$f(T) = f(\tau_1) + \{f(\tau_2) - f(\tau_1)\} + \cdots + \{f(T) - f(\tau_K)\},$$

so that the transformed time to the event evolves as the sum of the intervals between decisions on the transformed scale. A similar formulation is used by Goldberg and Kosorok (2012), discussed in Section 8.3.5.

Thus, at Decision K, posit a model for $Q_K^{R_d}(h_K, a_K)$ in (8.130),

$$Q_K^{R_d}(h_K, a_K; \beta_K),$$

in terms of a finite-dimensional parameter β_K; e.g., of the form

$$Q_K^{R_d}(h_K, a_K; \beta_K) = \exp\{g_K(h_K, a_K; \beta_K)\}$$

for some function $g_K(h_K, a_K; \beta_K)$, so that the model enforces strict positivity. Given such a model, estimate β_K by $\widehat{\beta}_K$ solving a suitable M-estimating equation; e.g., the OLS estimating equation

$$\sum_{i:\varkappa_i=K} \frac{\partial Q_K^{R_d}(H_{Ki}, A_{Ki}; \beta_K)}{\partial \beta_K} \left\{ f(T_i) - f(\mathcal{T}_{Ki}) - Q_K^{R_d}(H_{Ki}, A_{Ki}; \beta_K) \right\} = 0,$$

$$(8.131)$$

which involves only individuals who reached all K decision points.

Because, by construction, $Q_K^d(h_K, a_K) = f(\tau_K) + Q_K^{R_d}(h_K, a_K)$, a fitted model for $Q_K^d(h_K, a_K)$, which will be useful with the inverse probability weighted methods presented shortly, is obtained as

$$Q_K^d(h_K, a_K; \widehat{\beta}_K) = f(\tau_K) + Q_K^{R_d}(h_K, a_K; \widehat{\beta}_K),$$

and

$$V_K^d(h_K) = f(\tau_K) + Q_K^{R_d}\{h_K, d_K(h_K)\}.$$

Consequently, from above,

$$Q_{K-1}^d(h_{K-1}, a_{K-1}) = E\Big\{ \mathrm{I}(\varkappa = K-1)f(T)$$

$$+ \mathrm{I}(\varkappa = K)V_K^d(H_K) \mid H_{K-1} = h_{K-1}, A_{K-1} = a_{K-1}, \varkappa \geq K-1 \Big\}$$

$$= f(\tau_{K-1}) + E\Big(\mathrm{I}(\varkappa = K-1)f(T)$$

$$+ \mathrm{I}(\varkappa = K)[f(\tau_K) + Q_K^{R_d}\{h_K, d_K(h_K)\}]$$

$$- f(\tau_{K-1}) | H_{K-1} = h_{K-1}, A_{K-1} = a_{K-1}, \varkappa \geq K-1 \Big),$$

using the fact that, from (8.59), τ_{K-1} is a component of h_{K-1} when $\varkappa \geq K-1$. Thus, define

$$Q_{K-1}^{R_d}(h_{K-1}, a_{K-1})$$

$$= E\Big(\mathrm{I}(\varkappa = K-1)f(T) + \mathrm{I}(\varkappa = K)[f(\tau_K) + Q_K^{R_d}\{h_K, d_K(h_K)\}]$$

$$- f(\tau_{K-1}) | H_{K-1} = h_{K-1}, A_{K-1} = a_{K-1}, \varkappa \geq K-1 \Big), \quad (8.132)$$

so that

$$Q_{K-1}^{R_d}(h_{K-1}, a_{K-1}) = Q_{K-1}^d(h_{K-1}, a_{K-1}) - f(\tau_{K-1}).$$

These developments suggest positing a model

$$Q_{K-1}^{R_d}(h_{K-1}, a_{K-1}; \beta_{K-1})$$

for $Q_{K-1}^{R_d}(h_{K-1}, a_{K-1})$ in (8.132), enforcing strict positivity as above, in terms of a finite-dimensional parameter β_{K-1}. Then, defining the pseudo outcomes

$$\widetilde{V}_{Ki}^{R_d} = \mathrm{I}(\varkappa_i = K - 1)f(T_i)$$
$$+ \mathrm{I}(\varkappa_i = K)[f(\mathcal{T}_{Ki}) + Q_K^{R_d}\{H_{Ki}, d_K(H_{Ki}); \widehat{\beta}_K\}]$$
$$- f(\mathcal{T}_{K-1,i}) \quad \text{for } i : \varkappa_i \geq K - 1,$$

obtain the estimator $\widehat{\beta}_{K-1}$ for β_{K-1} by solving a suitable M-estimating equation, such as

$$\sum_{i:\varkappa_i \geq K-1} \left[\frac{\partial Q_{K-1}^{R_d}(H_{K-1,i}, A_{K-1,i}; \beta_{K-1})}{\partial \beta_{K-1}} \right.$$
$$\left. \times \left\{ \widetilde{V}_{Ki}^{R_d} - Q_{K-1}^{R_d}(H_{K-1,i}, A_{K-1,i}; \beta_{K-1}) \right\} \right] = 0,$$

involving individuals who reached Decision $K - 1$. Similar to $k = K$ above, obtain the fitted model

$$Q_{K-1}^d(h_{K-1}, a_{K-1}; \widehat{\beta}_{K-1}) = f(\tau_{K-1}) + Q_{K-1}^{R_d}(h_{K-1}, a_{K-1}; \widehat{\beta}_{K-1}),$$

and it follows that

$$V_{K-1}^d(h_{K-1}) = f(\tau_{K-1}) + Q_{K-1}^{R_d}\{h_{K-1}, d_{K-1}(h_{K-1})\}.$$

Thus, define the pseudo outcomes

$$\widetilde{V}_{K-1,i}^{R_d} = \mathrm{I}(\varkappa_i = K - 2)f(T_i)$$
$$+ \mathrm{I}(\varkappa_i \geq K - 1)[f(\mathcal{T}_{K-1,i}) + Q_{K-1}^{R_d}\{H_{K-1,i}, d_{K-1}(H_{K-1,i}); \widehat{\beta}_{K-1}\}]$$
$$- f(\mathcal{T}_{K-2,i}) \quad \text{for } i : \varkappa_i \geq K - 2.$$

Continuing in this fashion for $k = K - 1, \ldots, 1$, defining recursively

$$Q_k^{R_d}(h_k, a_k) = Q_k^d(h_k, a_k) - f(\tau_k),$$

and positing strictly positive models

$$Q_k^{R_d}(h_k, a_k; \beta_k)$$

in terms of finite-dimensional β_k, obtain the estimator $\widehat{\beta}_k$ for β_k by solving

$$\sum_{i:\varkappa_i \geq k} \frac{\partial Q_k^{R_d}(H_{ki}, A_{ki}; \beta_k)}{\partial \beta_k} \left\{ \widetilde{V}_{k+1,i}^{R_d} - Q_k^{R_d}(H_{ki}, A_{ki}; \beta_k) \right\} = 0,$$

where the pseudo outcomes

$$\widetilde{V}_{k+1,i}^{R_d} = I(\varkappa_i = k)f(T_i) + I(\varkappa_i \geq k+1)[f(\mathcal{T}_{k+1,i})$$
$$+ Q_{k+1}^{R_d}\{H_{k+1,i}, d_{k+1}(H_{k+1,i}); \widehat{\beta}_{k+1}\}] - f(\mathcal{T}_{k,i}) \quad \text{for } i : \varkappa_i \geq k,$$

$$V_k^d(h_k) = f(\tau_k) + Q_k^{R_d}\{h_k, d_k(h_k)\},$$

and

$$Q_k^d(h_k, a_k; \widehat{\beta}_k) = f(\tau_k) + Q_k^{R_d}(h_k, a_k; \widehat{\beta}_k).$$

Finally, let

$$\widetilde{V}_{1i}^d = f(\mathcal{T}_{1i}) + Q_1^{R_d}\{H_{1i}, d_1(H_{1i}); \widehat{\beta}_1\} = f(0) + Q_1^{R_d}\{H_{1i}, d_1(H_{1i}); \widehat{\beta}_1\},$$

where, ordinarily, $f(0) = 0$. The estimator for the value $\mathcal{V}(d) = E[f\{T^*(d)\}]$ is then given by

$$\widehat{\mathcal{V}}_Q(d) = n^{-1} \sum_{i=1}^{n} \widetilde{V}_{1i}^d. \tag{8.133}$$

Remark. When interest focuses on a truncated version of $f(t)$ such as restricted lifetime, $f(t) = \min(t, L)$, this formulation must be modified. Analogous to (8.85) in the case of censoring, define

$$\varkappa^L = \max_k\{k = 1, \ldots, \varkappa : \mathcal{T}_k \leq L\},$$

the largest decision point reached prior to the occurrence of the event or time L; and let $T^L = \min(T, L)$. In the above expressions, replace T by T^L and $\varkappa$ by $\varkappa^L$. From the definition of H_k in (8.59), it is not necessary to modify H_k, $k = 1, \ldots, K$, which is relevant only when $\varkappa \geq k$.

We now describe how the foregoing developments are revised to take censoring of the event time into account. As for the single decision case in Section 8.2.3, an obvious strategy is to use inverse probability of censoring estimating equations at each step of the backward recursive algorithm to estimate the parameters in models for appropriately defined functions $Q_k^{R_d}(h_k, a_k)$. Here, the observed data are as in (8.111), i.i.d.

$$(\kappa_i, \mathcal{T}_{1i}, X_{1i}, A_{1i}, \ldots, \mathcal{T}_{\kappa_i i}, X_{\kappa_i i}, A_{\kappa_i i}, U_i, \Delta_i), \quad i = 1, \ldots, n;$$

and, from (8.115), for each individual i and $k = 2, \ldots, K$, let

$$S_{ki}^\dagger = I(\kappa_i = k-1)U_i + I(\kappa_i \geq k)\mathcal{T}_{ki},$$
$$\Upsilon_{ki}^\dagger = 1 \quad \text{if } \kappa_i = k-1, \Delta_i = 1$$
$$= 0 \quad \text{if } \kappa_i = k-1, \Delta_i = 0$$
$$= -1 \quad \text{if } \kappa_i \geq k.$$

It is necessary to modify the recursive definitions in (8.124)–(8.127) as follows. Under the assumption of noninformative censoring, using (8.68), it is convenient to define for $k = 1, \ldots, K$ and $\kappa \geq k$

$$
\begin{aligned}
\mathcal{K}_k(u|h_k, a_k) &= \exp\left\{ -\int_{\tau_k}^{u} \lambda_C\{w \mid h(w)\} \, dw \right\} \\
&= \exp\left\{ -\int_{\tau_k}^{u} \lambda_C(w \mid h_k, a_k) \, dw \right\}, \quad \tau_k \leq u \leq S_{k+1}^{\dagger};
\end{aligned}
\tag{8.134}
$$

when $\kappa \geq k$, τ_k is a component of h_k.

For fixed $d \in \mathcal{D}$, now define for $\kappa = K$

$$
\begin{aligned}
&Q_K^d(h_K, a_K) \\
&= E\left\{ \frac{\Delta f(U)}{\mathcal{K}_K(U|h_K, a_K)} \,\bigg|\, H_K = h_K, A_K = a_K, \kappa = K \right\},
\end{aligned}
\tag{8.135}
$$

$$
V_K^d(h_K) = Q_K^d\{h_K, d_K(h_K)\}.
\tag{8.136}
$$

For $\kappa \geq K - 1$, let

$$
\begin{aligned}
&Q_{K-1}^d(h_{K-1}, a_{K-1}) \\
&= E\left\{ \frac{\mathrm{I}(\Upsilon_K^{\dagger} = 1)f(S_K^{\dagger}) + \mathrm{I}(\Upsilon_K^{\dagger} = -1)V_K^d(H_K)}{\mathcal{K}_{K-1}(S_K^{\dagger}|h_{K-1}, a_{K-1})} \right. \\
&\qquad\qquad \left. H_{K-1} = h_{K-1}, A_{K-1} = a_{K-1}, \kappa \geq K - 1 \right\},
\end{aligned}
$$

$$
V_{K-1}^d(h_{K-1}) = Q_{K-1}^d\{h_{K-1}, d_{K-1}(h_{K-1})\}.
$$

Continuing, for $\kappa \geq k$, $k = K - 1, \ldots, 1$, let

$$
\begin{aligned}
&Q_k^d(h_k, a_k) = \\
&= E\left\{ \frac{\mathrm{I}(\Upsilon_{k+1}^{\dagger} = 1)f(S_{k+1}^{\dagger}) + \mathrm{I}(\Upsilon_{k+1}^{\dagger} = -1)V_{k+1}^d(H_{k+1})}{\mathcal{K}_k(S_{k+1}^{\dagger}|h_k, a_k)} \right. \\
&\qquad\qquad \left. H_k = h_k, A_k = a_k, \kappa \geq k \right\},
\end{aligned}
\tag{8.137}
$$

$$
V_k^d(h_k) = Q_k^d\{h_k, d_k(h_k)\}.
\tag{8.138}
$$

It is shown in Section 8.5 that

$$
\mathcal{V}(d) = E[f\{T^*(d)\}] = E\{V_1^d(H_1)\}.
\tag{8.139}
$$

Analogous to the case of no censoring, this formulation suggests a backward recursive algorithm for estimating the value of a given regime $d \in \mathcal{D}$ using the data (8.111). As with the no censoring version, it is convenient to develop models $Q_k^{R_d}(h_k, a_k; \beta_k)$ for recursively defined

$$Q_k^{R_d}(h_k, a_k) = Q_k^d(h_k, a_k) - f(\mathcal{T}_k),$$

$k = K, \dots, 1$, in terms of finite-dimensional parameters β_k. The algorithm differs from that in the no censoring case in that the estimating equation at each step involves inverse probability of censoring weighting, as we now discuss.

As in the single decision case outlined in Section 8.2.3, $\mathcal{K}_k(u|h_k, a_k)$ is not known, $k = 1, \dots, K$, so an obvious approach is to posit a model for $\lambda_C\{u \mid h(u)\}$ in (8.69), which under the noninformative censoring assumption yields a model for $\lambda_C(u \mid h_k, a_k)$ in (8.134). A typical model for $\lambda_C\{u \mid h(u)\}$ is a proportional hazards model of the form

$$\lambda_C\{u \mid h(u); \beta_C\} = \lambda_{C0}(u) \exp[g_C\{u, h(u); \xi_C\}] \qquad (8.140)$$

for unspecified baseline hazard function $\lambda_{C0}(\cdot)$ and a function $g_C\{u, h(u); \xi_C\}$ of the history and finite-dimensional parameter ξ_C, and $\beta_C = \{\lambda_{0C}(t), \xi_C^T\}^T$. For example, for $K = 3$, from (8.61), writing $H_1 = (\mathcal{T}_1, X_1)$, $H_2 = (\mathcal{T}_1, X_1, A_1, \mathcal{T}_2, X_2)$ for $\kappa \geq 2$, and $H_3 = (\mathcal{T}_1, X_1, A_1, \mathcal{T}_2, X_2, A_2, \mathcal{T}_3, X_3)$ for $\kappa = 3$, one could take

$$g_C\{u, h(u); \xi_C\} = \xi_{C1}^T \widetilde{h}_1 + \xi_{C2} a_1 + \mathrm{I}(\kappa \geq 2, \tau_2 \leq u)(\xi_{C3}^T \widetilde{h}_2 + \xi_{C4} a_2)$$
$$+ \mathrm{I}(\kappa = 3, \tau_3 \leq u)(\xi_{C5}^T \widetilde{h}_3 + \xi_{C6} a_3),$$

where $\widetilde{h}_k$ are known functions of h_k, $k = 1, 2, 3$. The model $\lambda_C\{u \mid h(u); \beta_C\}$ can be fitted using standard software for fitting proportional hazards models with time dependent covariates applied to the "data"

$$\{H_i(U_i), U_i, 1 - \Delta_i\}, \quad i = 1, \dots, n, \qquad (8.141)$$

where $H_i(U_i)$ is the history to U_i for individual i defined in (8.62), to obtain $\widehat{\beta}_C$. Substituting the fitted hazard model in (8.134) then yields the estimators

$$\widehat{\mathcal{K}}_k(u|h_k, a_k) = \exp\left\{-\int_{\mathcal{T}_k}^u \lambda_C(w \mid h_k, a_k; \widehat{\beta}_C)\, dw\right\}, \quad k = 1, \dots, K. \qquad (8.142)$$

Remarks. (i) If the data are from a well conducted SMART, it is likely that censoring is primarily administrative; that is, due to the fact that a subject has not yet experienced the event at study termination. Here, it is reasonable to assume that censoring is not only noninformative as in

(8.68) but is in fact independent of treatment assignment, patient characteristics, and potential outcomes. In this case, we can write $\lambda_C\{u|h(u)\}$ in (8.69) as

$$\lambda_C\{u|h(u)\} = \lambda_C(u|h_k, a_k) = \lambda_C(u) \quad \text{for all } u \geq 0. \tag{8.143}$$

Under (8.143), with $\mathcal{K}(u) = \exp\{-\int_0^u \lambda_C(w)\, dw\}$, (8.134) can be written for $k = 1, \ldots, K$ as $\mathcal{K}_k(u|h_k, a_k) = \mathcal{K}_k(u) = \mathcal{K}(u)/\mathcal{K}(\tau_k)$ for $\tau_k \leq u \leq S_{k+1}^\dagger$. Thus, letting $\widehat{\mathcal{K}}^{KM}(u)$ denote the Kaplan-Meier estimator for the censoring distribution, which is obtained from standard software based on the "data"

$$\{U_i, 1 - \Delta_i\}, \quad i = 1, \ldots, n,$$

similar to (8.141), an estimator for $\mathcal{K}_k(u)$ is obtained as

$$\widehat{\mathcal{K}}_k(u) = \widehat{\mathcal{K}}^{KM}(u)/\widehat{\mathcal{K}}^{KM}(\tau_k) \quad k = 1, \ldots, K. \tag{8.144}$$

The estimator (8.144) can be used in place of (8.142) in this case.

(ii) Although, as noted in the discussion of the g-computation algorithm, we characterize "added life" via the cause-specific hazard functions (8.93), (8.94), and (8.96) and (8.117)–(8.119), we do not adopt such a formulation for the hazard of censoring. This is because the setting in Remark (i) above, in which censoring is primarily administrative, is common in practice. Here, we expect (8.143) to hold. Consistency of the estimators for $\mathcal{V}(d)$ discussed here and later in this chapter involving inverse weighting by estimators for $\mathcal{K}_k(u|h_k, a_k)$ is predicated on correct modeling of the <u>censoring hazard</u>. However, it is challenging if not impossible to obtain an estimator for the censoring hazard that respects (8.143) via an "added life" formulation; thus, such estimators would likely be incorrectly specified under this condition. Accordingly, we model the hazard of censoring directly as described above.

At Decision K, analogous to (8.131), estimate β_K by $\widehat{\beta}_K$ solving the <u>inverse probability of censoring</u> M-estimating equation

$$\sum_{i:\kappa_i=K} \left[\frac{\Delta_i}{\widehat{\mathcal{K}}_K(U_i|H_{ki}, A_{ki})} \frac{\partial Q_K^{R_d}(H_{Ki}, A_{Ki}; \beta_K)}{\partial \beta_K} \right.$$
$$\left. \times \left\{ f(U_i) - f(\mathcal{T}_{Ki}) - Q_K^{R_d}(H_{Ki}, A_{Ki}; \beta_K) \right\} \right] = 0, \tag{8.145}$$

which involves only individuals who reached all K decision points. In Section 8.5, we show that (8.145) is an unbiased estimating equation. A fitted model for $Q_K^d(h_K, a_K)$ is then obtained as

$$Q_K^d(h_K, a_K; \widehat{\beta}_K) = f(\tau_K) + Q_K^{R_d}(h_K, a_K; \widehat{\beta}_K).$$

As in the case of no censoring, define pseudo outcomes for individuals i for whom $\kappa_i \geq K - 1$ and $\Upsilon^\dagger_{K,i} \neq 0$ as

$$
\begin{aligned}
\tilde{V}^{R_d}_{K,i} = {} & I(\Upsilon^\dagger_{Ki} = 1) f(S^\dagger_{Ki}) \\
& + I(\Upsilon^\dagger_{Ki} = -1)[f(S^\dagger_{Ki}) + Q^{R_d}_K \{H_{Ki}, d_K(H_{Ki}); \widehat{\beta}_K\}] \\
& - f(\mathcal{T}_{K-1,i}) \quad \text{for } i : \kappa_i \geq K - 1, \Upsilon^\dagger_{K,i} \neq 0.
\end{aligned}
$$

Then estimate β_{K-1} in the model $Q^{R_d}_{K-1}(h_{K-1}, a_{K-1}; \beta_{K-1})$ by solving

$$
\sum_{i:\kappa_i \geq K-1} \left[\frac{I(\Upsilon^\dagger_{Ki} \neq 0)}{\widehat{\mathcal{K}}_{K-1}(S^\dagger_{Ki}|H_{K-1,i}, A_{K-1,i})} \frac{\partial Q^{R_d}_{K-1}(H_{K-1,i}, A_{K-1,i}; \beta_{K-1})}{\partial \beta_{K-1}} \right.
$$

$$
\left. \times \left\{ \tilde{V}^{R_d}_{Ki} - Q^{R_d}_{K-1}(H_{K-1,i}, A_{K-1,i}; \beta_{K-1}) \right\} \right] = 0, \qquad (8.146)
$$

based on individuals who reach Decision $K - 1$, to obtain $\widehat{\beta}_{K-1}$. That (8.146) is an unbiased estimating equation follows by an argument similar to that for (8.145). A fitted model for $Q^d_{K-1}(h_{K-1}, a_{K-1})$ is then

$$
Q^d_{K-1}(h_{K-1}, a_{K-1}; \widehat{\beta}_{K-1}) = f(\tau_{K-1}) + Q^{R_d}_{K-1}(h_{K-1}, a_{K-1}; \widehat{\beta}_{K-1}).
$$

In general, for $k = K - 1, \ldots, 1$, obtain the estimator $\widehat{\beta}_k$ for the parameter β_k in the model $Q^{R_d}_k(h_k, a_k; \beta_k)$ by solving

$$
\sum_{i:\kappa_i \geq k} \left[\frac{I(\Upsilon^\dagger_{k+1,i} \neq 0)}{\widehat{\mathcal{K}}_k(S^\dagger_{k+1,i}|H_{ki}, A_{ki})} \frac{\partial Q^{R_d}_k(H_{ki}, A_{ki}; \beta_k)}{\partial \beta_k} \right.
$$

$$
\left. \times \left\{ \tilde{V}^{R_d}_{k+1,i} - Q^{R_d}_k(H_{ki}, A_{ki}; \beta_k) \right\} \right] = 0, \qquad (8.147)
$$

where

$$
\begin{aligned}
\tilde{V}^{R_d}_{k+1,i} = {} & I(\Upsilon^\dagger_{k+1,i} = 1) f(S^\dagger_{k+1,i}) \\
& + I(\Upsilon^\dagger_{k+1,i} = -1)[f(S^\dagger_{k+1,i}) + Q^{R_d}_{k+1}\{H_{k+1,i}, d_{k+1}(H_{k+1,i}); \widehat{\beta}_{k+1}\}] \\
& - f(\mathcal{T}_{ki}) \quad \text{for } i : \kappa_i \geq k, \Upsilon^\dagger_{k+1,i} \neq 0.
\end{aligned}
$$

A fitted model for $Q^d_k(h_k, a_k)$ is given by

$$
Q^d_k(h_k, a_k; \widehat{\beta}_k) = f(\tau_k) + Q^{R_d}_k(h_k, a_k; \widehat{\beta}_k).
$$

At the final step, define

$$
\tilde{V}^d_{1i} = f(\mathcal{T}_{1i}) + Q^{R_d}_1 \{H_{1i}, d_1(H_{1i}); \widehat{\beta}_1\} = f(0) + Q^{R_d}_1 \{H_{1i}, d_1(H_{1i}); \widehat{\beta}_1\},
$$

and, analogous to (8.133), obtain the estimator for the value as

$$\widehat{\mathcal{V}}_Q(d) = n^{-1} \sum_{i=1}^{n} \widetilde{V}_{1i}^d.$$

Remarks. (i) As with no censoring, if interest focuses on $f(t)$ truncated at time L, define κ^L as in (8.85) to be the largest decision point reached before the event time, censoring time, or L, whichever comes first. Let

$$\begin{aligned} U^L &= \min(U, L), \\ \Delta^L &= \Delta \quad \text{if } U \leq L, \\ &= 1 \quad \text{if } U > L, \end{aligned} \tag{8.148}$$

so that U^L is the minimum of the event time, censoring time, and L; and $\Delta^L = 1$ if the event time or L is reached before an individual is censored, and $\Delta^L = 0$ otherwise. For $k = 2, \ldots, K$, let

$$\begin{aligned} S_k^{\dagger\, L} &= \mathrm{I}(\kappa^L = k - 1)U^L + \mathrm{I}(\kappa^L \geq k)\mathcal{T}_k, \\ \Upsilon_k^{\dagger\, L} &= 1 \quad \text{if } \kappa^L = k - 1, \Delta^L = 1 \\ &= 0 \quad \text{if } \kappa^L = k - 1, \Delta^L = 0 \\ &= -1 \quad \text{if } \kappa^L \geq k, \end{aligned} \tag{8.149}$$

$$S_{K+1}^{\dagger\, L} = \mathrm{I}(\kappa^L = K)U^L, \quad \Upsilon_{K+1}^{\dagger\, L} = \mathrm{I}(\kappa^L = K)\Delta^L.$$

Then in the estimating equations (8.145)–(8.147) and the definition of the pseudo outcomes at each step, replace κ, U, Δ, $S_k^\dagger$, and $\Upsilon_k^\dagger$ by κ^L, U^L, Δ^L, $S_k^{\dagger\, L}$, and $\Upsilon_k^{\dagger\, L}$, respectively. Because H_k, $k = 1, \ldots, K$, is relevant only for individuals for whom $\kappa \geq k$, no modification of the definition of H_k in (8.61) is necessary.

Fitting of the censoring hazard model $\lambda_C\{u|h(u); \beta_C\}$ should be carried out using the "data" (8.141).

(ii) As noted previously, in this chapter we do not present methodological developments with formal acknowledgment of feasible sets of treatment options, as in Section 6.2.2. In the case where there are feasible sets of options corresponding to different histories h_k at Decision k, $k = 1, \ldots, K$, specification of the models $Q_k^{R_d}(h_k, a_k; \beta_k)$, $k = 1, \ldots, K$, involves the same modeling strategies discussed in Remark (iii) of Section 6.4.2.

Hybrid Estimators

The regression-based approach via inverse probability of censoring weighted estimating equations presented above requires the analyst to develop models for the functions $Q_k^d(h_k, a_k)$ through models for

$Q_k^{R_d}(h_k, a_k)$ and, in the likely case of possible censoring of the event time, for the hazard of censoring $\lambda_C\{u|H(u)\}$. All of these models must be correctly specified to ensure consistent estimation of the value functions $V_k^d(h_k)$ and thus, ultimately, of the value $\mathcal{V}(d)$ for fixed $d \in \mathcal{D}$. Even if the models for $Q_k^{R_d}(h_k, a_k)$ are correct, when the event time is possibly censored, it is critical that the model for the censoring hazard upon which inverse weighting is based also is specified correctly. In principle, some robustness to model misspecification could be achieved by derivation of augmented inverse probability of censoring weighted estimating equations; however, this is quite involved and is not pursued here.

We now propose an alternative approach that involves developing models for the cause-specific hazard functions $\lambda_{Tk}(u|\overline{\tau}_k, \overline{x}_k, \overline{a}_k)$ and $\lambda_{\tau k}(u|\overline{\tau}_k, \overline{x}_k, \overline{a}_k)$, $k = 1, \dots, K-1$, and $\lambda_{TK}(u|\overline{\tau}_K, \overline{x}_K, \overline{a}_K)$ defined in (8.93), (8.94), and (8.96), which, as shown in Section 8.5, are equivalent to $\lambda_{Tk}^\dagger(u|\overline{\tau}_k, \overline{x}_k, \overline{a}_k)$ and $\lambda_{\tau k}^\dagger(u|\overline{\tau}_k, \overline{x}_k, \overline{a}_k)$, $k = 1, \dots, K-1$, and $\lambda_{TK}^\dagger(u|\overline{\tau}_K, \overline{x}_K, \overline{a}_K)$ given in (8.117)–(8.119), respectively, under the assumption of noninformative censoring (8.68). This approach does not require a model for the hazard of censoring, so that, relative to the regression-based approach, it may be less susceptible to model misspecification. However, this comes at the price of an increase in computational complexity. We refer to this strategy as a "hybrid" approach, as it integrates modeling tasks involved in the g-computation algorithm with a backward recursive scheme as in the regression-based approach.

We present first the rationale for the approach in the case of no censoring. Here, we reexpress the cause-specific hazards equivalently in terms of $(h_k, a_k) = (\overline{\tau}_k, \overline{x}_k, \overline{a}_k)$ for $\varkappa \geq k$, $k = 1, \dots, K$, as

$$\lambda_{Tk}(u|h_k, a_k) \tag{8.150}$$
$$= \lim_{du \to 0} du^{-1} P(\tau_k + u \leq S_{k+1} < \tau_k + u + du, \Upsilon_{k+1} = 1 \,|$$
$$S_{k+1} \geq \tau_k + u, H_k = h_k A_k = a_k, \varkappa \geq k),$$

$$\lambda_{\tau k}(u|h_k, a_k) \tag{8.151}$$
$$= \lim_{du \to 0} du^{-1} P(\tau_k + u \leq S_{k+1} < \tau_k + u + du, \Upsilon_{k+1} = -1 \,|$$
$$S_{k+1} \geq \tau_k + u, H_k = h_k, A_k = a_k, \varkappa \geq k),$$

for $k = 1, \dots, K-1$ and

$$\lambda_{TK}(u|h_K, a_K) \tag{8.152}$$
$$= \lim_{du \to 0} du^{-1} P(\tau_K + u \leq S_{K+1} < \tau_K + u + du, \Upsilon_{K+1} = 1 \,|$$
$$S_{K+1} \geq \tau_K + u, H_K = h_K, A_K = a_K, \varkappa = K).$$

As in (8.124), define

$$Q_K^d(h_K, a_K) = E\{f(T)|H_K = h_K, A_K = a_K, \varkappa = K\}.$$

It is straightforward that

$$Q_K^d(h_K, a_K) = \int_0^\infty f(\tau_K + w)\, dS_{TK}(w|h_K, a_K), \tag{8.153}$$

where, from (8.98) and (8.152)

$$S_{TK}(u|h_K, a_K) = \exp\left\{-\int_0^u \lambda_{TK}(w|h_K, a_K)\, dw\right\}. \tag{8.154}$$

Then, as in (8.125), define

$$V_K^d(h_K) = Q_K^d\{h_K, d_K(h_K)\}.$$

The next step is to compute

$$Q_{K-1}^d(h_{K-1}, a_{K-1}) = E\Big\{I(\varkappa = K-1)f(T)$$
$$+ I(\varkappa = K)V_K^d(H_K) \mid H_{K-1} = h_{K-1}, A_{K-1} = a_{K-1}, \varkappa \geq K-1\Big\}.$$

To this end, define

$$q_{K-1}^d(h_{K-1}, a_{K-1}, \tau_K) \tag{8.155}$$
$$= E\{V_K^d(H_K)|H_{K-1} = h_{K-1}, A_{K-1} = a_{K-1}, \mathcal{T}_K = \tau_K, \varkappa = K\},$$

which is the expected value of the event time given an individual reaches Decision K at time τ_K with history h_{K-1} and a_{K-1} and is a functional of the conditional distribution of X_K given $(H_{K-1}, A_{K-1}, \mathcal{T}_K)$ among individuals reaching Decision K. Then, using (8.155), it is straightforward to derive that

$$Q_{K-1}^d(h_{K-1}, a_{K-1}) = \int_0^\infty \Big\{f(\tau_{K-1} + w)\, S_{\bullet K-1}(w|h_{K-1}, a_{K-1})$$
$$\times \lambda_{T,K-1}(w|h_{K-1}, a_{K-1})\Big\}\, dw \tag{8.156}$$
$$+ \int_0^\infty \Big\{q_{K-1}^d(h_{K-1}, a_{K-1}, \tau_{K-1} + w)$$
$$\times S_{\bullet K-1}(w|h_{K-1}, a_{K-1})\lambda_{\tau,K-1}(w|h_{K-1}, a_{K-1})\Big\}\, dw,$$

where, from (8.97) and (8.150)–(8.151), for $k = 1, \ldots, K-1$,

$$S_{\bullet k}(u|h_k, a_k) = \exp\left[-\int_0^u \{\lambda_{Tk}(w|h_k, a_k) + \lambda_{\tau k}(w|h_k, a_k)\}\, dw\right]. \tag{8.157}$$

Let

$$V_{K-1}^d(h_{K-1}) = Q_{K-1}^d\{h_{K-1}, d_{K-1}(h_{K-1})\}.$$

Continue by iteratively defining for $k = K - 1, \ldots, 1$,

$$Q_k^d(h_k, a_k) = E\Big\{\mathrm{I}(\varkappa = k)f(T)$$
$$+ \mathrm{I}(\varkappa = k+1)V_{k+1}^d(H_{k+1}) \mid H_k = h_k, A_k = a_k, \varkappa \geq k\Big\},$$

and letting

$$q_k^d(h_k, a_k, \tau_{k+1}) \tag{8.158}$$
$$= E\{V_{k+1}^d(H_{k+1})|H_k = h_k, A_k = a_k, \mathcal{T}_{k+1} = \tau_{k+1}, \varkappa \geq k+1\}$$

for $k = 1, \ldots, K - 1$, which, as above, is a functional of the conditional distribution of X_{k+1} given $(H_k, A_k, \mathcal{T}_{k+1})$ among individuals reaching Decision $k + 1$. Then

$$Q_k^d(h_k, a_k) = \int_0^\infty f(\tau_k + w)\, \mathcal{S}_{\bullet k}(w|h_k, a_k)\lambda_{Tk}(w|h_k, a_k)\, dw$$
$$+ \int_0^\infty q_k^d(h_k, a_k, \tau_k + w)\mathcal{S}_{\bullet k}(w|h_k, a_k)\lambda_{\tau k}(w|h_k, a_k)\, dw, \tag{8.159}$$

and

$$V_k^d(h_k) = Q_k^d\{h_k, d_k(h_k)\}.$$

Then the value of a given regime $d \in \mathcal{D}$ is given by

$$\mathcal{V}(d) = E[f\{T^*(d)\}] = E\{V_1^d(H_1)\}. \tag{8.160}$$

These developments suggest the following backward recursive approach to estimation of $\mathcal{V}(d)$ based on (8.160), which we present in the case of possibly censored event times, where the observed data are as in (8.111), i.i.d.

$$(\kappa_i, \mathcal{T}_{1i}, X_{1i}, A_{1i}, \ldots, \mathcal{T}_{\kappa_i i}, X_{\kappa_i i}, A_{\kappa_i i}, U_i, \Delta_i), \quad i = 1, \ldots, n,$$

as that without censoring is a special case. As noted above, under the assumption of noninformative censoring (8.68), from Section 8.5, (8.150)–(8.152) are equivalent to

$$\lambda_{Tk}^\dagger(u|h_k, a_k) \tag{8.161}$$
$$= \lim_{du \to 0} du^{-1} P(\tau_k + u \leq S_{k+1}^\dagger < \tau_k + u + du, \Upsilon_{k+1}^\dagger = 1 \mid$$
$$S_{k+1}^\dagger \geq \tau_k + u, H_k = h_k A_k = a_k, \kappa \geq k),$$

$$\lambda_{\tau k}^{\dagger}(u|h_k, a_k) \tag{8.162}$$

$$= \lim_{du \to 0} du^{-1} P(\tau_k + u \le S_{k+1}^{\dagger} < \tau_k + u + du, \Upsilon_{k+1}^{\dagger} = -1 \,|$$

$$S_{k+1}^{\dagger} \ge \tau_k + u, H_k = h_k, A_k = a_k, \kappa \ge k),$$

for $k = 1, \ldots, K - 1$ and

$$\lambda_{TK}^{\dagger}(u|h_K, a_K) \tag{8.163}$$

$$= \lim_{du \to 0} du^{-1} P(\tau_K + u \le S_{K+1}^{\dagger} < \tau_K + u + du, \Upsilon_{K+1}^{\dagger} = 1 \,|$$

$$S_{K+1}^{\dagger} \ge \tau_K + u, H_K = h_K, A_K = a_K, \kappa = K).$$

As described in the context of the g-computation algorithm, parametric models

$$\lambda_{Tk}^{\dagger}(u|h_k, a_k; \beta_{Tk}), \quad k = 1, \ldots, K, \tag{8.164}$$

$$\lambda_{\tau k}^{\dagger}(u|h_k, a_k; \beta_{\tau k}), \quad k = 1, \ldots, K - 1 \tag{8.165}$$

as in (8.120)–(8.121) or semiparametric proportional hazards models

$$\lambda_{Tk}^{\dagger}(u|h_k, a_k; \beta_{Tk}) = \lambda_{Tk0}(u) \exp\{g_{Tk}(h_k, a_k; \xi_{Tk})\}, \tag{8.166}$$

$$\lambda_{\tau k}^{\dagger}(u|h_k, a_k; \beta_{\tau k}) = \lambda_{\tau k0}(u) \exp\{g_{\tau k}(h_k, a_k; \xi_{\tau k})\}, \tag{8.167}$$

with $\beta_{Tk} = \{\lambda_{Tk0}(\cdot), \xi_{Tk}^T\}^T$ and $\beta_{\tau k} = \{\lambda_{\tau k0}(\cdot), \xi_{\tau k}^T\}^T$, as in (8.122)–(8.123), for (8.161)–(8.163) in terms of parameters β_{Tk} and $\beta_{\tau k}$ can be posited and fitted via standard survival analysis methods, yielding estimators $\widehat{\beta}_{Tk}$, $k = 1, \ldots, K$, and $\widehat{\beta}_{\tau k}$, $k = 1, \ldots, K - 1$.

The algorithm proceeds as follows. From (8.154), now let

$$\mathcal{S}_{TK}(u|h_K, a_K; \widehat{\beta}_{TK}) = \exp\left\{-\int_0^u \lambda_{TK}^{\dagger}(w|h_K, a_K; \widehat{\beta}_{TK})\, dw\right\}.$$

Thus, by (8.153), a fitted model for $Q_K^d(h_K, a_K)$ is induced as

$$Q_K^d(h_K, a_K; \widehat{\beta}_{TK}) = \int_0^{\infty} f(\tau_K + w)\, d\mathcal{S}_{TK}(w|h_K, a_K; \widehat{\beta}_{TK}).$$

Because of the equivalence of (8.110) and (8.112) demonstrated in Section 8.5, it follows that, for $k = 1, \ldots, K - 1$, $q_k^d(h_k, a_k, \tau_{k+1})$ in (8.158) is equivalent to

$$E\{V_{k+1}^d(H_{k+1})|H_k = h_k, A_k = a_k, \mathcal{T}_{k+1} = \tau_{k+1}, \kappa \ge k + 1\}.$$

Consequently, modeling and fitting of $q_k^d(h_k, a_k, \tau_{k+1})$ can be carried out using the data from all individuals i for whom $\kappa_i \geq k+1$. Thus, we consider a model for

$$q_{K-1}^d(h_{K-1}, a_{K-1}, \mathcal{T}_K)$$
$$= E\{V_K^d(H_K)|H_{K-1} = h_{K-1}, A_{K-1} = a_{K-1}, \mathcal{T}_K = \mathcal{T}_K, \kappa = K\},$$

in (8.155). Because of the constraint

$$q_{K-1}^d(h_{K-1}, a_{K-1}, \mathcal{T}_K) \geq f(\mathcal{T}_K),$$

it is appropriate to develop a model instead for

$$q_{K-1}^{R_d}(h_{K-1}, a_{K-1}, \mathcal{T}_K) = q_{K-1}^d(h_{K-1}, a_{K-1}, \mathcal{T}_K) - f(\mathcal{T}_K)$$
$$= E\{V_K^d(H_K) - f(\mathcal{T}_K)|H_{K-1} = h_{K-1}, A_{K-1} = a_{K-1}, \mathcal{T}_K = \mathcal{T}_K, \kappa = K\},$$

$q_{K-1}^{R_d}(h_{K-1}, a_{K-1}, \mathcal{T}_K; \beta_{K-1})$, say, that enforces positivity as in the regression-based approach.

Now, based on the fitted model $\lambda_{TK}^\dagger(u|h_K, a_K; \widehat{\beta}_{TK})$ and (8.153), compute for all individuals i for whom $\kappa_i = K$, so who reached Decision K, the pseudo outcomes

$$\widetilde{V}_{Ki}^{R_d} = Q_K^d\{H_{Ki}, d_K(H_{Ki})\} - f(\mathcal{T}_{Ki})$$
$$= \int_0^\infty f(\mathcal{T}_{Ki} + w) \, d\mathcal{S}_{TK}\{w|H_{Ki}, d_K(H_{Ki}); \widehat{\beta}_{TK}\} - f(\mathcal{T}_{Ki}).$$

Then β_{K-1} can be estimated by solving a suitable M-estimating equation; e.g., the OLS equation

$$\sum_{i:\kappa_i=K} \left[\frac{\partial q_{K-1}^{R_d}(H_{K-1,i}, A_{K-1,i}, \mathcal{T}_{Ki}; \beta_{K-1})}{\partial \beta_{K-1}} \right.$$
$$\left. \times \left\{ \widetilde{V}_{Ki}^{R_d} - q_{K-1}^{R_d}(H_{K-1,i}, A_{K-1,i}, \mathcal{T}_{Ki}; \beta_{K-1}) \right\} \right] = 0$$

to obtain the estimator $\widehat{\beta}_{K-1}$, and

$$q_{K-1}^d(h_{K-1}, a_{K-1}, \mathcal{T}_K; \widehat{\beta}_{K-1}) = q_{K-1}^{R_d}(h_{K-1}, a_{K-1}, \mathcal{T}_K; \widehat{\beta}_{K-1}) + f(\mathcal{T}_K).$$

From (8.156) and (8.157), a fitted model for $Q_{K-1}^d(h_{K-1}, a_{K-1})$ is then

$$Q_{K-1}^d(h_{K-1}, a_{K-1}; \widehat{\beta}_{K-1}, \widehat{\beta}_{T,K-1}, \widehat{\beta}_{\tau,K-1})$$
$$= \int_0^\infty \left\{ f(\mathcal{T}_{K-1} + w) \, \mathcal{S}_{\bullet K-1}(w|h_{K-1}, a_{K-1}; \widehat{\beta}_{T,K-1}, \widehat{\beta}_{\tau,K-1}) \right.$$
$$\left. \times \lambda_{T,K-1}^\dagger(w|h_{K-1}, a_{K-1}; \widehat{\beta}_{T,K-1}) \right\} dw$$

$$+ \int_0^\infty \Big\{ q^d_{K-1}(h_{K-1}, a_{K-1}, \tau_{K-1} + w; \widehat{\beta}_{K-1})$$

$$\times \, \mathcal{S}_{\bullet K-1}(w | h_{K-1}, a_{K-1}; \widehat{\beta}_{T,K-1}, \widehat{\beta}_{\tau,K-1})$$

$$\times \, \lambda^\dagger_{\tau, K-1}(w | h_{K-1}, a_{K-1}; \widehat{\beta}_{\tau,K-1}) \Big\} \, dw,$$

where $\mathcal{S}_{\bullet K-1}(w | h_{K-1}, a_{K-1}; \widehat{\beta}_{T,K-1}, \widehat{\beta}_{\tau,K-1})$ is given by (8.157) with the fitted cause-specific hazard models substituted.

Next, using (8.156), compute for all individuals i for whom $\kappa_i \geq K-1$ the pseudo outcomes

$$\widetilde{V}^{R_d}_{K-1,i} = Q^d_{K-1}\{H_{K-1,i}, d_{K-1}(H_{K-1,i})\} - f(\mathcal{T}_{K-1,i})$$

$$= \int_0^\infty \Big[f(\mathcal{T}_{K-1,i} + w)$$

$$\times \, \mathcal{S}_{\bullet K-1}\{w | H_{K-1,i}, d_{K-1}(H_{K-1,i}); \widehat{\beta}_{T,K-1}, \widehat{\beta}_{\tau,K-1}\}$$

$$\times \, \lambda^\dagger_{T,K-1}\{w | H_{K-1,i}, d(H_{K-1,i}); \widehat{\beta}_{T,K-1}\} \Big] \, dw$$

$$+ \int_0^\infty \Big(\Big[q^{R_d}_{K-1}\{H_{K-1,i}, d_{K-1}(H_{K-1,i}), \mathcal{T}_{K-1,i} + w; \widehat{\beta}_{K-1}\}$$

$$+ f(\mathcal{T}_{K-1,i} + w) \Big]$$

$$\times \, \mathcal{S}_{\bullet K-1}\{w | H_{K-1,i}, d_{K-1}(H_{K-1,i}); \widehat{\beta}_{T,K-1}, \widehat{\beta}_{\tau,K-1}\}$$

$$\times \, \lambda^\dagger_{\tau,K-1}\{w | H_{K-1,i}, d_{K-1}(H_{K-1,i}); \widehat{\beta}_{\tau,K-1}\} \Big) \, dw - f(\mathcal{T}_{K-1,i}).$$

Develop a model $q^{R_d}_{K-2}(h_{K-2}, a_{K-2}, \tau_{K-1}; \beta_{K-2})$ for

$$q^{R_d}_{K-2}(h_{K-2}, a_{K-2}, \tau_{K-1}) = q^d_{K-2}(h_{K-2}, a_{K-2}, \tau_{K-1}) - f(\tau_{K-1})$$

$$= E\{V^d_{K-1}(H_{K-1}) - f(\tau_{K-1}) | H_{K-2} = h_{K-2}, A_{K-2} = a_{K-2},$$
$$\mathcal{T}_{K-1} = \tau_{K-1}, \kappa \geq K-1\},$$

and estimate β_{K-2} by solving an M-estimating equation such as

$$\sum_{i:\kappa_i \geq K-1} \left[\frac{\partial q^{R_d}_{K-2}(H_{K-2,i}, A_{K-2,i}, \mathcal{T}_{K-1,i}; \beta_{K-2})}{\partial \beta_{K-2}} \right.$$

$$\times \left. \Big\{ \widetilde{V}^{R_d}_{K-1,i} - q^{R_d}_{K-2}(H_{K-2,i}, A_{K-2,i}, \mathcal{T}_{K-1,i}; \beta_{K-2}) \Big\} \right] = 0.$$

Continuing in this fashion, for $k = K-1, \ldots, 1$, develop a model for

$$q^{R_d}_k(h_k, a_k, \tau_{k+1}) = q^d_k(h_k, a_k, \tau_{k+1}) - f(\tau_{k+1}) \tag{8.168}$$

$$= E\{V^d_{k+1}(H_{k+1}) - f(\tau_{k+1}) | H_k = h_k, A_k = a_k, \mathcal{T}_{k+1} = \tau_{k+1}, \kappa \geq k+1\},$$

$q_k^{R_d}(h_k, a_k, \tau_{k+1}; \beta_k)$, say; estimate β_k by solving

$$\sum_{i:\kappa_i \geq k+1} \left[\frac{\partial q_k^{R_d}(H_{ki}, A_{ki}, \mathcal{T}_{k+1,i}; \beta_k)}{\partial \beta_k} \right.$$

$$\left. \times \left\{ \widetilde{V}_{k+1,i}^{R_d} - q_k^{R_d}(H_{ki}, A_{ki}, \mathcal{T}_{k+1,i}; \beta_k) \right\} \right] = 0;$$

and let

$$q_k^d(h_k, a_k, \tau_{k+1}; \widehat{\beta}_k) = q_k^{R_d}(h_k, a_k, \tau_{k+1}; \widehat{\beta}_k) + f(\tau_{k+1}).$$

Then from (8.159) obtain the induced fitted model

$$Q_k^d(h_k, a_k; \widehat{\beta}_k, \widehat{\beta}_{Tk}, \widehat{\beta}_{\tau k}) = \int_0^\infty \left[f(\tau_k + w) \, \mathcal{S}_{\bullet k}(w|h_k, a_k; \widehat{\beta}_{Tk}, \widehat{\beta}_{\tau k}) \right.$$

$$\left. \times \lambda_{Tk}^\dagger(w|h_k, a_k; \widehat{\beta}_{Tk}) \right] dw$$

$$+ \int_0^\infty q_k^d(h_k, a_k, \tau_k + w; \widehat{\beta}_k) \mathcal{S}_{\bullet k}(w|h_k, a_k; \widehat{\beta}_{Tk}, \widehat{\beta}_{\tau k}) \lambda_{\tau k}^\dagger(w|h_k, a_k; \widehat{\beta}_{\tau k}) \, dw,$$

and define the pseudo outcomes for individuals i for whom $\kappa_i \geq k$ as

$$\widetilde{V}_{ki}^{R_d} = Q_k^d\{H_{ki}, d_k(H_{ki})\} - f(\mathcal{T}_{ki})$$

$$= \int_0^\infty \left[f(\mathcal{T}_{ki} + w) \, \mathcal{S}_{\bullet k}\{w|H_{ki}, d_k(H_{ki}); \widehat{\beta}_{Tk}, \widehat{\beta}_{\tau k}\} \right.$$

$$\left. \times \lambda_{Tk}^\dagger\{w|H_{ki}, d_k(H_{ki}); \widehat{\beta}_{Tk}\} \right] dw \tag{8.169}$$

$$+ \int_0^\infty \left([q_k^{R_d}\{H_{ki}, d_k(H_{ki}), \mathcal{T}_{ki} + w; \widehat{\beta}_k\} + f(\mathcal{T}_{ki} + w)] \right.$$

$$\times \mathcal{S}_{\bullet k}\{w|H_{ki}, d_k(H_{ki}); \widehat{\beta}_{Tk}, \widehat{\beta}_{\tau k}\}$$

$$\left. \times \lambda_{\tau k}^\dagger\{w|H_{ki}, d_k(H_{ki}); \widehat{\beta}_{\tau k}\} \right) dw - f(\mathcal{T}_{ki}),$$

where $\mathcal{S}_{\bullet k}(w|h_k, a_k; \widehat{\beta}_{Tk}, \widehat{\beta}_{\tau k})$ is given by (8.157) with the fitted cause-specific hazard models substituted.

For $k = 1$, from (8.169)

$$\widetilde{V}_{1i}^{R_d} = Q_1^d\{H_{1i}, d_1(H_{1i})\} - f(\mathcal{T}_{1i})$$

$$= \int_0^\infty \left[f(\mathcal{T}_{1i} + w) \, \mathcal{S}_{\bullet 1}\{w|H_{1i}, d_1(H_{1i}); \widehat{\beta}_{T1}, \widehat{\beta}_{\tau 1}\} \right.$$

$$\left. \times \lambda_{T1}^\dagger\{w|H_{1i}, d_1(H_{1i}); \widehat{\beta}_{T1}\} \right] dw$$

$$+ \int_0^\infty \Big([q_1^{R_d}\{H_{1i}, d_1(H_{1i}), \mathcal{T}_{1i} + w; \widehat{\beta}_1\} + f(\mathcal{T}_{1i} + w)]$$

$$\times \mathcal{S}_{\bullet 1}\{w|H_{1i}, d_1(H_{1i}); \widehat{\beta}_{T1}, \widehat{\beta}_{\tau1}\}$$

$$\times \lambda_{\tau 1}^\dagger\{w|H_{1i}, d_1(H_{1i}); \widehat{\beta}_{\tau 1}\} \Big) dw - f(\mathcal{T}_{1i}),$$

where $\mathcal{T}_{1i} = 0$, and ordinarily $f(0) = 0$. Defining

$$\widetilde{V}_{1i}^d = \widetilde{V}_{1i}^{R_d} + f(\mathcal{T}_{1i}),$$

from (8.160), the estimator for the value is then

$$\widehat{\mathcal{V}}_{HY}(d) = n^{-1} \sum_{i=1}^n \widetilde{V}_{1i}^d.$$

An advantage of this hybrid approach is that there is no need to develop models for the conditional densities

$$p_{X_k|\overline{\mathcal{T}}_{k-1}, \overline{X}_{k-1}, \overline{A}_{k-1}, \mathcal{T}_k, \kappa \geq k}(x_k|\overline{\mathcal{T}}_{k-1}, \overline{x}_{k-1}, \overline{a}_{k-1}, \tau_k)$$

in (8.112); instead, it suffices to posit models only for the functionals of these densities

$$q_k^d(h_k, a_k, \tau_{k+1})$$
$$= E\{V_k^d(H_k)|H_{k-1} = h_{k-1}, A_{k-1} = a_{k-1}, \mathcal{T}_k = \tau_k, \kappa \geq k\}.$$

Moreover, there is no need to model the hazard of censoring. Of course, these features come at the price of the added computational burden of deriving the pseudo outcomes (8.169).

Remarks. (i) As for the previous regression-based estimator, if interest focuses on $f(t)$ truncated at L, modifications are required. As in (8.85), define κ^L to be the largest decision point reached before the event time, censoring time, or L, whichever comes first. Define for $k = 1, \ldots, K-1$,

$$\lambda_{Tk}^{\dagger L}(u|h_k, a_k)$$
$$= \lim_{du \to 0} du^{-1} P(\tau_k + u \leq S_{k+1}^\dagger < \tau_k + u + du, \Upsilon_{k+1}^\dagger = 1 \,|$$
$$S_{k+1}^\dagger \geq \tau_k + u, H_k = h_k, A_k = a_k, \kappa^L \geq k),$$

$$\lambda_{TK}^{\dagger L}(u|h_K, a_K)$$
$$= \lim_{du \to 0} du^{-1} P(\tau_K + u \leq S_{K+1}^\dagger < \tau_K + u + du, \Upsilon_{K+1}^\dagger = 1 \,|$$
$$S_{K+1}^\dagger \geq \tau_K + u, H_K = h_K, A_K = a_K, \kappa^L = K),$$

and, from (8.162), define $\lambda_{\tau k}^{\dagger L}(u|h_k, a_k)$, $k = 1, \ldots, K-1$, similarly. Models $\lambda_{\tau k}^{\dagger L}(u|h_k, a_k; \beta_{\tau k})$ and $\lambda_{Tk}^{\dagger L}(u|h_k, a_k; \beta_{Tk})$ can then be fitted as described previously for each k based on the data for individuals i for whom $\kappa_i^L \geq k$, $k = 1, \ldots, K-1$, and $\kappa_i^L = K$ to obtain estimators $\widehat{\beta}_{\tau k}$ and $\widehat{\beta}_{Tk}$. In particular, fitting should be carried out directly using the data (8.111) with, for $k = 2, \ldots, K$,

$$S_{ki}^{\dagger} = I(\kappa_i = k - 1)U_i + I(\kappa_i \geq k)T_{ki},$$

$$\Upsilon_{ki}^{\dagger} = 1 \quad \text{if } \kappa_i = k - 1, \Delta_i = 1$$
$$= 0 \quad \text{if } \kappa_i = k - 1, \Delta_i = 0$$
$$= -1 \quad \text{if } \kappa_i \geq k,$$

with no modification, as noted in the context of the g-computation algorithm earlier. Then, with

$$S_{TK}^L(u|h_K, a_K; \widehat{\beta}_{TK}) = \exp\left\{-\int_0^u \lambda_{TK}^{\dagger L}(w|h_K, a_K; \widehat{\beta}_{TK})\, dw\right\},$$

obtain the fitted model for

$$Q_K^{d,L}(h_K, a_K) = E\{f(T)|H_K = h_K, A_K = a_K, \kappa^L = K\}$$

as

$$Q_K^{d,L}(h_K, a_K; \widehat{\beta}_{TK}) = \int_0^{L-\tau_K} f(\tau_K + w)\, dS_{TK}^L(w|h_K, a_K; \widehat{\beta}_{TK})$$
$$+ f(L)S_{TK}^L(L - \tau_K|h_K, a_K; \widehat{\beta}_{TK}), \qquad (8.170)$$

and define for individuals i for whom $\kappa_i^L = K$

$$\widetilde{V}_{Ki}^{R_d,L} = Q_K^{d,L}\{H_{Ki}, d_K(H_{Ki}); \widehat{\beta}_{TK}\} - f(T_{Ki}).$$

Given a model $q_{K-1}^{R_d,L}(h_{K-1}, a_{K-1}, \tau_K; \beta_{K-1})$ as before, estimate β_{K-1} by solving the estimating equation

$$\sum_{i:\kappa_i^L=K} \left[\frac{\partial q_{K-1}^{R_d,L}(H_{K-1,i}, A_{K-1,i}, T_{Ki}; \beta_{K-1})}{\partial \beta_{K-1}} \right.$$
$$\left. \times \left\{\widetilde{V}_{Ki}^{R_d,L} - q_{K-1}^{R_d,L}(H_{K-1,i}, A_{K-1,i}, T_{Ki}; \beta_{K-1})\right\} \right] = 0$$

to obtain the estimator $\widehat{\beta}_{K-1}$.

Continuing in this fashion for $k = K - 1, \ldots, 1$, develop models $q_k^{R_d, L}(h_k, a_k, \tau_{k+1}; \beta_k)$; estimate β_k by solving

$$\sum_{i:\kappa_i^L \geq k+1} \left[\frac{\partial q_k^{R_d, L}(H_{ki}, A_{ki}, \mathcal{T}_{k+1,i}; \beta_k)}{\partial \beta_k} \right.$$

$$\left. \times \left\{ \widetilde{V}_{k+1,i}^{R_d, L} - q_k^{R_d, L}(H_{ki}, A_{ki}, \mathcal{T}_{k+1,i}; \beta_k) \right\} \right] = 0;$$

let

$$q_k^{d, L}(h_k, a_k, \tau_{k+1}; \widehat{\beta}_k) = q_k^{R_d, L}(h_k, a_k, \tau_{k+1}; \widehat{\beta}_k) + f(\tau_{k+1});$$

and obtain fitted models for

$$Q_k^{d, L}(h_k, a_k) = E\Big\{ \mathrm{I}(\kappa^L = k) f(T)$$

$$+ \mathrm{I}(\varkappa = k + 1) V_{k+1}^d(H_{k+1}) \mid H_k = h_k, A_k = a_k, \kappa^L \geq k \Big\}$$

as

$$Q_k^{d, L}(h_k, a_k; \widehat{\beta}_k, \widehat{\beta}_{Tk}, \widehat{\beta}_{\tau k}) = \int_0^{L - \tau_k} \Big[f(\tau_k + w) \mathcal{S}_{\bullet k}^L(w | h_k, a_k; \widehat{\beta}_{Tk}, \widehat{\beta}_{\tau k})$$

$$\times \lambda_{Tk}^{\dagger L}\{w | h_k, d_k(h_k); \widehat{\beta}_{Tk}\} \Big] dw \qquad (8.171)$$

$$+ \int_0^{L - \tau_k} \Big[q_k^{d, L}(h_k, a_k, \tau_k + w; \widehat{\beta}_k) \mathcal{S}_{\bullet k}^L(w | h_k, a_k; \widehat{\beta}_{Tk}, \widehat{\beta}_{\tau k})$$

$$\times \lambda_{\tau k}^{\dagger L}\{w | h_k, d_k(h_k); \widehat{\beta}_{\tau k}\} \Big] dw + f(L) \mathcal{S}_{\bullet k}^L(L - \tau_k | h_k, a_k; \widehat{\beta}_{Tk}, \widehat{\beta}_{\tau k}).$$

In (8.171), $\mathcal{S}_{\bullet k}^L(u | h_k, a_k)$ is defined in the obvious way, and $\mathcal{S}_{\bullet k}^L(u | h_k, a_k; \widehat{\beta}_{Tk}, \widehat{\beta}_{\tau k})$ is found by substituting the fitted cause-specific hazard models. For individuals i for whom $\kappa_i^L \geq k$, the pseudo outcomes are defined as

$$\widetilde{V}_{ki}^{R_d, L} = Q_k^{d, L}\{H_{ki}, d_k(H_{ki}); \widehat{\beta}_k, \widehat{\beta}_{Tk}, \widehat{\beta}_{\tau k}\} - f(\mathcal{T}_{ki}).$$

Defining

$$\widetilde{V}_{1i}^{d, L} = \widetilde{V}_{1i}^{R_d, L} + f(\mathcal{T}_{1i}) = \widetilde{V}_{1i}^{R_d, L} + f(0),$$

from (8.160), the estimator for the value is then

$$\widehat{\mathcal{V}}_{HY}(d) = n^{-1} \sum_{i=1}^n \widetilde{V}_{1i}^{d, L}.$$

(ii) As for the regression-based approach, if there are feasible sets

$\Psi_k(h_k) \subseteq \mathcal{A}_k$ of treatment options corresponding to different histories h_k at Decision k, $k = 1, \ldots, K$, as discussed in Section 8.3.1, which we have downplayed here, specification of the models $q_k^{R_d}(h_k, a_k, \tau_{k+1}; \beta_k)$ or $q_k^{R_d, L}(h_k, a_k, \tau_{k+1}; \beta_k)$, $k = 1, \ldots, K-1$, involves the same modeling considerations discussed in Remark (iii) of Section 6.4.2.

Inverse Probability Weighted Estimators

In Sections 5.5.2, 6.4.3, and 6.4.4, we discuss simple inverse and augmented inverse probability weighted estimators for the value $\mathcal{V}(d) = E[f\{T^*(d)\}]$ of a fixed $d \in \mathcal{D}$. We now discuss how these approaches are adapted to the setting where the outcome is a possibly censored time to an event. We continue to assume that the appropriate versions (no censoring or censoring) of SUTVA, the SRA, and the noninformative censoring (if needed) and positivity assumptions hold.

Consider first the case of no censoring. Analogous to (6.83), using the recursive representation of d in (8.47), define the indicator that an individual receives treatment options consistent with those that would be selected by d through the first k decisions as

$$\mathcal{C}_{\overline{d}_k} = \mathrm{I}\{\overline{A}_k = \overline{d}_k(\overline{\mathcal{T}}_k, \overline{X}_k), \varkappa \geq k\}, \tag{8.172}$$

and define $\mathcal{C}_{d_0} \equiv 1$. From (8.65), similar to the definition of the densities of treatment received given past history in (5.54) and (6.85), write

$$p_{A_1|H_1,\varkappa \geq 1}(a_1|h_1) = P(A_1 = a_1|H_1 = h_1, \varkappa \geq 1),$$
$$= p_{A_1|\mathcal{T}_1,X_1,\varkappa \geq 1}(a_1|\tau_1, x_1)$$
$$p_{A_k|H_k,\varkappa \geq k}(a_k|h_k) = P(A_k = a_k|H_k = h_k, \varkappa \geq k) \tag{8.173}$$
$$= p_{A_k|\overline{\mathcal{T}}_k, \overline{X}_k, \overline{A}_{k-1},\varkappa \geq k}(a_k|\overline{\tau}_k, \overline{x}_k, \overline{a}_{k-1}),$$
$$k = 2, \ldots, K;$$

and, as in (5.56) and (6.86), let

$$\pi_{d,1}(\mathcal{T}_1, X_1) = p_{A_1|\mathcal{T}_1,X_1,\varkappa \geq 1}\{d_1(\mathcal{T}_1, X_1)|\mathcal{T}_1, X_1\},$$
$$\pi_{d,k}(\overline{\mathcal{T}}_k, \overline{X}_k) = p_{A_k|\overline{\mathcal{T}}_k, \overline{X}_k, \overline{A}_{k-1},\varkappa \geq k}[d_k\{\overline{\mathcal{T}}_k, \overline{X}_k, \overline{d}_{k-1}(\overline{\mathcal{T}}_{k-1}, \overline{X}_{k-1})\}|$$
$$\overline{\mathcal{T}}_k, \overline{X}_k, \overline{d}_{k-1}(\overline{\mathcal{T}}_{k-1}, \overline{X}_{k-1})],$$
$$k = 2, \ldots, K. \tag{8.174}$$

As in (6.110), let $\overline{\pi}_{d,1}(\mathcal{T}_1, X_1) = \pi_{d,1}(\mathcal{T}_1, X_1)$ and

$$\overline{\pi}_{d,k}(\overline{\mathcal{T}}_k, \overline{X}_k) = \left\{ \prod_{j=2}^{k} \pi_{d,j}(\overline{\mathcal{T}}_j, \overline{X}_j) \right\} \pi_{d,1}(\mathcal{T}_1, X_1), \quad k = 2, \ldots, K,$$

$$\tag{8.175}$$

with $\overline{\pi}_{d,0} \equiv 1$.

As in the discussion in Sections 5.5.2 and 6.4.3, suppose that we posit models for the propensities

$$\omega_k(h_k, a_k) = p_{A_k|H_k, \varkappa \geq k}(a_k|h_k)$$

in (8.173) in terms of parameters γ_k and denote these models as

$$\omega_k(h_k, a_k; \gamma_k) = \omega_k(\overline{\tau}_k, \overline{x}_k, \overline{a}_k; \gamma_k), \quad k = 1, \ldots, K.$$

Taking the parameters γ_k to be variationally independent across k, the models can be fitted as described in those sections for each $k = 1, \ldots, K$, where, for given k, this would be based on the data only from all individuals i for whom $\varkappa_i \geq k$, yielding estimators $\widehat{\gamma}_k$. Substituting these models in (8.174) induces models $\pi_{d,1}(\mathcal{T}_1, X_1; \gamma_1)$ and $\pi_{d,k}(\overline{\mathcal{T}}_k, \overline{X}_k; \gamma_k)$ and thus $\overline{\pi}_{d,k}(\overline{\mathcal{T}}_k, \overline{X}_k; \overline{\gamma}_k)$, $k = 1, \ldots, K$, where $\overline{\gamma}_k = (\gamma_1^T, \ldots, \gamma_k^T)^T$.

Analogous to (6.112), given estimators $\widehat{\gamma}_k$ for γ_k, and writing $\widehat{\overline{\gamma}}_k = (\widehat{\gamma}_1^T, \ldots, \widehat{\gamma}_k^T)^T$, $k = 1, \ldots, K$, it follows from semiparametric theory (Tsiatis, 2006) that all consistent and asymptotically normal estimators for $\mathcal{V}(d)$ are asymptotically equivalent to an augmented inverse probability weighted estimator of the form

$$\widehat{\mathcal{V}}_{AIPW}(d) = n^{-1} \sum_{i=1}^n \left(\frac{\mathcal{C}_{\overline{d}_{\varkappa_i}, i} f(T_i)}{\{\prod_{k=2}^{\varkappa_i} \pi_{d,k}(\overline{\mathcal{T}}_{ki}, \overline{X}_{ki}; \widehat{\overline{\gamma}}_k)\} \pi_{d,1}(\mathcal{T}_{1i}, X_{1i}; \widehat{\gamma}_1)} \right.$$

$$+ \sum_{k=1}^{\varkappa_i} \left[\left\{ \frac{\mathcal{C}_{\overline{d}_{k-1}, i}}{\overline{\pi}_{d,k-1}(\overline{\mathcal{T}}_{k-1,i}, \overline{X}_{k-1,i}; \widehat{\overline{\gamma}}_{k-1})} - \frac{\mathcal{C}_{\overline{d}_k, i}}{\overline{\pi}_{d,k}(\overline{\mathcal{T}}_{ki}, \overline{X}_{ki}, \widehat{\overline{\gamma}}_k)} \right\} \right.$$

$$\left. \left. \times L_k(\overline{\mathcal{T}}_{ki}, \overline{X}_{ki}) \right] \right), \tag{8.176}$$

where $L_k(\overline{\tau}_k, \overline{x}_k)$, $k = 1, \ldots, K$, are arbitrary functions of $(\overline{\tau}_k, \overline{x}_k)$. The estimator (8.176) differs from that in (6.112) in that the leading inverse weighted term in the summand of necessity depends on the consistency of treatment options received by individual i with those selected by d only through the last decision point $\varkappa_i$ reached by i. Moreover, the second augmentation term depends on information from i only through Decision $\varkappa_i$.

Taking the functions $L_k(\overline{\tau}_k, \overline{x}_k) \equiv 0$, $k = 1, \ldots, K$, yields the simple inverse probability weighted estimator

$$\widehat{\mathcal{V}}_{IPW}(d) = n^{-1} \sum_{i=1}^n \frac{\mathcal{C}_{\overline{d}_{\varkappa_i}, i} f(T_i)}{\{\prod_{k=2}^{\varkappa_i} \pi_{d,k}(\overline{\mathcal{T}}_{ki}, \overline{X}_{ki}; \widehat{\gamma}_k)\} \pi_{d,1}(\mathcal{T}_{1i}, X_{1i}; \widehat{\gamma}_1)}, \tag{8.177}$$

analogous to (5.64) and (6.100). As above, the contribution of each individual i to (8.177) depends on the consistency of the treatment options he received with those selected by d only through $\varkappa_i$. If all of the models $\omega_k(h_k, a_k; \gamma_k)$ for the propensities $p_{A_k|H_k, \varkappa \geq k}(a_k|h_k)$ in (8.173), $k = 1, \ldots, K$, are correctly specified, as for the previous estimators, (8.177) can be shown to be a consistent estimator for $\mathcal{V}(d)$ by an argument similar to those in Sections 5.5.2 and 6.4.3. However, as discussed in the remark near the end of Section 5.5.2, the inverse weighted estimator (8.177) is likely to be imprecise and unstable in practice. As in the discussion after (6.112), it can be shown under these conditions that the augmentation term converges in probability to zero for arbitrary $L_k(\overline{\mathcal{T}}_k, \overline{x}_k)$, so that (8.176) is also a consistent estimator. This term incorporates information from individuals whose actual treatment options received were not consistent with the rules in d up to their final decision times, and, through appropriate choice of the functions $L_k(\overline{\mathcal{T}}_k, \overline{x}_k)$, serves to increase efficiency. Accordingly, we focus on the class of augmented inverse probability weighted estimators of the form (8.176) henceforth.

It proves convenient, particularly when we consider modification of these developments in the case of censored outcome, to express (8.176) in an equivalent form, analogous to those in Section 7.4.4 and the discussion in Remark (ii) in Section 8.2.4. First, as in (7.109), let

$$\varpi_k(h_k, a_k) = \prod_{j=1}^{k} \omega_j(h_j, a_j), \quad k = 1, \ldots, K, \tag{8.178}$$

be the probability of receiving treatment options $\overline{a}_k$ through Decision k, given an individual reaches Decision k, and define $\varpi_0 \equiv 1$. As noted in the remark following (6.112) and shown in Section 7.4.4, because when $\mathcal{C}_{\overline{d}_k} = 1$ the treatments $A_1, \ldots, A_k$ actually received coincide with those dictated by the first k rules in d, from the recursive representation (8.47), $\mathcal{C}_{\overline{d}_k}$ can be reexpressed as

$$\mathcal{C}_{\overline{d}_k} = \mathrm{I}\{A_1 = d_1(H_1), \ldots, A_k = d_k(H_k), \varkappa \geq k\},$$

and

$$\overline{\pi}_{d,k}(\overline{\mathcal{T}}_k, \overline{X}_k; \widehat{\overline{\gamma}}_k) = \left\{ \prod_{j=2}^{k} \pi_{d,j}(\overline{\mathcal{T}}_j, \overline{X}_j; \widehat{\gamma}_j) \right\} \pi_{d,1}(\mathcal{T}_1, X_1; \widehat{\gamma}_1)$$

in (8.175) can be replaced in the denominators in (8.176) by the fitted induced model for (8.178) given by

$$\varpi_k(H_k, A_k; \widehat{\overline{\gamma}}_k) = \prod_{j=1}^{k} \omega_j(H_j, A_j; \widehat{\gamma}_j). \tag{8.179}$$

Making this substitution, it follows by further algebra and reasoning similar to that leading to (7.110) that (8.176) can be written as

$$
\begin{aligned}
\widehat{\mathcal{V}}_{AIPW}(d) = n^{-1} \sum_{i=1}^{n} & \left\{ \frac{\mathcal{C}_{\overline{d}_{\varkappa_i},i} f(T_i)}{\varpi_{\varkappa_i}(H_{\varkappa_i,i}, A_{\varkappa_i,i}; \widehat{\widehat{\gamma}}_{\varkappa_i})} \right. \\
& - \sum_{k=1}^{\varkappa_i} \left(\frac{\mathcal{C}_{\overline{d}_{k-1},i}}{\varpi_{k-1}(H_{k-1,i}, A_{k-1,i}; \widehat{\widehat{\gamma}}_{k-1})} \right. \\
& \times \left. \left. \left[\frac{I\{A_{ki} = d_k(H_{ki})\} - \omega_k(H_{ki}, A_{ki}; \widehat{\gamma}_k)}{\omega_k(H_{ki}, A_{ki}; \widehat{\gamma}_k)} \right] L_k(\overline{\mathcal{T}}_{ki}, \overline{X}_{ki}) \right) \right\}.
\end{aligned}
\tag{8.180}
$$

From the semiparametric theory, the optimal choice of $L_k(\overline{\tau}_k, \overline{x}_k)$, $k = 1, \ldots, K$, leading to the estimator of the form (8.176) or, equivalently, (8.180) with smallest asymptotic variance is

$$
L_k(\overline{\tau}_k, \overline{x}_k) = E[f\{T^*(d)\} | \overline{\mathcal{T}}_k^*(\overline{d}_{k-1}) = \overline{\tau}_k, \overline{X}_k^*(\overline{d}_{k-1}) = \overline{x}_k, \varkappa^*(d) \geq k],
$$
$$
k = 1, \ldots, K.
\tag{8.181}
$$

In Section 8.5, we argue that, under SUTVA, the SRA, and the positivity assumption, (8.181) implies that

$$
L_k(\overline{\tau}_k, \overline{x}_k) = V_k^d\{\overline{\tau}_k, \overline{x}_k, \overline{d}_{k-1}(\overline{\tau}_{k-1}, \overline{x}_{k-1})\}.
\tag{8.182}
$$

Thus, to obtain the optimal augmented estimator, substitute

$$
V_k^d\{\overline{\mathcal{T}}_{ki}, \overline{X}_{ki}, \overline{d}_{k-1}(\overline{\mathcal{T}}_{k-1,i}, \overline{X}_{k-1,i})\}
$$

for $L_k(\overline{\mathcal{T}}_{ki}, \overline{X}_{ki})$ in (8.180). In fact, because $\mathcal{C}_{\overline{d}_{k-1},i} = 1$ only when

$$
A_{1i} = d_1(H_{1i}), \ldots, A_{k-1,i} = d_{k-1}(H_{k-1,i}), \varkappa_i \geq k-1,
$$

and $L_k(\overline{\mathcal{T}}_{ki}, \overline{X}_{ki})$ enters the augmentation term only through the product $\mathcal{C}_{\overline{d}_{k-1},i} L_k(\overline{\mathcal{T}}_{ki}, \overline{X}_{ki})$, it follows from (8.182) that the optimal estimator can be obtained by substituting

$$
V_k^d(H_{ki}) = Q_k^d\{H_{ki}, d_k(H_{ki})\}, \quad k = 1, \ldots, K,
\tag{8.183}
$$

for $L_k(\overline{\mathcal{T}}_{ki}, \overline{X}_{ki})$ in (8.180).

The optimal choice in (8.183) implies that the optimal augmented inverse probability weighted estimator in practice can be obtained by developing models for $Q_k^d(h_k, a_k)$ and substituting these fitted models in (8.180). Such fitted models are induced in the course of the recursive regression-based or hybrid schemes for estimation of $\mathcal{V}(d)$ based on data with no censoring, as demonstrated earlier in this section. As shown there, the form of these models and their dependence on parameters is different for the two approaches. Accordingly, denote fitted models for $Q_k^d\{h_k, d_k(h_k)\}$ obtained via any of these approaches as

$$\widehat{\mathcal{Q}}_{d,k}(h_k), \quad k = 1, \ldots, K.$$

Remark. In the regression-based approach, models are developed for $Q_k^{R_d}(h_k, a_k) = Q_k^d(h_k, a_k) - f(\tau_k)$ rather than for $Q_k^d(h_k, a_k)$ directly. In the hybrid approach, models for $Q_k^d(h_k, a_k)$ are induced by posited models for $q_k^{R_d}(h_k, a_k, \tau_{k+1}) = q_k^d(h_k, a_k, \tau_{k+1}) - f(\tau_{k+1})$ and the cause-specific hazards $\lambda_{Tk}(u|\overline{\tau}_k, \overline{x}_k, \overline{a}_k)$, $k = 1, \ldots, K$, and $\lambda_{\tau k}(u|\overline{\tau}_k, \overline{x}_k, \overline{a}_k)$, $k = 1 \ldots, K-1$.

From the foregoing developments, it follows that the locally efficient estimator for $\mathcal{V}(d)$ is given by

$$\widehat{\mathcal{V}}_{LE}(d) = n^{-1} \sum_{i=1}^{n} \left\{ \frac{\mathcal{C}_{\overline{d}_{\varkappa_i}, i} f(T_i)}{\varpi_{\varkappa_i}(H_{\varkappa_i, i}, A_{\varkappa_i, i}; \widehat{\overline{\gamma}}_{\varkappa_i})} \right.$$
$$- \sum_{k=1}^{\varkappa_i} \left(\frac{\mathcal{C}_{\overline{d}_{k-1}, i}}{\varpi_{k-1}(H_{k-1, i}, A_{k-1, i}; \widehat{\overline{\gamma}}_{k-1})} \right. \tag{8.184}$$
$$\times \left. \left. \left[\frac{I\{A_{ki} = d_k(H_{ki})\} - \omega_k(H_{ki}, A_{ki}; \widehat{\gamma}_k)}{\omega_k(H_{ki}, A_{ki}; \widehat{\gamma}_k)} \right] \widehat{\mathcal{Q}}_{d,k}(H_{ki}) \right) \right\}.$$

The estimator (8.184) is doubly robust in that it is a consistent and asymptotically normal estimator for $\mathcal{V}(d)$ if either the models for the propensities $\omega_k(h_k, a_k)$ or the models for the $Q_k^d(h_k, a_k)$ are correctly specified for $k = 1, \ldots, K$. Moreover, if all of these models are correct, $\widehat{\mathcal{V}}_{LE}(d)$ is the efficient estimator among the class of semiparametric augmented inverse probability weighted estimators given in (8.180).

We now consider how these developments are revised when the outcome is censored, so that the observed data are as in (8.111),

$$(\kappa_i, \mathcal{T}_{1i}, X_{1i}, A_{1i}, \ldots, \mathcal{T}_{\kappa_i i}, X_{\kappa_i i}, A_{\kappa_i i}, U_i, \Delta_i), \quad i = 1, \ldots, n,$$

with $S_{ki}^{\dagger}$ and $\Upsilon_{ki}^{\dagger}$ defined as above, $k = 2, \ldots, K$. These developments are a generalization of those in Hager et al. (2018), who restrict attention to the case $K = 2$ and use a slightly different formulation that also makes explicit the possibility of feasible sets of treatment options.

Under the noninformative censoring assumption (8.68), as in (8.134), let

$$\mathcal{K}_k(u|h_k, a_k) = \exp\left\{ -\int_{\tau_k}^{u} \lambda_C(w \mid h_k, a_k)\, dw \right\}, \quad \tau_k \leq u \leq S_{k+1}^{\dagger},$$

when $\kappa \geq k$, $k = 1, \ldots, K$, and define $\mathcal{K}_0 \equiv 1$. We discussed previously in the context of the regression-based approach modeling of the $\mathcal{K}_k(u|h_k, a_k)$, $k = 1, \ldots, K$, via modeling of the hazard of censoring; e.g., by a proportional hazards model as in (8.140), yielding the estimators given in (8.142),

$$\widehat{\mathcal{K}}_k(u|h_k, a_k) = \exp\left\{-\int_{\tau_k}^{u} \lambda_C(w \mid h_k, a_k; \widehat{\beta}_C)\, dw\right\}, \quad k = 1, \ldots, K,$$

where we take $\widehat{\mathcal{K}}_0 \equiv 1$.

The modification of the estimator (8.184) to account for censoring incorporates the idea of inverse probability of censoring weighting as follows. Analogous to (8.172), define the indicator of consistency of treatment options received with those dictated by the first k rules in d for $k = 1, \ldots, K$ as

$$\mathcal{C}_{\overline{d}_k}^{\dagger} = \mathrm{I}\{\overline{A}_k = \overline{d}_k(\overline{\mathcal{T}}_k, \overline{X}_k), \kappa \geq k\},$$

with $\mathcal{C}_{\overline{d}_0}^{\dagger} \equiv 1$, so that $\mathcal{C}_{\overline{d}_k, i}^{\dagger}$ is defined for all individuals i for whom $\kappa_i \geq k$. From the development of the positivity assumption under censoring, similar to (8.173), write the propensities of treatment received given past history as

$$p_{A_1|H_1,\kappa\geq1}(a_1|h_1) = P(A_1 = a_1|H_1 = h_1, \kappa \geq 1),$$
$$= p_{A_1|\mathcal{T}_1,X_1,\kappa\geq1}(a_1|\tau_1, x_1)$$
$$p_{A_k|H_k,\kappa\geq k}(a_k|h_k) = P(A_k = a_k|H_k = h_k, \kappa \geq k) \qquad (8.185)$$
$$= p_{A_k|\overline{\mathcal{T}}_k,\overline{X}_k,\overline{A}_{k-1},\kappa\geq k}(a_k|\overline{\tau}_k, \overline{x}_k, \overline{a}_{k-1}),$$
$$k = 2, \ldots, K.$$

As in the case of no censoring, posit models for the propensities

$$\omega_k^{\dagger}(h_k, a_k) = p_{A_k|H_k,\kappa\geq k}(a_k|h_k), \quad k = 1, \ldots, K,$$

in (8.185) in terms of parameters γ_k, and denote these models by

$$\omega_k^{\dagger}(h_k, a_k; \gamma_k) = \omega_k^{\dagger}(\overline{\tau}_k, \overline{x}_k, \overline{a}_k; \gamma_k), \quad k = 1, \ldots, K. \qquad (8.186)$$

As above, assuming the parameters γ_k are variationally independent, the kth model is fitted and estimators $\widehat{\gamma}_k$ obtained by maximum likelihood based on the data from individuals i still at risk at Decision k; i.e., for whom $\kappa_i \geq k$.

Analogous to (8.178), denote the probability of receiving treatment options $\overline{a}_k$ through the kth decision point, without being censored prior to Decision k, so with $\kappa \geq k$, as

$$\varpi_k^\dagger(h_k, a_k) = \left\{ \prod_{j=1}^{k} \omega_j^\dagger(h_j, a_j) \right\} \left\{ \prod_{j=0}^{k-1} \mathcal{K}_j(\tau_{j+1}|h_j, a_j) \right\}, \quad k = 1, \ldots, K,$$

(8.187)

where, as above, $\mathcal{K}_0 \equiv 1$; and, for convenience below, define $\varpi_0^\dagger \equiv 1$. A model for (8.187) is induced by the models for $\omega_k^\dagger(h_k, a_k)$ and $\mathcal{K}_k(u|h_k, a_k)$; substituting fitted such models in (8.187) leads to the estimator

$$\widehat{\varpi}_k^\dagger(h_k, a_k) = \left\{ \prod_{j=1}^{k} \omega_j^\dagger(h_j, a_j; \widehat{\gamma}_k) \right\} \left\{ \prod_{j=0}^{k-1} \widehat{\mathcal{K}}_j(\tau_{j+1}|h_j, a_j) \right\}, \quad k = 1, \ldots, K,$$

where dependence on $\widehat{\overline{\gamma}}_k$ and $\widehat{\beta}_C$ is suppressed for brevity, with $\widehat{\varpi}_0^\dagger \equiv 1$.

Define $\Upsilon_1^\dagger \equiv 1$, so that $\mathrm{I}(\Upsilon_{1i}^\dagger \neq 0) = 1$ for all individuals i. With this and the above definitions, an augmented inverse probability weighted estimator for $\mathcal{V}(d)$ can be constructed as

$$\widehat{\mathcal{V}}_{AIPW}(d) = n^{-1} \sum_{i=1}^{n} \left\{ \frac{\mathcal{C}_{\overline{d}_{\kappa_i}, i}^\dagger \Delta_i f(U_i)}{\widehat{\varpi}_{\kappa_i}^\dagger(H_{\kappa_i, i}, A_{\kappa_i, i}) \widehat{\mathcal{K}}_{\kappa_i}(U_i|H_{\kappa_i, i}, A_{\kappa_i, i})} \right.$$

$$- \sum_{k=1}^{\kappa_i} \left(\frac{\mathcal{C}_{\overline{d}_{k-1}, i}^\dagger \mathrm{I}(\Upsilon_{ki}^\dagger \neq 0)}{\widehat{\varpi}_{k-1}^\dagger(H_{k-1,i}, A_{k-1,i}) \widehat{\mathcal{K}}_{k-1}(S_{ki}^\dagger|H_{ki}, A_{ki})} \right.$$

(8.188)

$$\left. \left. \times \left[\frac{\mathrm{I}\{A_{ki} = d_k(H_{ki})\} - \omega_k^\dagger(H_{ki}, A_{ki}; \widehat{\gamma}_k)}{\omega_k^\dagger(H_{ki}, A_{ki}; \widehat{\gamma}_k)} \right] \widehat{\mathcal{Q}}_{d,k}(H_{ki}) \right) \right\}.$$

The fitted models $\widehat{\mathcal{Q}}_{d,k}(h_k)$, $k = 1, \ldots, K$, are obtained through the regression-based or hybrid estimation approaches based on censored data presented earlier in this section.

In the leading term in (8.188), if $\mathcal{C}_{\overline{d}_{\kappa_i}, i}^\dagger \Delta_i = 1$, then the treatment options received by individual i are consistent with those selected by d through all κ_i decisions reached by i, after which i was observed to experience the event without being censored. Thus, similar to the estimator (8.40) in the single decision case, the leading term involves only individuals whose treatment experience is consistent with d through all decisions reached and for whom U is the event time. In this case, $f(U) = f\{T^*(d)\}$, and it can be shown that

$$E \left\{ \frac{\mathcal{C}_{\overline{d}_\kappa}^\dagger \Delta}{\varpi_\kappa^\dagger(H_\kappa, A_\kappa) \mathcal{K}_\kappa(U|H_\kappa, A_\kappa)} \right\} = 1$$

and

$$E\left\{\frac{\mathcal{C}_{\bar{d}_\kappa}^\dagger \Delta f(U)}{\varpi_\kappa^\dagger(H_\kappa, A_\kappa)\mathcal{K}_\kappa(U|H_\kappa, A_\kappa)}\right\} = E[f\{T^*(d)\}] = \mathcal{V}(d). \qquad (8.189)$$

In the augmentation term in (8.188), for $2 \leq k \leq \kappa_i$,

$$\mathcal{C}_{\bar{d}_{k-1},i}\mathrm{I}(\Upsilon_{ki} \neq 0) = 1$$

indicates that individual i's treatment options actually received are consistent with those dictated by the first $k - 1$ rules in d and that the individual subsequently reached Decision k without being censored. Accordingly, all individuals i whose treatment options received are consistent with d for a subset of the κ_i decision points reached by i contribute to this term. Thus, the augmentation term, which has mean zero when evaluated at the true propensities and hazard of censoring, can be interpreted as recovering information from uncensored individuals whose realized treatment experience was only partially consistent with d.

The estimator (8.188) is a consistent estimator for $\mathcal{V}(d)$ as long as the model for the hazard of censoring, and thus the models for $\mathcal{K}_k(u|h_k, a_k)$, $k = 1, \ldots, K$, are correctly specified and at least one of (i) the models for the propensities $\omega_k^\dagger(h_k, a_k)$ in (8.187), $k = 1, \ldots, K$, or (ii) those for the $Q_k^d(h_k, a_k)$, $k = 1, \ldots, K$, are correctly specified. From (8.188), a simple inverse probability weighted estimator for $\mathcal{V}(d)$ is obtained as

$$\widehat{\mathcal{V}}_{IPW}(d) = n^{-1}\sum_{i=1}^n \frac{\mathcal{C}_{\bar{d}_{\kappa_i},i}^\dagger \Delta_i f(U_i)}{\widehat{\varpi}_{\kappa_i}^\dagger(H_{\kappa_i,i}, A_{\kappa_i,i})\widehat{\mathcal{K}}_{\kappa_i}(U_i|H_{\kappa_i,i}, A_{\kappa_i,i})}. \qquad (8.190)$$

The result (8.189) demonstrates that, as long as both the models for the propensities and for the hazard of censoring are correctly specified, (8.190) is a consistent estimator for $\mathcal{V}(d)$. However, as in the case of no censoring, this estimator is inefficient relative to (8.188) and potentially unstable in practice.

Remark. If the observed data are from a SMART, so that each subject is randomly assigned to receive one of the feasible treatment options given his history at each decision point he reaches, then the SRA is automatically satisfied. Moreover, the probabilities associated with assignment to feasible treatment options are known, so that the propensities $\omega_k^\dagger(h_k, a_k)$, $k = 1, \ldots, K$, in (8.187) are known and thus can be correctly specified. As noted in the remark following (8.142), in a well conducted SMART, censoring is primarily administrative and can be assumed to be not only noninformative as in (8.68) but in fact independent of treatment assignment, patient characteristics, and potential outcomes, so that $\mathcal{K}_k(u|h_k, a_k) = \mathcal{K}_k(u)$, $k = 1, \ldots, K$. In this case, as noted in the remark at the end of Section 8.2.4 in the single decision case, as long as $g_C\{h(u); \xi_C\} = 0$ for some ξ_C, a posited proportional hazards model for censoring as in (8.140) is correctly specified. Alternatively, $\widehat{\mathcal{K}}_k(u|h_k, a_k)$ can be replaced wherever it appears in (8.190) and (8.188) by (8.144) based on the Kaplan-Meier estimator for the censoring distribution. Both (8.190) and (8.188) are consistent estimators for $\mathcal{V}(d)$ under these conditions.

The simple inverse weighted estimator (8.190), which is also the leading term in the augmented inverse probability weighted estimator (8.188), bases estimation of $\mathcal{V}(d)$ on data only from individuals whose treatment options received are consistent with those dictated by d through all decisions reached and for whom the time-to-event outcome is observed. The augmented estimator seeks to gain efficiency over the simple inverse weighted estimator by recovering information from individuals who received treatment options consistent with d up to a certain decision before possibly deviating from d at subsequent decisions. Neither estimator incorporates the additional information that is lost to censoring. We now consider how (8.188) can be augmented further to recover this additional information for efficiency gain.

In the augmentation term in (8.188), when $\mathcal{C}_{\overline{d}_{k-1}}^\dagger \, \mathrm{I}(\Upsilon_k^\dagger \neq 0) = 1$, information is retrieved from individuals who receive treatment options consistent with those selected by the first $k - 1$ decision points and are not censored prior to the kth decision point. However, information from individuals whose treatment experience is consistent with d through Decision $k - 1$ but are then censored prior to Decision k is lost. The lost information on the event time for such an individual if he were to have continued to receive treatment consistent with d and was not censored can be viewed as monotone missing data.

Similar to (8.41) in the single decision case, define the martingale increment for censoring at time u for $S_k^\dagger \leq u < S_{k+1}^\dagger$, conditional on H_k, A_k, as

$$dM_{C,k}(u|h_k, a_k) = dN_C(u) - \lambda_C(u|h_k, a_k)Y(u)\, du, \qquad (8.191)$$

with $N_C(u) = \mathrm{I}(U \leq u, \Delta = 0)$, $Y(u) = \mathrm{I}(U \geq u)$, and $\lambda_C(u|h_k, a_k)$ the hazard function for censoring under the noninformative censoring assumption. Using semiparametric theory for monotone coarsening at random in Chapters 7–11 of Tsiatis (2006), it follows that all consistent and asymptotically normal semiparametric estimators for $\mathcal{V}(d)$ are asymptotically equivalent to an estimator of the form

$$
\widehat{\mathcal{V}}_{CAIPW}(d) = n^{-1} \sum_{i=1}^{n} \Bigg\{ \frac{\mathcal{C}^{\dagger}_{\overline{d}_{\kappa_i},i} \Delta_i f(U_i)}{\widehat{\varpi}^{\dagger}_{\kappa_i}(H_{\kappa_i,i}, A_{\kappa_i,i}) \widehat{\mathcal{K}}_{\kappa_i}(U_i | H_{\kappa_i,i}, A_{\kappa_i,i})}
$$

$$
- \sum_{k=1}^{\kappa_i} \Bigg(\frac{\mathcal{C}^{\dagger}_{\overline{d}_{k-1},i} \mathrm{I}(\Upsilon^{\dagger}_{ki} \neq 0)}{\widehat{\varpi}^{\dagger}_{k-1}(H_{k-1,i}, A_{k-1,i}) \widehat{\mathcal{K}}_{k-1}(S^{\dagger}_{ki} | H_{k-1,i}, A_{k-1,i})} \tag{8.192}
$$

$$
\times \left[\frac{\mathrm{I}\{A_{ki} = d_k(H_{ki})\} - \omega^{\dagger}_k(H_{ki}, A_{ki}; \widehat{\gamma}_k)}{\omega^{\dagger}_k(H_{ki}, A_{ki}; \widehat{\gamma}_k)} \right] L_k(\overline{\mathcal{T}}_{ki}, \overline{X}_{ki}) \Bigg)
$$

$$
+ \sum_{k=1}^{\kappa_i} \frac{\mathcal{C}^{\dagger}_{\overline{d}_k i}}{\widehat{\varpi}^{\dagger}_k(H_{ki}, A_{ki})} \int_{S^{\dagger}_{ki}}^{S^{\dagger}_{k+1,i}} \frac{d\widehat{M}_{C,k}(u | H_{ki}, A_{ki})}{\widehat{\mathcal{K}}_k(u | H_{ki}, A_{ki})} D_k(\overline{\mathcal{T}}_{ki}, \overline{X}_{ki}, u) \Bigg\},
$$

where

$$
d\widehat{M}_{C,k}(u | h_k, a_k) = dN_C(u) - \lambda_C(u | h_k, a_k; \widehat{\beta}_C) Y(u) \, du;
$$

as before, $L_k(\overline{\mathcal{T}}_k, \overline{x}_k)$, $k = 1, \dots, K$, are arbitrary functions of $\overline{\mathcal{T}}_k, \overline{x}_k$; and $D_k(\overline{\mathcal{T}}_k, \overline{x}_k, u)$, $k = 1, \dots, K$, are arbitrary functions of $\overline{\mathcal{T}}_k, \overline{x}_k$, and time u. In the final augmentation term in (8.192), $S^{\dagger}_{\kappa_i+1,i} = U_i$ by definition. This additional augmentation term recovers information from individuals who received treatment options consistent with those selected by the rules in d up to a <u>certain point</u> and then were censored, as discussed above.

From semiparametric theory, the optimal estimator in the class (8.192) is found by taking for $k = 1, \dots, K$

$$
L_k(\overline{\mathcal{T}}_k, \overline{x}_k) = E[f\{T^*(d)\} | \overline{\mathcal{T}}^*_k(\overline{d}_{k-1}) = \overline{\mathcal{T}}_k, \overline{X}^*_k(\overline{d}_{k-1}) = \overline{x}_k, \varkappa^*(d) \geq k]
$$

as in (8.181) and

$$
D_k(\overline{\mathcal{T}}_k, \overline{x}_k, u) = E[f\{T^*(d)\} | \overline{\mathcal{T}}^*_k(\overline{d}_{k-1}) = \overline{\mathcal{T}}_k, \tag{8.193}
$$
$$
\overline{X}^*_k(\overline{d}_{k-1}) = \overline{x}_k, \varkappa^*(d) \geq k, S^*_{k+1}(\overline{d}_k) \geq u].
$$

Here, $S^*_{k+1}(\overline{d}_k)$ is the potential event time if an individual would reach Decision k but then achieve the event before Decision $k + 1$ or is the potential time of $(k+1)$th decision point otherwise if she were to follow the rules in d, defined similar to (8.51) in terms of the potential outcomes (8.52). As in (8.183), it follows that the optimal estimator can be constructed by substituting

$$
V^d_k(H_{ki}) = Q^d_k\{H_{ki}, d_k(H_{ki})\}, \quad k = 1, \dots, K,
$$

for $L_k(\overline{\mathcal{T}}_{ki}, \overline{X}_{ki})$, which can be estimated via fitted models

$$\widehat{\mathcal{Q}}_{d,k}(h_k), \quad k = 1, \ldots, K,$$

as discussed earlier. We thus consider how to estimate the optimal $D_k(\overline{\tau}_k, \overline{x}_k, u)$ in (8.193).

Using arguments similar to those used to demonstrate (8.128), (8.139), and (8.182) in Section 8.5, it can be shown that the optimal choice of $D_k(\overline{\tau}_k, \overline{x}_k, u)$ in (8.193) is equivalent to

$$E\{f(T)|\overline{\mathcal{T}}_K = \overline{\tau}_K, \overline{X}_K = \overline{x}_K, \overline{A}_K = \overline{d}_K(\overline{\tau}_K, \overline{x}_K), \varkappa = K, T \geq u\} \tag{8.194}$$

for $k = K$ and $u > \tau_K$; and, for $k = 1, \ldots, K - 1$ and $u > \tau_k$,

$$E\{I(\varkappa = k)f(T) + I(\varkappa \geq k + 1)V_k^d(H_{k+1})|\overline{\mathcal{T}}_k = \overline{\tau}_k, \overline{X}_k = \overline{x}_k,$$
$$\overline{A}_k = \overline{d}_k(\overline{\tau}_k, \overline{x}_k), \varkappa \geq k, S_{k+1} \geq u\}, \tag{8.195}$$

expressed in terms of the data that could be observed if there were no censoring. When $k = K$, (8.194) can be expressed as

$$\int_{u-\tau_K}^{\infty} f(\tau_K + w) \left[-\frac{d\mathcal{S}_{TK}\{w|\overline{\tau}_K, \overline{x}_K, \overline{d}_K(\overline{\tau}_K, \overline{x}_K)\}}{\mathcal{S}_{TK}\{u - \tau_K|\overline{\tau}_K, \overline{x}_K, \overline{d}_K(\overline{\tau}_K, \overline{x}_K)\}} \right]. \tag{8.196}$$

For $k = 1, \ldots, K - 1$, the first conditional expectation in (8.195) can be written as

$$E\{I(\Upsilon_{k+1} = 1)f(S_{k+1})|\overline{\mathcal{T}}_k = \overline{\tau}_k, \overline{X}_k = \overline{x}_k, \overline{A}_k = \overline{d}_k(\overline{\tau}_k, \overline{x}_k),$$
$$\varkappa \geq k, S_{k+1} \geq u\}$$
$$= \int_{u-\tau_k}^{\infty} \left[f(\tau_k + w) \frac{\mathcal{S}_{\bullet k}\{w|\overline{\tau}_k, \overline{x}_k, \overline{d}_k(\overline{\tau}_k, \overline{x}_k)\}}{\mathcal{S}_{\bullet k}\{u - \tau_k|\overline{\tau}_k, \overline{x}_k, \overline{d}_k(\overline{\tau}_k, \overline{x}_k)\}} \right. \tag{8.197}$$
$$\left. \times \lambda_{Tk}\{w|\overline{\tau}_k, \overline{x}_k, \overline{d}_k(\overline{\tau}_k, \overline{x}_k)\} \right] dw.$$

The second conditional expectation in (8.195) is equal to

$$E[I(\Upsilon_{k+1} = -1)q_k^d\{\overline{\tau}_k, \overline{x}_k, \overline{d}_k(\overline{\tau}_k, \overline{x}_k), S_{k+1}\}|$$
$$\overline{\mathcal{T}}_k = \overline{\tau}_k, \overline{X}_k = \overline{x}_k, \overline{A}_k = \overline{d}_k(\overline{\tau}_k, \overline{x}_k), \varkappa \geq k, S_{k+1} \geq u] \tag{8.198}$$
$$= \int_{u-\tau_k}^{\infty} \left[q_k^d\{\overline{\tau}_k, \overline{x}_k, \overline{d}_k(\overline{\tau}_k, \overline{x}_k), \tau_k + w\} \frac{\mathcal{S}_{\bullet k}\{w|\overline{\tau}_k, \overline{x}_k, \overline{d}_k(\overline{\tau}_k, \overline{x}_k)\}}{\mathcal{S}_{\bullet k}\{u - \tau_k|\overline{\tau}_k, \overline{x}_k, \overline{d}_k(\overline{\tau}_k, \overline{x}_k)\}} \right.$$
$$\left. \times \lambda_{\tau k}\{w|\overline{\tau}_k, \overline{x}_k, \overline{d}_k(\overline{\tau}_k, \overline{x}_k)\} \right] dw.$$

In (8.196)–(8.198), the cause-specific hazards $\lambda_{Tk}(u|\overline{\tau}_k, \overline{x}_k, \overline{a}_k)$, $k = 1, \ldots, K$, and $\lambda_{\tau k}(u|\overline{\tau}_k, \overline{x}_k, \overline{a}_k)$, $k = 1 \ldots, K - 1$, are defined in (8.93), (8.94), and (8.96) and in (8.150)–(8.152); $\mathcal{S}_{TK}(u|\overline{\tau}_k, \overline{x}_k, \overline{a}_k)$ is defined in terms of $\lambda_{TK}(u|\overline{\tau}_k, \overline{x}_k, \overline{a}_k)$ in (8.98) and (8.154); $\mathcal{S}_{\bullet k}(u|\overline{\tau}_k, \overline{x}_k, \overline{a}_k)$, $k = 1, \ldots, K$, is defined in terms of the cause-specific hazards in (8.97) and (8.157); and $q_k^d(\overline{\tau}_k, \overline{x}_k, \overline{a}_k, \tau_{k+1})$ is defined in (8.158) in the context of the hybrid estimation scheme.

From (8.196)–(8.198), define

$$\mathfrak{Q}_{d,K}(h_K, a_K, u) = \int_{u-\tau_K}^{\infty} f(\tau_K + w) \left[-\frac{d\mathcal{S}_{TK}(w|h_K, a_K)}{\mathcal{S}_{TK}(u - \tau_K|h_K, a_K)} \right]; \quad (8.199)$$

and, for $k = 1, \ldots, K - 1$,

$$\mathfrak{Q}_{d,k}(h_k, a_k, u) = \int_{u-\tau_k}^{\infty} f(\tau_k + w) \frac{\mathcal{S}_{\bullet k}(w|h_k, a_k)}{\mathcal{S}_{\bullet k}(u - \tau_k|h_k, a_k)} \lambda_{Tk}(w|h_k, a_k) \, dw$$
$$+ \int_{u-\tau_k}^{\infty} q_k^d(h_k, a_k, \tau_k + w) \frac{\mathcal{S}_{\bullet k}(w|h_k, a_k)}{\mathcal{S}_{\bullet k}(u - \tau_k|h_k, a_k)} \lambda_{\tau k}(w|h_k, a_k) \, dw, \quad (8.200)$$

where the dependence of $\mathfrak{Q}_{d,k}(h_k, a_k, u)$ on d is through $q_k^d(h_k, a_k, \tau_{k+1})$ in the second integral in (8.200). Then, because, in the additional augmentation term in (8.192), when $C_{d_k}^{\dagger} = 1$, the treatment options $A_1, \ldots, A_k$ coincide with those dictated by the first k rules in d, the optimal estimator of the form (8.192) can be obtained by substituting

$$\mathfrak{Q}_{d,k}(H_{ki}, A_{ki}, u), \quad k = 1, \ldots, K, \quad (8.201)$$

for $D_k(\overline{\mathcal{T}}_{ki}, \overline{X}_{ki}, u)$ for each individual i in this term.

In practice, as in the first augmentation term, fitted models for $\mathfrak{Q}_{d,k}(h_k, a_k, u)$ are required. From (8.199)–(8.200), models for (8.201) are induced by models for the cause-specific hazards $\lambda_{Tk}(u|h_k, a_k)$ and $\lambda_{\tau k}(u|h_k, a_k)$ in (8.150)–(8.152) and for $q_k^d(h_k, a_k, \tau_{k+1})$ in (8.158). As discussed previously, under the noninformative censoring assumption (8.68), these hazards are equivalent to $\lambda_{Tk}^{\dagger}(u|h_k, a_k)$ and $\lambda_{\tau k}^{\dagger}(u|h_k, a_k)$ in (8.161)–(8.163), and parametric or semiparametric models

$$\lambda_{Tk}^{\dagger}(u|h_k, a_k; \beta_{Tk}), \quad k = 1, \ldots, K,$$
$$\lambda_{\tau k}^{\dagger}(u|h_k, a_k; \beta_{\tau k}), \quad k = 1, \ldots, K - 1$$

as in (8.164)–(8.165) or (8.166)–(8.167) can be posited and fitted based on the censored data using standard survival analysis methods, yielding estimators $\widehat{\beta}_{Tk}$ and $\widehat{\beta}_{\tau k}$. Given models for $q_k^d(h_k, a_k, \tau_{k+1}; \beta_k)$ for $q_k^d(h_k, a_k, \tau_{k+1})$, $k = 1, \ldots, K - 1$, which follow from the models for $q_k^{R_d}(h_k, a_k, \tau_{k+1})$ defined in (8.168), the fitted cause-specific hazard models can be used in the backward hybrid estimation algorithm presented earlier, yielding fitted models $q_k^d(h_k, a_k, \tau_{k+1}; \widehat{\beta}_k)$. Substituting these models in (8.199)–(8.200) then yields the induced models

$$\mathfrak{Q}_{d,k}(h_k, a_k, u; \beta_k, \beta_{Tk}, \beta_{\tau k}), \quad k = 1, \ldots, K,$$

say, where it is understood from (8.199) that the model for $k = K$ depends only on β_{TK} (and not on d). Denote the resulting fitted models for (8.199)–(8.200) for brevity by

$$\widehat{\mathfrak{Q}}_{d,k}(h_k, a_k, u) = \mathfrak{Q}_k(h_k, a_k, u; \widehat{\beta}_k, \widehat{\beta}_{Tk}, \widehat{\beta}_{\tau k}), \quad k = 1, \ldots, K.$$

Substituting the fitted models for the optimal choices for $L_k(\overline{\tau}_k, \overline{x}_k)$ and $D_k(\overline{\tau}_k, \overline{x}_k, u)$ in (8.192) yields the locally efficient estimator for $\mathcal{V}(d)$ in the presence of censoring given by

$$
\begin{aligned}
\widehat{\mathcal{V}}_{LE}(d) = n^{-1} \sum_{i=1}^{n} \Bigg\{ & \frac{\mathcal{C}_{d_{\kappa_i},i}^\dagger \Delta_i f(U_i)}{\widehat{\varpi}_{\kappa_i}^\dagger(H_{\kappa_i,i}, A_{\kappa_i,i})\widehat{\mathcal{K}}_{\kappa_i}(U_i | H_{\kappa_i,i}, A_{\kappa_i,i})} \\
& - \sum_{k=1}^{\kappa_i} \Bigg(\frac{\mathcal{C}_{d_{k-1},i}^\dagger \mathrm{I}(\Upsilon_{ki}^\dagger \neq 0)}{\widehat{\varpi}_{k-1}^\dagger(H_{k-1,i}, A_{k-1,i})\widehat{\mathcal{K}}_{k-1}(S_{ki}^\dagger | H_{k-1,i}, A_{k-1,i})} \\
& \qquad\qquad \times \left[\frac{\mathrm{I}\{A_{ki} = d_k(H_{ki})\} - \omega_k^\dagger(H_{ki}, A_{ki}; \widehat{\gamma}_k)}{\omega_k^\dagger(H_{ki}, A_{ki}; \widehat{\gamma}_k)} \right] \widehat{\mathfrak{Q}}_{d,k}(H_{ki}) \Bigg) \\
& + \sum_{k=1}^{\kappa_i} \frac{\mathcal{C}_{d_k i}^\dagger}{\widehat{\varpi}_k^\dagger(H_{ki}, A_{ki})} \int_{S_{ki}^\dagger}^{S_{k+1,i}^\dagger} \frac{d\widehat{M}_{C,k}(u | H_{ki}, A_{ki})}{\widehat{\mathcal{K}}_k(u | H_{ki}, A_{ki})} \widehat{\mathfrak{Q}}_{d,k}(H_{ki}, A_{ki}, u) \Bigg\}.
\end{aligned}
$$

(8.202)

Remark. Intuitively, the fitted models $\widehat{\mathfrak{Q}}_{d,k}(h_k)$ substituted in the first augmentation term in (8.202) should be obtained from the hybrid estimation strategy based on (8.153) and (8.159) rather than via the earlier regression-based approach, so that these models are compatible with the induced fitted models $\widehat{\mathfrak{Q}}_{d,k}(h_k, a_k, u; \beta_k, \beta_{Tk}, \beta_{\tau k})$ used in the final augmentation term in (8.202).

Deducing the models for $\mathcal{Q}_{d,k}(h_k, a_k)$ as in the preceding remark, the estimator (8.202) is a consistent estimator for the value $\mathcal{V}(d)$ as long as either (i) the model for the hazard of censoring, and thus the models for $\mathcal{K}_k(u | h_k, a_k)$, $k = 1, \ldots, K$, and the models for the propensities $\omega_k^\dagger(h_k, a_k)$, $k = 1, \ldots, K$, are correctly specified; or (ii) the models $\lambda_{Tk}(u | h_k, a_k)$, $k = 1, \ldots, K$, and $\lambda_{\tau k}(u | h_k, a_k)$, $k = 1, \ldots, K - 1$, or, equivalently, for $\lambda_{Tk}^\dagger(u | h_k, a_k)$ and $\lambda_{\tau k}^\dagger(u | h_k, a_k)$, and the models for $q_k^d(h_k, a_k, \tau_{k+1})$, $k = 1, \ldots, K - 1$, are correctly specified. In this sense the estimator is doubly robust.

Of course, taking $\widehat{\mathfrak{Q}}_{d,k}(h_k, a_k, u) \equiv 0$, $k = 1, \ldots, K$, in (8.202) yields the augmented inverse probability weighted estimator $\widehat{\mathcal{V}}_{AIPW}(d)$ in (8.192), which does not recover information from censored individuals to improve efficiency. The addition of the final augmentation term in (8.202) comes at the price of a nontrivial increase in computational burden. Simulation studies reported by Hager et al. (2018) in the case $K = 2$ show the potential for substantial gains in efficiency of $\widehat{\mathcal{V}}_{LE}(d)$ over $\widehat{\mathcal{V}}_{AIPW}(d)$, suggesting that this extra effort may be worthwhile.

Implementation of either $\widehat{\mathcal{V}}_{AIPW}(d)$ or $\widehat{\mathcal{V}}_{LE}(d)$ requires the analyst to obtain the fitted models $\widehat{\mathcal{Q}}_{d,k}(h_k)$ by carrying out the hybrid or regression-based algorithm (preferably the former, as in the remark above), and for $\widehat{\mathfrak{Q}}_{d,k}(h_k, a_k, u; \beta_k, \beta_{Tk}, \beta_{\tau k})$, $k = 1, \ldots, K$, by carrying out the hybrid algorithm, which in itself is computationally demanding. Given that these algorithms yield estimators $\widehat{\mathcal{V}}_{HY}(d)$ or $\widehat{\mathcal{V}}_Q(d)$ for $\mathcal{V}(d)$, it is natural to question the need to appeal to these inverse weighted methods. As in simpler settings, the former methods are predicated on correct specification of all required models, whereas $\widehat{\mathcal{V}}_{AIPW}(d)$ or $\widehat{\mathcal{V}}_{LE}(d)$ rely on these models only to gain efficiency. These methods also enjoy some robustness to model misspecification, as outlined above.

Remarks. (i) As for the previous estimators, modifications are necessary if interest focuses on $f(t)$ truncated at L, as for restricted lifetime $f(t) = \min(t, L)$. We note these for the case of censoring and the estimators (8.188), (8.190), and (8.202).

With κ^L as in (8.85), and U^L, Δ^L, $S_k^{\dagger L}$, and $\Upsilon_k^{\dagger L}$ as defined in (8.148) and (8.149), with $S_{K+1}^{\dagger L} = U^L$, replace κ, U, Δ, $S_k^\dagger$, and $\Upsilon_k^\dagger$ by κ^L, U^L, Δ^L, $S_k^{\dagger L}$, and $\Upsilon_k^{\dagger L}$, respectively. As for the regression-based approach, no modification is necessary to H_k, $k = 1, \ldots, K$, and the censoring hazard model $\lambda_C\{u|h(u); \beta_C\}$ should be fitted using the "data" (8.141).

If using the hybrid approach as recommended above, $Q_k^d\{h_k, d_k(h_k)\}$ should be replaced by $Q_k^{d,L}\{h_k, d_k(h_k)\}$ defined in the remark at the end of the description of the hybrid scheme and fitted as described there. For the locally efficient estimator, $\mathfrak{Q}_{d,k}(h_k, a_k, u)$ in (8.199) and (8.200) must also be replaced as follows. With $\lambda_{Tk}^{\dagger L}(u|h_k, a_k)$, $\lambda_{\tau k}^{\dagger L}(u|h_k, a_k)$, $S_{\bullet k}^L(u|h_k, a_k)$, and $q_k^{d,L}(h_k, a_k, \tau_{k+1})$ defined as for the hybrid scheme, let

$$
\mathfrak{Q}_{d,K}^L(h_K, a_K, u) = \int_{u-\tau_K}^{L-\tau_K} f(\tau_K + w) \left[-\frac{dS_{TK}^L(w|h_K, a_K)}{S_{TK}^L(u - \tau_K|h_K, a_K)} \right]
$$
$$
+ f(L) \frac{S_{TK}^L(L - \tau_K|h_K, a_K)}{S_{TK}^L(u - \tau_K|h_K, a_K)}; \tag{8.203}
$$

and, for $k = 1, \ldots, K - 1$,

$$\mathfrak{Q}_{d,k}^L(h_k, a_k, u) = \int_{u - \tau_k}^{L - \tau_k} f(\tau_k + w) \frac{\mathcal{S}_{\bullet k}^L(w | h_k, a_k)}{\mathcal{S}_{\bullet k}^L(u - \tau_k | h_k, a_k)} \lambda_{\tau k}^{\dagger L}(w | h_k, a_k) \, dw$$

$$+ \int_{u - \tau_k}^{L - \tau_k} q_k^{d,L}(h_k, a_k, \tau_k + w) \frac{\mathcal{S}_{\bullet k}^L(w | h_k, a_k)}{\mathcal{S}_{\bullet k}^L(u - \tau_k | h_k, a_k)} \lambda_{\tau k}^{\dagger L}(w | h_k, a_k) \, dw$$

$$+ f(L) \frac{\mathcal{S}_{\bullet k}^L(L - \tau_k | h_k, a_k)}{\mathcal{S}_{\bullet k}^L(u - \tau_k | h_k, a_k)}. \tag{8.204}$$

The induced models for $\mathfrak{Q}_{d,k}^L(h_k, a_k, u)$ can be fitted using the same strategy used to fit the models for $Q_k^{d,L}\{h_k, d_k(h_k)\}$, as referenced above.

(ii) As for the previous approaches, when there are feasible sets of treatment options $\Psi_k(h_k) \subseteq \mathcal{A}_k$ for individuals who reach Decision k with history h_k, $k = 1, \ldots, K$, development of the propensity and other models required to construct the estimators $\widehat{\mathcal{V}}_{IPW}(d)$, $\widehat{\mathcal{V}}_{AIPW}(d)$, and $\widehat{\mathcal{V}}_{LE}(d)$ follows the same strategies outlined in Remark (iii) of Section 6.4.2 and at the end of Section 6.4.3.

8.3.4   Characterization of an Optimal Regime

As in previous chapters, a major objective is to estimate an optimal treatment regime $d^{opt} \in \mathcal{D}$, where, in the present context with a time-to-event outcome, d^{opt} is such that

$$E[f\{T^*(d^{opt})\}] \geq E[f\{T^*(d)\}] \quad \text{for all } d \in \mathcal{D}. \tag{8.205}$$

In Sections 5.6 and 7.2, we discuss characterization of an optimal regime in the case where the outcome of interest is ascertained for all individuals following the final, Kth decision point under SUTVA, the SRA, and the positivity assumption. The characterization of an optimal regime in Section 5.6 is informal, downplaying the notion of feasible sets of treatment regimes at each decision point, and is presented in terms of the observed data. That in Section 7.2 is more technical, incorporating the careful definition of feasible sets given in Section 6.2.2 and used throughout Chapters 6 and 7, and is in terms of potential outcomes, along with a detailed proof that the regime so characterized is indeed optimal. The reader may wish to review the first of or both of these accounts before proceeding.

We now give an analogous characterization of d^{opt} satisfying (8.205) when the outcome is a time to an event, where we continue to assume that the appropriate versions of SUTVA, the SRA, the noninformative censoring (if needed) and positivity assumptions given earlier in this chapter hold. This account is not at the level of technical detail in Section 7.2 in terms of potential outcomes, so that the presentation is as in Section 5.6 in terms of the observed data, which may involve censoring, and we do not provide a formal proof of optimality. Formal such developments would follow along lines similar to those in Section 7.2 and in Section 8.5. We do acknowledge the possibility of feasible sets of treatment options at each decision point; namely, as discussed at the end of Section 8.3.1, for history h_k at Decision k, let $\Psi_k(h_k) \subseteq \mathcal{A}_k$ denote the set of treatment options in $\mathcal{A}_k$ that are feasible for an individual who reaches Decision k with realized history h_k, $k = 1, \ldots, K$.

We first discuss the case of no censoring of the event time. Backward inductive reasoning as in Section 5.6 can be used, so that d^{opt} and its value can be defined recursively in a manner similar to (5.78)–(5.84) and the development of the regression-based approach for estimation $\mathcal{V}(d)$ for a fixed regime $d \in \mathcal{D}$, as follows.

For $\varkappa = K$, similar to (8.124), define

$$Q_K(h_K, a_K) = E\{f(T)|H_K = h_K, A_K = a_K, \varkappa = K\}, \qquad (8.206)$$

and let

$$d_K^{opt}(h_K) = \underset{a_K \in \Psi_K(h_K)}{\arg\max} \; Q_K(h_K, a_K). \qquad (8.207)$$

Let

$$V_K(h_K) = \underset{a_K \in \Psi_K(h_K)}{\max} \; Q_K(h_K, a_K) = Q_K\{h_K, d_K^{opt}(h_K)\}. \qquad (8.208)$$

Then for $\varkappa \geq K - 1$, define

$$Q_{K-1}(h_{K-1}, a_{K-1}) = E\Big\{I(\varkappa = K - 1)f(T)$$
$$+ I(\varkappa = K)V_K(H_K) \mid H_{K-1} = h_{K-1}, A_{K-1} = a_{K-1}, \varkappa \geq K - 1\Big\}$$

and

$$d_{K-1}^{opt}(h_{K-1}) = \underset{a_{K-1} \in \Psi_{K-1}(h_{K-1})}{\arg\max} \; Q_{K-1}(h_{K-1}, a_{K-1}),$$

and let

$$V_{K-1}(h_{K-1}) = \underset{a_{K-1} \in \Psi_{K-1}(h_{K-1})}{\max} \; Q_{K-1}(h_{K-1}, a_{K-1})$$
$$= Q_{K-1}\{h_{K-1}, d_{K-1}^{opt}(h_{K-1})\}.$$

Continuing, for $\varkappa \geq k$, $k = K - 1, \ldots, 1$, let

$$Q_k(h_k, a_k) = E\Big\{I(\varkappa = k)f(T) \qquad (8.209)$$
$$+ I(\varkappa \geq k + 1)V_{k+1}(H_{k+1}) \mid H_k = h_k, A_k = a_k, \varkappa \geq k\Big\},$$

$$d_k^{opt}(h_k) = \underset{a_k \in \Psi_k(h_k)}{\arg\max} \; Q_k(h_k, a_k), \tag{8.210}$$

and

$$V_k(h_k) = \max_{a_k \in \Psi_k(h_k)} Q_k(h_k, a_k) = Q_k\{h_k, d_k^{opt}(h_k)\}. \tag{8.211}$$

As in (8.209), the definition of $Q_k(h_k, a_k)$ accounts for the possibility that the event may be achieved following Decision k, so that subsequent decision points are not reached.

Then it can be shown that an optimal treatment regime in $\mathcal{D}$ satisfying (8.205) is given by

$$d^{opt} = (d_1^{opt}, \ldots, d_K^{opt}),$$

and the value of an optimal regime is

$$\mathcal{V}(d^{opt}) = E\{V_1(H_1)\}. \tag{8.212}$$

When the event time is censored, d^{opt} is characterized in terms of the observed data in a similar manner, with minor modifications to (8.206)–(8.211) as in (8.135)–(8.138) that take censoring into account and with $\mathcal{K}_k(u|h_k, a_k)$ defined as in (8.134). For $\kappa = K$, analogous to (8.206), let

$$Q_K(h_K, a_K)$$
$$= E\left\{ \frac{\Delta f(U)}{\mathcal{K}_K(U|h_K, a_K)} \middle| H_K = h_K, A_K = a_K, \kappa = K \right\}, \tag{8.213}$$

and let

$$d_K^{opt}(h_K) = \underset{a_K \in \Psi_K(h_K)}{\arg\max} \; Q_K(h_K, a_K). \tag{8.214}$$

Let

$$V_K(h_K) = \max_{a_K \in \Psi_K(h_K)} Q_K(h_K, a_K) = Q_K\{h_K, d_K^{opt}(h_K)\}. \tag{8.215}$$

Then for $\kappa \geq K - 1$, define

$$Q_{K-1}(h_{K-1}, a_{K-1})$$
$$= E\left\{ \frac{\mathrm{I}(\Upsilon_K^\dagger = 1)f(S_K^\dagger) + \mathrm{I}(\Upsilon_K^\dagger = -1)V_K(H_K)}{\mathcal{K}_{K-1}(S_K^\dagger|h_{K-1}, a_{K-1})} \middle| \right.$$
$$\left. H_{K-1} = h_{K-1}, A_{K-1} = a_{K-1}, \kappa \geq K - 1 \right\},$$

$$d_{K-1}^{opt}(h_{K-1}) = \underset{a_{K-1} \in \Psi_{K-1}(h_{K-1})}{\arg\max} \; Q_{K-1}(h_{K-1}, a_{K-1}),$$

and let

$$V_{K-1}(h_{K-1}) = \max_{a_{K-1} \in \Psi_{K-1}(h_{K-1})} Q_{K-1}(h_{K-1}, a_{K-1})$$

$$= Q_{K-1}\{h_{K-1}, d_{K-1}^{opt}(h_{K-1})\}.$$

Continuing for $\kappa \geq k$, $k = K - 1, \ldots, 1$, let

$$Q_k(h_k, a_k) =$$

$$= E\left\{ \frac{\mathrm{I}(\Upsilon_{k+1}^\dagger = 1)f(S_{k+1}^\dagger) + \mathrm{I}(\Upsilon_{k+1}^\dagger = -1)V_{k+1}(H_{k+1})}{\mathcal{K}_k(S_{k+1}^\dagger | h_k, a_k)} \right.$$

$$\left. H_k = h_k, A_k = a_k, \kappa \geq k \right\}, \tag{8.216}$$

$$d_k^{opt}(h_k) = \arg\max_{a_k \in \Psi_k(h_k)} Q_k(h_k, a_k), \tag{8.217}$$

and

$$V_k(h_k) = \max_{a_k \in \Psi_k(h_k)} Q_k(h_k, a_k) = Q_k\{h_k, d_k^{opt}(h_k)\}. \tag{8.218}$$

Then it can be shown that an optimal treatment regime in $\mathcal{D}$ satisfying (8.205) is given by $d^{opt} = (d_1^{opt}, \ldots, d_K^{opt})$, and, analogous to (8.212), the value of an optimal regime is

$$\mathcal{V}(d^{opt}) = E\{V_1(H_1)\}. \tag{8.219}$$

8.3.5 Estimation of an Optimal Regime

Parallel to the developments in Sections 5.7 and 7.4, we now discuss several approaches to estimation of an optimal regime d^{opt} as characterized in the previous section, and its value $\mathcal{V}(d^{opt})$. For brevity, we present the methods for the case where the observed data are as in (8.111), i.i.d.

$$(\kappa_i, \mathcal{T}_{1i}, X_{1i}, A_{1i}, \ldots, \mathcal{T}_{\kappa_i i}, X_{\kappa_i i}, A_{\kappa_i i}, U_i, \Delta_i), \quad i = 1, \ldots, n,$$

so involving censoring of the outcome. The methods are modified in the obvious ways when there is no censoring.

Q-learning

As in Sections 5.7.1 and 7.4.1, the foregoing characterization of an optimal regime $d^{opt} \in \mathcal{D}$ given by (8.213)–(8.218) and of its value (8.219) suggest modification of the method of Q-learning to the case of possibly censored, time-to-event outcome.

We first discuss such a Q-learning approach based on a modification of the regression-based algorithm for estimation of the value of a fixed regime. Analogous to the development for that method, define

$$Q_k^R(h_k, a_k) = Q_k(h_k, a_k) - f(\tau_k), \quad k = K, \ldots, 1,$$

and note that $d_k^{opt}(h_k)$ defined in (8.214) and (8.217) can be written equivalently as

$$d_k^{opt}(h_k) = \underset{a_k \in \Psi_k(h_k)}{\arg \max} \; Q_k^R(h_k, a_k), \quad k = K, \ldots, 1. \tag{8.220}$$

The Q-learning algorithm then proceeds as follows.

First, obtain estimators

$$\widehat{\mathcal{K}}_k(u|h_k, a_k) = \exp \left\{ - \int_{\tau_k}^u \lambda_C(w \mid h_k, a_k; \widehat{\beta}_C) \, dw \right\}, \quad k = 1, \ldots, K,$$

as in (8.142) based on the model for the hazard of censoring. Posit parametric models

$$Q_k^R(h_k, a_k; \beta_k), \quad k = K, \ldots, 1,$$

for $Q_k^R(h_k, a_k)$ in terms of finite-dimensional parameters β_k, $k = K, \ldots, 1$.

At Decision K, estimate β_K by $\widehat{\beta}_K$ solving, analogous to (8.145), the inverse probability of censoring M-estimating equation involving individuals i who reach all decision points given by

$$\sum_{i: \kappa_i = K} \left[\frac{\Delta_i}{\widehat{\mathcal{K}}_K(U_i|H_{Ki}, A_{Ki})} \frac{\partial Q_K^R(H_{Ki}, A_{Ki}; \beta_K)}{\partial \beta_K} \right.$$

$$\left. \times \left\{ f(U_i) - f(\mathcal{T}_{Ki}) - Q_K^R(H_{Ki}, A_{Ki}; \beta_K) \right\} \right] = 0. \tag{8.221}$$

Then, substituting $Q_k^R(h_k, a_k; \beta_k)$ in (8.220) for $k = K$, obtain the estimator for d_K^{opt} given by

$$\widehat{d}_{Q,K}^{opt}(h_K) = \underset{a_K \in \Psi_K(h_K)}{\arg \max} \; Q_K^R(h_K, a_K; \widehat{\beta}_K). \tag{8.222}$$

Form pseudo outcomes for individuals i for whom $\kappa_i \geq K - 1$ and $\Upsilon_{Ki}^{\dagger} \neq 0$ as

$$\widetilde{V}_{Ki}^R = \mathrm{I}(\Upsilon_{Ki}^{\dagger} = 1) f(S_{Ki}^{\dagger})$$
$$+ \mathrm{I}(\Upsilon_{Ki}^{\dagger} = -1)[f(S_{Ki}^{\dagger}) + Q_K^R\{H_{Ki}, \widehat{d}_{Q,K}^{opt}(H_{Ki}); \widehat{\beta}_K\}]$$
$$- f(\mathcal{T}_{K-1,i}) \quad \text{for } i : \kappa_i \geq K - 1, \Upsilon_{K,i}^{\dagger} \neq 0;$$

and, based on individuals i who reach Decision $K - 1$, estimate β_{K-1} by $\widehat{\beta}_{K-1}$ solving

$$
\sum_{i:\kappa_i \geq K-1} \left[\frac{I(\Upsilon^\dagger_{Ki} \neq 0)}{\widehat{\mathcal{K}}_{K-1}(S^\dagger_{Ki}|H_{K-1,i}, A_{K-1,i})} \frac{\partial Q^R_{K-1}(H_{K-1,i}, A_{K-1,i}; \beta_{K-1})}{\partial \beta_{K-1}} \right.
$$

$$
\left. \times \left\{ \widetilde{V}^R_{Ki} - Q^R_{K-1}(H_{K-1,i}, A_{K-1,i}; \beta_{K-1}) \right\} \right] = 0.
$$

Obtain from (8.220) for $k = K - 1$ the estimator for d^{opt}_{K-1} given by

$$
\widehat{d}^{opt}_{Q,K-1}(h_{K-1}) = \underset{a_{K-1} \in \Psi_{K-1}(h_{K-1})}{\arg\max} Q^R_{K-1}(h_{K-1}, a_{K-1}; \widehat{\beta}_{K-1}).
$$

In general, for $k = K - 1, \ldots, 1$, obtain the estimator $\widehat{\beta}_k$ for the parameter β_k in the model $Q^R_k(h_k, a_k; \beta_k)$ by solving

$$
\sum_{i:\kappa_i \geq k} \left[\frac{I(\Upsilon^\dagger_{k+1,i} \neq 0)}{\widehat{\mathcal{K}}_k(S^\dagger_{k+1,i}|H_{ki}, A_{ki})} \frac{\partial Q^R_k(H_{ki}, A_{ki}; \beta_k)}{\partial \beta_k} \right.
$$

$$
\left. \times \left\{ \widetilde{V}^R_{k+1,i} - Q^R_k(H_{ki}, A_{ki}; \beta_k) \right\} \right] = 0, \qquad (8.223)
$$

where

$$
\widetilde{V}^R_{k+1,i} = I(\Upsilon^\dagger_{k+1,i} = 1) f(S^\dagger_{k+1,i})
$$

$$
+ I(\Upsilon^\dagger_{k+1,i} = -1)[f(S^\dagger_{k+1,i}) + Q^R_{k+1}\{H_{k+1,i}, \widehat{d}^{opt}_{Q,k+1}(H_{k+1,i}); \widehat{\beta}_{k+1}\}]
$$

$$
- f(\mathcal{T}_{ki}) \quad \text{for } i: \kappa_i \geq k, \Upsilon^\dagger_{k+1,i} \neq 0;
$$

and obtain from (8.220) the estimator for d^{opt}_k

$$
\widehat{d}^{opt}_{Q,k}(h_k) = \underset{a_k \in \Psi_k(h_k)}{\arg\max} Q^R_k(h_k, a_k; \widehat{\beta}_k).
$$

Denote the estimated optimal regime resulting from this recursive scheme as

$$
\widehat{d}^{opt}_Q = \{\widehat{d}^{opt}_{Q,1}(h_1), \ldots, \widehat{d}^{opt}_{Q,K}(h_K)\}; \qquad (8.224)
$$

and, with

$$
\widetilde{V}_{1i} = f(\mathcal{T}_{1i}) + Q^R_1\{H_{1i}, \widehat{d}^{opt}_{Q,1}(H_{1i}); \widehat{\beta}_1\} = f(0) + Q^R_1\{H_{1i}, \widehat{d}^{opt}_{Q,1}(H_{1i}); \widehat{\beta}_1\},
$$

obtain the estimator for the value $\mathcal{V}(d^{opt}) = E[f\{T^*(d^{opt})\}]$ as

$$
\widehat{\mathcal{V}}_Q(d^{opt}) = n^{-1} \sum_{i=1}^n \widetilde{V}_{1i}. \qquad (8.225)
$$

This regression-based Q-learning algorithm leading to the estimator for an optimal regime d^{opt} in (8.224) and the corresponding estimator (8.225) for the value is a generalization of that proposed by Goldberg and Kosorok (2012). These authors assume that censoring is independent of treatment assignment, patient characteristics, and potential outcomes and thus base inverse weighting on the Kaplan-Meier estimator for the censoring distribution as in (8.144). The formulation here requires only the weaker assumption of noninformative censoring (8.68).

An alternative Q-learning algorithm for estimation of an optimal regime d^{opt} is based on the hybrid estimation scheme. Given fitted parametric or semiparametric models

$$\lambda_{Tk}^{\dagger}(u|h_k, a_k; \widehat{\beta}_{Tk}), \quad k = 1, \ldots, K,$$
$$\lambda_{\tau k}^{\dagger}(u|h_k, a_k; \widehat{\beta}_{\tau k}), \quad k = 1, \ldots, K-1,$$

for the cause-specific hazards (8.161)–(8.163) as discussed previously, inducing fitted models

$$\mathcal{S}_{TK}(u|h_K, a_K; \widehat{\beta}_{TK}), \quad \mathcal{S}_{\bullet k}(w|h_k, a_k; \widehat{\beta}_{Tk}, \widehat{\beta}_{\tau k}), \quad k = 1, \ldots, K-1,$$

the algorithm proceeds as follows.

At Decision K, a fitted model for $Q_K(h_K, a_K)$ is induced as

$$Q_K(h_K, a_K; \widehat{\beta}_{TK}) = \int_0^\infty f(\tau_K + w) \, d\mathcal{S}_{TK}(w|h_K, a_K; \widehat{\beta}_{TK}).$$

Substituting in (8.217) for $k = K$ leads to the estimator for d_K^{opt} given by

$$\widehat{d}_{HY,K}^{opt}(h_K) = \underset{a_K \in \Psi_K(h_K)}{\arg\max} \; Q_K(h_K, a_K; \widehat{\beta}_{TK}).$$

Then form pseudo outcomes for all individuals i for whom $\kappa_i = K$ as

$$\widetilde{V}_{Ki}^R = Q_K\{H_{Ki}, \widehat{d}_{HY,K}^{opt}(H_{Ki})\} - f(\mathcal{T}_{Ki}),$$

posit a model $q_{K-1}^R(h_{K-1}, a_{K-1}, \tau_K; \beta_{K-1})$ for

$$q_{K-1}^R(h_{K-1}, a_{K-1}, \tau_K) = E\{V_K(H_K) - f(\tau_K)|H_{K-1} = h_{K-1},$$
$$A_{K-1} = a_{K-1}, \mathcal{T}_K = \tau_K, \kappa = K\}$$

that enforces positivity, and estimate β_{K-1} by $\widehat{\beta}_{k-1}$ solving

$$\sum_{i:\kappa_i = K} \left[\frac{\partial q_{K-1}^R(H_{K-1,i}, A_{K-1,i}, \mathcal{T}_{Ki}; \beta_{K-1})}{\partial \beta_{K-1}} \right.$$
$$\left. \times \left\{ \widetilde{V}_{Ki}^R - q_{K-1}^R(H_{K-1,i}, A_{K-1,i}, \mathcal{T}_{Ki}; \beta_{K-1}) \right\} \right] = 0.$$

At Decision $K - 1$, define

$$Q_{K-1}(h_{K-1}, a_{K-1}; \widehat{\beta}_{K-1}, \widehat{\beta}_{T,K-1}, \widehat{\beta}_{\tau,K-1})$$

$$= \int_0^\infty \left\{ f(\tau_{K-1} + w)\, \mathcal{S}_{\bullet K-1}(w|h_{K-1}, a_{K-1}; \widehat{\beta}_{T,K-1}, \widehat{\beta}_{\tau,K-1}) \right.$$

$$\left. \times \lambda^\dagger_{T,K-1}(w|h_{K-1}, a_{K-1}; \widehat{\beta}_{T,K-1}) \right\} dw$$

$$+ \int_0^\infty \left[\{ q^R_{K-1}(h_{K-1}, a_{K-1}, \tau_{K-1} + w; \widehat{\beta}_{K-1}) + f(\tau_{K-1} + w) \} \right.$$

$$\times \mathcal{S}_{\bullet K-1}(w|h_{K-1}, a_{K-1}; \widehat{\beta}_{T,K-1}, \widehat{\beta}_{\tau,K-1})$$

$$\left. \times \lambda^\dagger_{\tau,K-1}(w|h_{K-1}, a_{K-1}; \widehat{\beta}_{\tau,K-1}) \right] dw.$$

Then, from (8.217) with $k = K-1$, obtain the estimator for the $(K-1)$th optimal rule given by

$$\widehat{d}^{opt}_{HY,K-1}(h_{K-1})$$

$$= \operatorname*{arg\,max}_{a_{K-1} \in \Psi_{K-1}(h_{K-1})} Q_{K-1}(h_{K-1}, a_{K-1}; \widehat{\beta}_{K-1}, \widehat{\beta}_{T,K-1}, \widehat{\beta}_{\tau,K-1}).$$

For all individuals i for whom $\kappa_i \geq K-1$, construct the pseudo outcomes

$$\widetilde{V}^R_{K-1,i}$$

$$= Q_K\{ H_{K-1,i}, \widehat{d}^{opt}_{HY,K-1}(H_{K-1,i}); \widehat{\beta}_{K-1}, \widehat{\beta}_{T,K-1}, \widehat{\beta}_{\tau,K-1} \} - f(\mathcal{T}_{K-1,i}).$$

Continuing in this fashion for $k = K - 1, \dots, 1$, posit a model $q^R_k(h_k, a_k, \tau_{k+1}; \beta_k)$ that enforces positivity for

$$q^R_k(h_k, a_k, \tau_{k+1})$$

$$= E\{ V_{k+1}(H_{k+1}) - f(\tau_{k+1}) | H_k = h_k, A_k = a_k, \mathcal{T}_{k+1} = \tau_{k+1}, \kappa \geq k+1 \},$$

and estimate β_k by $\widehat{\beta}_k$ solving

$$\sum_{i: \kappa_i \geq k+1} \left[\frac{\partial q^R_k(H_{ki}, A_{ki}, \mathcal{T}_{k+1,i}; \beta_k)}{\partial \beta_k} \right.$$

$$\left. \times \left\{ \widetilde{V}^R_{k+1,i} - q^R_k(H_{ki}, A_{ki}, \mathcal{T}_{k+1i}; \beta_k) \right\} \right] = 0.$$

Then, from (8.159), obtain the induced fitted model

$$Q_k(h_k, a_k; \widehat{\beta}_k, \widehat{\beta}_{Tk}, \widehat{\beta}_{\tau k}) = \int_0^\infty f(\tau_k + w)\, \mathcal{S}_{\bullet k}(w|h_k, a_k; \widehat{\beta}_{Tk}, \widehat{\beta}_{\tau k})$$

$$\times \lambda^\dagger_{Tk}(w|h_k, a_k; \widehat{\beta}_{Tk})\, dw \qquad (8.226)$$

$$+ \int_0^\infty \left[\{ q^R_k(h_k, a_k, \tau_k + w; \widehat{\beta}_k) + f(\tau_k + w) \} \mathcal{S}_{\bullet k}(w|h_k, a_k; \widehat{\beta}_{Tk}, \widehat{\beta}_{\tau k}) \right.$$

$$\left. \times \lambda^\dagger_{\tau k}(w|h_k, a_k; \widehat{\beta}_{\tau k}) \right] dw,$$

and obtain the estimator for d_k^{opt} by substituting in (8.217); namely

$$\widehat{d}_{HY,k}^{opt}(h_k) = \underset{a_k \in \Psi_k(h_k)}{\arg\max} \ Q_k(h_k, a_k; \widehat{\beta}_k, \widehat{\beta}_{Tk}, \widehat{\beta}_{\tau k}).$$

Form the pseudo outcomes

$$\widetilde{V}_{ki}^R = Q_k\{H_{ki}, \widehat{d}_{HY,k}^{opt}(H_{ki}); \widehat{\beta}_k, \widehat{\beta}_{Tk}, \widehat{\beta}_{\tau k}\} - f(\mathcal{T}_{ki})$$

for all individuals i for whom $\kappa_i = k$.

By analogy to the regression-based Q-learning algorithm above, denote the estimated optimal regime as

$$\widehat{d}_{HY}^{opt} = \{\widehat{d}_{HY,1}^{opt}(h_1), \dots, \widehat{d}_{HY,K}^{opt}(h_K)\}. \tag{8.227}$$

Letting

$$\widetilde{V}_{1i} = \widetilde{V}_{1i}^R + f(\mathcal{T}_{1i}),$$

where, ordinarily, $f(\mathcal{T}_{1i}) = f(0) = 0$, the corresponding estimator for the value of d^{opt} is

$$\widehat{\mathcal{V}}_{HY}(d^{opt}) = n^{-1} \sum_{i=1}^n \widetilde{V}_{1i}.$$

Remarks. (i) If interest focuses on $f(t)$ truncated at L, both the regression-based and hybrid Q-learning algorithms must be modified in accordance with the needed changes discussed for estimation of the value of a fixed regime.

For the regression-based scheme, from (8.148) and (8.149), replace κ, U, Δ, $S_k^\dagger$, and $\Upsilon_k^\dagger$ by κ^L, U^L, Δ^L, $S_k^{\dagger L}$, and $\Upsilon_k^{\dagger L}$, respectively, in the estimating equations (8.221) and (8.223). The modifications required for the hybrid Q-learning scheme are more involved and follow in the obvious way from Remark (i) at the end of the discussion of hybrid estimators for the value of a fixed regime in Section 8.3.3.

(ii) As for estimation of the value of a fixed regime, estimation of an optimal regime via the hybrid Q-learning algorithm has the advantage over the regression-based approach of not requiring modeling of the hazard of censoring, but can be computationally more burdensome.

In the regression-based approach, the estimated rules $\widehat{d}_{Q,k}^{opt}(h_k)$ in the estimated optimal regime $\widehat{d}_Q^{opt}$ in (8.224) have a closed form dictated by the estimated parameters $\widehat{\beta}_k$ in the fitted models $Q_k^R(h_k, a_k; \widehat{\beta}_k)$ for $Q_k^R(h_k, a_k)$. In contrast, the estimated rules $\widehat{d}_{HY,k}^{opt}(h_k)$ in $\widehat{d}_{HY}^{opt}$ in (8.227) are defined by a complex combination of the estimated parameters in the models $\lambda_{Tk}^\dagger(u|h_k, a_k; \beta_{Tk})$, $\lambda_{\tau k}^\dagger(u|h_k, a_k; \beta_{\tau k})$, and $q_k^R(h_k, a_k, \tau_{k+1}; \beta_k)$ and thus do not have a closed form. Accordingly, $\widehat{d}_{HY,k}^{opt}(h_k)$ must be determined by evaluating (8.226) for each value of h_k when selecting treatment for an arbitrary patient and for each individual i when constructing pseudo outcomes.

Value Search Estimation

From the discussion in Sections 5.7.2 and 7.4.3, methods like those just outlined for estimation of an optimal multiple decision regime, which are based on direct or indirect specification of models for $Q_k(h_k, a_k)$, $k = 1, \ldots, K$, effectively induce a restricted class of regimes indexed by the collection of parameters involved in the relevant models. Thus, these methods limit the search for $d^{opt} \in \mathcal{D}$ to that induced class, and misspecification of the required models can lead to an induced class that does not contain d^{opt} and thus to poor estimation of d^{opt}. This motivates alternative methods that are predicated on restricting attention deliberately to a class $\mathcal{D}_\eta \subset \mathcal{D}$ of regimes of interest whose rules are indexed by a parameter η, where $\mathcal{D}_\eta$ is specified on the basis of interpretability, cost, ease of implementation, and so on. We now discuss this approach in the context of a possibly censored time-to-event outcome.

As in Sections 5.7.2 and 7.4.3, a regime $d_\eta \in \mathcal{D}_\eta$ comprises K rules; i.e.,

$$d_\eta = \{d_1(h_1; \eta_1), \ldots, d_K(h_K; \eta_K)\}, \quad \eta = (\eta_1^T, \ldots, \eta_K^T)^T,$$

where the rule at Decision k is indexed by a parameter η_k and for brevity is often written as

$$d_{\eta,k}(h_k) = d_k(h_k; \eta_k), \quad k = 1, \ldots, K.$$

The form of the rules $d_k(h_k; \eta_k)$, $k = 1, \ldots, K$, should respect the nature of the feasible sets $\Psi_k(h_k)$, as discussed in detail in those sections. An optimal regime d_η^{opt} in $\mathcal{D}_\eta$ is then given by

$$d_\eta^{opt} = \{d_1(h_1; \eta_1^{opt}), \ldots, d_K(h_K; \eta_K^{opt})\},$$
$$\eta^{opt} = (\eta_1^{opt\,T}, \ldots, \eta_K^{opt\,T})^T = \arg\max_\eta \mathcal{V}(d_\eta), \tag{8.228}$$

where, here,

$$\mathcal{V}(d_\eta) = E[f\{T^*(d_\eta)\}].$$

If $\widehat{\mathcal{V}}(d)$ is an estimator for the value of a fixed regime d, (8.228) suggests obtaining

$$\widehat{\eta}^{opt} = (\widehat{\eta}_1^{opt\,T}, \ldots, \widehat{\eta}_K^{opt\,T})^T = \arg\max_\eta \widehat{\mathcal{V}}(d_\eta).$$

An obvious estimator for d_η^{opt} is then the value search (or direct or policy search) estimator

$$\widehat{d}_\eta^{opt} = \{d_1(h_1, \widehat{\eta}_1^{opt}), \ldots, d_K(h_K, \widehat{\eta}_K^{opt})\}. \tag{8.229}$$

As for the Q-learning methods, we continue to focus on the case where the observed data involve censoring of the outcome as in (8.111), i.i.d.

$$(\kappa_i, \mathcal{T}_{1i}, X_{1i}, A_{1i}, \ldots, \mathcal{T}_{\kappa_i i}, X_{\kappa_i i}, A_{\kappa_i i}, U_i, \Delta_i), \quad i = 1, \ldots, n.$$

By analogy to the developments in Sections 5.7.2 and 7.4.3, a natural strategy for estimation of d_η^{opt} from these data is to maximize in η any one of $\widehat{\mathcal{V}}_{IPW}(d_\eta)$, $\widehat{\mathcal{V}}_{AIPW}(d_\eta)$, or $\widehat{\mathcal{V}}_{LE}(d_\eta)$ given in (8.188), (8.190), and (8.202), for example,

$$
\begin{aligned}
\widehat{\mathcal{V}}_{LE}(d_\eta) = n^{-1} \sum_{i=1}^{n} & \left\{ \frac{\mathcal{C}_{d_\eta,\kappa_i,i}^\dagger \Delta_i f(U_i)}{\widehat{\varpi}_{\kappa_i}^\dagger (H_{\kappa_i,i}, A_{\kappa_i,i}) \widehat{\mathcal{K}}_{\kappa_i}(U_i | H_{\kappa_i,i}, A_{\kappa_i,i})} \right. \\
& - \sum_{k=1}^{\kappa_i} \left(\frac{\mathcal{C}_{d_\eta,k-1,i}^\dagger \mathrm{I}(\Upsilon_{ki}^\dagger \neq 0)}{\widehat{\varpi}_{k-1}^\dagger (H_{k-1,i}, A_{k-1,i}) \widehat{\mathcal{K}}_{k-1}(S_{ki}^\dagger | H_{k-1,i}, A_{k-1,i})} \right. \\
& \times \left. \left[\frac{\mathrm{I}\{A_{ki} = d_{\eta,k}(H_{ki})\} - \omega_k^\dagger (H_{ki}, A_{ki}; \widehat{\gamma}_k)}{\omega_k^\dagger (H_{ki}, A_{ki}; \widehat{\gamma}_k)} \right] \widehat{\mathcal{Q}}_{d_\eta,k}(H_{ki}) \right) \\
& \left. + \sum_{k=1}^{\kappa_i} \frac{\mathcal{C}_{d_\eta,ki}^\dagger}{\widehat{\varpi}_k^\dagger (H_{ki}, A_{ki})} \int_{S_{ki}^\dagger}^{S_{k+1,i}^\dagger} \frac{d\widehat{M}_{C,k}(u | H_{ki}, A_{ki})}{\widehat{\mathcal{K}}_k(u | H_{ki}, A_{ki})} \widehat{\mathfrak{Q}}_{d_\eta,k}(H_{ki}, A_{ki}, u) \right\};
\end{aligned}
\tag{8.230}
$$

and substitute the resulting maximizer in (8.229).

Of course, as outlined at the end of Section 7.4.3, although this approach is conceptually straightforward, it involves considerable computational challenges that are almost certain to render it infeasible in practice. First, maximization of any of $\widehat{\mathcal{V}}_{IPW}(d_\eta)$, $\widehat{\mathcal{V}}_{AIPW}(d_\eta)$, or $\widehat{\mathcal{V}}_{LE}(d_\eta)$ is a nonsmooth optimization problem, requiring specialized techniques, such as use of a genetic algorithm, even if the dimension of η is small enough to make direct maximization of one of these value estimators computationally tractable. In most problems, as in Section 7.4.3, the dimension of η is sufficiently large to make optimization via such an approach formidable. In addition, analogous to the second main issue discussed in detail in Section 7.4.3, focusing on (8.230), obtaining the fitted models $\widehat{\mathcal{Q}}_{d_\eta,k}(H_{ki})$ and $\widehat{\mathfrak{Q}}_{d_\eta,k}(H_{ki}, A_{ki}, u)$ for each individual i in the augmentation terms in (8.230) via the previous backward recursive schemes depends on the regime d_η and thus on η. Accordingly, at each internal iteration of the optimization algorithm used to maximize $\widehat{\mathcal{V}}_{LE}(d_\eta)$

in η, these models must be refitted using the current iterate of η, so that both backward recursive schemes must be carried out anew. Clearly, the computational burden involved is substantial. Although maximization of $\widehat{\mathcal{V}}_{IPW}(d_\eta)$ in η does not involve this complication, the instability and inefficiency of this estimator for $\mathcal{V}(d_\eta)$ noted previously translates into likely unstable and inefficient estimation of d_η^{opt}.

As discussed at the end of Section 7.4.3, an ad hoc strategy to avoid this issue is to carry out Q-learning based on the hybrid estimation approach once as described above and substitute the resulting fitted models in (8.230), recognizing that these do not represent fitted models for the desired quantities, the hope being that they are "close enough." However, as noted there, even with such a simplification, the high dimension of η may make global maximization in η of any of these value estimators simply untenable in practice.

Backward Iterative Estimation

The foregoing considerations are one motivation for the backward iterative implementation of value search estimation we now discuss, which is analogous to that presented in Section 7.4.4, adapted to the case where the outcome is a possibly censored time to an event. The reader may wish to review the developments in Section 7.4.4 before proceeding.

We continue to assume that interest focuses on estimating an optimal regime $d_\eta^{opt} \in \mathcal{D}_\eta$ as in (8.228), where $\mathcal{D}_\eta$ is a restricted class of regimes of the form $d_\eta = \{d_1(h_1; \eta_1), \ldots, d_K(h_K; \eta_K)\} = \{d_{\eta,1}(h_1), \ldots, d_{\eta,K}(h_K)\}$. Consider the case where the observed data involve possible censoring of the outcome, so are as in (8.111),

$$(\kappa_i, \mathcal{T}_{1i}, X_{1i}, A_{1i}, \ldots, \mathcal{T}_{\kappa_i i}, X_{\kappa_i i}, A_{\kappa_i i}, U_i, \Delta_i), \quad i = 1, \ldots, n,$$

i.i.d. across i, with, for $k = 2, \ldots, K$,

$$S_{ki}^\dagger = I(\kappa_i = k - 1)U_i + I(\kappa_i \geq k)\mathcal{T}_{ki},$$

$$\Upsilon_{ki}^\dagger = 1 \quad \text{if } \kappa_i = k - 1, \Delta_i = 1$$
$$= 0 \quad \text{if } \kappa_i = k - 1, \Delta_i = 0$$
$$= -1 \quad \text{if } \kappa_i \geq k;$$

and $S_{K+1,i}^\dagger = I(\kappa_i = K)U_i$ and $\Upsilon_{K+1,i}^\dagger = I(\kappa_i = K)\Delta_i$.

We consider value search estimation of an optimal regime based on maximizing in η the locally efficient estimator $\widehat{\mathcal{V}}_{LE}(d_\eta)$ given in (8.230). The backward scheme we now describe can be adapted to maximization of $\widehat{\mathcal{V}}_{IPW}(d_\eta)$ or $\widehat{\mathcal{V}}_{AIPW}(d_\eta)$ in (8.188) or (8.190) in the obvious way.

As in Section 7.4.4, let

$$\underline{d}_{\eta,k} = (d_{\eta,k}, d_{\eta,k+1}, \ldots, d_{\eta,K}), \quad k = 1, \ldots, K,$$

so $\underline{d}_{\eta,1} = d_\eta$. Analogous to (7.111) and similar to (8.187), for an individual for whom $\kappa \geq r$, so who reaches Decision r and whose event time is not censored prior to Decision r, denote the probability of receiving options $a_\ell, \ldots, a_r$ at Decisions ℓ to r as

$$\underline{\omega}_{\ell,r}^\dagger(h_r, a_r) = \left\{ \prod_{j=\ell}^r \omega_j^\dagger(h_j, a_j) \right\} \left\{ \prod_{j=\ell}^{r-1} \mathcal{K}_j(\tau_{j+1}|h_j, a_j) \right\}, \quad r \geq \ell + 1$$

$$= \omega_\ell^\dagger(h_\ell, a_\ell), \quad r = \ell,$$

for $r \geq \ell = 1, \ldots, K$. Given models $\omega_k^\dagger(h_k, a_k; \gamma_k)$ as in (8.186) and models for $\mathcal{K}_k(u|h_k, a_k)$ depending on a parameter β_C, $k = 1, \ldots, K$, models for $\underline{\omega}_{\ell,r}^\dagger(h_r, a_r)$, $r \geq \ell + 1$, are induced as

$$\underline{\omega}_{\ell,r}^\dagger(h_r, a_r; \underline{\gamma}_{\ell,r}, \beta_C) = \left\{ \prod_{j=\ell}^r \omega_j^\dagger(h_j, a_j; \gamma_j) \right\} \left\{ \prod_{j=\ell}^{r-1} \mathcal{K}_j(\tau_{j+1}|h_j, a_j; \beta_C) \right\},$$

where $\underline{\gamma}_{\ell,r} = (\gamma_\ell^T, \ldots, \gamma_r^T)^T$. Assume that models for $Q_k^{d_\eta}(h_k, a_k)$ and $\mathfrak{Q}_{d_\eta,k}(h_k, a_k, u)$, $k = 1, \ldots, K$, are induced by the hybrid strategy and thus are of the form

$$Q_k^{d_\eta}(h_k, a_k; \beta_k, \beta_{Tk}, \beta_{\tau k}) \quad \text{and} \quad \mathfrak{Q}_{d_\eta,k}(h_k, a_k, u; \beta_k, \beta_{Tk}, \beta_{\tau k})$$

as before, where the models for $k = K$ depend only on β_{TK} and not on d_η. Define $\underline{\gamma}_k = (\gamma_k^T, \ldots, \gamma_K^T)^T$; define $\underline{\beta}_{Tk}$ similarly for $k = 1, \ldots, K$, and $\underline{\beta}_k = (\beta_k^T, \ldots, \beta_{K-1}^T)^T$ and $\underline{\beta}_{\tau k} = (\beta_{\tau 1}^T, \ldots, \beta_{\tau,K-1}^T)^T$ for $k = 1, \ldots, K - 1$; and denote estimated versions as $\widehat{\underline{\gamma}}_k$, $\widehat{\underline{\beta}}_k$, $\widehat{\underline{\beta}}_{Tk}$, and $\widehat{\underline{\beta}}_{\tau k}$. Finally, analogous to (7.112), define the indicator that the treatment options actually received by an individual for whom $\kappa \geq r$ are consistent with those dictated by d_η at Decisions ℓ through r, $r \geq \ell = 1, \ldots, K$, as

$$\mathfrak{C}_{d_\eta,\ell,r}^\dagger = \mathrm{I}\{A_\ell = d_{\eta,\ell}(H_\ell), \ldots, A_r = d_{\eta,r}(H_r), \kappa \geq r\}. \tag{8.231}$$

With these definitions, analogous to (7.113), let

$$\mathcal{G}_{LE,k}(\underline{d}_{\eta,k}; \underline{\gamma}_k, \beta_C, \underline{\beta}_k, \underline{\beta}_{Tk}, \underline{\beta}_{\tau k})$$

$$= \mathrm{I}(\kappa \geq k) \left\{ \frac{\mathfrak{C}_{d_\eta,k,\kappa}^\dagger \Delta f(U)}{\underline{\omega}_{k,\kappa}^\dagger(H_\kappa, A_\kappa; \underline{\gamma}_{k,\kappa}, \beta_C) \mathcal{K}_\kappa(U|H_\kappa, A_\kappa; \beta_C)} \right.$$

$$\left. - \left[\frac{\mathrm{I}\{A_k = d_{\eta,k}(H_k)\} - \omega_k^\dagger(H_k, A_k; \gamma_k)}{\omega_k^\dagger(H_k, A_k; \gamma_k)} \right] Q_k^{d_\eta}\{H_k, d_{\eta,k}(H_k); \beta_k, \beta_{Tk}, \beta_{\tau k}\} \right.$$

$$
\begin{aligned}
-\sum_{r=k+1}^{\kappa} &\left(\frac{\mathrm{I}(\kappa > k)\mathfrak{C}^{\dagger}_{d_\eta,k,r-1}\mathrm{I}(\Upsilon^{\dagger}_r \neq 0)}{\underline{\omega}^{\dagger}_{k,r-1}(H_{r-1}, A_{r-1}; \underline{\gamma}_{k,r-1}, \beta_C)\mathcal{K}_{r-1}(S^{\dagger}_r | H_{r-1}, A_{r-1}; \beta_C)} \right. \\
&\times \left[\frac{\mathrm{I}\{A_r = d_{\eta,r}(H_r)\} - \omega^{\dagger}_r(H_r, A_r; \gamma_r)}{\omega^{\dagger}_r(H_r, A_r; \gamma_r)} \right] \qquad (8.232)\\
&\left. \times Q^{d_\eta}_r \{H_r, d_{\eta,r}(H_r); \beta_r, \beta_{Tr}, \beta_{rr}\} \right) \\
+\sum_{r=k}^{\kappa} &\left[\frac{\mathfrak{C}^{\dagger}_{d_\eta,k,r}}{\underline{\omega}^{\dagger}_{k,r}(H_r, A_r; \underline{\gamma}_{k,r})} \right. \\
&\left. \left. \times \int_{S^{\dagger}_r}^{S^{\dagger}_{r+1}} \frac{dM_{C,r}(u|H_r, A_r; \beta_C)}{\mathcal{K}_r(u|H_r, A_r; \beta_C)} \mathfrak{Q}_{d_\eta,r}(H_r, A_r, u; \beta_r, \beta_{Tr}, \beta_{rr}) \right] \right\}.
\end{aligned}
$$

In (8.232), as in (7.113), dependence on the observed data is suppressed, the third term on the right-hand side of (8.232) is equal to zero for $k = \kappa$, and $\mathcal{G}_{LE,ki}(\underline{d}_{\eta,k}; \underline{\gamma}_k, \beta_C, \underline{\beta}_k, \underline{\beta}_{Tk}, \underline{\beta}_{rk})$ denotes evaluation at the data for individual i given above.

Similar to (7.114), it is straightforward to demonstrate that $\widehat{\mathcal{V}}_{LE}(d_\eta)$ in (8.230) can be written as

$$
\widehat{\mathcal{V}}_{LE}(d_\eta) = n^{-1} \sum_{i=1}^{n} \mathcal{G}_{LE,1i}(\underline{d}_{\eta,1}; \widehat{\underline{\gamma}}_1, \widehat{\beta}_C, \widehat{\underline{\beta}}_1, \widehat{\underline{\beta}}_{T1}, \widehat{\underline{\beta}}_{r1}), \qquad (8.233)
$$

where in fact $\widehat{\underline{\gamma}}_1 = \widehat{\overline{\gamma}}_K$, $\widehat{\underline{\beta}}_1 = \widehat{\overline{\beta}}_{K-1} = (\widehat{\beta}^T_1, \ldots, \widehat{\beta}^T_{K-1})^T$, $\widehat{\underline{\beta}}_{T1} = \widehat{\overline{\beta}}_{TK} = (\widehat{\beta}^T_{T1}, \ldots, \widehat{\beta}^T_{TK})^T$, and $\widehat{\underline{\beta}}_{r1} = \widehat{\overline{\beta}}_{r,K-1} = (\widehat{\beta}^T_{r1}, \ldots, \widehat{\beta}^T_{r,K-1})^T$.

The backward iterative strategy we now present follows the same principle as that in Section 7.4.4. For definiteness, we consider $f(t)$ involving truncation at a restricted time L, so incorporating the modifications for this case discussed previously, and describe implementation in some detail. Recall from (8.85), (8.148), and (8.149) that

$$
\kappa^L = \max_k \{k = 1, \ldots, \kappa : \mathcal{T}_k \leq L\};
$$

$$
U^L = \min(U, L), \quad \Delta^L = \Delta \quad \text{if } U \leq L,
$$
$$
= 1 \quad \text{if } U > L;
$$

$$
S^{\dagger L}_k = \mathrm{I}(\kappa^L = k-1)U^L + \mathrm{I}(\kappa^L \geq k)\mathcal{T}_k,
$$
$$
\Upsilon^{\dagger L}_k = 1 \quad \text{if } \kappa^L = k-1, \Delta^L = 1,
$$
$$
= 0 \quad \text{if } \kappa^L = k-1, \Delta^L = 0,
$$
$$
= -1 \quad \text{if } \kappa^L \geq k
$$

for $k = 2, \ldots, K$, with $S_{K+1}^{\dagger L} = I(\kappa^L = K)U^L$ and $\Upsilon_{K+1}^{\dagger L} = I(\kappa^L = K)\Delta^L$. Analogous to (8.231), define

$$\mathfrak{C}_{d_\eta,\ell,r}^{\dagger L} = I\{A_\ell = d_{\eta,\ell}(H_\ell), \ldots, A_r = d_{\eta,r}(H_r), \kappa^L \geq r\}. \qquad (8.234)$$

For an individual who reaches Decision K without achieving the event or being censored, selection of a treatment option at Decision K is effectively equivalent to a single decision problem where he presents with baseline history H_K. Using the data from individuals i for whom $\kappa_i^L = K$, posit and fit a model $\lambda_{TK}^{\dagger L}(u|h_K, a_K; \beta_{TK})$ for $\lambda_{TK}^{\dagger L}(u|h_K, a_K)$ as in Remark (i) in the description of the hybrid estimation scheme in Section 8.3.3, inducing a model $S_{TK}^L(u|h_K, a_K; \beta_{TK})$. As in (8.170) and (8.203), write

$$Q_K^{d_\eta, L}(h_K, a_K; \beta_{TK}) = \int_0^{L-\tau_K} f(\tau_K + w)\{-dS_{TK}^L(w|h_K, a_K; \beta_{TK})\}$$
$$+ f(L)S_{TK}^L(L - \tau_K|h_K, a_K; \beta_{TK})$$

and

$$\mathfrak{Q}_{d_\eta,K}^L(h_K, a_K, u; \beta_{TK})$$
$$= \int_{u-\tau_K}^{L-\tau_K} f(\tau_K + w)\left[-\frac{dS_{TK}^L(w|h_K, a_K; \beta_{TK})}{S_{TK}^L(u - \tau_K|h_K, a_K; \beta_{TK})}\right]$$
$$+ f(L)\frac{S_{TK}^L(L - \tau_K|h_K, a_K; \beta_{TK})}{S_{TK}^L(u - \tau_K|h_K, a_K; \beta_{TK})},$$

which, as in (8.170) and (8.203), do not depend on d_η. Then, from (8.232) with $k = K$, in obvious notation reflecting truncation of $f(t)$ at L; with κ^L, U^L, Δ^L, and $S_K^{\dagger L}$ defined above; and using $\underline{\omega}_{K,K}^\dagger(h_K, a_K; \underline{\gamma}_{K,K}, \beta_C) = \omega_K(h_K, a_K; \gamma_K)$ and $S_{K+1}^{\dagger L} = U^L$,

$$\mathcal{G}_{LE,K}^L(d_{\eta,K}; \gamma_K, \beta_C, \beta_{TK})$$
$$= I(\kappa^L = K)\left(\frac{\mathfrak{C}_{d_\eta,K,K}^{\dagger L}\Delta^L f(U^L)}{\omega_K^\dagger(H_K, A_K; \gamma_K)\mathcal{K}_K(U^L|H_K, A_K; \beta_C)}\right.$$
$$- \left[\frac{I\{A_K = d_{\eta,K}(H_K)\} - \omega_K^\dagger(H_K, A_K; \gamma_K)}{\omega_K^\dagger(H_K, A_K; \gamma_K)}\right]Q_K^{d_\eta, L}\{H_K, d_{\eta,K}(H_K); \beta_{TK}\}$$

$$\qquad (8.235)$$

$$+ \left\{\frac{\mathfrak{C}_{d_\eta,K,K}^{\dagger L}}{\omega_K^\dagger(H_K, A_K; \gamma_K)}\right.$$
$$\left.\left. \times \int_{S_K^{\dagger L}}^{U^L} \frac{dM_{C,K}(u|H_K, A_K; \beta_C)}{\mathcal{K}_K(u|H_K, A_K; \beta_C)}\mathfrak{Q}_{d_\eta,K}^L(H_K, A_K, u; \beta_{TK})\right\}\right),$$

where, from (8.234),

$$\mathfrak{C}^{\dagger L}_{d_\eta, K, K} = I\{A_K = d_{\eta, K}(H_K), \kappa^L = K\}.$$

With $\widehat{\beta}_{TK}$ the estimator for β_{TK} obtained as described above, let

$$\widehat{\mathcal{V}}^{(K)}_{LE}(d_{\eta, K}) = n^{-1} \sum_{i=1}^{n} \mathcal{G}^L_{LE, Ki}(d_{\eta, K}; \widehat{\gamma}_K, \widehat{\beta}_C, \widehat{\beta}_{TK}), \qquad (8.236)$$

where the subscript i indicates evaluation at κ^L_i, U^L_i, Δ^L_i, $S^{\dagger L}_{Ki}$, H_{Ki}, and A_{Ki}. From (8.235), $\widehat{\mathcal{V}}^{(K)}_{LE}(d_{\eta, K})$ is based only on the data for individuals i for whom $\kappa^L_i = K$, so who reached all K decisions prior to L. Also, upon substitution of $\widehat{\gamma}_K$, $\widehat{\beta}_C$, and $\widehat{\beta}_K$ in (8.235), $\mathcal{K}_K(u|H_K, A_K; \widehat{\beta}_C) = \widehat{\mathcal{K}}_K(u|H_K, A_K)$, $Q^{d_\eta, L}_K\{H_K, d_{\eta, K}(H_K); \widehat{\beta}_{TK}\} = \widehat{\mathcal{Q}}^L_{d_\eta, K}(H_K)$, $\mathfrak{Q}^L_{d_\eta, K}(H_K, A_K, u; \widehat{\beta}_{TK}) = \widehat{\mathfrak{Q}}^L_{d_\eta, K}(H_K, A_K, u)$, and the martingale increment $dM_{C, K}(u|H_K, A_K; \widehat{\beta}_C) = d\widehat{M}(u|H_K, A_K)$ in the previous notation.

Similar to the developments in Sections 6.4.2, 7.2.3, and 7.4.4 and as discussed in Section 8.5, let

$$T^*(\overline{a}_{k-1}, d_{\eta, k}, \ldots, d_{\eta, K}) = T^*(\overline{a}_{k-1}, \underline{d}_{\eta, k}), \quad k = 1, \ldots, K, \qquad (8.237)$$

be the potential event time for an individual who reaches Decision k if she were to receive options $a_1, \ldots, a_{k-1}$ at Decisions 1 to $k-1$ and then be treated according to the rules $d_{\eta, k}, \ldots, d_{\eta, K}$ at the remaining decision points, where it is understood that (8.237) depends on the rules $d_{\eta, k}, \ldots, d_{\eta, K}$ only through those that are not null. For $\widehat{\gamma}_K$, $\widehat{\beta}_C$, and $\widehat{\beta}_{TK}$ in (8.236), let γ^*_K, β^*_C, and β^*_{TK} be the limits in probability of these estimators. Then if either (i) the models $\lambda_C(u|h_K, a_K; \beta_C)$, and thus $\mathcal{K}_K(u|h_K, a_K; \beta_C)$, and $\omega^\dagger_K(h_K, a_K; \gamma_K)$ are correctly specified; or (ii) $\lambda^\dagger_{TK}(u|h_K, a_K; \beta_{TK})$ is correctly specified, so that β^*_C or γ^*_K and β^*_{TK} are equal to the true values of these parameters, using the double robustness property of $\widehat{\mathcal{V}}^{(K)}_{LE}(d_{\eta, K})$, analogous to (7.117), from (8.237),

$$E\{\mathcal{G}^L_{LE, K}(d_{\eta, K}; \gamma^*_K, \beta^*_C, \beta^*_{TK})|H_K\}$$
$$= I(\kappa^L = K)E[f\{T^*(\overline{A}_{K-1}, d_{\eta, K})\} \,|\, H_K]$$
$$= E[I(\kappa^L = K)f\{T^*(\overline{A}_{K-1}, d_{\eta, K})\} \,|\, H_K].$$

Taking expectation with respect to the distribution of H_K yields, analogous to (7.118),

$$E\{\mathcal{G}^L_{LE, K}(d_{\eta, K}; \gamma^*_K, \beta^*_C, \beta^*_{TK})\} = E[I(\kappa^L = K)f\{T^*(\overline{A}_{K-1}, d_{\eta, K})\}]. \qquad (8.238)$$

From (8.238), for fixed $d_{\eta,K}$, under these conditions, $\widehat{\mathcal{V}}_{LE}^{(K)}(d_{\eta,K})$ is thus a consistent estimator for $E[\mathrm{I}(\kappa^L = K)f\{T^*(\overline{A}_{K-1}, d_{\eta,K})\}]$, which plays the role of the value of the "single decision regime" $d_{\eta,K}$. Accordingly, as in (7.119), define

$$
\begin{aligned}
d_{\eta,K,B}^{opt}(h_K) &= d_K(h_K; \eta_{K,B}^{opt}), \\
\eta_{K,B}^{opt} &= \arg\max_{\eta_K} E[\mathrm{I}(\kappa^L = K)f\{T^*(\overline{A}_{K-1}, d_{\eta,K})\}],
\end{aligned}
\tag{8.239}
$$

where, as in Section 7.4.4, $\eta_{K,B}^{opt}$ defined in (8.239) is probably not the same as the component η_K^{opt} of η^{opt} globally maximizing $\mathcal{V}(d_\eta)$ in η as in (8.228).

Thus, the first step of the backward iterative algorithm is, analogous to (7.120), to maximize $\widehat{\mathcal{V}}_{LE}^{(K)}(d_{\eta,K})$ in η_K to obtain $\widehat{\eta}_{K,B,LE}^{opt}$, an estimator for $\eta_{K,B}^{opt}$, and the estimator

$$
\widehat{d}_{\eta,K,B}^{opt}(h_K) = d_K(h_K; \widehat{\eta}_{K,B,LE}^{opt})
$$

for $d_{\eta,K,B}^{opt}(h_K)$ in (8.239). Because $Q_K^{d_\eta,L}\{H_K, d_{\eta,K}(H_K); \widehat{\beta}_{TK}\}$ in this maximization depends on η_K only through substitution of $d_{\eta,K}(h_K)$, this model need be fitted only once.

As for the algorithm in Section 7.4.4, now consider Decision $K-1$. For all individuals i for whom $\kappa_i^L = K$, obtain the pseudo outcomes

$$
\widetilde{V}_{Ki}^{R_{d_\eta},L} = Q_K^{d_\eta,L}\{H_{Ki}, \widehat{d}_{\eta,K,B}^{opt}(H_{Ki}); \widehat{\beta}_{TK}\} - f(\mathcal{T}_{Ki});
$$

and, given a model $q_{K-1}^{R_{d_\eta},L}(h_{K-1}, a_{K-1}, \tau_K; \beta_{K-1})$, where

$$
q_{K-1}^{d_\eta,L}(h_{K-1}, a_{K-1}, \tau_K; \beta_{K-1}) = q_{K-1}^{R_{d_\eta},L}(h_{K-1}, a_{K-1}, \tau_K; \beta_{K-1}) + f(\mathcal{T}_K),
$$

use these to obtain the estimator $\widehat{\beta}_{K-1}$ as described in Remark (i) at the end of the description of the hybrid estimation scheme in Section 8.3.3. Posit cause-specific hazard models $\lambda_{T,K-1}^{\dagger L}(u|h_{K-1}, a_{K-1}; \beta_{T,K-1})$ and $\lambda_{\tau,K-1}^{\dagger L}(u|h_{K-1}, a_{K-1}; \beta_{\tau,K-1})$, which can be fitted based on the data from individuals i for whom $\kappa_i^L \geq K-1$ to yield $\widehat{\beta}_{T,K-1}$ and $\widehat{\beta}_{\tau,K-1}$ and imply the model $\mathcal{S}_{\bullet K-1}^L(u|h_{K-1}, a_{K-1}; \beta_{T,K-1}, \beta_{\tau,K-1})$. Then, from (8.171) and (8.204) with $k = K-1$,

$$
\begin{aligned}
Q_{K-1}^{d_\eta,L}&(h_{K-1}, a_{K-1}; \beta_{K-1}, \beta_{T,K-1}, \beta_{\tau,K-1}) = \\
&\int_0^{L-\tau_{K-1}} \Big\{ f(\tau_{K-1} + w)\mathcal{S}_{\bullet K-1}^L(w|h_{K-1}, a_{K-1}; \beta_{T,K-1}, \beta_{\tau,K-1}) \\
&\qquad \times \lambda_{T,K-1}^{\dagger L}(w|h_{K-1}, a_{K-1}; \beta_{T,K-1}) \Big\} dw
\end{aligned}
$$

$$+ \int_0^{L-\tau_{K-1}} \left\{ q_{K-1}^{d_\eta, L}(h_{K-1}, a_{K-1}, \tau_{K-1} + w; \beta_{K-1}) \right.$$

$$\times \mathcal{S}_{\bullet K-1}^L(w | h_{K-1}, a_{K-1}; \beta_{T,K-1}, \beta_{\tau,K-1})$$

$$\left. \times \lambda_{\tau,K-1}^{\dagger L}(w | h_{K-1}, a_{K-1}; \beta_{\tau,K-1}) \right\} dw$$

$$+ f(L) \mathcal{S}_{\bullet K-1}^L(L - \tau_{K-1} | h_{K-1}, a_{K-1}; \beta_{T,K-1}, \beta_{\tau,K-1}),$$

and

$$\mathfrak{Q}_{d_\eta, K-1}^L(h_{K-1}, a_{K-1}, u; \beta_{K-1}, \beta_{T,K-1}, \beta_{\tau,K-1})$$

$$= \int_{u-\tau_{K-1}}^{L-\tau_{K-1}} \left\{ f(\tau_{K-1} + w) \frac{\mathcal{S}_{\bullet K-1}^L(w | h_{K-1}, a_{K-1}; \beta_{T,K-1}, \beta_{\tau,K-1})}{\mathcal{S}_{\bullet K-1}^L(u - \tau_{K-1} | h_{K-1}, a_{K-1}; \beta_{T,K-1}, \beta_{\tau,K-1})} \right.$$

$$\left. \times \lambda_{T,K-1}^{\dagger L}(w | h_{K-1}, a_{K-1}; \beta_{T,K-1}) \right\} dw$$

$$+ \int_{u-\tau_{K-1}}^{L-\tau_{K-1}} \left\{ q_k^{d_\eta, L}(h_{K-1}, a_{K-1}, \tau_{K-1} + w; \beta_{K-1}) \right.$$

$$\times \frac{\mathcal{S}_{\bullet K-1}^L(w | h_{K-1}, a_{K-1}; \beta_{T,K-1}, \beta_{\tau,K-1})}{\mathcal{S}_{\bullet K-1}^L(u - \tau_{K-1} | h_{K-1}, a_{K-1}; \beta_{T,K-1}, \beta_{\tau,K-1})}$$

$$\left. \times \lambda_{\tau,K-1}^{\dagger L}(w | h_{K-1}, a_{K-1}; \beta_{\tau,K-1}) \right\} dw$$

$$+ f(L) \frac{\mathcal{S}_{\bullet K-1}^L(L - \tau_{K-1} | h_{K-1}, a_{K-1}; \beta_{T,K-1}, \beta_{\tau,K-1})}{\mathcal{S}_{\bullet K-1}^L(u - \tau_{K-1} | h_{K-1}, a_{K-1}; \beta_{T,K-1}, \beta_{\tau,K-1})}.$$

From (8.234) with $\ell = K - 1$ and $r = \kappa^L = K - 1$ or K,

$$\mathfrak{C}_{d_\eta, K-1, \kappa^L}^{\dagger L} = \mathrm{I}\{A_{K-1} = d_{\eta, K-1}(H_{K-1}), \kappa^L \geq K - 1\}$$

$$\times \mathrm{I}\{A_K = d_{\eta, K}(H_K), \kappa^L = K\},$$

and

$$\mathfrak{C}_{d_\eta, K-1, K-1}^{\dagger L} = \mathrm{I}\{A_{K-1} = d_{\eta, K-1}(H_{K-1}), \kappa^L \geq K - 1\}.$$

Then, from (8.232) with $k = K - 1$, $\underline{d}_{\eta, K-1} = (d_{\eta, K-1}, d_{\eta, K})$, and incorporating truncation of $f(T)$ at L,

$$\mathcal{G}_{LE, K-1}^L(d_{\eta, K-1}, d_{\eta, K}; \underline{\gamma}_{K-1}, \beta_C, \underline{\beta}_{K-1}, \underline{\beta}_{T,K-1}, \underline{\beta}_{\tau,K-1})$$

$$= \mathrm{I}(\kappa^L \geq K - 1)$$

$$\times \left\{ \frac{\mathfrak{C}_{d_\eta, K-1, \kappa^L}^{\dagger L} \Delta^L f(U^L)}{\underline{\omega}_{K-1, \kappa^L}^\dagger(H_{\kappa^L}, A_{\kappa^L}; \underline{\gamma}_{K-1, \kappa^L}, \beta_C) \mathcal{K}_{\kappa^L}(U^L | H_{\kappa^L}, A_{\kappa^L}; \beta_C)} \right.$$

$$-\left(\left[\frac{I\{A_{K-1} = d_{\eta,K-1}(H_{K-1})\} - \omega_{K-1}^{\dagger}(H_{K-1}, A_{K-1}; \gamma_{K-1})}{\omega_{K-1}^{\dagger}(H_{K-1}, A_{K-1}; \gamma_{K-1})}\right]\right.$$

$$\left. \times Q_{K-1}^{d_{\eta},L}\{H_{K-1}, d_{\eta,K-1}(H_{K-1}); \beta_{K-1}, \beta_{T,K-1}, \beta_{\tau,K-1}\}\right)$$

$$-\left(\frac{I(\kappa^L = K)\, \mathfrak{C}_{d_{\eta},K-1,K-1}^{\dagger\, L}\, I(\Upsilon_K^{\dagger\, L} \neq 0)}{\underline{\omega}_{K-1,K}^{\dagger}(H_{K-1}, A_{K-1}; \underline{\gamma}_{K-1,K-1}, \beta_C)\mathcal{K}_{K-1}(S_K^{\dagger\, L}|H_{K-1}, A_{K-1}; \beta_C)}\right.$$

$$\times \left[\frac{I\{A_K = d_{\eta,K}(H_K)\} - \omega_K^{\dagger}(H_K, A_K; \gamma_K)}{\omega_K^{\dagger}(H_K, A_K; \gamma_K)}\right] \qquad (8.240)$$

$$\left. \times Q_K^{d_{\eta},L}\{H_K, d_{\eta,K}(H_K); \beta_{TK}\}\right)$$

$$+ \sum_{r=K-1}^{\kappa^L}\left[\frac{\mathfrak{C}_{d_{\eta},K-1,r}^{\dagger\, L}}{\underline{\omega}_{K-1,r}^{\dagger}(H_r, A_r; \underline{\gamma}_{K-1,r}, \beta_C)}\right.$$

$$\left.\left. \times \int_{S_r^{\dagger\, L}}^{S_{r+1}^{\dagger\, L}} \frac{dM_{C,r}(u|H_r, A_r; \beta_C)}{\mathcal{K}_r(u|H_r, A_r; \beta_C)}\, \mathfrak{Q}_{d_{\eta},r}^{L}(H_r, A_r, u; \beta_r, \beta_{Tr}, \beta_{\tau r})\right]\right\},$$

where, in the final term on the right-hand side, when $r = K$, $\mathfrak{Q}_{d_{\eta},r}^{L}(H_r, A_r, u; \beta_r, \beta_{Tr}, \beta_{\tau r})$ depends only on β_{TK}.

In (8.240), $\mathcal{G}_{LE,K-1}^{L}(d_{\eta,K-1}, d_{\eta,K}; \underline{\gamma}_{K-1}, \beta_C, \underline{\beta}_{K-1}, \underline{\beta}_{T,K-1}, \underline{\beta}_{\tau,K-1})$ depends on $d_{\eta,K}$ where indicated explicitly and through $\mathfrak{C}_{d_{\eta},K-1,\kappa^L}^{\dagger\, L}$, which is important next.

Analogous to (7.121) in Section 7.4.4, define

$$\widehat{\mathcal{V}}_{LE}^{(K-1)}(\underline{d}_{\eta,K}) = \widehat{\mathcal{V}}_{LE}^{(K-1)}(d_{\eta,K-1}, d_{\eta,K})$$

$$= n^{-1}\sum_{i=1}^{n} \mathcal{G}_{LE,K-1,i}^{L}(d_{\eta,K-1}, d_{\eta,K}; \underline{\widehat{\gamma}}_{K-1}, \widehat{\beta}_C, \underline{\widehat{\beta}}_{K-1}, \underline{\widehat{\beta}}_{T,K-1}, \underline{\widehat{\beta}}_{\tau,K-1}),$$

where the subscript i indicates evaluation at κ_i^L, U_i^L, Δ_i^L, $S_{K-1,i}^{\dagger\, L}$, $S_{Ki}^{\dagger\, L}$, $\Upsilon_{Ki}^{\dagger\, L}$, H_{Ki}, and A_{Ki}. Then, by analogy to a two-decision problem, with Decisions $K - 1$ and K playing the roles of Decisions 1 and 2 and "baseline" information H_{K-1}, and by reasoning similar to that above, for fixed $\underline{d}_{\eta,K-1}$, $\widehat{\mathcal{V}}_{LE}^{(K-1)}(\underline{d}_{\eta,K-1})$ is a doubly robust estimator for

$$E[I(\kappa^L \geq K - 1)f\{T^*(\overline{A}_{K-2}, d_{\eta,K-1}, d_{\eta,K})\}]. \qquad (8.241)$$

Thus, as in (8.239), define

$$d_{\eta,K-1,B}^{opt}(h_{K-1}) = d_{K-1}(h_{K-1}; \eta_{K-1,B}^{opt}), \qquad (8.242)$$

$$\eta^{opt}_{K-1,B} = \arg\max_{\eta_{K-1}} E[\mathrm{I}(\kappa^L \geq K - 1)f\{T^*(\overline{A}_{K-2}, d_{\eta,K-1}, d^{opt}_{\eta,K,B})\}].$$

In (8.242), $d_{\eta,K}$ is fixed at $d^{opt}_{\eta,K,B}$, so that $\eta^{opt}_{K-1,B}$ is not necessarily the global maximizer of (8.241) in $(\eta^T_{K-1}, \eta^T_K)^T$, nor is $\eta^{opt}_{K-1,B}$ necessarily equal to η^{opt}_{K-1} globally maximizing $\mathcal{V}(d_\eta)$.

It follows that $\widehat{\mathcal{V}}^{(K-1)}_{LE}(d_{\eta,K-1}, d^{opt}_{\eta,K,B})$ is a doubly robust estimator for $E[\mathrm{I}(\kappa^L \geq K - 1)f\{T^*(\overline{A}_{K-2}, d_{\eta,K-1}, d^{opt}_{\eta,K,B})\}]$. Thus, an obvious estimator for $\eta^{opt}_{K-1,B}$ in (8.242) is obtained by maximizing in η_{K-1}

$$\widehat{\mathcal{V}}^{(K-1)}_{LE}(d_{\eta,K-1}, \widehat{d}^{opt}_{\eta,K,B}),$$

yielding $\widehat{\eta}^{opt}_{K-1,B,LE}$ and the estimator for $d^{opt}_{\eta,K-1,B}(h_{K-1})$ given by

$$\widehat{d}^{opt}_{\eta,K-1,B}(h_{K-1}) = d_{K-1}(h_{K-1}; \widehat{\eta}^{opt}_{K-1,B,LE}).$$

Note that, by the substitution of $\widehat{d}^{opt}_{\eta,K,B}$ for $d_{\eta,K}$, in the third term of (8.240), $Q^{d_\eta}_K\{H_{Ki}, \widehat{d}^{opt}_{\eta,K,B}(H_{Ki}); \widehat{\beta}_{TK}\}$ is fixed for each i.

The algorithm then continues to Decision $K-2$, where the first step is to obtain for all individuals i for whom $\kappa^L_i \geq K-1$ the pseudo outcomes

$$\widetilde{V}^{R_{d_\eta},L}_{K-1,i} = Q^{d_\eta,L}_{K-1}\{H_{K-1,i}, \widehat{d}^{opt}_{\eta,K-1,B}(H_{K-1,i}); \widehat{\beta}_{K-1}, \widehat{\beta}_{T,K-1}, \widehat{\beta}_{\tau,K-1}\}$$
$$- f(\mathcal{T}_{K-1,i})$$

and then proceed as above.

In general, at Decision k, $k = K - 1, \ldots, 1$,

$$Q^{d_\eta,L}_\ell(h_\ell, a_\ell; \widehat{\beta}_\ell, \widehat{\beta}_{T\ell}, \widehat{\beta}_{\tau\ell}), \quad \text{and} \quad \mathfrak{Q}^L_{d_\eta,\ell}(h_\ell, a_\ell, u; \widehat{\beta}_\ell, \widehat{\beta}_{T\ell}, \widehat{\beta}_{\tau\ell})$$

have already been obtained for $\ell = k + 1, \ldots, K$ and depend only on $\widehat{\beta}_{TK}$ when $\ell = K$. Likewise, $\widehat{d}^{opt}_{\eta,\ell,B}(h_\ell)$ have already been obtained for $\ell = k + 1, \ldots, K$, where

$$d^{opt}_{\eta,\ell,B}(h_\ell) = d_\ell(h_\ell; \eta^{opt}_{\ell,B}),$$
$$\eta^{opt}_{\ell,B} = \arg\max_{\eta_\ell} E[\mathrm{I}(\kappa^L \geq \ell)f\{T^*(\overline{A}_{\ell-1}, d_{\eta,\ell}, d^{opt}_{\eta,\ell+1,B})\}],$$

along with pseudo outcomes

$$\widetilde{V}^{R_{d_\eta},L}_{k+1,i} = Q^{d_\eta,L}_{k+1}\{H_{k+1,i}, \widehat{d}^{opt}_{\eta,k+1,B}(H_{k+1,i}); \widehat{\beta}_{k+1}, \widehat{\beta}_{T,k+1}, \widehat{\beta}_{\tau,k+1}\}$$
$$- f(\mathcal{T}_{k+1,i})$$

for individuals i for whom $\kappa_i^L \geq k + 1$. Then, given a model $q_k^{R_{d_\eta},L}(h_k, a_k, \tau_{k+1}; \beta_k)$, with

$$q_k^{d_\eta,L}(h_k, a_k, \tau_{k+1}; \beta_k) = q_k^{R_{d_\eta},L}(h_k, a_k, \tau_{k+1}; \beta_k) + f(\tau_{k+1}),$$

obtain $\widehat{\beta}_k$ as in Remark (i) at the end of the description of the hybrid estimation scheme in Section 8.3.3. Positing hazard models $\lambda_{T,k}^{\dagger L}(u|h_k, a_k; \beta_{T,k})$ and $\lambda_{\tau,k}^{\dagger L}(u|h_k, a_k; \beta_{\tau,k})$ inducing a model $\mathcal{S}_{\bullet k}^L(u|h_k, a_k; \beta_{T,k}, \beta_{\tau,k})$, and fitting these based on the data from individuals i for whom $\kappa_i^L \geq k$, obtain $\widehat{\beta}_{T,k}$ and $\widehat{\beta}_{\tau,k}$. From (8.171) and (8.204), let

$$Q_k^{d_\eta,L}(h_k, a_k; \beta_k, \beta_{T,k}, \beta_{\tau,k}) = \int_0^{L-\tau_k} \left\{ f(\tau_k + w) \mathcal{S}_{\bullet k}^L(w|h_k, a_k; \beta_{T,k}, \beta_{\tau,k}) \right.$$

$$\left. \times \lambda_{T,k}^{\dagger L}(w|h_k, a_k; \beta_{T,k}) \right\} dw$$

$$+ \int_0^{L-\tau_k} \left\{ q_k^{d_\eta,L}(h_k, a_k, \tau_k + w; \beta_k) \mathcal{S}_{\bullet k}^L(w|h_k, a_k; \beta_{T,k}, \beta_{\tau,k}) \right.$$

$$\left. \times \lambda_{\tau,k}^{\dagger L}(w|h_k, a_k; \beta_{\tau,k}) \right\} dw$$

$$+ f(L) \mathcal{S}_{\bullet k}^L(L - \tau_k|h_k, a_k; \beta_{T,k}, \beta_{\tau,k}),$$

and

$$\mathfrak{Q}_{d_\eta,k}^L(h_k, a_k, u; \beta_k, \beta_{T,k}, \beta_{\tau,k})$$

$$= \int_{u-\tau_k}^{L-\tau_k} \left\{ f(\tau_k + w) \frac{\mathcal{S}_{\bullet k}^L(w|h_k, a_k; \beta_{T,k}, \beta_{\tau,k})}{\mathcal{S}_{\bullet k}^L(u - \tau_k|h_k, a_k; \beta_{T,k}, \beta_{\tau,k})} \right.$$

$$\left. \times \lambda_{T,k}^{\dagger L}(w|h_k, a_k; \beta_{T,k}) \right\} dw$$

$$+ \int_{u-\tau_k}^{L-\tau_k} \left\{ q_k^{d_\eta,L}(h_k, a_k, \tau_k + w; \beta_k) \frac{\mathcal{S}_{\bullet k}^L(w|h_k, a_k; \beta_{T,k}, \beta_{\tau,k})}{\mathcal{S}_{\bullet k}^L(u - \tau_k|h_k, a_k; \beta_{T,k}, \beta_{\tau,k})} \right.$$

$$\left. \times \lambda_{\tau,k}^{\dagger L}(w|h_k, a_k; \beta_{\tau,k}) \right\} dw$$

$$+ f(L) \frac{\mathcal{S}_{\bullet k}^L(L - \tau_k|h_k, a_k; \beta_{T,k}, \beta_{\tau,k})}{\mathcal{S}_{\bullet k}^L(u - \tau_k|h_k, a_k; \beta_{T,k}, \beta_{\tau,k})}.$$

Then, from (8.232),

$$\mathcal{G}_{LE,k}(\underline{d}_{\eta,k}; \underline{\gamma}_k, \beta_C, \underline{\beta}_k, \underline{\beta}_{Tk}, \underline{\beta}_{\tau k})$$

$$= \mathcal{G}_{LE,k}(d_{\eta,k}, \underline{d}_{\eta,k+1}; \underline{\gamma}_k, \beta_C, \underline{\beta}_k, \underline{\beta}_{Tk}, \underline{\beta}_{\tau k})$$

$$= \mathrm{I}(\kappa^L \geq k) \left\{ \frac{\mathfrak{C}^{\dagger L}_{d_\eta, k, \kappa^L} \Delta^L f(U^L)}{\underline{\omega}^{\dagger}_{k, \kappa^L}(H_{\kappa^L}, A_{\kappa^L}; \underline{\gamma}_{k, \kappa^L}, \beta_C) \mathcal{K}_{\kappa^L}(U^L | H_\kappa, A_\kappa; \beta_C)} \right.$$

$$- \left[\frac{\mathrm{I}\{A_k = d_{\eta, k}(H_k)\} - \omega^{\dagger}_k(H_k, A_k; \gamma_k)}{\omega^{\dagger}_k(H_k, A_k; \gamma_k)} \right]$$

$$\times Q^{d_\eta, L}_k \{H_k, d_{\eta, k}(H_k); \beta_k, \beta_{Tk}, \beta_{\tau k}\}$$

$$- \sum_{r=k+1}^{\kappa^L} \left(\frac{\mathrm{I}(\kappa^L > k) \mathfrak{C}^{\dagger L}_{d_\eta, k, r-1} \mathrm{I}(\Upsilon^{\dagger L}_r \neq 0)}{\underline{\omega}^{\dagger}_{k, r-1}(H_{r-1}, A_{r-1}; \underline{\gamma}_{k, r-1}, \beta_C) \mathcal{K}_{r-1}(S^{\dagger L}_r | H_{r-1}, A_{r-1}; \beta_C)} \right.$$

$$\times \left[\frac{\mathrm{I}\{A_r = d_{\eta, r}(H_r)\} - \omega^{\dagger}_r(H_r, A_r; \gamma_r)}{\omega^{\dagger}_r(H_r, A_r; \gamma_r)} \right] \qquad (8.243)$$

$$\left. \times Q^{d_\eta, L}_r \{H_r, d_{\eta, r}(H_r); \beta_r, \beta_{Tr}, \beta_{\tau r}\} \right)$$

$$+ \sum_{r=k}^{\kappa^L} \left[\frac{\mathfrak{C}^{\dagger L}_{d_\eta, k, r}}{\underline{\omega}^{\dagger}_{k, r}(H_r, A_r; \underline{\gamma}_{k, r})} \right.$$

$$\left. \left. \times \int_{S^{\dagger L}_r}^{S^{\dagger L}_{r+1}} \frac{dM_{C, r}(u | H_r, A_r; \beta_C)}{\mathcal{K}_r(u | H_r, A_r; \beta_C)} \mathfrak{Q}^L_{d_\eta, r}(H_r, A_r, u; \beta_r, \beta_{Tr}, \beta_{\tau r}) \right] \right\},$$

where, as before, $\mathfrak{Q}^L_{d_\eta, r}(H_r, A_r, u; \beta_r, \beta_{Tr}, \beta_{\tau r})$ depends only on $\widehat{\beta}_{TK}$ when $r = \kappa^L = K$.

As for (8.240), $\mathcal{G}_{LE, k}(d_{\eta, k}, \underline{d}_{\eta, k+1}; \underline{\gamma}_k, \beta_C, \underline{\beta}_k, \underline{\beta}_{Tk}, \underline{\beta}_{\tau k})$ in (8.243) depends on $\underline{d}_{\eta, k+1}$ where indicated explicitly and through $\mathfrak{C}^{\dagger L}_{d_\eta, k, r}$ for $r = k+1, \ldots, K$.

Now define

$$\widehat{\mathcal{V}}^{(k)}_{LE}(d_{\eta, k}, \underline{d}_{\eta, k+1}) \qquad (8.244)$$

$$= n^{-1} \sum_{i=1}^n \mathcal{G}^L_{LE, ki}(d_{\eta, k}, \underline{d}_{\eta, k+1}; \widehat{\underline{\gamma}}_k, \widehat{\beta}_C, \widehat{\underline{\beta}}_k, \widehat{\underline{\beta}}_{Tk}, \widehat{\underline{\beta}}_{\tau k}),$$

where the subscript i indicates evaluation at κ^L_i; U^L_i; Δ^L_i; $S^{\dagger L}_{ri}$ and $\Upsilon^{\dagger L}_{ri}$, $r = k, \ldots, K$; H_{Ki}; and A_{Ki}, which can be viewed as a doubly robust estimator for $E[\mathrm{I}(\kappa^L \geq k) f\{T^*(\overline{A}_{k-1}, d_{\eta, k}, \underline{d}_{\eta, k+1})\}]$. As above, define

$$d^{opt}_{\eta, k, B}(h_k) = d_k(h_k; \eta^{opt}_{k, B}),$$

$$\eta^{opt}_{k, B} = \arg\max_{\eta_k} E[\mathrm{I}(\kappa^L \geq k) f\{T^*(\overline{A}_{k-1}, d_{\eta, k}, \underline{d}^{opt}_{\eta, k+1, B})\}], \qquad (8.245)$$

where, with $\underline{d}_{\eta,k+1}^{opt}$ fixed at $\underline{d}_{\eta,k+1,B}^{opt}$, $\eta_{k,B}^{opt}$ is not necessarily the global maximizer of $E[\mathrm{I}(\kappa^L \geq k)f\{T^*(\overline{A}_{k-1}, d_{\eta,k}, \underline{d}_{\eta,k+1})\}]$ nor equal to η_k^{opt} globally maximizing $\mathcal{V}(d_\eta)$. Then obtain $\widehat{\eta}_{k,B,LE}^{opt}$ and thus

$$\widehat{d}_{\eta,k,B}^{opt}(h_k) = d_k(h_k; \widehat{\eta}_{k,B,LE}^{opt}).$$

by maximizing in η_k

$$\widehat{\mathcal{V}}_{LE}^{(k)}(d_{\eta,k}, \widehat{\underline{d}}_{\eta,k+1,B}^{opt}), \quad \widehat{\underline{d}}_{\eta,k+1,B}^{opt} = (\widehat{d}_{\eta,k+1,B}^{opt}, \ldots, \widehat{d}_{\eta,K,B}^{opt}).$$

As in Section 7.4.4, continuing to Decision 1, the estimator for

$$d_{\eta,B}^{opt} = \{d_{\eta,1,B}^{opt}(h_1), \ldots, d_{\eta,K,B}^{opt}(h_K)\},$$

where $d_{\eta,k,B}^{opt}(h_k)$, $k = 1, \ldots, K$, are defined in (8.239), (8.242), and (8.245), is given by

$$\widehat{d}_{\eta,B,LE}^{opt} = \{d_1(h_1; \widehat{\eta}_{1,B,LE}^{opt}), \ldots, d_K(h_K; \widehat{\eta}_{K,B,LE}^{opt})\}. \tag{8.246}$$

An estimator for $\mathcal{V}(d_{\eta,B}^{opt})$ is then obtained by substituting $\widehat{d}_{\eta,B,LE}^{opt}$ in $\widehat{\mathcal{V}}_{LE}(d_\eta)$ in (8.230) or, equivalently, in (8.233).

Remark. As in the remark at the end of the description of the backward iterative implementation of value search estimation in Section 7.4.4, it is critical to recognize that it is not necessarily the case that $\widehat{d}_{\eta,B,LE}^{opt}$ in (8.246) is an estimator for $d_\eta^{opt} \in \mathcal{D}_\eta$, as $\eta_{k,B}^{opt}$, $k = 1, \ldots, K$, do not globally maximize $\mathcal{V}(d_\eta)$ in η. By reasoning analogous to that given in this remark, which is not repeated here, it can be argued that $\widehat{d}_{\eta,B,LE}^{opt}$ is a valid estimator for d_η^{opt} if the restricted class $\mathcal{D}_\eta$ in fact contains the globally optimal regime $d^{opt} \in \mathcal{D}$, the class of all possible regimes involving the associated specification of feasible sets of treatment options at each decision point. If $d^{opt} \notin \mathcal{D}_\eta$, then it is not necessarily the case that $\widehat{d}_{\eta,B,LE}^{opt}$ need estimate an optimal restricted regime $d_\eta^{opt} \in \mathcal{D}_\eta$. In the context of a possibly censored time-to-event outcome and with $K = 2$, Hager et al. (2018) present simulation results showing that a version of the foregoing iterative implementation can yield estimators that perform similarly to a true optimal restricted regime d_η^{opt} in practice.

Classification Perspective

Although the backward iterative implementation of value search estimation replaces the insurmountable global optimization $\widehat{\mathcal{V}}_{LE}(d_\eta)$ or other value estimator in possibly high-dimensional η by a series of lower-dimensional optimization problems in $\eta_K, \ldots, \eta_1$, respectively, the latter can still pose computational challenges, as they still involve nonsmooth objective functions. As in Section 7.4.5, one approach to circumventing these difficulties in the case where all feasible sets involve two treatment options is to characterize the optimization task at each step as a weighted classification problem and exploit well-studied approaches for optimization of a nonsmooth, nonconvex objective function used in this context. Because the development is entirely analogous to that in Section 7.4.5, we sketch the basic formulation and refer the reader to that section for further details and discussion.

Consider the backward iterative strategy outlined above in the case of $f(t)$ involving truncation at L, and assume for simplicity that, for $k = 1, \ldots, K$, $\mathcal{A}_k$ comprises exactly two treatment options coded as 0 and 1; i.e., $\mathcal{A}_k = \{0, 1\}$, that are feasible for all individuals who reach Decision k regardless of history. At Decision K, from (8.236), the first step of the algorithm is to maximize in η_K

$$\widehat{\mathcal{V}}_{LE}^{(K)}(d_{\eta,K}) = n^{-1} \sum_{i=1}^{n} \mathcal{G}_{LE,Ki}^{L}(d_{\eta,K}; \widehat{\gamma}_K, \widehat{\beta}_C, \widehat{\beta}_{TK})$$

to obtain $\widehat{\eta}_{K,B,LE}^{opt}$ and thus $\widehat{d}_{\eta,K,B}^{opt}(h_K) = d_K(h_K; \widehat{\eta}_{K,B,LE}^{opt})$. Letting $\mathcal{G}_{LE,Ki}^{L}(a; \widehat{\gamma}_K, \widehat{\beta}_C, \widehat{\beta}_{TK})$ denote $\mathcal{G}_{LE,Ki}^{L}(d_{\eta,K}; \widehat{\gamma}_K, \widehat{\beta}_C, \widehat{\beta}_{TK})$ with $d_{\eta,K}(H_{Ki})$ replaced by option a, $a = 0, 1$ wherever it appears and defining

$$\widehat{C}_{Ki} = \mathcal{G}_{LE,Ki}^{L}(1; \widehat{\gamma}_K, \widehat{\beta}_C, \widehat{\beta}_{TK}) - \mathcal{G}_{LE,Ki}^{L}(0; \widehat{\gamma}_K, \widehat{\beta}_C, \widehat{\beta}_{TK}),$$

analogous to (7.155), by algebra identical to that leading to (7.156), maximizing $\widehat{\mathcal{V}}_{LE}^{(K)}(d_{\eta,K})$ is equivalent to maximizing

$$n^{-1} \sum_{i=1}^{n} d_K(H_{Ki}; \eta_K) \widehat{C}_{Ki}.$$

By further manipulations, which are presented in detail in Section 4.2.2, maximizing this quantity in η_K can be shown to be equivalent to minimizing the weighted classification error

$$n^{-1} \sum_{i=1}^{n} |\widehat{C}_{Ki}| \left\{ \mathrm{I}(\widehat{C}_{Ki} > 0) - d_K(H_{Ki}; \eta_K) \right\}^2$$

$$= n^{-1} \sum_{i=1}^{n} |\widehat{C}_{Ki}| \, \mathrm{I}\left\{ \mathrm{I}(\widehat{C}_{Ki} > 0) \neq d_K(H_{Ki}; \eta_K) \right\}. \tag{8.247}$$

Then, as discussed in Sections 4.2.2 and 7.4.5, if the restricted class is chosen to comprise regimes whose rules $d_{\eta,k}(h_k)$ $k = 1, \ldots, K$, are induced by a particular choice of classifier, such as support vector machines (Cortes and Vapnik, 1995) or classification and regression trees (Breiman et al., 1984), standard algorithms and software can be used to minimize (8.247) in η_K and thus maximize $\widehat{\mathcal{V}}_{LE}^{(K)}(d_{\eta,K})$, leading to $\widehat{\eta}_{K,B,LE}^{opt}$ and $\widehat{d}_{\eta,K,B}^{opt}(h_K) = d_K(h_K; \widehat{\eta}_{K,B,LE}^{opt})$.

The same argument applies for Decision k, $k = K - 1, \ldots, 1$. At Decision k, from (8.244), the goal is to maximize in η_k

$$\widehat{\mathcal{V}}_{LE}^{(k)}(d_{\eta,k}, \widehat{\underline{d}}_{\eta,k+1,B}^{opt})$$
$$= n^{-1} \sum_{i=1}^{n} \mathcal{G}_{LE,ki}^{L}(d_{\eta,k}, \widehat{\underline{d}}_{\eta,k+1,B}^{opt}; \widehat{\underline{\gamma}}_k, \widehat{\beta}_C, \widehat{\underline{\beta}}_k, \widehat{\underline{\beta}}_{Tk}, \widehat{\underline{\beta}}_{\tau k}),$$

where $\widehat{\underline{d}}_{\eta,k+1,B}^{opt} = (\widehat{\underline{d}}_{\eta,k+1,B}^{opt}, \ldots, \widehat{\underline{d}}_{\eta,K,B}^{opt})$ have been obtained at previous steps. Using obvious notation and defining analogous to (7.160)

$$\widehat{C}_{ki}(\underline{d}_{\eta,k+1}) = \mathcal{G}_{LE,ki}(1, \underline{d}_{\eta,k+1}; \widehat{\underline{\gamma}}_k, \widehat{\beta}_C, \widehat{\underline{\beta}}_k, \widehat{\underline{\beta}}_{Tk}, \widehat{\underline{\beta}}_{\tau k})$$
$$- \mathcal{G}_{LE,ki}(0, \underline{d}_{\eta,k+1}; \widehat{\underline{\gamma}}_k, \widehat{\beta}_C, \widehat{\underline{\beta}}_k, \widehat{\underline{\beta}}_{Tk}, \widehat{\underline{\beta}}_{\tau k}),$$

by manipulations like to those leading to (8.247), maximizing $\widehat{\mathcal{V}}_{LE}^{(k)}(d_{\eta,k}, \widehat{\underline{d}}_{\eta,k+1,B}^{opt})$ in η_k is equivalent to maximizing

$$n^{-1} \sum_{i=1}^{n} d_k(H_{ki}; \eta_k) \widehat{C}_{ki}(\widehat{\underline{d}}_{\eta,k+1,B}^{opt}),$$

which in turn is equivalent to minimizing in η_k the weighted classification error

$$n^{-1} \sum_{i=1}^{n} |\widehat{C}_{ki}(\widehat{\underline{d}}_{\eta,k+1,B}^{opt})| \, \mathrm{I}\left[\mathrm{I}\{\widehat{C}_{ki}(\widehat{\underline{d}}_{\eta,k+1,B}^{opt}) > 0\} \neq d_k(H_{ki}; \eta_k)\right]. \quad (8.248)$$

As above, with the restricted class $\mathcal{D}_\eta$ induced by a particular choice of classifier, standard algorithms and software can be used to minimize (8.248), and thus maximize $\widehat{\mathcal{V}}_{LE}^{(k)}(d_{\eta,k}, \widehat{\underline{d}}_{\eta,k+1,B}^{opt})$, in η_k, leading to $\widehat{\eta}_{k,B,LE}^{opt}$ and $\widehat{d}_{\eta,k,B}^{opt}(h_k) = d_k(h_k; \widehat{\eta}_{k,B,LE}^{opt})$.

A specific implementation of this approach is presented by Hager et al. (2018) for $K = 2$, which we now generalize. At Decision K, writing

$$d_K(h_K; \eta_K) = \mathrm{I}\{f_K(h_K; \eta_K) > 0\}$$

for some decision function $f_K(h_K; \eta_K)$ as in Section 7.4.5, the objective function (8.247) can be written in terms of the nonconvex 0-1 loss function $\ell_{0\text{-}1}(x) = I(x \leq 0)$ as

$$n^{-1} \sum_{i=1}^{n} |\widehat{C}_{Ki}| \, \ell_{0\text{-}1}\left[\left\{2\mathrm{I}(\widehat{C}_{Ki} > 0) - 1\right\} f_K(H_{Ki}; \eta_K)\right]. \quad (8.249)$$

As proposed by Zhao et al. (2015a) and discussed in Section 7.4.5, replace the nonconvex 0-1 loss function in (8.249) by the convex surrogate hinge loss function

$$\ell_{hinge}(x) = (1-x)^+, \quad x^+ = \max(0, x).$$

This suggests minimizing a penalized version of (8.247) or equivalently (8.249), namely,

$$n^{-1} \sum_{i=1}^{n} |\widehat{C}_{Ki}| \, \ell_{hinge}\left[\left\{2I(\widehat{C}_{Ki} > 0) - 1\right\} f_K(H_{Ki}; \eta_K)\right] + \lambda_{K,n} \|f_K\|^2,$$

(8.250)

where $\lambda_{K,n}$ is a penalty controlling the complexity of f_K in η_K, and $\| \cdot \|$ is a suitable norm. Note that, from the definition of $\mathcal{G}_{LE,K}^L(d_{\eta,K}; \gamma_K, \beta_C, \beta_{TK})$ in (8.235), the sum over $i = 1, \ldots, n$ in any of the above equivalent objective functions involves individuals i for whom $\kappa_i^L = K$. As noted in Section 7.4.5, minimization of (8.250) does not necessarily lead to the same estimator for $d_{\eta,K}$ as minimization of (8.249), or, equivalently, (8.247). Accordingly, denote the resulting estmator as $\widehat{\eta}_{K,B,CS}^{opt}$ and $\widehat{d}_{\eta,K,CS}^{opt}(h_K) = d_K(h_K; \widehat{\eta}_{K,B,CS}^{opt})$, where CS indicates the use of the convex surrogate hinge loss function.

Similarly, for $k = K - 1, \ldots, 1$, analogous to (8.249), writing $d_k(h_k; \eta_k) = I\{f_k(h_k; \eta_k) > 0\}$ for decision function $f_k(h_k; \eta_k)$, (8.248) can be written in terms of the 0-1 loss function $\ell_{0\text{-}1}(x)$ as

$$n^{-1} \sum_{i=1}^{n} |\widehat{C}_{ki}(\underline{\widehat{d}}_{\eta,k+1,B}^{opt})| \, \ell_{0\text{-}1}\left(\left[2I\{\widehat{C}_{ki}(\underline{\widehat{d}}_{\eta,k+1,B}^{opt}) > 0\} - 1\right] f_k(H_{ki}; \eta_k)\right).$$

Replacing the nonconvex 0-1 loss function by the convex surrogate hinge loss and imposing a complexity penalty suggests minimizing

$$n^{-1} \sum_{i=1}^{n} \left\{ |\widehat{C}_{ki}(\underline{\widehat{d}}_{\eta,k+1,CS}^{opt}) \right.$$

(8.251)

$$\left. \times \ell_{hinge}\left(\left[2I\{\widehat{C}_{ki}(\underline{\widehat{d}}_{\eta,k+1,CS}^{opt}) > 0\} - 1\right] f_k(H_{ki}; \eta_k)\right) \right\} + \lambda_{k,n} \|f_k\|^2$$

in η_k, leading to $\widehat{\eta}_{k,B,CS}^{opt}$ and thus $\widehat{d}_{\eta,k,CS}^{opt}(h_k)$, where, in obvious notation, $\underline{\widehat{d}}_{\eta,k+1,CS}^{opt} = (\widehat{d}_{\eta,k+1,CS}^{opt}, \ldots, \widehat{d}_{\eta,K,CS}^{opt})$.

In summary, parallel to the developments in Section 7.4.5, if there are two feasible treatment options at each decision point, taking $\mathcal{D}_\eta$ to be the restricted class of regimes whose rules $d_{\eta,k}(h_k)$, $k = 1, \ldots, K$, are induced by a specific classifier, an optimal regime within $\mathcal{D}_\eta$ can be estimated by casting the optimization at each step of the backward iterative implementation of value search estimation as a weighted classification problem, allowing the analyst to exploit computational tools and strategies for such problems. In the generalization to the situation where there are different feasible sets depending on h_k, each comprising two treatment options, for $K = 2$, Hager et al. (2018) evaluate the performance of the strategy based on (8.250) and (8.251) when the chosen classifier is linear support vector machines with penalty chosen by cross validation.

8.3.6 Discussion

While, as noted in Section 7.4.8, the literature on multiple decision treatment regimes and estimation of optimal regimes in particular based on a noncensored outcome is vast and continues to expand, that on methodology for treatment regimes based on a possibly censored time-to-event outcome is evolving. We have focused here on providing a foundation for advances in this area, including formulation of a formal potential outcomes framework and associated assumptions and description of representative methodological approaches. We refer the reader to the emerging literature for further developments. A brief list of existing work includes Goldberg and Kosorok (2012), Huang et al. (2014), Jiang et al. (2017a), Jiang et al. (2017b), Shen et al. (2017), and Hager et al. (2018).

All of the estimators for the value of a fixed regime $d \in \mathcal{D}$ discussed in Section 8.3.3 are in principle regular and asymptotically linear. Thus, as for the single decision case in Section 8.2.5, measures of uncertainty for the estimators $\widehat{\mathcal{V}}_Q(d)$ and $\widehat{\mathcal{V}}_{HY}(d)$ of the value of a fixed regime $d \in \mathcal{D}$ discussed here could be derived by appealing to the theory of M-estimation if all relevant models, including those for the hazard of censoring and cause-specific hazards such as (8.117)–(8.119) are fully parametric. However, even in this ideal situation, because these estimators involve iterative development and fitting of models, either directly or, in the case of $\widehat{\mathcal{V}}_{AIPW}(d)$ and $\widehat{\mathcal{V}}_{LE}(d)$, indirectly, carrying out the required derivations would be a formidable task. In practice, it is likely that analysts will posit proportional hazards or other semiparametric models for these hazard functions, which involve infinite-dimensional components. As noted in Section 8.2.5, although the asymptotic theory for estimators for $\mathcal{V}(d)$ could in principle be formulated, this would be a significantly greater challenge. Accordingly, we recommend that measures of uncertainty for estimators for the value of a fixed regime be obtained via a standard nonparametric bootstrap. This could be prohibitive for the g-computation estimator $\widehat{\mathcal{V}}_{GC}(d)$, which is simulation-based, as noted earlier.

As in the single decision case, all of the estimators for the value of an optimal regime discussed in Section 8.3.5, $\widehat{\mathcal{V}}_Q(d^{opt})$ and $\widehat{\mathcal{V}}_{HY}(d^{opt})$ for the value of $d^{opt} \in \mathcal{D}$ and the inverse weighed estimators for $\mathcal{V}(d_\eta^{opt})$ for d_η^{opt} in a restricted class $\mathcal{D}_\eta$, are nonregular. Thus, principled inference on the true value of an optimal or restricted optimal regime is challenging, and little empirical evidence of practical performance of ad hoc strategies, such as use of a standard nonparametric bootstrap, is available. For value search estimation based on the inverse probability weighted locally efficient estimator $\widehat{\mathcal{V}}_{LE}(d_\eta)$ implemented via the backward iterative algorithm under the classification perspective, Hager et al. (2018) present simulation evidence suggesting that, similar to that in Bai et al. (2017) in the single decision case, obtaining reliable standard errors and associated confidence intervals for $\widehat{\mathcal{V}}_{LE}(d_\eta^{opt})$ when $K = 2$ and all models are correctly specified is possible using the sandwich technique; see Web Appendix B of the supplementary material for this paper.

8.4 Application

Implementations of some of the methods introduced in this chapter are demonstrated on the book's companion website given in the Preface. All codes used to generate simulated data and to implement each method are available on the website.

8.5 Technical Details

In this section, we present arguments justifying results given in earlier sections.

We start by demonstrating claims of equivalence under the noninformative censoring assumption (8.68). We first state a lemma of which we make considerable use.

Lemma 8.5.1. Let $\mathfrak{f}(W^*)$ be any function or vector of functions of the potential outcomes W^*. Then under the assumption of noninformative censoring (8.68),

$$P\{U \geq u \mid S^*_{k+1}(\bar{a}_k) \geq u, H_k = h_k, A_k = a_k, \mathfrak{f}(W^*), \kappa \geq k\} \quad (8.252)$$

$$= \exp\left\{-\int_{\tau_k}^{u} \lambda_C(w|H_k = h_k, A_k = a_k)\, dw\right\} > 0.$$

Proof. We present a heuristic argument. As in Section 8.3.2, using the notion of a product integral as in Andersen et al. (1993), (8.252) can be written as

$$\prod_{\tau_k \leq w < u} P\{U \geq w + dw | U \geq w, S^*_{k+1}(\bar{a}_k) \geq u,$$

$$H_k = h_k, A_k = a_k, \mathfrak{f}(W^*), \kappa \geq k\}$$

$$= \prod_{\tau_k \leq w < u} P\{U \geq w + dw | U \geq w, S^*_{k+1}(\overline{a}_k) \geq u,$$

$$H_k = h_k, A_k = a_k, \mathfrak{f}(W^*)\} \qquad (8.253)$$

$$= \prod_{\tau_k \leq w < u} \left[1 - P\{w \leq u < w + dw | U \geq w, S^*_{k+1}(\overline{a}_k) \geq u, \right.$$

$$\left. H_k = h_k, A_k = a_k, \mathfrak{f}(W^*)\} \right]$$

$$= \prod_{\tau_k \leq w < u} \left[1 - P\{w \leq U < w + dw, \Delta = 0 | U \geq w, S^*_{k+1}(\overline{a}_k) \geq u, \right.$$

$$\left. H_k = h_k, A_k = a_k, \mathfrak{f}(W^*)\} \right] \qquad (8.254)$$

$$= \prod_{\tau_k \leq w < u} \left[1 - \lambda_C\{w \mid h(w), S^*_{k+1}(\overline{a}_k) \geq u, \mathfrak{f}(W^*)\} \, dw \right] \qquad (8.255)$$

$$= \prod_{\tau_k \leq w < u} \left[1 - \lambda_C\{w \mid h(w)\} \, dw \right], \qquad (8.256)$$

$$= \prod_{\tau_k \leq w < u} \left\{ 1 - \lambda_C(w \mid h_k, a_k) \, dw \right\}, \qquad (8.257)$$

$$= \exp\left\{ -\int_{\tau_k}^u \lambda_C(w | h_k, a_k) \, dw \right\},$$

where (8.253) follows because $U \geq w$ and $\tau_k \leq w$ implies that $\kappa \geq k$; (8.254) holds because, with $w < u$ and $S^*_{k+1}(\overline{a}_k) \geq u$, $w \leq U < w + dw$ if and only if $\Delta = 0$; (8.256) follows from the noninformative censoring assumption (8.68); and (8.255) and (8.257) follow because $\tau_k \leq w \leq S^*_{k+1}(\overline{a}_k)$, so that the history $H(w)$ through time w is given by $H_k = h_k, A_k = a_k$. $\qquad \square$

Demonstration of Equivalence of (8.110) and (8.112)

We wish to show that, for $k = 2, \ldots, K$, the conditional density in (8.110),

$$p_{X_k | \overline{T}_{k-1}, \overline{X}_{k-1}, \overline{A}_{k-1}, T_k, \varkappa \geq k}(x_k | \overline{T}_{k-1}, \overline{x}_{k-1}, \overline{a}_{k-1}, \tau_k), \qquad (8.258)$$

when there is no censoring is equivalent to the conditional density

$$p_{X_k | \overline{T}_{k-1}, \overline{X}_{k-1}, \overline{A}_{k-1}, T_k, \kappa \geq k}(x_k | \overline{T}_{k-1}, \overline{x}_{k-1}, \overline{a}_{k-1}, \tau_k) \qquad (8.259)$$

in (8.112) under SUTVA, the SRA, the assumption of noninformative censoring in (8.68), and the positivity assumption characterized by (8.70)–(8.84).

Proof. This is accomplished by demonstrating that both (8.258) and

(8.259) are equal to

$$p_{X_k^*(\bar{a}_{k-1})|\overline{\mathcal{T}}_{k-1}^*(\bar{a}_{k-2}),\overline{X}_{k-1}^*(\bar{a}_{k-2}),\mathcal{T}_k^*(\bar{a}_{k-1}),\varkappa_k^*(\bar{a}_{k-1})=1}(x_k|\overline{\tau}_{k-1},\overline{x}_{k-1},\tau_k),$$
(8.260)

where, by definition, the events $\varkappa^*(\bar{a}) \geq k$ and $\varkappa_k^*(\bar{a}_{k-1}) = 1$ are equivalent.

We first show that (8.259) is equal to (8.260). Because the situation of no censoring of the event time is a special case of censoring, it follows immediately from this result that (8.258) is also equivalent to (8.260). As in previous chapters, we carry out the argument taking all random variables to be discrete and thus write (8.259) as

$$P(X_k = x_k|\overline{\mathcal{T}}_{k-1} = \overline{\tau}_{k-1}, \overline{X}_{k-1} = \overline{x}_{k-1}, \overline{A}_{k-1} = \bar{a}_{k-1}, \mathcal{T}_k = \tau_k, \kappa \geq k),$$

which is equivalent to

$$P(X_k = x_k|\overline{\mathcal{T}}_{k-1} = \overline{\tau}_{k-1}, \overline{X}_{k-1} = \overline{x}_{k-1}, \overline{A}_{k-1} = \bar{a}_{k-1}, \mathcal{T}_k = \tau_k,$$
$$\kappa \geq k, U \geq \tau_k)$$
$$= P(X_k = x_k|H_{k-1} = h_{k-1}, A_{k-1} = a_{k-1}, \mathcal{T}_k = \tau_k, \kappa \geq k, U \geq \tau_k),$$
(8.261)

as $(H_{k-1} = h_{k-1}) = (\overline{\mathcal{T}}_{k-1} = \overline{\tau}_{k-1}, \overline{X}_{k-1} = \overline{x}_{k-1}, \overline{A}_{k-2} = \bar{a}_{k-2})$ when $\kappa \geq k$. By SUTVA (8.66), (8.261) is equal to

$$P\{X_k^*(\bar{a}_{k-1}) = x_k|H_{k-1} = h_{k-1}, A_{k-1} = a_{k-1}, \mathcal{T}_k^*(\bar{a}_{k-1}) = \tau_k,$$
$$\varkappa_k^*(\bar{a}_{k-1}) = 1, U \geq \tau_k\}.$$
(8.262)

We now argue that (8.262) is equal to

$$P\{X_k^*(\bar{a}_{k-1}) = x_k|H_{k-1} = h_{k-1}, A_{k-1} = a_{k-1}, \mathcal{T}_k^*(\bar{a}_{k-1}) = \tau_k,$$
$$\varkappa_k^*(\bar{a}_{k-1}) = 1, U \geq \tau_{k-1}\},$$
(8.263)

which, by the definition of U, is equal to

$$P\{X_k^*(\bar{a}_{k-1}) = x_k|H_{k-1} = h_{k-1}, A_{k-1} = a_{k-1}, \mathcal{T}_k^*(\bar{a}_{k-1}) = \tau_k,$$
$$\varkappa_k^*(\bar{a}_{k-1}) = 1, \kappa \geq k - 1\}.$$
(8.264)

It is straightforward to write (8.262) as $\mathcal{B}_1/\mathcal{B}_2$, where

$$\mathcal{B}_1 = P\{U \geq \tau_k|U \geq \tau_{k-1}, H_{k-1} = h_{k-1}, A_{k-1} = a_{k-1}, \mathcal{T}_k^*(\bar{a}_{k-1}) = \tau_k,$$
$$\varkappa_k^*(\bar{a}_{k-1}) = 1, \overline{X}_k^*(\bar{a}_{k-1}) = x_k\}$$
(8.265)
$$\times P\{U \geq \tau_{k-1}, H_{k-1} = h_{k-1}, A_{k-1} = a_{k-1}, \mathcal{T}_k^*(\bar{a}_{k-1}) = \tau_k,$$
$$\varkappa_k^*(\bar{a}_{k-1}) = 1, \overline{X}_k^*(\bar{a}_{k-1}) = x_k\}$$
(8.266)

and

$$\mathcal{B}_2 = P\{U \geq \tau_k | U \geq \tau_{k-1}, H_{k-1} = h_{k-1}, A_{k-1} = a_{k-1}, T_k^*(\overline{a}_{k-1}) = \tau_k,$$
$$\varkappa_k^*(\overline{a}_{k-1}) = 1\} \tag{8.267}$$
$$\times P\{U \geq \tau_{k-1}, H_{k-1} = h_{k-1}, A_{k-1} = a_{k-1}, T_k^*(\overline{a}_{k-1}) = \tau_k,$$
$$\varkappa_k^*(\overline{a}_{k-1}) = 1\}. \tag{8.268}$$

By arguments similar to those used to show that (8.71) is equal to (8.77) and more generally the equality in (8.82), under the positivity and non-informative censoring assumptions, it is straightforward to deduce that both (8.265) and (8.267) are equal to

$$\exp\left\{-\int_{\tau_{k-1}}^{\tau_k} \lambda_C(w \mid h_{k-1}, a_{k-1}) \, dw\right\} > 0,$$

so that these terms cancel from the quotient $\mathcal{B}_1/\mathcal{B}_2$. It follows that (8.262) is equal to (8.266) divided by (8.268), which is easily seen to be equal to (8.263) and thus (8.264).

By the SRA, it is straightforward that (8.264) is equal to

$$P\{X_k^*(\overline{a}_{k-1}) = x_k | H_{k-1} = h_{k-1}, T_k^*(\overline{a}_{k-1}) = \tau_k,$$
$$\varkappa_k^*(\overline{a}_{k-1}) = 1, \kappa \geq k-1\}$$
$$= P\{X_k^*(\overline{a}_{k-1}) = x_k | \overline{T}_{k-2} = \overline{\tau}_{k-2}, \overline{X}_{k-2} = \overline{x}_{k-2}, X_{k-1} = x_{k-1},$$
$$\overline{A}_{k-2} = \overline{a}_{k-2}, T_{k-1} = \tau_{k-1}, T_k^*(\overline{a}_{k-1}) = \tau_k, \varkappa_k^*(\overline{a}_{k-1}) = 1, \kappa \geq k-1\}$$
$$= P\{X_k^*(\overline{a}_{k-1}) = x_k | \overline{T}_{k-2} = \overline{\tau}_{k-2}, \overline{X}_{k-2} = \overline{x}_{k-2}, X_{k-1}^*(\overline{a}_{k-2}) = x_{k-1},$$
$$\overline{A}_{k-2} = \overline{a}_{k-2}, T_{k-1}^*(\overline{a}_{k-2}) = \tau_{k-1}, T_k^*(\overline{a}_{k-1}) = \tau_k,$$
$$\varkappa_k^*(\overline{a}_{k-1}) = 1, \kappa \geq k-1\}, \tag{8.269}$$

where (8.269) follows by SUTVA. Repeating the above argument for $\kappa \geq k-1$, we obtain that (8.269) is equal to

$$P\{X_k^*(\overline{a}_{k-1}) = x_k | \overline{T}_{k-3} = \overline{\tau}_{k-3}, \overline{X}_{k-3} = \overline{x}_{k-3}, X_{k-2}^*(\overline{a}_{k-3}) = x_{k-2},$$
$$X_{k-1}^*(\overline{a}_{k-2}) = x_{k-1}, \overline{A}_{k-3} = \overline{a}_{k-3}, T_{k-2}^*(\overline{a}_{k-3}) = \tau_{k-2},$$
$$T_{k-1}^*(\overline{a}_{k-2}) = \tau_{k-1}, T_k^*(\overline{a}_{k-1}) = \tau_k, \varkappa_k^*(\overline{a}_{k-1}) = 1, \kappa \geq k-2\}.$$

Continuing backward in this fashion, for $\kappa \geq j, j = k, k-1, \ldots, 1$, yields the desired result that (8.259) is equal to (8.260) and thus (8.258) is also equal to (8.260). $\square$

Equivalence of (8.93) and (8.117), (8.94) and (8.118), and (8.96) and (8.119)

It is possible to demonstrate the equivalence of the cause-specific hazard functions with and without censoring by showing the equivalence of each to the corresponding cause-specific hazard functions (8.103), (8.104), and (8.105). Namely, it can be shown that $(8.93) = (8.117) = (8.103)$, $(8.94) = (8.118) = (8.104)$, and $(8.96\ ) = (8.119) = (8.105)$. The proof follows along the same lines as that for the conditional densities (8.258) and (8.259) above and is omitted.

Proof of (8.128) (No Censoring)

If we define recursively as in (8.124)–(8.127)

$$Q_K^d(h_K, a_K) = E\{f(T) | H_K = h_K, A_K = a_K, \varkappa = K\},$$

$$V_K^d(h_K) = Q_K^d\{h_K, d_K(h_K)\},$$

for $\varkappa = K$ and, for $\varkappa \geq k$, $k = K - 1, \ldots, 1$,

$$Q_k^d(h_k, a_k) = E\Big\{\mathrm{I}(\varkappa = k)f(T) +$$

$$\mathrm{I}(\varkappa = k + 1)V_{k+1}^d(H_{k+1}) \mid H_k = h_k, A_k = a_k, \varkappa \geq k\Big\},$$

$$V_k^d(h_k) = Q_k^d\{h_k, d_k(h_k)\},$$

then we demonstrate (8.128), namely, that

$$\mathcal{V}(d) = E[f\{T^*(d)\}] = E\{V_1^d(H_1)\}.$$

Proof. Similar to the proof of (6.53), we show that for $\varkappa \geq k$

$$V_k^d(h_k) = E[f\{T^*(\bar{a}_{k-1}, d_k, \ldots, d_K)\} \mid H_k = h_k, \varkappa \geq k]. \qquad (8.270)$$

In (8.270), as in (8.237), $T^*(\bar{a}_{k-1}, d_k, \ldots, d_K)$ is the potential event time for an individual who reaches Decision k if she were to receive options $a_1, \ldots, a_k$ at Decisions 1 to $k - 1$ and then be treated according to the rules $d_k, \ldots, d_K$ at the remaining decision points. As for $T^*(d)$ defined in Section 8.3.2. it is understood that $T^*(\bar{a}_{k-1}, d_k, \ldots, d_K)$ depends on the rules $d_k, \ldots, d_K$ only through those that are not null; that is, as in Section 8.3.1, treatment options corresponding to Decisions $j > \varkappa$ are considered null. The desired result (8.128) follows immediately from (8.270) with $k = 1$, using the fact that $\varkappa \geq 1$ is superfluous. The proof is by induction.

When $\varkappa = K$, it is straightforward that

$$
\begin{aligned}
V_K^d(h_K) &= E\{f(T)|H_K = h_K, A_K = d_K(h_K), \varkappa = K\} \\
&= E[f\{T^*(\overline{a}_{K-1}, d_K)\}|H_K = h_K, A_K = d_K(h_K), \varkappa = K] \\
&= E[f\{T^*(\overline{a}_{K-1}, d_K)\}|H_K = h_K, \varkappa = K],
\end{aligned}
$$

where the second equality follows by SUTVA (8.63) and the third by the SRA (8.64). This demonstrates that (8.270) holds for $\varkappa = K$.

It thus suffices for the induction proof to show that, if for $\varkappa \geq k+1$

$$
V_{k+1}^d(h_{k+1}) = E[f\{T^*(\overline{a}_k, d_{k+1}, \dots, d_K)\} \mid H_{k+1} = h_{k+1}, \varkappa \geq k+1], \tag{8.271}
$$

then (8.270) holds. Now (8.271) implies that

$$
\begin{aligned}
I(\varkappa = k)f(T) + I(\varkappa \geq k+1)V_{k+1}^d(H_{k+1}) &= I(\varkappa = k)f(T) + I(\varkappa \geq k+1) \\
\times E[f\{T^*(\overline{A}_k, d_{k+1}, \dots, d_K)\} &\mid H_{k+1}, \varkappa \geq k+1]. \tag{8.272}
\end{aligned}
$$

By (8.59), if $\varkappa = k$, H_{k+1} contains T, and (8.272) can be written as

$$
E[I(\varkappa = k)f(T) + I(\varkappa \geq k+1)f\{T^*(\overline{A}_k, d_{k+1}, \dots, d_K)\} \mid H_{k+1}]. \tag{8.273}
$$

Moreover, by SUTVA, when $\varkappa = k$, conditional on H_{k+1}, $f(T) = f\{T^*(\overline{A}_k, d_{k+1}, \dots, d_K)\}$. It follows by substitution of this result in (8.273) that (8.273) can be written as

$$
E[I(\varkappa \geq k)f\{T^*(\overline{A}_k, d_{k+1}, \dots, d_K)\}|H_{k+1}]. \tag{8.274}
$$

Thus, (8.272) is equal to (8.274). It then follows from the definition of $Q_k^d(h_k, a_k)$ above that

$$
\begin{aligned}
Q_k^d(h_k, a_k) &= E\Big(E[I(\varkappa \geq k)f\{T^*(\overline{A}_k, d_{k+1}, \dots, d_K)\} \\
&\qquad \Big| H_{k+1}]|H_k = h_k, A_k = a_k, \varkappa \geq k\Big) \\
&= E[f\{T^*(\overline{a}_k, d_{k+1}, \dots, d_K)\}|H_k = h_k, A_k = a_k, \varkappa \geq k].
\end{aligned}
$$

This yields, using SUTVA and the SRA,

$$
\begin{aligned}
V_k^d(h_k) &= Q_k^d\{h_k, d_k(h_k)\} \\
&= E[f\{T^*(\overline{a}_k, d_{k+1}, \dots, d_K)\}|H_k = h_k, A_k = d_k(h_k), \varkappa \geq k] \\
&= E[f\{T^*(\overline{a}_{k-1}, d_k, \dots, d_K)\}|H_k = h_k, A_k = d_k(h_k), \varkappa \geq k] \\
&= E[f\{T^*(\overline{a}_{k-1}, d_k, \dots, d_K)\}|H_k = h_k, \varkappa \geq k],
\end{aligned}
$$

which is (8.270), demonstrating the result. $\qquad \square$

Proof of (8.139) (Censoring)

Proof. Analogous to the proof of (8.128) in the case of no censoring, we show that for $\kappa \geq k$

$$V_k^d(h_k) = E[f\{T^*(\overline{A}_{k-1}, d_k, \ldots, d_K)\} \mid H_k = h_k, \kappa \geq k]. \qquad (8.275)$$

As in the preceding argument, the proof is by induction. For $\kappa = K$,

$$V_K^d(h_K) = E\left\{ \frac{\Delta f(U)}{\mathcal{K}_K(U|h_K, a_K)} \middle| H_K = h_K, A_K = d_K(h_K), \kappa = K \right\}$$

$$= E\left[\frac{\Delta f\{T^*(\overline{a}_{K-1}, d_K)\}}{\mathcal{K}_K\{T^*(\overline{a}_{K-1}, d_K)|h_K, a_K\}} \middle| H_K = h_K, A_K = d_K(h_K), \kappa = K \right],$$

$$(8.276)$$

where (8.276) follows by SUTVA. Now (8.276) can be written using iterative conditional expectations as

$$E\left\{ G(h_K, K, W^*)|H_K = h_K, A_K = d_K(h_K), \kappa = K \right\} \qquad (8.277)$$

where W^* is the set of potential outcomes (8.50), and

$$G(h_K, K, W^*) = E\left[\frac{\Delta f\{T^*(\overline{a}_{K-1}, d_K)\}}{\mathcal{K}_K\{T^*(\overline{a}_{K-1}, d_K)|h_K, d_K(h_K)\}} \right.$$

$$\left. \middle| H_K = h_K, A_K = d_K(h_K), \kappa = K, W^* \right]$$

$$(8.278)$$

$$= \frac{f\{T^*(\overline{a}_{K-1}, d_K)\}}{\mathcal{K}_K\{T^*(\overline{a}_{K-1}, d_K)|h_K, d_K(h_K)\}}$$

$$\times E\{\Delta|H_K = h_K, A_K = d_K(h_K), \kappa = K, W^*\}.$$

It is straightforward that

$$E\{\Delta|H_K = h_K, A_K = d_K(h_K), \kappa = K, W^*\}$$

$$= P\{U \geq T^*(\overline{a}_{K-1}, d_K)|H_K = h_K, A_K = d_K(h_K), \kappa = K, W^*\}$$

$$= \mathcal{K}_K\{T^*(\overline{a}_{K-1}, d_K)|h_K, d_K(h_K)\}, \qquad (8.279)$$

where the last equality follows by Lemma 8.5.1. Substituting this in (8.278) shows that

$$G(h_K, K, W^*) = f\{T^*(\overline{a}_{K-1}, d_K)\}.$$

Thus, (8.277) becomes

$$E\left[f\{T^*(\overline{a}_{K-1}, d_K)\}|H_K = h_K, A_K = d_K(h_K), \kappa = K \right]$$

$$= E\left[f\{T^*(\overline{a}_{K-1}, d_K)\}|H_K = h_K, \kappa = K \right]$$

by the SRA, thus demonstrating (8.275) for $k = K$.

To complete the induction proof, we now show that if (8.275) holds for $k + 1$, so that

$$V_{k+1}^d(h_{k+1}) = E[f\{T^*(\overline{A}_k, d_{k+1}, \ldots, d_K)\} \mid H_{k+1} = h_{k+1}, \kappa \geq k + 1], \tag{8.280}$$

then it holds for k.

Consider $Q_k^d(h_k, a_k)$ defined in (8.137), which we write as

$$Q_k^d(h_k, a_k) =$$

$$= E\left\{ \frac{\mathrm{I}(\Upsilon_{k+1}^\dagger = 1)\mathrm{I}(\kappa = k)f(S_{k+1}^\dagger)}{\mathcal{K}_k(S_{k+1}^\dagger \mid H_k, A_k)} \middle| H_k = h_k, A_k = a_k, \kappa \geq k \right\} \tag{8.281}$$

$$+ E\left\{ \frac{\mathrm{I}(\Upsilon_{k+1}^\dagger = -1)\mathrm{I}(\kappa \geq k + 1)V_{k+1}^d(H_{k+1})}{\mathcal{K}_k(S_{k+1}^\dagger \mid H_k, A_k)} \right. \tag{8.282}$$

$$\left. \middle| H_k = h_k, A_k = a_k, \kappa \geq k \right\}.$$

Using (8.280), the quantity inside the expectation in (8.282) can be written as

$$\frac{\mathrm{I}(\Upsilon_{k+1}^\dagger = -1)\mathrm{I}(\kappa \geq k + 1)}{\mathcal{K}_k(S_{k+1}^\dagger \mid H_k, A_k)}$$

$$\times E[f\{T^*(\overline{A}_k, d_{k+1}, \ldots, d_K)\} \mid H_{k+1}, \kappa \geq k + 1]$$

which is a well-defined random variable as a function of H_{k+1}, so can be rewritten as

$$E\left[\frac{\mathrm{I}(\Upsilon_{k+1}^\dagger = -1)\mathrm{I}(\kappa \geq k + 1)f\{T^*(\overline{A}_k, d_{k+1}, \ldots, d_K)\}}{\mathcal{K}_k(S_{k+1}^\dagger \mid H_k, A_k)} \middle| H_{k+1} \right].$$

Applying an iterative conditioning argument to (8.282) and substituting this expression yields that (8.282) is equal to

$$E\left[\frac{\mathrm{I}(\Upsilon_{k+1}^\dagger = -1)\mathrm{I}(\kappa \geq k + 1)f\{T^*(\overline{A}_k, d_{k+1}, \ldots, d_K)\}}{\mathcal{K}_k(S_{k+1}^\dagger \mid h_k, a_k)} \right.$$

$$\left. \middle| H_k = h_k, A_k = a_k, \kappa \geq k \right].$$

By SUTVA, this can be written equivalently as

$$E\left[\frac{\mathrm{I}\{U \geq S_{k+1}^*(\overline{a}_k)\}\mathrm{I}\{\Upsilon_{k+1}^*(\overline{a}_k) = -1\}\mathrm{I}\{\varkappa_{k+1}^*(\overline{a}_k) = 1\}}{\mathcal{K}_k\{S_{k+1}^*(\overline{a}_k) \mid h_k, a_k\}} \right.$$

$$\times f\{T^*(\overline{A}_k, d_{k+1}, \ldots, d_K)\}\Big| H_k = h_k, A_k = a_k, \kappa \geq k\Big]$$

$$= E[\mathrm{I}\{\Upsilon^*_{k+1}(\overline{a}_k) = -1\}\mathrm{I}\{\varkappa^*_{k+1}(\overline{a}_k) = 1\}$$
$$\times f\{T^*(\overline{A}_k, d_{k+1}, \ldots, d_K)\}|H_k = h_k, A_k = a_k, \kappa \geq k], \quad (8.283)$$

where (8.283) follows from using the assumption of noninformative censoring as above and Lemma 8.5.1. By similar manipulations, it can be shown that (8.281) can be written as

$$E[\mathrm{I}\{\Upsilon^*_{k+1}(\overline{a}_k) = 1\}\mathrm{I}\{\varkappa^*_k(\overline{a}_{k-1}) = 1, \varkappa^*_{k+1}(\overline{a}_k) = 0\}$$
$$\times f\{T^*(\overline{A}_k, d_{k+1}, \ldots, d_K)\}|H_k = h_k, A_k = a_k, \kappa \geq k]. \quad (8.284)$$

Thus, $Q^d_k(h_k, a_k)$ in (8.137) can written as the sum of (8.283) and (8.284), which is given by

$$E\Big([\mathrm{I}\{\Upsilon^*_{k+1}(\overline{a}_k) = 1\}\mathrm{I}\{\varkappa^*_k(\overline{a}_{k-1}) = 1, \varkappa^*_{k+1}(\overline{a}_k) = 0\}$$
$$+ \mathrm{I}\{\Upsilon^*_{k+1}(\overline{a}_k) = -1\}\mathrm{I}\{\varkappa^*_{k+1}(\overline{a}_k) = 1\}]$$
$$\times f\{T^*(\overline{A}_k, d_{k+1}, \ldots, d_K)\}|H_k = h_k, A_k = a_k, \kappa \geq k\Big)$$
$$= E[\mathrm{I}\{\varkappa^*_k(\overline{a}_{k-1}) = 1\}f\{T^*(\overline{A}_k, d_{k+1}, \ldots, d_K)\}$$
$$|H_k = h_k, A_k = a_k, \kappa \geq k] \quad (8.285)$$
$$= E[\mathrm{I}(\kappa \geq k)f\{T^*(\overline{A}_k, d_{k+1}, \ldots, d_K)\}|H_k = h_k, A_k = a_k, \kappa \geq k]$$
$$= E[f\{T^*(\overline{A}_k, d_{k+1}, \ldots, d_K)\}|H_k = h_k, A_k = a_k, \kappa \geq k], \quad (8.286)$$

where (8.285) follows by SUTVA. Now, from (8.138), substituting (8.286) and using SUTVA and then the SRA,

$$V^d_k(h_k) = Q^d_k\{h_k, d_k(h_k)\}$$
$$= E[f\{T^*(\overline{A}_k, d_{k+1}, \ldots, d_K)\}|H_k = h_k, A_k = d_k(h_k), \kappa \geq k]$$
$$= E[f\{T^*(\overline{A}_{k-1}, d_k, \ldots, d_K)\}|H_k = h_k, A_k = d_k(h_k), \kappa \geq k]$$
$$= E[f\{T^*(\overline{A}_{k-1}, d_k, \ldots, d_K)\}|H_k = h_k, \kappa \geq k],$$

demonstrating that (8.275) holds for k, completing the induction proof. $\square$

Remark. Via arguments similar to those used to establish the equivalence of (8.110) and (8.112) earlier in this section, making use of Lemma 8.5.1, it can be shown that

$$V^d_k(h_k) = E[f\{T^*(\overline{A}_{k-1}, d_k, \ldots, d_K)\}|H_k = h_k, \kappa \geq k]$$
$$= E[f\{T^*(\overline{A}_{k-1}, d_k, \ldots, d_K)\}|H_k = h_k, \varkappa \geq k].$$

Note that (8.279) implies that

$$E\left\{\frac{\Delta}{\mathcal{K}_K(U|h_K,a_K)}\middle|H_K = h_K, A_K = a_K, \kappa = K\right\} = 1. \qquad (8.287)$$

By a similar argument,

$$E\left\{I(\Upsilon_{k+1}^\dagger \neq 0)|H_k = h_k, A_k = a_k, \kappa \geq k, W^*\right\}$$
$$= P\{U \geq S_{k+1}^*(\bar{a}_k)|H_k = h_k, A_k = a_k, \kappa \geq k, W^*\}$$
$$= \mathcal{K}_k\{S_{k+1}^*(\bar{a}_k)|h_k, a_k\}$$

so that

$$E\left\{\frac{I(\Upsilon_{k+1}^\dagger \neq 0)}{\mathcal{K}_k(S_{k+1}^\dagger|h_k,a_k)}\middle|H_k = h_k, A_k = a_k, \kappa \geq k\right\} = 1. \qquad (8.288)$$

The results (8.287) and (8.288) are used to show that the estimating equations (8.145)–(8.147) in Section 8.3.3 are unbiased.

Demonstration that (8.145) Is Unbiased

To show that (8.145) is an unbiased estimating equation, we must demonstrate that

$$E\left[\frac{I(\kappa = K)\Delta}{\mathcal{K}_K(U|H_K,A_K)}\frac{\partial Q_K^{R_d}(H_K,A_K;\beta_K)}{\partial \beta_K}\right.$$
$$\qquad\qquad\qquad\qquad\qquad\qquad\qquad (8.289)$$
$$\left.\times\left\{f(U) - f(\mathcal{T}_i) - Q_K^{R_d}(H_K,A_K;\beta_K)\right\}\right] = 0.$$

Proof. This is accomplished via an iterative conditional expectation argument. The conditional expectation of (8.289) given $(H_K, A_K, \kappa = K)$ is easily seen to be

$$I(\kappa = K)\frac{\partial Q_K^{R_d}(H_K,A_K;\beta_K)}{\partial \beta_K}\left[E\left\{\frac{\Delta f(U)}{\mathcal{K}_K(U|H_K,A_K)}\middle|H_K,A_K,\kappa = K\right\}\right.$$
$$\left. - E\left\{\frac{\Delta}{\mathcal{K}_K(U|H_K,A_K)}\middle|H_K,A_K,\kappa = K\right\}\right. \qquad (8.290)$$
$$\left.\times\left\{-f(\mathcal{T}_K) - Q_K^{R_d}(H_K,A_K;\beta_K)\right\}\right].$$

By definition, from (8.135)

$$E\left\{\frac{\Delta f(U)}{\mathcal{K}_K(U|H_K,A_K)}\middle|H_K,A_K,\kappa = K\right\} = Q_K^d(H_K,A_K).$$

Substituting this and (8.287) above in (8.290) yields that (8.290) is equal to

$$
\begin{aligned}
I(\kappa = K) &\frac{\partial Q_K^{R_d}(H_K, A_K; \beta_K)}{\partial \beta_K} \\
&\times \{Q_K^d(H_K, A_K) - f(\mathcal{T}_K) - Q_K^{R_d}(H_K, A_K; \beta_K)\}.
\end{aligned}
\tag{8.291}
$$

Because by definition

$$
Q_K^{R_d}(H_K, A_K) = Q_K^d(H_K, A_K) - f(\mathcal{T}_K),
$$

it follows that (8.291) is equal to zero. It thus follows that (8.290) is equal to zero, which implies (8.289), demonstrating the result. $\square$

The argument to show that the estimating equations (8.147), $k = K - 1, \ldots, 1$, are unbiased is similar to that for $k = K$ using the definition of $Q_k^d(H_k, A_k)$ in (8.137) and (8.288) above, and is omitted.

Demonstration of (8.182)

We argue that

$$
\begin{aligned}
V_k^d &\{\overline{\tau}_k, \overline{x}_k, \overline{d}_{k-1}(\overline{\tau}_{k-1}, \overline{x}_{k-1})\} \\
&= E[f\{T^*(d)\}|\overline{T}_k^*(d_{k-1}) = \overline{\tau}_{k-1}, \overline{X}_k^*(d_{k-1}) = \overline{x}_k, \varkappa^*(d) \geq k],
\end{aligned}
$$

so that the result follows.

Proof. In the proof of (8.128) earlier in this section, we show (8.270),

$$
V_k^d(h_k) = E[f\{T^*(\overline{a}_{k-1}, d_k, \ldots, d_K)\} \mid H_k = h_k, \varkappa \geq k], \quad k = 1, \ldots, K.
$$

It thus follows that

$$
\begin{aligned}
V_k^d &\{\overline{\tau}_k, \overline{x}_k, \overline{d}_{k-1}(\overline{\tau}_{k-1}, \overline{x}_{k-1})\} \\
&= E[f\{T^*(d)\}|\overline{T}_k = \overline{\tau}_k, \overline{X}_k = \overline{x}_k, \overline{A}_{k-1} = \overline{d}_{k-1}(\overline{\tau}_{k-1}, \overline{x}_{k-1}), \varkappa^*(d) \geq k].
\end{aligned}
$$

The result follows by SUTVA, SRA, and the positivity assumption. $\square$

Chapter 9

Sequential Multiple Assignment Randomized Trials

9.1 Introduction

As noted in Sections 5.3.2 and 5.3.3, the sequential multiple assignment randomized trial (SMART, Lavori and Dawson, 2000, 2004; Murphy, 2005) is the gold standard study design for estimation and evaluation of multistage treatment regimes. In this chapter, we present an overview of considerations for the conception, design, and analysis of SMARTs.

In a SMART, at each of $K \geq 2$ stages, each participant is randomly assigned to one of the treatment options that are feasible given his history to that point, where each stage corresponds to a key decision point in the disease or disorder process of interest. Thus, SMARTs seek to mimic clinical practice in that treatment is adjusted when and if needed; however, in a SMART, such adjustments may be randomly assigned.

Figure 9.1 shows the schematic for a SMART with $K = 2$ stages designed to study sequences of doses of behavioral interventions for management of pain in cancer patients (Kelleher et al., 2017). At the first stage, patients are randomized to receive Pain Coping Skills Training (PCST) at full dose (PCST-Full) or low dose (PCST-Brief), and whether or not a patient responds, defined as whether or not the percent reduction from baseline of a patient reported pain score exceeds a given threshold, is ascertained at the end of stage one. At the second stage, responders to PCST-Full are randomized to receive PCST-Full maintenance therapy or no further treatment, and nonresponders to PCST-Full are randomized to a more intensive training regimen, PCST-Plus, or to PCST-Full maintenance. Responders to PCST-Brief are randomized to PCTS-Brief maintenance therapy or no further intervention, and nonresponders to PCST-Brief are randomized to PCST-Full or PCST-Brief maintenance. Thus, the feasible treatment options at the second stage are different depending on a participant's history, so that randomization at the second stage depends on first-stage treatment and response status. The (continuous) outcome, percent reduction in pain from baseline, is recorded at the end of stage two.

This example illustrates a key feature of SMARTs, which is that they may include multiple randomized treatment assignments, where the tim-

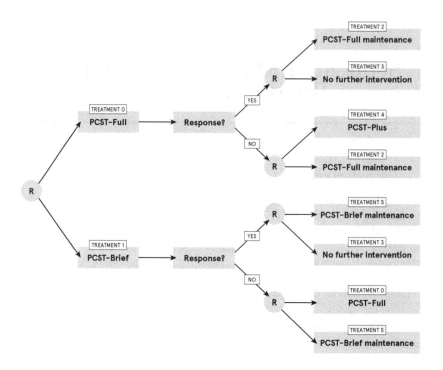

Figure 9.1 *SMART for the study of behavioral interventions for cancer pain management. In this and subsequent figures in this chapter, the symbol* Ⓡ *denotes randomization.*

ing, number, and nature of these randomizations depend on the evolving health status of each participant. Consequently, SMART designs are highly flexible and vary as widely as the diseases and disorders that they are used to study. This flexibility can be daunting to researchers designing a SMART, as there are often significantly more design choices than in a conventional k-arm randomized clinical trial. However, as demonstrated in this chapter, these design choices are in many cases dictated by the underlying clinical science.

As a result of these choices, a number of simple, fixed treatment regimes are *embedded* in the design of a SMART. For example, in the SMART in Figure 9.1, there will be participants who, by virtue of randomization, have realized treatment experience consistent with having followed the regime "Give PCST-Full initially followed by PCST-Full maintenance if response or PCST-Plus if nonresponse," which of course could be expressed formally as a fixed regime d with rules d_1 and d_2.

Consideration of Figure 9.1 shows that there are eight such regimes embedded in this design, which represent "treatment sequences" reflecting the motivating clinical considerations.

A common concern that arises upon seeing a SMART schematic like that in Figure 9.1 is that "sample splitting" will result in low precision or power for detecting meaningful differences. However, many primary comparisons of interest involve pooling subjects across multiple terminal nodes of the design. For example, comparison of first-stage treatments in terms of response rate can be carried out using a standard two-sample test of proportions based on the data from all subjects assigned to the first-stage treatments of interest, regardless of the treatments assigned to them at later stages. In this chapter, we discuss this and other primary comparisons commonly of interest in SMART designs that may involve pooling of subjects, as well as comparison of the fixed treatment regimes embedded in a SMART on the basis of outcomes measured at the end of the final stage, including accompanying power calculations for these comparisons. We also discuss the scientific considerations involved in selecting the primary, secondary, and exploratory analyses of interest.

We also present sample size estimation procedures for SMARTs when the goal is to estimate and evaluate an optimal treatment regime using Q-learning with posited parametric models for the Q-functions as in Section 5.7.1. Estimation of an optimal regime is typically a secondary or exploratory analysis; one reason for this is that it is widely regarded as being excessively expensive to collect enough samples to ensure high-quality estimation of an optimal regime with high probability. Thus, these sample size procedures can be used to characterize how much additional information is needed to estimate an optimal regime relative to carrying out a simple comparison, such as testing for a difference in mean outcome under two fixed treatment regimes. We show that if one is willing to make parametric assumptions, then sample size formulæ are available in a closed form and resemble those for simpler comparisons. Without such parametric assumptions, however, sample size calculations for estimation of an optimal regime depend on nuisance parameters that are difficult to elicit from domain experts and therefore must be estimated from historical or pilot data.

SMARTs are sometimes confused with adaptive clinical trial designs with a single point of randomization for which the randomization probabilities are adjusted over time as information about treatment effects accrues (e.g., Berry and Fristedt, 1985; Whitehead, 1997). However, although SMARTs comprise a sequence of randomizations, these randomizations are *within* a subject over time and are conducted for the purpose of evaluating treatment sequences. In contrast, an adaptive clinical trial applies a sequence of randomizations *across* participants, driven by the perspective that randomization probabilities should be informed by current evidence from previous participants of each candidate treatment's efficacy. SMARTs also may be confused with crossover designs, as both involve randomly assigning treatment sequences to each patient (Jones and Kenward, 2014). However, the primary goal of a crossover trial is the identification of a single best treatment option, and such designs use assignment of the same subject to multiple treatments as a mechanism to control for subject-specific characteristics and thereby reduce variance. Thus, in a crossover design, treatment sequences are a means to compare fixed treatments efficiently rather than a reflection of clinical interest in such sequences.

We begin our overview of SMARTs in Section 9.2 by discussing core components of a SMART design and how the underlying clinical science should be used to inform these components. This material and that in Section 9.3 on primary comparisons commonly used to power a SMART is fundamental for a reader seeking a broad appreciation of considerations and methods involved in routine deployment of SMARTs in practice. This reader will also benefit from reviewing the introduction to Section 9.4 and Section 9.4.2, which discuss additional comparisons of interest; and the introduction to Section 9.5, which describes the framework for sample size formulæ for estimation of an optimal regime. The subsequent material on sample size procedures for more complex comparisons in Section 9.4 and for estimation of an optimal regime in Section 9.5 is more technical. Readers interested in the theoretical underpinnings will wish also to study these sections in detail. All readers will wish to review the brief discussion of extensions in Section 9.6.

Throughout, we focus for definiteness mainly on SMARTs with $K = 2$ stages, which are most common in practice. This case is sufficient to illustrate the key considerations involved; extension of most of the methods discussed to $K > 2$ stages is possible, albeit at the expense of additional complexity.

9.2   Design Considerations

9.2.1   Basic SMART Framework, $K = 2$

We first describe a SMART with $K = 2$ stages. Considerations for determining of the timing and nature of the decision points that dictate the stages of the SMART are discussed in Section 9.2.2.

As in Chapters 5–7, assume that for each participant entering the SMART, baseline information X_1 is to be collected, so that each participant has baseline history $H_1 = X_1$ at the outset of the study. Assume that there are sets of candidate treatment options $\mathcal{A}_1$ and $\mathcal{A}_2$ that could be implemented at the first and second decision points, respectively. As demonstrated shortly, there can be overlap between the options in each of $\mathcal{A}_1$ and $\mathcal{A}_2$, and it is likely that not all options are feasible for all individuals, particularly at the second stage.

An important design consideration, reviewed in detail in Section 9.2.3 below, is to determine the sets of feasible treatment options from among those in $\mathcal{A}_1$ and $\mathcal{A}_2$ to be included in the SMART at each stage; the reader may wish to review Section 6.2.2 for an introduction to the notion of feasible sets before proceeding. From (6.7) in Section 6.2.2, at the first stage, the set of feasible options for a subject with realized baseline history h_1 is $\Psi_1(h_1) \subseteq \mathcal{A}_1$, which must be defined for each possible h_1. In many SMARTs, such as that depicted in Figure 9.1 and others presented later in this section, all treatment options in $\mathcal{A}_1$ are feasible for all individuals, so that $\Psi_1(h_1) = \mathcal{A}_1$ for all h_1, although this is not necessary in general.

For a subject with baseline history H_1, an option A_1 is assigned from the set $\Psi_1(H_1)$; and additional, intervening information X_2 is to be collected during the first stage. Thus, at the beginning of the second stage, a participant has history $H_2 = (X_1, A_1, X_2)$. With $\Psi_2(h_2) \subseteq \mathcal{A}_2$ the set of feasible options for a subject with realized history h_2, a subject with history H_2 is assigned an option A_2 from the set $\Psi_2(H_2)$. As in Section 6.2.2 and demonstrated shortly, $\Psi_2(h_2)$ is often a strict subset of $\mathcal{A}_2$ determined by a component or function of components of h_2. It may well be the case that, for certain histories h_2, $\Psi_2(h_2)$ may comprise a single option, so that subjects with such histories are assigned that option with certainty and thus are not randomized (or can be viewed as being randomized to that option with probability 1).

For illustration, consider the SMART in Figure 9.1. As above, using the coding of the treatment options given in the design schematic, $\Psi_1(h_1) = \{0, 1\}$ for all h_1. The feasible sets at stage two depend on response status r_2, which in general can be an explicit component or function of components of h_2, as discussed in Section 6.2.2, where $r_2 = 0\,(1)$ indicates nonresponse (response). Then

$$\Psi_2(h_2) = \begin{cases} \{2,3\} & \text{if } r_2 = 1 \text{ and } a_1 = 0 \\ \{2,4\} & \text{if } r_2 = 0 \text{ and } a_1 = 0 \\ \{3,5\} & \text{if } r_2 = 1 \text{ and } a_1 = 1 \\ \{0,5\} & \text{if } r_2 = 0 \text{ and } a_1 = 1. \end{cases}$$

The eight regimes embedded in the design are determined by these specifications and are given by the following:

(e_1) Give PCST-Full initially followed by PCST-Full maintenance if response or PCST-Plus if nonresponse.

(e_2) Give PCST-Full initially followed by PCST-Full maintenance regardless of response status

(e_3) Give PCST-Full initially, followed by no further treatment if response or PCST-Plus if nonresponse

(e_4) Give PCST-Full initially followed by no further treatment if response or PCST-Full maintenance if nonresponse

(e_5) Give PCST-Brief initially followed by PCST-Brief maintenance if response or PCST-Full if nonresponse

(e_6) Give PCST-Brief initially followed by PCST-Brief maintenance regardless of response status

(e_7) Give PCST-Brief initially followed by no further treatment if response or PCST-Full if nonresponse

(e_8) Give PCST-Brief initially followed by no further treatment if response or PCST-Brief maintenance if nonresponse.

In many SMARTs, particularly for the study of treatment of behavioral disorders, the outcome of interest, Y, coded so that larger values are preferred, is ascertained at the end of the second stage. The observed data to be collected in a SMART involving n subjects are then as in (5.16); namely,

$$(X_{1i}, A_{1i}, X_{2i}, A_{2i}, Y_i), \quad i = 1, \ldots, n. \tag{9.1}$$

Alternatively, in SMARTs focused on treatment of a chronic disease such as cancer, the outcome of interest might be a time to an event, as in Chapter 8, which may be possibly censored. For definiteness, we focus primarily on the former setting where the outcome is ascertained for all participants at the end of the second stage.

9.2.2 Critical Decision Points

A key design principle for SMARTs is that the design should mimic the clinical decision-making process in that treatment adjustments are made if and when they are needed. Thus, provided that the timing of treatment adjustments is dictated by the nature of the treatments or established by the science, the timing of treatment changes in a SMART should match, as closely as possible, what is done in clinical practice. For example, in the cancer pain management SMART depicted in Figure 9.1, response status is assessed approximately 35 days after completion of the first-stage treatment, as this was deemed by the investigators to be sufficient time for patients to assess whether or not assigned treatment has had an appreciable effect on pain coping. However, treatment change need not be fixed in calendar time but instead can be driven by interim patient outcomes, as illustrated by the following example.

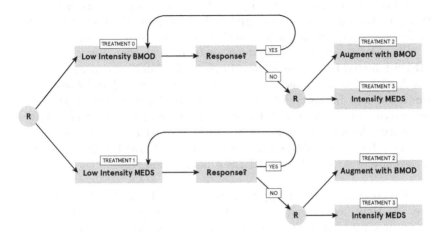

Figure 9.2 *SMART for the study of behavioral and medical interventions for school-aged children with ADHD.*

SMART for Treatment of ADHD in School-Aged Children

Figure 9.2 depicts a SMART for the study of treatment of attention deficit hyperactivity disorder (ADHD) among school-aged children; see Section 1.2.2. At the first stage, participants are randomized to receive low intensity behavioral modification therapy (Low Intensity BMOD) or low intensity medication (Low Intensity MEDS). Over the next twelve weeks, an interim measure of the outcome, a clinical assessment of ADHD severity, is made at weekly clinic visits. The first time that a child is deemed nonresponsive based on this interim measure, he enters stage two of the trial as a nonresponder and is randomly assigned to either augment or intensify stage one treatment. Nonresponders assigned to Low Intensity BMOD at stage one are randomized to augment that intervention with Low Intensity MEDS (Augment with MEDs) or to increase the frequency of BMOD therapy sessions (Intensify BMOD), while those assigned initially to Low Intensity MEDS are randomized to either augment that treatment with Low Intensity BMOD (Augment with BMOD) or to increase the dose of medication (Intensify MEDS). At the final clinic visit at week twelve, any participant who has not yet been determined to be nonresponsive during stage one is deemed a responder and enters stage two, continuing on the treatment assigned in stage one. Thus, subjects remain on their initial treatments until they become nonresponsive, as there is no clinical justification to switch a child from a treatment that appears to be working. In this example, then, the timing of the second critical decision point defining stage two varies across patients according to their interim outcome trajectories.

Here, there are four embedded regimes: (e_1) Give Low Intensity MEDS followed by continued Low Intensity MEDS if response or Intensify MEDS if nonresponse; (e_2) give Low Intensity MEDS followed by continued Low Intensity MEDS if response or Augment with BMOD if nonresponse; (e_3) give Low Intensity BMOD followed by continued Low Intensity BMOD if response or Intensify BMOD if nonresponse; (e_4) give Low Intensity BMOD followed by continued Low Intensity BMOD if response or Augment with MEDS if nonresponse.

Similar considerations apply in the acute leukemia SMART in Figure 5.1. Here, as typically is the case in clinical practice as discussed in Section 1.2.1, after one cycle of first-stage induction chemotherapy, a bone marrow biopsy is performed to assess whether or not a subject has achieved remission (response). If so, the subject enters stage two and is randomized to a maintenance option. If not, she receives a second cycle of induction therapy, after which response status is again ascertained, and she enters stage two; if deemed a responder (nonresponder) at this point, she is randomly assigned to a maintenance (salvage) option. Thus, as in the ADHD example, the timing of the second decision point at which selection of maintenance or salvage therapy is made, as appropriate, varies across patients with interim assessment of remission.

In some contexts, the timing and/or conditions that should dictate treatment changes are of primary interest; e.g., it is of interest to determine how long post-treatment one should wait before changing treatment or how much of a change in symptom severity should be used to deem a patient a nonresponder. The next example reflects this situation.

SMART for mHealth Interventions in HIV Positive Young Men

Figure 9.3 shows a SMART to study mobile health (mHealth) interventions to increase antiretroviral therapy (ART) use among HIV positive young men who have sex with men. The trial involves two novel interventions: AllyQuest, a mHealth medication adherence and social support application, and AllyQuest+, an intensified version of AllyQuest. Participants are randomized at the first stage to one of these two interventions or a control condition with equal probabilities, and response status is assessed for all subjects at three months following initiation of first-stage treatment, where response is defined as a function of interim measures of adherence to stage one treatment and viral suppression. Among participants initially assigned to AllyQuest+, nonresponders are assigned to continue AllyQuest+, and responders are randomly assigned

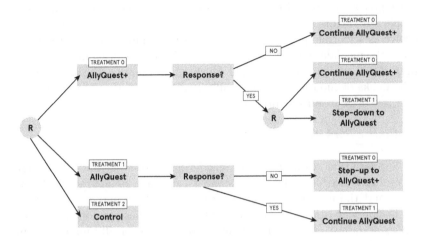

Figure 9.3 *SMART for the study of mHealth interventions to enhance adherence to ART among HIV positive young men who have sex with men.*

to continue AllyQuest+ or to step down to the less intensive AllyQuest. Among subjects initially assigned to AllyQuest, nonresponders are assigned to step up to the more intensive AllyQuest+, and responders are assigned to continue AllyQuest. Those assigned to the control condition do not change treatment during the follow-up period. The primary outcome is a measure of viral suppression at six months. See Muessig (2019) for further details.

In addition to the control condition, there are three embedded regimes: (e_1) Give AllyQuest+ initially, and continue AllyQuest+ regardless of response status; (e_2) give AllyQuest+ initially, and continue AllyQuest+ if nonresponse or step down to AllyQuest if response; and (e_3) give AllyQuest initially, and continue AllyQuest if response or step up to AllyQuest+ if nonresponse.

One of the key questions motivating this design is whether or not individuals who are responsive to AllyQuest+ can be stepped down to the less intensive AllyQuest at three months or if they should be kept on AllyQuest+ to maintain response. Thus, the timing of treatment deescalation is a primary focus in this design.

In many settings, the optimal timing for treatment change is unknown. However, as with any trial, one must choose a design that allows efficient study of those scientific questions that are the most pressing or potentially impactful and leave some (or potentially many) questions to secondary analyses or follow-up studies. We now present a simplified example illustrating how critical decision points in a SMART design might evolve as scientific questions are prioritized. We have tried to preserve a bit of the meandering that is inherent to this process, with many designs postulated, evaluated, and refined. However, in practice, this process can take weeks or months, making a fully realistic rendering of this process as a textbook example impractical.

Illustrative SMART Example 1

Suppose that researchers are considering a two-stage SMART design to evaluate two candidate first-stage treatments, a new active treatment and the current standard of care; a single maintenance therapy for responders; and two candidate salvage therapies for nonresponders. Under standard of care, treatment changes are typically made at four weeks after treatment initiation. Without additional information, one might consider a SMART design like that in Figure 9.4. At the first stage, participants are randomized with equal probability to the new active treatment or to standard of care. After four weeks, subjects are deemed as responders or nonresponders and transition into the second stage, wherein responders are assigned to maintenance therapy and nonresponders are randomized to one of two candidate salvage therapies.

This design facilitates head-to-head comparisons of the new active treatment, coded as 0, with standard of care, coded as 1, in terms of response status and the terminal outcome. With $A_1 = 0$ or 1 as a participant is assigned to the new or standard treatment, let R_2 be a subject's observed response status at the end of stage one, where $R_2 = 0\,(1)$ indicates nonresponse (response). Then, from Section 2.3.2,

$$\frac{\sum_{i=1}^{n} A_{1i}R_{2i}}{\sum_{i=1}^{n} A_{1i}} - \frac{\sum_{i=1}^{n}(1 - A_{1i})R_{2i}}{\sum_{i=1}^{n}(1 - A_{1i})} \tag{9.2}$$

is the estimated difference in response rate at four weeks between standard of care and the new active treatment, and

$$\frac{\sum_{i=1}^{n} A_{1i}Y_{i}}{\sum_{i=1}^{n} A_{1i}} - \frac{\sum_{i=1}^{n}(1 - A_{1i})Y_{i}}{\sum_{i=1}^{n}(1 - A_{1i})} \tag{9.3}$$

is the estimated difference in the mean terminal outcome, marginalizing over the second-stage treatment. Standard test statistics based on these quantities are well known to be asymptotically standard normal so can

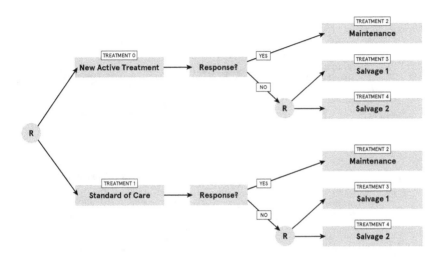

Figure 9.4 *Potential design for illustrative SMART example 1.*

be compared against an appropriate t or standard normal critical value; we discuss testing more formally in Sections 9.3 and 9.4.

Suppose that, over the course of discussions among the researchers, concern is raised that a fixed, four-week follow-up period for both first-stage treatments is unsatisfactory. Although four weeks is typical under standard of care, there is not strong evidence for how long one should wait to assess response under the new active treatment; in particular, there is disagreement in the clinical community about whether the follow-up time should be approximately four weeks or eight weeks.

With these additional considerations, one approach is to consider a trinary first-stage randomization under which subjects are randomized at the first stage to one of new active treatment, with response assessed at four weeks; new active treatment, with response assessed at eight weeks; or standard of care, with response assessed at four weeks. After response status is assessed, subjects enter the second stage, in which responders are assigned to maintenance therapy, and nonresponders are randomized to one of two candidate salvage therapies. See Figure 9.5 for a schematic of this design.

This design allows for more comparisons than that in Figure 9.4, including the timing of responder assessment under the new active treatment. However, this flexibility comes at the price of a potential loss in

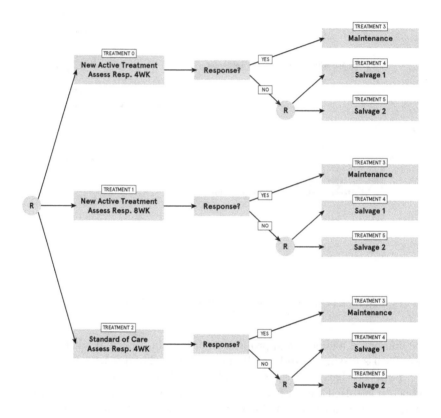

Figure 9.5 *Potential SMART design for illustrative SMART example 1 in which the timing of response assessment for the new treatment is also of interest.*

power. Researchers must decide if this additional comparison is worth the added expense of running a larger and more complex trial.

Some alternative designs and corresponding (hypothetical) scientific justification are as follows.

(T1) It might be determined that optimal timing for treatment change under the new treatment is unlikely to be fixed across patients and not easily operationalized as a deterministic rule based on patient outcome trajectories. In this setting, one might consider a SMART like that in Figure 9.4, except that the clinician and subject decide jointly at each clinical evaluation whether or not the subject should be deemed a responder or a nonresponder or if this determination should be postponed to a later evaluation. See Swartz et al. (2003) for an example of a SMART in which participants and clinicians jointly decided on treatment discontinuation.

(T2) It might be determined that evaluation of candidate salvage therapies under the standard of care arm is of less interest than the comparison of responder assessment at four and eight weeks under the new active treatment. In this case, one might consider a design in which patients are initially randomized among new active treatment with a four-week follow-up period, new active treatment with an eight-week follow-up period, or a control condition in which treatment changes are made at the discretion of the clinician (or some other standard of care). See Figure 9.6(a) for a schematic. In this design, one might consider unequal randomization at the first stage to increase power for comparisons among the regimes embedded in the trial, as discussed later in Section 9.3.2.

(T3) An optimal treatment regime estimated from (T2) would use patient baseline information to dictate if and for how long a patient should receive the new treatment. For example, it could recommend that patients with more severe symptoms at baseline should receive the new active treatment for eight weeks and all others should receive the new treatment for only four weeks. However, in considering (T2), suppose that the researchers would like to decide at four weeks whether or not to change treatment or continue the first-stage treatment for another four weeks. Thus, they might consider a design in which patients are initially randomized to either the new active treatment or control, and, after four weeks, those assigned to the new active treatment are subsequently randomized to either being assessed immediately or staying on the new treatment for another four weeks. A schematic of this design is given in Figure 9.6(b). Note that although this design involves three stages, it is effectively equivalent to (T2), provided that in (T2) subjects assigned to be assessed for response at eight weeks are evaluated for response (but do not change treatment) at four weeks; and the randomization probabilities are chosen in (T2) and (T3) so that the proportions assigned to be assessed at four and eight weeks are equal across trials.

The preceding narrative provides a glimpse into how critical decision points in a SMART design can evolve as clinical questions are prioritized and refined. There are many more ways in which the initial design in Figure 9.4 can be modified. During the design process, the focus should be on identifying pressing clinical questions and from these deriving a design, rather than the reverse, in which one postulates candidate

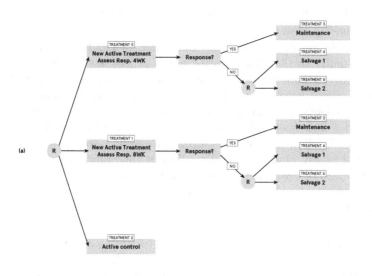

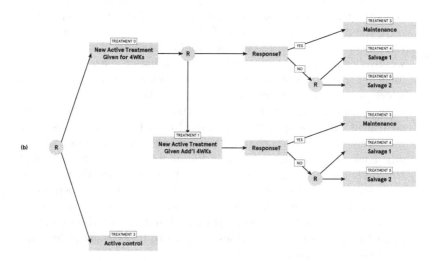

Figure 9.6 *Potential designs for (a) variant (T2) and (b) variant (T3) of illustrative SMART example 1.*

designs and then derives the clinical questions that potentially could be addressed using the design.

9.2.3 Feasible Treatment Options

Perhaps the most obvious design consideration in a SMART is the set of feasible treatments at each stage. In some settings, the sets of feasible treatments are well established by current science and the questions motivating the trial, and no further consideration of the treatment options is necessary. We focus on cases where the sets of feasible treatments are not well established at the onset of the design process.

Switch away from the Loser Designs

One motivation for conducting a SMART is to develop a principled, evidence-based treatment strategy for patients who fail to respond to a standard treatment. In such settings, all subjects may be assigned initially to a standard treatment in a "run-in" period, and nonresponders are then randomized to potential follow-up treatments.

An example is provided by the SMART depicted in the schematic in Figure 9.7, which was designed to evaluate treatment sequences for HIV prevention among adolescent men who have sex with men. From this schematic, it can be seen that there are eight distinct interventions, coded as follows: (0) Queer Sex Ed (QSE), an established web-based sexual education program; (1) Keep it Up! (KIU), a new web-based sexual health intervention; (2) Attention Control (AC), a static informational website serving as a control; (3) KIU booster; (4) AC booster; (5) KIU booster plus the Young Men's Health Program (YMHP), which involves viewing a motivational video; (6) YMHP alone; or (7) no intervention. Initially, all subjects receive QSE, and responders to QSE receive no further treatment, where response is defined as reported 100% condom use or intention for use. Nonresponders to QSE transition into the first stage of the trial in which participants are randomly assigned to either KIU or AC. At the second stage, responders to KIU or AC receive a booster designed to maintain response. Nonresponders to KIU are randomized to either the KIU booster or the KIU booster plus YMHP, and nonresponders to AC are assigned to either KIU or or YMHP. In addition to condom use, primary outcomes following the final stage include measures of sexual risk and self-reported HIV testing. See Mustanski (2018) for further trial details and scientific background and Fava et al. (2003) and Rush et al. (2004) for another example of a SMART in which subjects were all assigned to the same first-line treatment before randomization. Because all subjects are first assigned to an established treatment, QSE, in an initial "run-in" period, and only nonresponders are randomized to

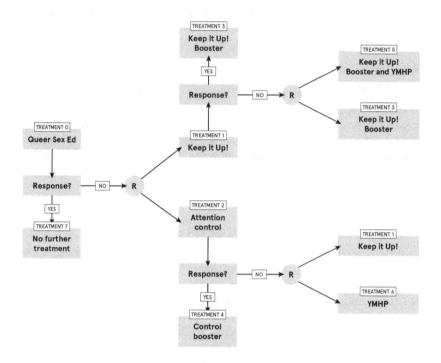

Figure 9.7 *SMART for the study of HIV prevention among adolescent men who have sex with men.*

follow-up interventions, this SMART facilitates evaluation of these interventions within the target population of adolescent men who have sex with men *who do not respond to QSE* (so for whom QSE is a "loser"). It is straightforward that, for such individuals, there are four regimes embedded in the design.

The sets of feasible treatment options in this SMART are as follows. Define R_1 to be the indicator that a subject is a responder to QSE, where $R_1 = 0$ (1) indicates nonresponse (response). Among subjects with $R_1 = 0$, so who enter stage one and are randomized to KIU (treatment 1) or AC (treatment 2), define R_2 to be the indicator that a subject is a responder to first-stage assigned treatment, where $R_2 = 0$ (1) indicates nonresponse (response) and may be a function of H_2; R_2 need not be defined for responders to QSE not entering stage one. The sets of feasible treatments at stage one are then

$$\Psi_1(h_1) = \begin{cases} \{7\} & \text{if } r_1 = 1 \\ \{1, 2\} & \text{if } r_1 = 0, \end{cases}$$

and the sets of feasible treatments at the second stage are

$$\Psi_2(h_2) = \begin{cases} \{7\} & \text{if } r_1 = 1 \\ \{3, 5\} & \text{if } r_1 = 0, \ r_2 = 0, \text{ and } a_1 = 1 \\ \{3\} & \text{if } r_1 = 0, \ r_2 = 1, \text{ and } a_1 = 1 \\ \{1, 6\} & \text{if } r_1 = 0, \ r_2 = 0, \text{ and } a_1 = 2 \\ \{4\} & \text{if } r_1 = 0, \ r_2 = 1, \text{ and } a_1 = 2. \end{cases}$$

Because participants for whom $R_1 = 1$ are assigned no further treatment (7), we take $A_1 = A_2 = 7$ for these subjects.

Another common SMART design that is based on discontinuing unsatisfactory treatments arises when there are several candidate treatments that will be tried in sequence until a patient becomes responsive. An optimal treatment regime in this setting minimizes the mean time to response. Figure 9.8 shows a generic such "switch away from the loser" SMART design in which there are three candidate treatments coded as 0, 1, and 2. At the first stage, subjects are randomly assigned to 0, 1 or 2. Responders to assigned first-stage treatment receive no further treatment adjustments, whereas nonresponders are randomized among the treatments that they have not yet received. Responders at the second stage receive no further treatment adjustments, and nonresponders are assigned to the remaining treatment not received. Thus, if a participant is not responsive to current treatment, he switches to a heretofore untried treatment and away from an ineffective treatment (loser). The design facilitates comparison of six candidate treatment sequences, $(0, 1, 2), (0, 2, 1), (1, 0, 2), (1, 2, 0), (2, 0, 1), (2, 1, 0)$, as well as estimation of an optimal treatment regime that uses baseline patient information to choose an initial treatment and intervening patient information to choose a follow-up treatment for nonresponders. Interim patient information among nonresponders might include measures of adherence, reasons for nonresponse, and changes in symptom severity.

As in the preceding example, define R_2 to be the indicator that a subject is a responder at the end of the first stage. The set of feasible treatments at the first stage is $\Psi_1(h_1) = \{0, 1, 2\}$ for all h_1, and the sets of feasible treatments at the second stage are

$$\Psi_2(h_2) = \begin{cases} \{a_1\} & \text{if } r_2 = 1 \\ \{0, 1, 2\} \setminus \{A_1\} & \text{if } r_2 = 0, \end{cases}$$

where, for two sets A and B, $A \setminus B$ is the set of elements in A but not in B. Nonresponders to second-stage treatment are assigned deterministically to the treatment comprising the set $\{0, 1, 2\} \setminus \{a_1, a_2\}$. Because this

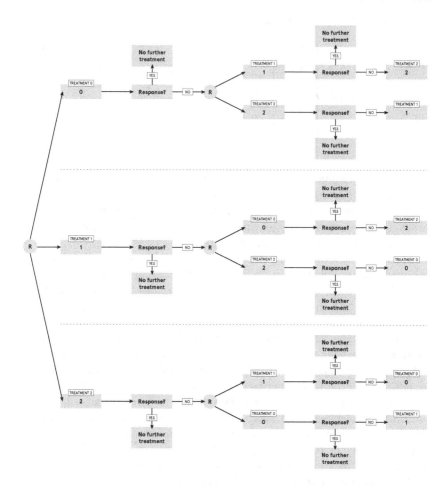

Figure 9.8 *SMART design to identify the optimal sequencing of treatments coded as 0, 1, and 2.*

assignment is deterministic, there is no third stage of randomization nor the need to define the set of feasible third-stage treatments.

Stepped Care Designs

A natural goal is to develop cost-effective treatment regimes under which "expensive" treatments are only given if, to whom, and for how long they are needed. "Cost" might refer to resource expenditures, risk of adverse events, treatment burden, or any other undesirable feature associated with a given treatment; thus, the term "expensive" refers to a treatment that has a high cost relative to other treatment options, however cost is defined. Stepped care SMARTs attempt to identify treatment regimes that produce a large mean outcome at low cost. We present templates for two common stepped care SMART designs. The conceptual framework for these designs can be used to create a wide range of novel alternative such designs.

Figure 9.9(a) shows a template for a two-stage stepped care SMART design. In stage one, each subject is randomly assigned to one of two candidate inexpensive treatments. In the second stage, responders continue on their initially assigned treatments, while nonresponders are randomized to two expensive treatments; i.e., they are "stepped up." Using the numbering scheme in the design schematic, the sets of feasible treatments are $\Psi_1(h_1) = \{0, 1\}$ for all h_1 at the first stage and, with r_2 indicating response,

$$\Psi_2(h_2) = \begin{cases} \{a_1\} & \text{if } r_2 = 1 \\ \{2, 3\} & \text{if } a_1 = 0 \text{ and } r_2 = 0 \\ \{4, 5\} & \text{if } a_1 = 1 \text{ and } r_2 = 0. \end{cases}$$

The regimes embedded in this design are (e_1) give inexpensive treatment I initially, and continue inexpensive treatment I if response or step up to expensive treatment I if nonresponse; (e_2) give inexpensive treatment I initially, and continue inexpensive treatment I if response or step up to expensive treatment II if nonresponse; (e_3) give inexpensive treatment II initially, and continue inexpensive treatment II if response or step up to expensive treatment III if nonresponse; and (e_4) give inexpensive treatment II initially, and continue inexpensive treatment II if response or step up to expensive treatment IV if nonresponse. These embedded regimes represent step-up strategies in which expensive treatment is given only if and when it is necessary, thereby potentially reducing cost. An optimal treatment regime similarly would step up treatment only as needed but would furthermore tailor the choice of inexpensive and expensive treatment according to individual patient characteristics.

In the alternative design in Figure 9.9(b), subjects are randomized in stage one to either an expensive or an inexpensive treatment. In stage two, responders to the inexpensive treatment continue, whereas nonresponders are randomly assigned to two candidate expensive treatments, so are stepped up. Responders to stage one expensive treatment are randomized to either continuing on stage one treatment or being "stepped down" to an inexpensive treatment; nonresponders are randomized to two expensive treatment options. Thus, this design allows for the comparison of both step-up and step-down strategies. Using the numbering of treatments in the diagram and letting r_2 indicate response, the sets

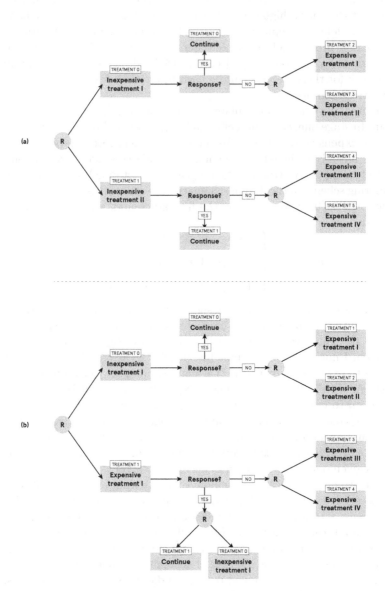

Figure 9.9 *Canonical stepped care SMART designs. (a): A step-up SMART design wherein patients are initially randomized among two candidate inexpensive treatments. (b): A stepped care SMART design that includes both step-up and step-down treatment sequences.*

of feasible treatments are $\Psi_1(h_1) = \{0, 1\}$ for all h_1 and

$$
\Psi_2(h_2) = \begin{cases}
\{0\} & \text{if } a_1 = 0 \text{ and } r_2 = 1 \\
\{1, 2\} & \text{if } a_1 = 0 \text{ and } r_2 = 0 \\
\{0, 1\} & \text{if } a_1 = 1 \text{ and } r_2 = 1 \\
\{3, 4\} & \text{if } a_1 = 1 \text{ and } r_2 = 0.
\end{cases}
$$

There are six embedded regimes: (e_1) give inexpensive treatment I initially, and continue inexpensive treatment I if response or step up to expensive treatment I if nonresponse; (e_2) give inexpensive treatment I initially, and continue inexpensive treatment I if response or step up to expensive treatment II if nonresponse; (e_3) give expensive treatment I initially, and continue expensive treatment I if response or switch to expensive treatment III if nonresponse; (e_4) give expensive treatment I initially, and continue expensive treatment I if response or switch to expensive treatment IV if nonresponse; (e_5) give expensive treatment I initially, and step down to inexpensive treatment I if response or switch to expensive treatment III if nonresponse; and (e_6) give expensive treatment I initially, and step down to inexpensive treatment I if response or switch to expensive treatment IV if nonresponse. The comparison among e_1, the least costly embedded regime, and the most costly regimes, e_3 and e_4, may be of primary interest in a cost-benefit analysis. An estimated optimal treatment regime based on the data from this design could provide insight into if, how, when, and for whom expensive treatment should be provided.

In both designs in Figure 9.9, the dichotomy of expensive and inexpensive oversimplifies what might be more nuanced notions of treatment cost in practice.

Dose Adjustment Designs

In some contexts, the treatment options may be doses of a drug or other intervention, and SMARTs can be designed to identify optimal dosing regimes. If the number of possible doses is small; e.g., high versus low dose, then one can apply the preceding considerations, treating each dose as a distinct treatment. However, in some cases, the number of candidate doses may be large or even infinite. Here, one must make additional assumptions to support analyses of the data collected without requiring massive sample sizes. We illustrate through two examples.

In the first example, we consider the design of a two-stage SMART to identify an optimal dose adjustment strategy, where each candidate dose/treatment option is dictated by the presence or absence of several binary factors. For example, in the context of treatment of bipolar disorder, suppose that a dose comprises administration of an antidepressant medication along with zero or more of cognitive behavioral therapy (CBT), group therapy (GT), mood stabilizer drug A (MS-A), and mood stabilizer drug B (MS-B). That is, considering four binary factors corresponding to presence/absence of CBT, GT, MS-A, and MS-B, there are $2^4 = 16$ possible doses, where, for example, dose $(1, 1, 0, 0)$ corresponds to receiving CBT and GT (but not MS-A or MS-B). A natural strategy is to select an initial dose and possibly adjust that dose depending on a patient's response.

In general, let L denote the number of binary factors dictating dose, so that there are 2^L possible doses. There need not be a meaningful notion of distance between dose levels; however, for moderate L, regarding the 2^L doses as completely separate treatments would require a potentially enormous sample size to support comparisons among doses. Thus, additional assumptions about the treatment effect are generally needed. Encode each dose as a binary vector of length L as above, so that the jth component is equal to 1 if the jth factor is present and 0 otherwise. Then the set of possible treatments at each stage is $\mathcal{A} = \mathcal{A}_1 = \mathcal{A}_2 = \{0, 1\}^L$, and a possible option at stage k is $a_k = (a_{k1}, \ldots, a_{kL})^T$, $k = 1, 2$, where $a_{k\ell}$, $\ell = 1, \ldots, L$, is equal to 0 (1) if the ℓth binary factor is absent (present). In describing a candidate SMART design, we assume that all doses are feasible for all individuals, so that $\Psi_1(h_1) = \mathcal{A}$ and $\Psi_2(h_2) = \mathcal{A}$ for all h_1 and h_2; and interest focuses on strategies in which a patient who responds to her initial dose continues on that dose and otherwise is switched to another dose. Of course, other designs are possible, such as the step-up designs as discussed above.

Let $R_2^*(a_1)$ be the indicator that a randomly chosen patient would respond to initial dose $a_1 \in \mathcal{A}$, where $R_2^*(a_1) = 0\,(1)$ if nonresponse (response); and let $Y^*(a_1, a_2)$ denote the outcome a patient would have under the dose sequence $(a_1, a_2) \in \mathcal{A} \times \mathcal{A}$. Let $\mu(a_1, a_2) = E\{Y^*(a_1, a_2)\}$ denote the mean potential outcome under the sequence (regime) (a_1, a_2) for given $a_1, a_2 \in \mathcal{A}$. One might posit a model of the form

$$\mu(a_1, a_2; \alpha) = \alpha_0 + \sum_{\ell=1}^{L} \alpha_{1\ell} a_{1\ell} + \sum_{\ell < k} \alpha_{2,\ell k} a_{1\ell} a_{1k}$$

$$+ \{1 - R_2^*(a_1)\} \left(\sum_{\ell=1}^{L} \alpha_{3\ell} a_{2\ell} + \sum_{\ell < k} \alpha_{4,\ell k} a_{2\ell} a_{2k} \right. \tag{9.4}$$

$$\left. + \sum_{\ell=1}^{L} \sum_{k=1}^{L} \alpha_{5,\ell k} a_{1\ell} a_{2k} \right).$$

In (9.4), which can be viewed as a marginal structural model for the value of the fixed regime (a_1, a_2) as in Section 6.4.5, it is assumed that third- and higher-order interaction effects are zero, so that $\alpha = (\alpha_0, \alpha_{11}, \ldots, \alpha_{5,LL})^T$ is the collection of parameters indexing main effects and second-order interactions among factors. Thus, the model contains $O(L^2)$ parameters, compared with the $O(2^{2L})$ parameters required to index all possible treatment combinations at the first and second stages (i.e., in a saturated model). Of course, higher-order interactions could be included as appropriate.

To estimate the parameters indexing such a posited model, a full factorial design (Wu and Hamada, 2011) can be embedded into a SMART as follows. At the first stage, assign the factors dictating treatment according to a full factorial design with L binary factors. Responders are kept on their initial treatment, and nonresponders are randomized among the factors dictating treatment again using full factorial design with L binary factors. Figure 9.10 depicts such a design in the example of bipolar disorder above, with four binary factors. This design allows participants to receive the same treatment during the first and second stage even if they do not respond to that treatment during the first stage; an alternative design would randomize a nonresponder at stage two to the feasible set of all possible doses save for the one he received initially. Because, as discussed in Section 6.2.4, the SRA (6.17) and the positivity assumption (6.23) hold in a SMART, assuming SUTVA (6.16) and that the model is correctly specified, the model can be fitted using methods similar to those used to implement marginal structural models in Section 6.4.5.

Given that the postulated model for the mean potential outcome does not contain interactions of all orders, one could reduce the number of possible treatment combinations by using a fractional factorial design at each stage (Wu and Hamada, 2011; Dean et al., 2015). One only need ensure that the parameters indexing the posited mean model are identifiable under the chosen design.

Although in previous chapters we have not considered treatment options in a continuous range of options, in our second example we briefly consider this case. Assume that interest focuses on a continuous range of doses, so doses taking values in an interval $[d_{\min}, d_{\max}]$, and the ultimate goal is to develop regimes in which patient characteristics are used to choose an initial dose from this range, which might then be adjusted if needed. Assume that for each h_k, $k = 1, 2$, the feasible set of treatment options is an allowable subinterval of safe doses in this range, so that $\Psi_k(h_k) \subseteq [d_{\min}, d_{\max}]$. A SMART suited to this goal is as follows. At the first stage, a subject with baseline history $H_1 = h_1$ receives dose A_1 drawn from a distribution with density $p_{A_1|H_1}(a_1|h_1)$ satisfying $p_{A_1|H_1}(a_1|h_1) \geq \epsilon$ for all $a_1 \in \Psi_1(h_1)$, where $\epsilon > 0$ does not depend on h_1. Here, $\Psi_1(h_1)$ may depend on a patient's age, weight, and other baseline factors in h_1. At the end of the first stage, response status is ascertained. Responders continue on their initial doses, whereas nonre-

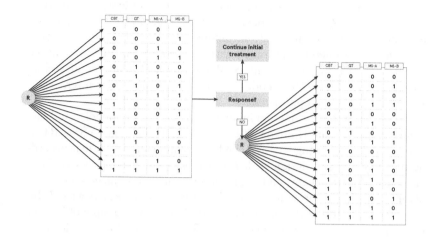

Figure 9.10 *SMART factorial dosing design for bipolar depression with four binary factors.*

sponders are randomized to a second dose, A_2, which for a subject with $H_2 = h_2$ is drawn from a distribution with density $p_{A_2|H_2}(a_2|h_2)$ satisfying $p_{A_2|H_2}(a_2|h_2) \geq \epsilon$ for all $a_2 \in \Psi_2(h_2)$. The history h_2 at the second stage may include reasons for nonresponse, such as lack of efficacy or intolerable side effects, and thus $\Psi_2(h_2)$ may vary widely across these reasons. For example, if nonresponse to the initial dose a_1 is due to lack of efficacy, $\Psi_2(h_2)$ may lie completely above a_1, while if it is due to intolerable side effects, $\Psi_2(h_2)$ might lie completely below a_1. An optimal regime can be estimated from such a design using variants of Q-learning and value search estimation for treatment options in a continuous range (Rich et al., 2014; Laber and Zhao, 2015; Chen et al., 2016).

9.2.4 Interim Outcomes, Randomization, and Stratification

The last three design components we discuss are grouped together as commonly being challenging to those first encountering SMARTs. As in previous cases, the choices surrounding these components should be dictated by scientific or cost considerations.

Choosing an Interim Outcome

In a SMART where second-stage treatment assignment depends on a subject's response status, one must choose an interim outcome(s) characterizing the response criterion, as in the preceding examples. We consider three cases: (C1) there are no cost or resource constraints, and there is strong scientific theory or clinical consensus supporting when and if a treatment change should be made; (C2) there are no cost or resource constraints, but there is not strong scientific theory or clinical consensus regarding treatment change; and (C3) there are cost or resource constraints that could prevent a treatment change for all subjects.

In (C1), the response criterion should be chosen to mimic actual clinical decision making; in this way, treatment switches occurring in the trial will reflect clinical practice. In (C2), if identification of a high-quality response criterion is of central scientific interest, then one can configure the SMART design to facilitate estimation of treatment regimes across a range of response criteria. The most straightforward approach is to randomly assign participants to different response criteria along with their initial treatment assignments. For example, if there are two initial candidate treatments and two candidate response criteria, then one could randomize patients at stage one among the four possible combinations. Such an approach requires specification of a small number of response criteria a priori to avoid excessive sample splitting, although one could marginalize over response criteria for some analyses.

Alternatively, one might consider response criteria in which an individual with history h_2 at the beginning of stage two is deemed a responder if $\tilde{h}_2 > \tau(h_1; c)$ and a nonresponder otherwise, where $\tilde{h}_2$ is some function (feature) of elements of h_2; and $\tau(h_1; c)$ is some real-valued function of baseline history h_1 that is known up to a parameter $c \in \mathcal{C}$. As a simple example, in a SMART to study antiretroviral therapy for HIV infected individuals, as in Section 1.2.3, if h_2 includes CD4 T-cell count (cells/mm^3) measured immediately prior to the second decision, CD4$_2$, one might take $\tilde{h}_2 =$ CD4$_2$ and $\tau(h_1; c) = c$, leading to the response criterion of CD4 count exceeding a threshold value.

Suppose that, for simplicity, response status is assessed at a fixed time after baseline that does not depend on the response criterion and that all treatment options in $\mathcal{A} = \mathcal{A}_1 = \mathcal{A}_2$ are feasible for all individuals. In this case, a potential SMART is as follows. At the first stage, each subject is randomly assigned to a treatment-response criterion pair $(A_1, C) \in \mathcal{A} \times \mathcal{C}$; and, at the end of the first stage, a subject with $\tilde{H}_2 > \tau(H_1; C)$ is deemed a responder and continues his first-stage treatment. A subject with $\tilde{H}_2 \le \tau(H_1; C)$ is deemed a nonresponder and is randomly assigned a second-stage treatment $A_2 \in \mathcal{A}$. The outcome is ascertained at the end of stage two.

For any triple $(a_1, c, a_2) \in \mathcal{A} \times \mathcal{C} \times \mathcal{A}$, there is an associated embedded regime of the form "administer treatment a_1 at baseline, and, if $\tilde{h}_2 > \tau(h_1; c)$, deem patient a responder and continue a_1; else, if $\tilde{h}_2 \le \tau(h_1; c)$, deem patient a nonresponder and give treatment a_2." It can be seen that the data (H_1, A_1, C, H_2, A_2) for a subject who has completed the trial are consistent with having followed regime (a_1, c, a_2) if either

(i) $A_1 = a_1$, $\widetilde{H}_2 > \max\{\tau(H_1; c), \tau(H_1; C)\}$, and $A_2 = a_1$; or

(ii) $A_1 = a_1$, $\widetilde{H}_2 \leq \min\{\tau(H_1; c), \tau(H_1; C)\}$, and $A_2 = a_2$.

The reasoning is similar to that in the discussion of marginal structural models in Section 6.4.5 in a somewhat more complex context. If the data satisfy (i), then the subject was deemed a responder because $\widetilde{H}_2 > \tau(H_1; C)$ and would still be a responder if also $\widetilde{H}_2 > \tau(H_1; c)$. Otherwise, if the data satisfy (ii), the subject was deemed a nonresponder because $\widetilde{H}_2 \leq \tau(H_1; C)$ and would also be a nonresponder if $\widetilde{H}_2 \leq \tau(H_1; c)$. This shows that there will be some subjects whose data are consistent with following candidate regimes with different response criteria, so that the data collected in a SMART can be used to evaluate such regimes. Moreover, the methods discussed in Section 5.7 and Chapter 7 can be applied to the data to estimate an optimal regime, which includes optimization over candidate response criteria.

In (C3), there are constraints that may limit treatment changes for all subjects. To discuss this case, we assume that the "response criterion" is being used to identify those patients who are in most need of a treatment change; were resources unlimited, all subjects would receive a treatment change. For example, all subjects might begin on an initial treatment, with responders assigned to an inexpensive follow-up treatment and nonresponders assigned to an expensive (but more effective) follow-up treatment; if cost were not a concern, it might be preferable to assign all subjects to the more expensive treatment.

As in the preceding example, suppose that there exists a feature $\widetilde{h}_2$ and threshold $\tau(h_1; c)$ indexed by $c \in \mathcal{C}$ that will be used to dictate responder status. Assume further that $\mathcal{C} = [0, 1]$, for each h_1 the threshold $\tau(h_1; c)$ is monotone increasing in c, and that switching treatment always leads to outcomes that are no worse than staying on current treatment. In this case, one should choose c to be as large as possible subject to the constraint $P\{\widetilde{H}_2 \leq \tau(H_1; c)\} \leq \omega$, where $\omega \in [0, 1]$ encodes what proportion of subjects can be assigned to the expensive treatment given available resources. An estimator for $P\{\widetilde{H}_2 \leq \tau(H_1; c)\}$ can be constructed using historical data or an internal pilot study.

Randomization Probabilities

Standard practice in SMARTs is to randomize participants to the feasible treatment options with equal probability at each stage. However, depending on the goals of the planned analyses, it may be advantageous to use unequal randomization. For example, consider the SMART for evaluation of mHealth interventions in Figure 9.3. Suppose a primary analysis of interest is comparison of each of the embedded regimes (e_1) give AllyQuest+ initially, and continue AllyQuest+ regardless of response status; and (e_3) give AllyQuest initially, and continue AllyQuest if response or step up to AllyQuest+ if nonresponse, to the control condition. With n subjects and equal randomization at each stage, the expected number of patients assigned to control and (e_3) is $n/3$, whereas the expected number assigned to (e_1) is $(1-\rho)n/3 + \rho n/6$, where ρ is the probability of response to AllyQuest+. Thus, one might wish to adjust the randomization probabilities to ensure equal sample sizes (on average) in the comparison groups or to maximize power given additional information, e.g., postulated variances for a continuous outcome under each of (e_1), (e_3), and the control; see Section 9.3.

Stratification

As with any clinical trial, there may be scientific, statistical, or logistical reasons for wanting to stratify randomization in a SMART. In a conventional stratified randomized trial, a finite number of strata is identified on the basis of baseline characteristics thought to be associated with outcome. Subjects within each stratum are then randomized to the treatment options according to a separate randomization scheme for each stratum. An objective is to ensure approximate balance of the treatment groups with respect to the strata, which cannot be guaranteed with simple randomization that does not take the strata into account.

For a SMART, suppose that strata have been specified depending on baseline characteristics. The simplest way to carry out stratified randomization is to randomly assign subjects to the regimes embedded in the SMART within each stratum. Although this seems counter to the notion that randomization in a SMART should take place when and if needed, as we now show, it is mathematically equivalent to randomize subjects once at baseline, so "up front," to the embedded regimes.

To see this, consider again the SMART depicted in Figure 9.1, with eight embedded regimes enumerated in Section 9.2.1. If, at each point of randomization, equal randomization is used, it is straightforward to demonstrate that this is equivalent to randomizing at baseline to the eight embedded regimes with equal probability in that the treatment assignment probabilities at each stage are the same under sequential randomization or randomization to the embedded regimes. Let (A_1, A_2) denote the options assigned under the design where randomization is carried out sequentially, let $\widetilde{E}$ denote a regime selected uniformly at random from the eight embedded regimes, and let $(\widetilde{A}_1, \widetilde{A}_2)$ denote the options assigned under $\widetilde{E}$. Then $P(\widetilde{E} = e_j) = 1/8$, $j = 1, \ldots, 8$; and, under equal randomization at the first stage, $P(A_1 = a_1|H_1) = P(A_1 = a_1) = 1/2$ for $a_1 = \Psi_1(h_1) = \mathcal{A}_1$. It is straightforward that $P(\widetilde{A}_1 = a_1|\widetilde{E} = e_j) = \mathrm{I}(\widetilde{A}_1 = a_1, \widetilde{E} = e_j)$, $j = 1, \ldots, 8$; half of the embedded regimes begin with each of the two treatment options at stage one, so four of these probabilities are equal to 1 and four to 0. Then

$$P(\widetilde{A}_1 = a_1) = \sum_{j=1}^{8} P(\widetilde{A}_1 = a_1|\widetilde{E} = e_j)P(\widetilde{E} = e_j) = 1/2 = P(A_1 = a_1).$$

Under either scheme, stage two treatment assignment depends on history only through stage one treatment and response status; thus, for any h_2, write $\Psi_2(h_2) = \Psi_2(a_1, r_2)$, where $r_2 = 0(1)$ indicates nonresponse (response). Letting R_2 and $\widetilde{R}_2$ denote response status following stage one assignment under sequential randomization or by embedded regime, respectively, we show that, for all $a_1 \in \mathcal{A}_1$, $a_2 \in \mathcal{A}_2$, and $r_2 = 0, 1$,

$$P(\widetilde{A}_2 = a_2|\widetilde{R}_2 = r_2, \widetilde{A}_1 = a_1) = P(A_2 = a_2|R_2 = r_2, A_1 = a_1).$$

Under SUTVA, letting $R_2^*(a_1)$ be potential response status under $a_1 \in \mathcal{A}_1$, it is immediate that $P(A_2 = a_2|R_2 = r_2, A_1 = a_1) = P\{A_2 = a_2|R_2^*(a_1) = r_2, A_1 = a_1\} = \mathrm{I}\{a_2 \in \Psi(a_1, r_2)\}/2$. Similarly, $P(\widetilde{A}_2 = a_2|\widetilde{R}_2 = r_2, \widetilde{A}_1 = a_1) = P\{\widetilde{A}_2 = a_2|R_2^*(a_1) = r_2, \widetilde{A}_1 = a_1\}$, which is equal to zero if $a_2 \notin \Psi(a_1, r_2)$. For $a_2 \in \Psi(a_1, r_2)$, letting E_{a_1} and $\mathsf{E}_{a_1}^{a_2}$ denote the sets of embedded regimes involving a_1 at the first stage and (a_1, a_2) at the first and second stages, respectively, using $\mathsf{E}_{a_1}^{a_2} \subset \mathsf{E}_{a_1}$,

$$P\{\widetilde{A}_2 = a_2 \mid R_2^*(a_1) = r_2, \widetilde{A}_1 = a_1\} = P\{\widetilde{E} = \mathsf{E}_{a_1}^{a_2} \mid R_2^*(a_1) = r_2, \widetilde{E} = \mathsf{E}_{a_1}\}$$
$$= \frac{P\{\widetilde{E} = \mathsf{E}_{a_1}^{a_2} \mid R_2^*(a_1) = r_2\}}{P\{\widetilde{E} = \mathsf{E}_{a_1} \mid R_2^*(a_1) = r_2\}} = 1/2.$$

It follows that $P(\widetilde{A}_2 = a_2|\widetilde{R}_2 = r_2, \widetilde{A}_1 = a_1) = \mathrm{I}\{a_2 \in \Psi(a_1, r_2)\}/2 = P(A_2 = a_2|R_2 = r_2, A_1 = a_1)$, as required.

An advantage of randomizing to embedded regimes with each stratum rather than sequentially is that this stratified randomization can be carried out using existing tools and software for this purpose for conventional clinical trials. For example, if the SMART will have rolling enrollment, then one can use a permuted block scheme to ensure balanced allocation to regimes within strata even though the sample sizes within each stratum are not known a priori (Matts and Lachin, 1988). The preceding derivations show that randomizing to embedded regimes within strata will ensure balance across first-stage treatments and second-stage treatments within responder status within strata.

Although the treatment assignment probabilities at each stage are equivalent under randomization sequentially or to embedded regimes at baseline, the latter has the potential for bias in some settings induced by anticipatory effects if proper blinding procedures are not followed or if blinding is infeasible. For example, suppose that response status is a function of patient reported outcomes and that nonresponders are randomized to two candidate salvage therapies, one of which is associated with significant side effects. If a subject knows she has been assigned to an embedded regime involving this salvage therapy, she may be optimistic in reporting her outcome to avoid being deemed a nonresponder. Proper blinding mitigates such effects.

9.2.5 Other Candidate Designs

As we have seen, there is great flexibility in the design of a SMART through which researchers can address a variety of scientific and policy questions. However, SMARTs are not a panacea for addressing complex questions, nor are they the only choice for evaluating treatment sequences. In some settings, interest may focus on evaluating entire treatment "packages" comprising individual components that are administered sequentially, where the timing of the components within a package is well supported by existing evidence. In such cases, a standard k-arm trial randomizing participants to the competing treatment packages may be the most appropriate design. Alternatively, the nature of treatments may dictate another design approach. For example, with mHealth interventions, treatment decisions may occur on a fine time scale, as in the case of real-time control of a condition such as diabetes. In this case, informative study of these interventions may require multiple randomizations per day, making a so-called microrandomized trial more appropriate (Klasnja et al., 2015; Liao et al., 2016).

Thus, in considering a SMART, researchers should ask if there are any alternative designs that would address the motivating scientific questions more effectively.

9.3 Power and Sample Size for Simple Comparisons

A SMART generates a rich data resource that can be used to support a variety of analyses, including secondary, hypothesis-generating analyses such as estimation of an optimal treatment regime. However, in practice, the primary analyses in a SMART on which power and sample size calculations are based are typically simple. For example, the primary analysis specified in the protocol for many SMARTs is comparison of response rates among first-stage treatment options or comparison of fixed treatment regimes embedded in the SMART (treatment sequences). As we now discuss, the sample size formulæ required for these primary analyses are known or straightforward. We defer considerations for more specialized analyses, including sample size calculations to ensure high-quality estimation of an optimal treatment regime, to Sections 9.4 and 9.5.

9.3.1 Comparing Response Rates

Consider a SMART in which each participant is deemed to be either a responder or nonresponder at the end of the first stage, as in many of the examples in this chapter. Perhaps the simplest primary analysis for a SMART is the comparison of response rates associated with first-stage treatment options.

Suppose that the set of candidate stage one treatments $\mathcal{A}_1$ comprises m_1 options, and suppose first that all options are feasible for all individuals and are assigned with known randomization probabilities that do not depend on baseline characteristics, so that, for each option $a_1 \in \mathcal{A}_1$, using the definitions (3.96) and (5.65)

$$\omega_1(H_1, a_1) = P(A_1 = a_1 | H_1) = P(A_1 = a_1) = \omega_1(a_1) \qquad (9.5)$$

is a known constant. Let $R_2^*(a_1)$ be potential response status under $a_1 \in \mathcal{A}_1$, with $R_2^*(a_1) = 0\,(1)$ indicating nonresponse (response), so that $E\{R_2^*(a_1)\} = p_{a_1}$, say, is the expected response rate under a_1. Letting $a_1, a_1' \in \mathcal{A}_1$ be two distinct first-stage options of interest, one might size a SMART to ensure that a level α test of H_0 : $E\{R_2^*(a_1)\} = E\{R_2^*(a_1')\}\,(p_{a_1} = p_{a_1'})$ against the two-sided alternative $H_1 : E\{R_2^*(a_1)\} \neq E\{R_2^*(a_1')\}\,(p_{a_1} \neq p_{a_1'})$ has sufficient power to detect

$$|E\{R_2^*(a_1)\} - E\{R_2^*(a_1')\}| = |p_{a_1} - p_{a_1'}| \geq \delta, \qquad (9.6)$$

where in this chapter we use $\delta > 0$ to denote a clinically meaningful difference. Of course, under (9.5), from the discussion of randomized studies in Section 2.3.2, $R_2^*(a_1) \perp\!\!\!\perp A_1$ as in (2.11), and the difference in (9.6) is just the average causal treatment effect based on the response outcome, so that this is a formal statement of the usual hypotheses for the comparison of two response rates. As in Figure 9.1 and many of the other foregoing examples of SMARTs, $m_1 = 2$, and this is the comparison of response rates for the two first-stage treatments.

From Section 2.3.2, under SUTVA, observed response status $R_2 = R_2^*(A_1) = \sum_{a_1 \in \mathcal{A}_1} R_2^*(a_1)\mathrm{I}(A_1 = a_1)$, and it is well known that, analogous to (9.2), a test of H_0 versus H_1 can be based on the difference of sample response rates $T_n = \widehat{p}_{a_1} - \widehat{p}_{a_1'}$, where

$$\widehat{p}_a = \frac{\sum\limits_{i=1}^{n} \mathrm{I}(A_{1i} = a) R_{2i}}{\sum\limits_{i=1}^{n} \mathrm{I}(A_{1i} = a)},$$

which is a consistent estimator for the true difference

$$p_{a_1} - p_{a_1'} = E\{R_2^*(a_1)\} - E\{R_2^*(a_1')\} = E(R_2|A_1 = a_1) - E(R_2|A_1 = a_1').$$

Based on large sample theory, standard power and sample size calculations are readily available for this comparison, which we now present as background for the derivation of those for other, more complex analyses of interest.

It is straightforward to show that, as $n \to \infty$, $n^{1/2}\{T_n - (p_{a_1} - p_{a_1'})\} \xrightarrow{D} \mathcal{N}(0, \sigma_{a_1, a_1'}^2)$, where

$$\sigma_{a_1, a_1'}^2 = \frac{E[\{R_2^*(a_1) - p_{a_1}\}^2]}{\omega_1(a_1)} + \frac{E[\{R_2^*(a_1') - p_{a_1'}\}^2]}{\omega_1(a_1')}$$

$$= \frac{p_{a_1}(1 - p_{a_1})}{\omega_1(a_1)} + \frac{p_{a_1'}(1 - p_{a_1'})}{\omega_1(a_1')}.$$

Thus, under H_0, $n^{1/2} T_n / \widehat{\sigma}_{a_1, a_1'}$ converges in distribution to a standard normal random variable, where

$$\widehat{\sigma}_{a_1, a_1'}^2 = \frac{\widehat{p}_{a_1}(1 - \widehat{p}_{a_1})}{\omega_1(a_1)} + \frac{\widehat{p}_{a_1'}(1 - \widehat{p}_{a_1'})}{\omega_1(a_1')}$$

is a consistent estimator for $\sigma_{a_1, a_1'}^2$. Let z_u be the $u \times 100$ percentile of the standard normal distribution; and, as in Chapter 3, let $\Phi(\cdot)$ denote the cumulative distribution function of a standard normal random variable. Then the test that rejects H_0 when $|T_n|/(\widehat{\sigma}_{a_1, a_1'}/n^{1/2}) > z_{1-\alpha/2}$ has approximate type I error probability α under H_0 and power at least

$$\Phi(-z_{1-\alpha/2} - n^{1/2}\delta/\sigma_{a_1, a_1'}) + \Phi(-z_{1-\alpha/2} + n^{1/2}\delta/\sigma_{a_1, a_1'}) \qquad (9.7)$$

under the alternative H_1 with $|p_{a_1} - p_{a_1'}| \geq \delta$. Thus, to ensure type II error probability of no more than β; i.e., power of at least $(1 - \beta) \times 100\%$ to detect a difference of δ or greater, one should solve for the sample size n such that (9.7) is $\geq 1 - \beta$. (In discussing sample size calculations, as conventional in the literature, we use α and β to denote type I and II error probability, respectively.) In practice, to simplify this calculation, it is conventional to ignore the first term in (9.7), which is typically very small relative to the second, and solve for n satisfying $\Phi(-z_{1-\alpha/2} + n^{1/2}\delta/\sigma_{a_1, a_1'}) = z_{1-\beta}$, which leads to the sample size formula

$$n = \frac{\sigma_{a_1, a_1'}^2 (z_{1-\alpha/2} + z_{1-\beta})^2}{\delta^2}. \qquad (9.8)$$

Thus, for example, if the SMART involves equal randomization to the m_1 options in $\mathcal{A}_1$ at stage one, so that $\omega_1(a_1) = \omega_1(a_1') = 1/m_1$, then the required sample size is $n = m_1\{p_{a_1}(1-p_{a_1}) + p_{a_1'}(1-p_{a_1'})\}(z_{1-\alpha/2} + z_{1-\beta})^2/\delta^2$. A common variant is to replace $\hat{\sigma}^2_{a_1,a_1'}$ in the test statistic by the alternative estimator

$$\overline{p}_{a_1,a_1'}(1 - \overline{p}_{a_1,a_1'})\left\{\frac{1}{\omega_1(a_1)} + \frac{1}{\omega_1(a_1')}\right\}$$

based on the pooled sample proportion (under the null hypothesis)

$$\overline{p}_{a_1,a_1'} = \frac{\sum\limits_{i=1}^{n} R_{2i}\mathrm{I}(A_{1i} = a_1 \text{ or } A_{1i} = a_1')}{\sum\limits_{i=1}^{n} \mathrm{I}(A_{1i} = a_1 \text{ or } A_{1i} = a_1')}.$$

Inspection of (9.8) shows that, for desired level α and power $(1-\beta) \times 100\%$, one must postulate response rates for each of a_1 and a_1', which then imply the desired meaningful difference δ. Note that (9.8) involves a standardized effect size $\delta/\sigma_{a_1,a_1'}$; see Cohen (1988). Thus, alternatively, the sample size calculation can be based on a posited standardized effect size, which, in practice, can be chosen based on domain expertise or estimated from historical data. Basing sample size determination on postulated response rates is the dominant approach in medical applications, while it is common to base this on a standardized effect size in the behavioral and educational sciences.

The preceding developments focus on the comparison of two fixed first-stage treatments. To power a SMART for all pairwise comparisons among the m_1 first-stage treatment options while controlling the family-wise type I error rate, one can apply a Bonferroni correction; i.e., adjust the critical value from $z_{1-\alpha/2}$ to $z_{1-\alpha/(2m^*)}$, where, with m_1 treatment options, there are $m^* = m_1(m_1 - 1)/2$ distinct pairs.

We now consider the case where the randomization probabilities at the first stage depend on baseline history h_1; i.e., in contrast to (9.5),

$$\omega_1(H_1, a_1) = P(A_1 = a_1|H_1),$$

and the goal is again to base sample size on the comparison of response rates for options $a_1, a_1' \in \mathcal{A}_1$. With $\mathcal{A}_1$ comprising m_1 stage one treatment options that are feasible for all individuals, there may be a scientific rationale for randomizing subjects to these options with different probabilities depending on a component or function of components of h_1. For example, with $m_1 = 2$, while subjects whose age is below a threshold are randomized with equal probability to the two options, there may be ethical or logistical reasons to randomize older participants to one of the options preferentially. Alternatively, as in Section 6.2.2, there may be a small number of subsets of $\mathcal{A}_1$ that are feasible sets $\Psi_1(h_1)$, where the numbers of options in each differ. For example, for $\mathcal{A}_1$ comprising three options coded as 0, 1, and 2, it may be that $\Psi_1(h_1) = \{0, 1, 2\}$, with $m_{11} = 3$ options, when h_1 indicates that a subject's age is below the threshold; and $\Psi_1(h_1) = \{0, 1\}$, with $m_{12} = 2$ options, when it is above. Here, as formalized at the end of Section 6.4.3, there are separate sets of randomization probabilities for each feasible set; e.g., for equal randomization to the options within each feasible set, $\omega_1(h_1, a_1) = 1/m_{11} = 1/3$ if h_1 is such that age is below the threshold for $a_1 \in \{0, 1, 2\} = \mathcal{A}_1$, and $\omega_1(h_1, a_1) = 1/m_{12} = 1/2$ for $a_1 \in \{0, 1\} \subset \mathcal{A}_1$ if h_1 indicates age above the threshold. The options a_1, a_1' that are the focus of the comparison should appear in both feasible sets. Here, because randomization depends on H_1, we now have $R_2^*(a_1) \perp\!\!\!\perp A_1 | H_1$.

We base sample size calculations on an inverse probability weighted estimator for response rate in the spirit of that in the alternative form in (3.25), which can have considerably smaller sampling variation than the usual, simple inverse probability weighted estimator; that is, we use the estimator for p_{a_1} given by

$$\widehat{p}_{a_1} = \left\{ \sum_{i=1}^{n} \frac{\mathrm{I}(A_{1i} = a_1)}{\omega_1(H_{1i}, a_1)} \right\}^{-1} \sum_{i=1}^{n} \frac{\mathrm{I}(A_{1i} = a_1)R_{2i}}{\omega_1(H_{1i}, a_1)} \tag{9.9}$$

rather than $n^{-1} \sum_{i=1}^{n} \{\mathrm{I}(A_{1i} = a_1)R_{2i}/\omega_1(H_{1i}, a_1)\}$. This estimator is consistent for p_{a_1} if $\omega_1(h_1, a_1)$ are the true randomization probabilities. Note that if $\omega_1(h_1, a_1)$ does not depend on h_1, the estimator (9.9) reduces to the usual sample proportion above.

In the context of a SMART, the probabilities $\omega_1(h_1, a_1)$ are known. As discussed at the end of Section 2.6.3, inverse probability weighted estimators such as (9.9) with $\omega_1(h_1, a_1)$ estimated by the observed sample proportions of subjects randomized to each option for each h_1 are also consistent and have smaller large sample variance than when the known probabilities are used, so that one may prefer to base the primary analysis on (9.9) with these estimated randomization probabilities. In fact, as noted in the remark at the end of Section 2.7, an augmented inverse probability weighted estimator is also consistent under these conditions and can be relatively more efficient than either of these estimators, even if based on incorrect posited outcome regression models. However, basing sample size calculation on (9.9) with known probabilities leads to sample size formulæ that are more straightforward for practical use (basing this calculation on an augmented estimator would require that outcome regression models also be specified). More importantly, this strategy has the advantage of leading to a conservative sample size estimate. This principle persists for the more complex analyses considered

in the sequel. Accordingly, the sample size calculations we present here
and for subsequent analyses are based on alternative inverse probability
weighted estimators as in (9.9), taking the randomization probabilities
to be known.

As in Sections 2.6.3 and 3.3.2, the estimator $T_n = \widehat{p}_{a_1} - \widehat{p}_{a_1'}$ based
on (9.9) with $\omega_1(h_1, a_1)$ equal to the known randomization probabilities
can be cast as an M-estimator. By appealing to the general theory for
M-estimation reviewed in Section 2.5, it can be shown that $n^{1/2}\{T_n -$
$(p_{a_1} - p_{a_1'})\} \xrightarrow{D} \mathcal{N}(0, \sigma^2_{a_1,a_1'})$, where now

$$\sigma^2_{a_1,a_1'} = E\left[\frac{\{R_2^*(a_1) - p_{a_1}\}^2}{\omega_1(H_1, a_1)}\right] + E\left[\frac{\{R_2^*(a_1') - p_{a_1'}\}^2}{\omega_1(H_1, a_1')}\right]. \qquad (9.10)$$

Using SUTVA, from (2.40), a consistent estimator for $\sigma^2_{a_1,a_1'}$ in (9.10) is

$$\widehat{\sigma}^2_{a_1,a_1'}$$

$$= n^{-1} \sum_{i=1}^{n} \left[\left\{\frac{(R_{2i} - \widehat{p}_{a_1})\mathrm{I}(A_{1i} = a_1)}{\omega_1(H_{1i}, a_1)}\right\}^2 + \left\{\frac{(R_{2i} - \widehat{p}_{a_1'})\mathrm{I}(A_{1i} = a_1')}{\omega_1(H_{1i}, a_1')}\right\}^2\right],$$

and the test that rejects H_0 when $|T_n|/(\widehat{\sigma}_{a_1,a_1'}/n^{1/2}) > z_{1-\alpha/2}$ has ap-
proximate type I error probability α under H_0 and power at least

$$\Phi(-z_{1-\alpha/2} - n^{1/2}\delta/\sigma_{a_1,a_1'}) + \Phi(-z_{1-\alpha/2} + n^{1/2}\delta/\sigma_{a_1,a_1'}) \qquad (9.11)$$

when $|p_{a_1} - p_{a_1'}| > \delta$.

In principle, to ensure power of at least $(1 - \beta) \times 100\%$ to detect
a difference of δ or greater, one should solve for n such that (9.11) is
$\geq 1 - \beta$. Because (9.10) is complicated by dependence on $\omega_1(H_1, a_1)$
and $\omega_1(H_1, a_1')$, similar to Murphy (2005), one strategy for the purpose of deriving a sample size formula is to use a simple upper bound
on (9.10). Replacing $\omega_1(H_1, a_1)$ and $\omega_1(H_1, a_1')$ by $\min_{h_1} \omega_1(h_1, a_1)$ and
$\min_{h_1} \omega_1(h_1, a_1')$, respectively, in (9.10), an upper bound on $\sigma^2_{a_1,a_1'}$ is

$$\widetilde{\sigma}^2_{a_1,a_1'} = \frac{p_{a_1}(1 - p_{a_1})}{\min_{h_1} \omega_1(h_1, a_1)} + \frac{p_{a_1'}(1 - p_{a_1'})}{\min_{h_1} \omega_1(h_1, a_1')}.$$

Then a conservative sample size calculation is to solve for n such that

$$\Phi(-z_{1-\alpha/2} - n^{1/2}\delta/\widetilde{\sigma}_{a_1,a_1'}) + \Phi(-z_{1-\alpha/2} + n^{1/2}\delta/\widetilde{\sigma}_{a_1,a_1'}) \geq 1 - \beta.$$

As in the simpler case above, analogous to (9.8), one can disregard the
first term, which leads to the sample size formula

$$n = \frac{\widetilde{\sigma}^2_{a_1,a_1'}(z_{1-\alpha/2} + z_{1-\beta})^2}{\delta^2}.$$

To use this formula, because $\widetilde{\sigma}_{a_1, a_1'}$ depends on p_{a_1} and $p_{a_1'}$, one can postulate (marginal) response rates for a_1 and a_1', which imply the desired difference δ. As an illustration, consider the example above where $\Psi_1(h_1) = \{0, 1, 2\}$ when h_1 indicates age below a threshold and $\Psi_1(h_1) = \{0, 1\}$ when it is above, and suppose $a_1 = 0$ and $a_1' = 1$. In this case, $\min_{h_1} \omega_1(h_1, 0) = \min_{h_1} \omega_1(h_1, 1) = 1/m_{11} = 1/3$. Then, for posited rates p_0 and p_1, $\widetilde{\sigma}_{0,1}^2 = 3\{p_0(1-p_0)+p_1(1-p_1)\}$, and $\delta = p_1 - p_0$. Alternatively, as above, the calculation can be based on a specified value for the standardized effect size $\delta/\sigma_{a_1, a_1'}$.

Remark. Sizing a SMART for the comparison of first-stage response rates is equivalent to sizing a standard k-arm randomized trial with binary outcomes, and therefore the calculations are familiar to clinical and intervention scientists. This familiarity may help to allay concerns about the complexity of SMARTs; e.g., among grant reviewers. However, a SMART should be sized for the comparison of first-stage response rates only if such a comparison is genuinely of primary scientific interest. For example, in the SMART depicted in Figure 9.1, the primary analysis was chosen to be comparison of the response rates to PCST-Full and PCST-Brief because no substantial prior study comparing these two interventions had been conducted. If the primary interest is in comparing treatment *sequences*, then comparison of first-stage treatments is only meaningful within the context of the treatment regimes in which they are embedded; e.g., it is easy to construct an example in which the initial first-stage treatment that produces the highest response rate yet is embedded in a regime that is worst among all embedded regimes with respect to the final outcome of interest. We consider sizing a SMART when the primary analysis of interest is comparison of fixed treatment regimes in the next section.

9.3.2 Comparing Fixed Regimes

We first consider the comparison of two fixed regimes that differ in the first-stage treatment option (Murphy, 2005), so can be considered to be "nonoverlapping," where the comparison is with respect to the terminal outcome. In most cases, both of these fixed regimes will be embedded in the SMART, although this does not affect the sample size calculations. Having the initial treatment differ across the two fixed regimes is convenient statistically, as the sets of subjects whose realized treatment experience is consistent with each regime are disjoint and therefore independent, simplifying the formulation. Moreover, such comparisons are often of great clinical interest; e.g., it is common to compare the most intensive or expensive embedded regime (with respect to cost, resource utilization, patient burden, and so on) to the least intensive or expensive embedded regime. We consider the general problem of comparing any two fixed regimes at the end of this section.

Let $d = \{d_1, d_2\}$ and $d' = \{d'_1, d'_2\}$ encode two fixed, nonoverlapping regimes; formally, d and d' satisfy

$$d_1(h_1) \neq d'_1(h_1) \text{ for all } h_1 \in \mathcal{H}_1,$$

so that the regimes do not recommend the same first-stage treatment option for any possible baseline history. With $Y^*(d)$ and $Y^*(d')$ the potential terminal outcomes under regimes d and d', with values $\mathcal{V}(d) = E\{Y^*(d)\}$ and $\mathcal{V}(d') = E\{Y^*(d')\}$, the goal is to choose a sample size n to ensure that a level α test of $\mathsf{H}_0 : \mathcal{V}(d) = \mathcal{V}(d')$ against $\mathsf{H}_1 : \mathcal{V}(d) \neq \mathcal{V}(d')$ has sufficient power provided that $|\mathcal{V}(d) - \mathcal{V}(d')| \geq \delta$, where δ is a clinically meaningful difference.

Analogous to the comparison of response rates above, we base the calculation on the alternative inverse probability weighted estimator for $\mathcal{V}(d)$ in (5.67) and (6.101) given by

$$
\begin{aligned}
\widehat{\mathcal{V}}(d) &= \left[\sum_{i=1}^n \frac{I\{A_{1i} = d_1(H_{1i})\}I\{A_{2i} = d_2(H_{2i})\}}{\omega_1\{H_{1i}, d_1(H_{1i})\}\,\omega_2\{H_{2i}, d_2(H_{2i})\}} \right]^{-1} \\
&\quad \times \sum_{i=1}^n \frac{I\{A_{1i} = d_1(H_{1i})\}I\{A_{2i} = d_2(H_{2i})\}\,Y_i}{\omega_1\{H_{1i}, d_1(H_{1i})\}\,\omega_2\{H_{2i}, d_2(H_{2i})\}} \\
&= \left[\sum_{i=1}^n \frac{I\{A_{1i} = d_1(H_{1i})\}I\{A_{2i} = d_2(H_{2i})\}}{\omega_1(H_{1i}, A_{1i})\,\omega_2(H_{2i}, A_{2i})} \right]^{-1} \\
&\quad \times \sum_{i=1}^n \frac{I\{A_{1i} = d_1(H_{1i})\}I\{A_{2i} = d_2(H_{2i})\}\,Y_i}{\omega_1(H_{1i}, A_{1i})\,\omega_2(H_{2i}, A_{2i})},
\end{aligned}
\tag{9.12}
$$

where the second equality follows as discussed below (6.101), and we regard the randomization probabilities $\omega_k(h_k, a_k)$, $k = 1, 2$ as known; define $\widehat{\mathcal{V}}(d')$ similarly. Under these conditions, $\widehat{\mathcal{V}}(d)$ and $\widehat{\mathcal{V}}(d')$ are consistent estimators for $\mathcal{V}(d)$ and $\mathcal{V}(d')$.

It follows that

$$T_n = \widehat{\mathcal{V}}(d) - \widehat{\mathcal{V}}(d')$$

is a consistent estimator for the difference in values and, as above, can be cast as an M-estimator. Applying the general theory of M-estimation in Section 2.5, it can be shown that $n^{1/2}[T_n - \{\mathcal{V}(d) - \mathcal{V}(d')\}] \xrightarrow{D} \mathcal{N}(0, \sigma_{d,d'}^2)$ (Murphy, 2005, Equation (10)), where

$$
\begin{aligned}
\sigma_{d,d'}^2 = E&\left[\frac{\{Y^*(d) - \mathcal{V}(d)\}^2}{\omega_1\{H_1, d_1(H_1)\}\,\omega_2\{H_2, d_2(H_2)\}} \right] \\
&+ E\left[\frac{\{Y^*(d') - \mathcal{V}(d')\}^2}{\omega_1\{H_1, d'_1(H_1)\}\,\omega_2\{H_2, d'_2(H_2)\}} \right],
\end{aligned}
\tag{9.13}
$$

and the lack of a cross-product term in (9.13) is a consequence of the fact that the regimes d and d' are nonoverlapping. A consistent estimator for $\sigma^2_{d,d'}$ is given by

$$\widehat{\sigma}^2_{d,d'} = n^{-1} \sum_{i=1}^{n} \left[\frac{\{Y_i - \widehat{\mathcal{V}}(d)\}\mathrm{I}\{A_{1i} = d_1(H_{1i})\}\mathrm{I}\{A_{2i} = d_2(H_{2i})\}}{\omega_1(H_{1i}, A_{1i})\,\omega_2(H_{2i}, A_{2i})} \right]^2$$
$$+ n^{-1} \sum_{i=1}^{n} \left[\frac{\{Y_i - \widehat{\mathcal{V}}(d')\}\mathrm{I}\{A_{1i} = d'_1(H_{1i})\}\mathrm{I}\{A_{2i} = d'_2(H_{2i})\}}{\omega_1(H_{1i}, A_{1i})\,\omega_2(H_{2i}, A_{2i})} \right]^2.$$

Thus, under H_0, $n^{1/2}T_n/\widehat{\sigma}_{d,d'}$ converges in distribution to a standard normal random variable, so that a test that rejects H_0 when $n^{1/2}|T_n|/\widehat{\sigma}_{d,d'} \geq z_{1-\alpha/2}$ will have type I error $\alpha + o(1)$ under H_0 and power exceeding

$$\Phi(-z_{1-\alpha/2} - n^{1/2}\delta/\sigma_{d,d'}) + \Phi(-z_{1-\alpha/2} + n^{1/2}\delta/\sigma_{d,d'}) + o(1) \quad (9.14)$$

under H_1 provided that $|\mathcal{V}(d) - \mathcal{V}(d')| \geq \delta$. Thus, to ensure power of at least $(1 - \beta) \times 100\%$, one should choose n so that $(9.14) \geq 1 - \beta$. Analogous to the preceding results, disregarding the first term in (9.14) leads to the approximate formula

$$n = \frac{\sigma^2_{d,d'}(z_{1-\alpha/2} + z_{1-\beta})^2}{\delta^2}. \quad (9.15)$$

As before, a conservative sample size calculation can be obtained by using an upper bound on $\sigma^2_{d,d'}$. From (9.13) and using $E[\{Y^*(d) - \mathcal{V}(d)\}^2] = \mathrm{var}\{Y^*(d)\}$ and similarly for d', a simple upper bound is

$$\widetilde{\sigma}^2_{d,d'} = \frac{\mathrm{var}\{Y^*(d)\}}{\min_{\overline{x}_2} \omega_1\{x_1, d_1(x_1)\}\,\omega_2\{\overline{x}_2, \overline{d}_2(\overline{x}_2)\}}$$
$$+ \frac{\mathrm{var}\{Y^*(d')\}}{\min_{\overline{x}_2} \omega_1\{x_1, d'_1(x_1)\}\,\omega_2\{\overline{x}_2, \overline{d}'_2(\overline{x}_2)\}}. \quad (9.16)$$

In (9.16), we use $h_1 = x_1$ and $h_2 = (\overline{x}_2, a_1)$ and the recursive representation in Section 5.2 to emphasize that the minimization is over the randomization probabilities associated with following each of the regimes d and d'. See Murphy (2005) for a similar formulation.

To use these formulæ, based on knowledge of the outcome or preliminary data, the analyst can posit $\mathcal{V}(d)$ and $\mathcal{V}(d')$ for regimes d and d', which imply δ, or specify δ directly; and specify $\mathrm{var}\{Y^*(d)\}$ and $\mathrm{var}\{Y^*(d')\}$, where it may be reasonable to take these variances to be the same for both regimes. Alternatively, as above, n can be chosen based on a given standardized effect size of $\delta/\sigma_{d,d'}$. We demonstrate both approaches in the following example.

Illustrative SMART Example 2

To illustrate how the preceding sample size formulæ might be applied, consider again the SMART shown in Figure 9.1. Suppose that interest focuses on comparing the most and least intensive embedded regimes, which, from Section 9.2.1, are as follows:

(e_1) Give PCST-Full initially followed by PCST-Full maintenance if response or PCST-Plus if nonresponse

(e_8) Give PCST-Brief initially followed by no further treatment if response or PCST-Brief maintenance if nonresponse.

Let d encode embedded regime e_1 so that, using the treatment coding from the schematic in Figure 9.1, $d_1(h_1) \equiv 0$ for all h_1 and $d_2(h_2) = 2r_2 + 4(1-r_2)$, where, as in Section 9.2.1, $r_2 = 0$ (1) if response (nonresponse). Similarly, let d' encode e_8, so that $d'_1(h_1) \equiv 1$ for all h_1 and $d'_2(h_2) = 3r_2 + 5(1 - r_2)$. The requisite statistics are

$$T_n = \widehat{\mathcal{V}}(d) - \widehat{\mathcal{V}}(d')$$

$$= \frac{\sum_{i=1}^{n} Y_i \mathrm{I}(A_{1i} = 0)\mathrm{I}(A_{2i} = 4 - 2R_{2i})}{\sum_{i=1}^{n} \mathrm{I}(A_{1i} = 0)\mathrm{I}(A_{2i} = 4 - 2R_{2i})}$$

$$- \frac{\sum_{i=1}^{n} Y_i \mathrm{I}(A_{1i} = 1)\mathrm{I}(A_{2i} = 5 - 2R_{2i})}{\sum_{i=1}^{n} \mathrm{I}(A_{1i} = 1)\mathrm{I}(A_{2i} = 5 - 2R_{2i})},$$

$$\widehat{\sigma}^2_{d,d'} = 16 \sum_{i=1}^{n} \{Y_i - \widehat{\mathcal{V}}(d)\}^2 \mathrm{I}(A_{1i} = 0)\mathrm{I}(A_{2i} = 4 - 2R_{2i})$$

$$+ 16 \sum_{i=1}^{n} \{Y_i - \widehat{\mathcal{V}}(d')\}^2 \mathrm{I}(A_{1i} = 1)\mathrm{I}(A_{2i} = 5 - 2R_{2i}),$$

where we have used $\omega_k\{h_k, d_k(h_k)\} \equiv 1/2$ and similarly for d'_k, $k = 1, 2$, in this trial. In fact, $\omega_k(h_k, a_k) \equiv 1/2$ for all h_k and $a_k \in \Psi_k(h_k)$.

The terminal (continuous) outcome is percent reduction in pain from baseline. Based on information on this outcome from prior studies, suppose that the researchers are willing to specify that the standard deviation of this outcome is 30% under each regime, so that $\mathrm{var}\{Y^*(d)\} = \mathrm{var}\{Y^*(d')\} = 30^2$. Under these conditions, from (9.13) and using the fact that all randomization probabilities are equal to $1/2$, $\sigma_{d,d'}^2$ can be calculated directly as

$$\sigma_{d,d'}^2 = 4[\text{var}\{Y^*(d)\} + \text{var}\{Y^*(d')\}] = 8(30^2). \qquad (9.17)$$

Suppose first that the stated goal is to detect a $\delta = 10\%$ difference in mean percent reduction in pain between the two regimes with 80% power using an $\alpha = 0.05$ level test. Then, using the approximate formula (9.15) and rounding up to the nearest even integer, the sample size required is $n = 566$. The sample size required to detect a difference of $\delta = 12.73\%$ is approximately $n = 350$, which will be of interest momentarily.

Suppose instead that the stated goal is to detect a standardized effect size of $e = \delta/\sigma_{d,d'} = 0.15$ with 80% power using a 0.05 level test. Under these conditions, from (9.15), the approximate sample size required is $n = 350$. Readers familiar with classical standardized effect sizes such as Cohen's d (Cohen, 1988) might view an effect size of $e = 0.15$ to be exceptionally small. However, in the definition of e, the standardization is according to the sum of the asymptotic variances of the inverse probability weighted estimators for $\mathcal{V}(d)$ and $\mathcal{V}(d')$, while in its most familiar form Cohen's d is defined as $d = \delta/\sigma$, where in the present context σ^2 is the variance of the outcome (assumed similar for d and d'). Because the asymptotic variance of the inverse probability weighted estimator is larger than σ^2, the standardized effect size e as we have defined it is smaller. To see this, note from (9.17) that in this example $\sigma_{d,d'}^2 = 4[\text{var}\{Y^*(d)\} + \text{var}\{Y^*(d')\}] = 8\sigma^2$, so that, under the assumption that $\sigma = 30\%$ as above, Cohen's $d = (8)^{1/2}e$, so $e = 0.15$ corresponds to $d \approx 0.42$, which corresponds to a "small" to "medium" effect size as defined by Cohen (1988) and others. Here, then, $e = 0.15$ corresponds to $\delta \approx 12.73\%$, as above.

In general, when $\sigma_{d,d'}^2$ is a constant multiple of the outcome variance σ^2, which will be the case for many SMARTs, specifying effect size as defined here is analogous to specifying the variance of the outcome, which is more clinically meaningful – and thereby more easily elicited – than the variance of the difference in inverse probability weighted estimators.

Comparison of nonoverlapping regimes involves no subjects who have treatment experience in the trial consistent with having followed both regimes, which simplifies the foregoing sample size calculations and makes them more accessible to domain scientists. However, depending on the context, there may be interest in comparison of overlapping regimes; that is, regimes $d = \{d_1, d_2\}$ and $d' = \{d_1', d_2'\}$, say, whose first-stage rules can assign the same stage one treatment option, so for which it is possible for $d_1(h_1) = d_1'(h_1)$ for some $h_1 \in \mathcal{H}_1$. Here, there will be subjects whose realized treatment experience is consistent with having received treatment according to both d and d'.

To see this, for definiteness, consider the simplest case where $d_1(h_1)$ and $d'_1(h_1)$ assign the same treatment option in $\mathcal{A}_1$ for all h_1, as is the case for the embedded regimes in most of the previous examples in this chapter. For example, in the SMART depicted in Figure 9.4, two of the embedded regimes assign new active treatment (coded as 0): (e_1) give new active treatment initially followed by maintenance if response or salvage therapy 1 if nonresponse, and (e_2) give new active treatment initially followed by maintenance if response or salvage therapy 2 if nonresponse. Suppose that interest focuses on comparison of these two regimes. Denoting e_1 as d and e_2 as d', note that a subject in this trial who is assigned new active treatment at stage one, responds, and receives maintenance treatment at stage two has experience consistent with having followed the rules in either of d and d'. Accordingly, from (9.12), such a subject contributes to both $\widehat{\mathcal{V}}(d)$ and $\widehat{\mathcal{V}}(d')$, so that these estimators are no longer based on disjoint groups of subjects and thus are correlated. This correlation complicates calculation of sample size formulæ analogous to that above.

To demonstrate, define for any fixed regime d

$$W(d) = \frac{\mathrm{I}\{A_1 = d_1(H_1)\}\mathrm{I}\{A_2 = d_2(H_2)\}}{\omega_1\{H_1, d_1(H_1)\}\omega_2\{H_2, d_2(H_2)\}}$$
$$= \frac{\mathrm{I}\{A_1 = d_1(H_1)\}\mathrm{I}\{A_2 = d_2(H_2)\}}{\omega_1(H_1, A_1)\omega_2(H_2, A_2)}.$$

Then, with again $T_n = \widehat{\mathcal{V}}(d) - \widehat{\mathcal{V}}(d')$, appealing to the general theory of M-estimation in Section 2.5, it can be shown that, for any two possibly overlapping fixed regimes d and d'

$$n^{1/2}[T_n - \{\mathcal{V}(d) - \mathcal{V}(d')\}] \overset{D}{\longrightarrow} \mathcal{N}(0, \varsigma^2_{d,d'}),$$

where now

$$\varsigma^2_{d,d'} = \sigma^2_{d,d'} - 2E[W(d)\{Y^*(d) - \mathcal{V}(d)\}W(d')\{Y^*(d') - \mathcal{V}(d')\}], \quad (9.18)$$

and $\sigma^2_{d,d'}$ is as in (9.13). If the regimes are nonoverlapping, it is straightforward that $W(d)W(d') \equiv 0$ with probability one, and thus (9.18) reduces to $\sigma^2_{d,d'}$, and sample size formulæ are as above. In the case of overlapping regimes, $\varsigma^2_{d,d'}$ can be estimated by

$$\widehat{\varsigma}^2_{d,d'} = \widehat{\sigma}^2_{d,d'} - 2n^{-1}\sum_{i=1}^{n} W_i(d)W_i(d')\{Y_i - \widehat{\mathcal{V}}(d)\}\{Y_i - \widehat{\mathcal{V}}(d')\},$$

where the subscript i on $W(d)$ denotes evaluation at $A_{ki}, H_{ki}, k = 1, 2$.

Note that the product $W_i(d)W_i(d')$ is nonzero only for subjects for whom d and d' lead to the same treatment experience.

Under H_0, $n^{1/2}T_n/\widehat{\varsigma}_{d,d'}^2$ converges in distribution to a standard normal random variable and in principle can form the basis for a test as before. However, the power calculation depends on $\varsigma_{d,d'}^2$, which involves both $\sigma_{d,d'}^2$ and the unknown covariance term in (9.18), where this term depends on the nature of the overlap between d and d'. Thus, a general expression for $\varsigma_{d,d'}^2$ is not readily available. If specification of the standardized effect size $\delta/\varsigma_{d,d'}$ is possible, the sample size calculation can be carried out as for nonoverlapping regimes with $\delta/\sigma_{d,d'}$ replaced by this quantity; however, $\varsigma_{d,d'}$ may be substantially different from $\sigma_{d,d'}$ and may also be difficult to elicit from domain experts.

Remark. In the example above, embedded regimes e_1 and e_2 differ only in the recommendation of a salvage therapy option to nonresponders. Thus, comparison of these two embedded regimes effectively reduces to comparison of the two salvage therapies among nonresponders to new active treatment. Accordingly, sample size can be based on a conventional two-sample test statistic appropriate for the final outcome of interest. For example, suppose that, for a continuous outcome, interest is in a "medium" effect size (Cohen's d) of 0.50, corresponding to δ/σ, where σ is the standard deviation of the outcome (assumed the same for both salvage therapies among nonresponders to new active treatment). Then the number of nonresponders to new active treatment required to detect this effect with a two-sided $\alpha = 0.05$ level test with 80% power, assuming equal randomization of nonresponders to the two salvage therapies at stage two, is $4(1.96 + 0.84)^2/(0.5)^2 \approx 126$ based on a conventional sample size calculation for a two-sample comparison of means. This sample size must be inflated, however, to account for the fact that, of a total of n subjects in the SMART, roughly $n/2$ will be assigned to new active treatment (assuming equal randomization at stage one), and, of these, a proportion θ will be nonresponders. This leads to $n = 2(126)/\theta$. To determine sample size, the analyst must posit the nonresponse probability θ.

See Kidwell and Wahed (2013) for an alternative approach to sizing a SMART for comparison of overlapping embedded regimes. Instead of considering comparison of embedded regimes, Ertefaie et al. (2016) and Artman et al. (2018) base sample size methodology on identifying an optimal embedded regime(s) from among those represented in the SMART.

9.4   Power and Sample Size for More Complex Comparisons

9.4.1   Marginalizing versus Maximizing

Researchers interested in conducting a SMART often indicate that they wish to use the data to "compare first-stage treatments" or to "identify the optimal first-stage treatment" on the basis of a final, terminal outcome. These questions as stated are imprecise and thus are not well posed statistically, as there are several quantities, or *estimands*, that are related to the "goodness" of a given first-stage treatment $a_1 \in \mathcal{A}_1$. To illustrate, we consider three different estimands that could be considered as relevant to these questions. Each addresses a different issue, and which is the most appropriate depends on the scientific goals of the trial.

To define the first two estimands, it is useful to write $Y^*\{a_1, \mu_2(H_2)\}$ to denote the potential outcome for a randomly chosen individual in the population who receives option $a_1 \in \mathcal{A}_1$ at the first stage and then is assigned stage two treatment $\mu_2(H_2)$ depending on her history, where H_2 is understood to be equal to $(\overline{X}_2, a_1)$ (so with stage one treatment fixed at a_1). Here, $\mu_2(h_2)$ is a stochastic process indexed by $h_2 \in \mathcal{H}_2$ that takes values $a_2 \in \mathcal{A}_2$ according to a probability distribution satisfying

$$\mu_2(h_2) = a_2 \text{ with probability } \omega_{\mu,2}(h_2, a_2), \qquad (9.19)$$

where $\sum_{a_2 \in \mathcal{A}_2} \omega_{\mu,2}(h_2, a_2) = 1$ for $h_2 = (\overline{x}_2, a_1) \in \mathcal{H}_2$. In (9.19), for given a_2 and such h_2, $\omega_{\mu,2}(h_2, a_2)$ is the probability of assignment to option a_2 at second stage under an assignment mechanism that is possibly different from that in the SMART. The specific probability distribution of $\mu_2(h_2)$ reflects the situation of interest, as discussed in each case below.

Marginalizing over the Second Stage

As noted after (9.3), interest may focus on comparison of the mean terminal outcomes associated with two or more first-stage treatment options, marginalizing over second-stage treatment received in the trial. In the SMART, stage-two treatments are assigned according to the specified, known randomization probabilities $\omega_2(h_2, a_2)$. Thus, these mean outcomes reflect a "world" in which second-stage treatments are administered in the population with probabilities identical to these randomization probabilities; that is, for $a_2 \in \mathcal{A}_2$ and $h_2 = (\overline{x}_2, a_1)$,

$$\mu_2(h_2) = a_2 \text{ with probability } \omega_{\mu,2}(h_2, a_2) = \omega_2(h_2, a_2). \qquad (9.20)$$

Then, using the definition of $Y^*\{a_1, \mu_2(H_2)\}$ above, the mean terminal outcome of interest for stage one treatment a_1, marginalizing over second-stage treatment received, is

$$\mathcal{E}_1(a_1) = E[Y^*\{a_1, \mu_2(H_2)\}],$$

where $\mu_2(h_2)$ is as in (9.20). This can be interpreted as the mean outcome if all individuals in the population were to receive option a_1 at stage one and then receive an option in $\mathcal{A}_2$ according to the same probabilities used to randomize subjects in the SMART; see below for discussion. For two stage-one treatment options a_1 and a_1', interest is then in the difference $\mathcal{E}_1(a_1) - \mathcal{E}_1(a_1')$. This difference may be relevant in settings where the second-stage treatment options have effects that are qualitatively similar across first-stage treatments.

Marginalizing with Respect to Standard of Care

Let $\mu_2(h_2)$ instead have probability distribution reflecting how stage-two treatments are assigned in actual clinical practice; i.e., under the current standard of care in the population. Here, the probabilities $\omega_{\mu,2}(h_2, a_2)$ are those with which individuals in the population with history h_2 are assigned to receive option a_2 under standard of care. The estimand

$$\mathcal{E}_2(a_1) = E[Y^*\{a_1, \mu_2(H_2)\}]$$

is thus the mean outcome if all individuals in the population were to receive option a_1 at the first decision point and then be treated according to standard of care thereafter, so reflects a "world" in which second-stage treatments are administered in the population according to the standard of care; see below. For two stage-one treatments a_1 and a_1', the difference $\mathcal{E}_2(a_1) - \mathcal{E}_2(a_1')$ is then of interest if one wishes to recommend a stage-one treatment option assuming that the standard of care will be followed subsequently.

Maximizing over the Second Stage

Consider the embedded regimes in the SMART that assign a particular option $a_1 \in \mathcal{A}_1$ at stage one; denote these regimes by $e_1^{a_1}, \ldots, e_{J_{a_1}}^{a_1}$. For the jth such regime, $Y^*(e_j^{a_1})$ is the potential outcome if a randomly chosen individual in the population were to receive treatments at both stages according to regime $e_j^{a_1}$, and thus $E\{Y^*(e_j^{a_1})\}$ is the mean outcome if all individuals in the population were to be treated according to regime $e_j^{a_1}$. Then, for given $a_1 \in \mathcal{A}_1$, the estimand

$$\mathcal{E}_3(a_1) = \max_{j=1,\ldots,J_{a_1}} E\{Y^*(e_j^{a_1})\}, \tag{9.21}$$

reflects the mean terminal outcome if all individuals in the population were to receive a_1 initially and then receive stage two treatment according to the optimal decision that could be made based on their histories h_2, among all those represented in the SMART, in the future. Typically, as in the examples in this chapter, this decision would depend on h_2 only through response status. For two stage-one treatments a_1 and a_1', interest is then in the difference $\mathcal{E}_3(a_1) - \mathcal{E}_3(a_1')$.

Preliminaries

In the next three sections, for distinct $a_1, a_1' \in \mathcal{A}_1$, we derive sample size procedures for testing $\mathsf{H}_0 : \mathcal{E}_j(a_1) = \mathcal{E}_j(a_1')$ against the two-sided alternative $\mathsf{H}_1 : \mathcal{E}_j(a_1) \neq \mathcal{E}_j(a_1')$ for $j = 1, 2, 3$. The development is similar for the first two estimands, which involve marginalizing, so before we present these results, we first discuss estimation of $E[Y^*\{a_1, \mu_2(H_2)\}]$, which is relevant to both. The derivation for the third estimand is more complex, owing to the maximization operation in (9.21), as discussed further in Section 9.4.4.

It can be shown (Murphy et al., 2001) that $E[Y^*\{a_1, \mu_2(H_2)\}]$ can be expressed in terms of the observed data from a SMART as

$$E[Y^*\{a_1, \mu_2(H_2)\}] = E\left\{\frac{\mathrm{I}(A_1 = a_1)\,\omega_{\mu,2}(H_2, A_2)Y}{\omega_1(H_1, A_1)\,\omega_2(H_2, A_2)}\right\} \qquad (9.22)$$

and that

$$E\left\{\frac{\mathrm{I}(A_1 = a_1)\,\omega_{\mu,2}(H_2, A_2)}{\omega_1(H_1, A_1)\,\omega_2(H_2, A_2)}\right\} = 1,$$

provided that $\omega_{\mu,2}(h_2, a_2) = 0$ whenever $\omega_2(h_2, a_2) = 0$ (so that probability under the treatment assignment mechanism associated with $\mu_2(h_2)$ is absolutely continuous with respect to that for the SMART). It is instructive to contrast (9.22) with the analogous expression for a fixed regime $d = (d_1, d_2)$ that assigns $d_1(h_1) \equiv a_1$ for all h_1; namely

$$E\{Y^*(d)\} = E\left[\frac{\mathrm{I}(A_1 = a_1)\,\mathrm{I}\{A_2 = d_2(H_2)\}Y}{\omega_1(H_1, A_1)\,\omega_2(H_2, A_2)}\right].$$

While this expression places point mass at the options recommended by d, (9.22) also places point mass at a_1 but recognizes that stage-two treatment is assigned with probabilities dictated by $\mu_2(h_2)$. Thus, this expression can be viewed as implementing a reweighting of the information from the SMART to reflect the hypothetical "world" in which stage two treatment is assigned according to the probability distribution of $\mu_2(h_2)$.

The regime that assigns a_1 at stage one and stage two treatment according to $\mu_2(h_2)$ is an example of a random treatment regime, as discussed in Section 1.4.1. See Murphy et al. (2001) for a formal framework and methodology for random regimes that lead to the above results.

Based on these developments, an estimator for $E[Y^*\{a_1, \mu_2(H_2)\}]$ is

$$\left\{\sum_{i=1}^{n} \frac{I(A_{1i}=a_1)\,\omega_{\mu,2}(H_{2i},A_{2i})}{\omega_1(H_{1i},A_{1i})\,\omega_2(H_{2i},A_{2i})}\right\}^{-1} \sum_{i=1}^{n} \frac{I(A_{1i}=a_1)\,\omega_{\mu,2}(H_{2i},A_{2i})Y_i}{\omega_1(H_{1i},A_{1i})\,\omega_2(H_{2i},A_{2i})}.$$

$$(9.23)$$

The estimator (9.23) is consistent for $E[Y^*\{a_1,\mu_2(H_2)\}]$ if the randomization probabilities and the probabilities $\omega_{\mu,2}(h_2,a_2)$ are known.

We now use this formulation to derive sample size formulæ for the first two estimands.

9.4.2 *Marginalizing over the Second Stage*

Operationally, inference on $\mathcal{E}_1(a_1)-\mathcal{E}_1(a_1')$ mimics that for the difference of two mean outcomes in a conventional k-arm randomized trial. This is shown by appealing to the results at the end of the last section, as follows. With $\mu_2(h_2)$ as in (9.20); i.e., $\omega_{\mu,2}(h_2,a_2) = \omega_2(h_2,a_2)$, from (9.23), it is immediate that an estimator for $\mathcal{E}_1(a_1)$ for given $a_1 \in \mathcal{A}_1$ is

$$\widehat{\mathcal{E}}_1(a_1) = \left\{\sum_{i=1}^{n} \frac{I(A_{1i}=a_1)}{\omega_1(H_{1i},A_{1i})}\right\}^{-1} \sum_{i=1}^{n} \frac{I(A_{1i}=a_1)\,Y_i}{\omega_1(H_{1i},A_{1i})}.$$

Then for $a_1,a_1' \in \mathcal{A}_1$, an estimator for $\mathcal{E}_1(a_1) - \mathcal{E}_1(a_1')$ is given by $T_n = \widehat{\mathcal{E}}_1(a_1) - \widehat{\mathcal{E}}_1(a_1')$; note that this estimator reduces to an expression analogous to (9.3) if the stage one randomization probabilities do not depend on h_1.

As in Section 9.3, applying M-estimation theory, it follows that $n^{1/2}[T_n - \{\mathcal{E}_1(a_1) - \mathcal{E}_1(a_1')\}] \xrightarrow{D} \mathcal{N}(0,\sigma_{a_1,a_1'}^2)$, where

$$\sigma_{a_1,a_1'}^2 = E\left(\left[\frac{\{Y-\mathcal{E}_1(a_1)\}I(A_1=a_1)}{\omega_1(H_1,a_1)}\right]^2\right)$$

$$+ E\left(\left[\frac{\{Y-\mathcal{E}_1(a_1')\}I(A_1=a_1')}{\omega_1(H_1,a_1')}\right]^2\right),$$

$$(9.24)$$

which can be estimated consistently by the plug-in estimator

$$\widehat{\sigma}_{a_1,a_1'}^2 = n^{-1} \sum_{i=1}^{n}\left(\left[\frac{\{Y_i-\widehat{\mathcal{E}}_1(a_1)\}I(A_{1i}=a_1)}{\omega_1(H_{1i},a_1)}\right]^2\right.$$

$$\left.+ \left[\frac{\{Y_i-\widehat{\mathcal{E}}_1(a_1')\}I(A_{1i}=a_1')}{\omega_1(H_{1i},a_1')}\right]^2\right).$$

Then, as in the preceding cases, under the null hypothesis $H_0 : \mathcal{E}_1(a_1) = \mathcal{E}_1(a_1')$, the test that rejects H_0 when $n^{1/2}|T_n|/\widehat{\sigma}_{a_1,a_1'} \geq z_{1-\alpha/2}$ has type I error $\alpha + o(1)$ under H_0 and power at least $\Phi(-z_{1-\alpha/2} - n^{1/2}\delta/\sigma_{a_1,a_1'}) + \Phi(-z_{1-\alpha/2} + n^{1/2}\delta/\sigma_{a_1,a_1'}) + o(1)$ under H_1 provided that $|\mathcal{E}_1(a_1) - \mathcal{E}_1(a_1')| \geq \delta$. Ignoring the very small first term in the expression for power yields the approximate sample size formula

$$n = \frac{\sigma_{a_1,a_1'}^2 (z_{1-\alpha/2} + z_{1-\beta})^2}{\delta^2}.$$

Similar to the tests in Section 9.3.1, using this result is complicated by the form of $\sigma_{a_1,a_1'}^2$. First consider the case where randomization at the first stage of the SMART does not depend on baseline history, so that for each $a_1 \in \mathcal{A}_1$, $\omega_1(h_1, a_1) = \omega_1(a_1)$ as in (9.5), which is a known constant. Under these conditions, it is straightforward from (9.22) that

$$\mathcal{E}_1(a_1) = \omega_1^{-1}(a_1)E\{YI(A_1 = a_1)\} = E(Y|A_1 = a_1)$$

and similarly for a_1', so that

$$\sigma_{a_1,a_1'}^2 = \frac{\text{var}(Y|A_1 = a_1)}{\omega_1(a_1)} + \frac{\text{var}(Y|A_1 = a_1')}{\omega_1(a_1')}.$$

Thus, for the purpose of sample size calculation, one can posit values for $\text{var}(Y|A_1 = a_1)$ and $\text{var}(Y|A_1 = a_1')$ along with specified values for $\mathcal{E}_1(a_1)$ and $\mathcal{E}_1(a_1')$ (or for δ directly). For example, assuming that the variances are the same and equal to some σ^2 for a_1, a_1' and that a_1 and a_1' are assigned with probability $1/m_1$, one is led to the familiar sample size formula for a two-sample comparison

$$n = \frac{2m_1\sigma^2(z_{1-\alpha/2} + z_{1-\beta})^2}{\delta^2},$$

where $2m_1 = 4$ if there are two stage-one options.

If $\omega_1(h_1, a_1)$ depend on h_1, it can be shown that

$$E\left[\frac{\{Y - \mathcal{E}_1(a_1)\}^2 I(A_1 = a_1)}{\omega_1^2(H_1, a_1)}\right] = E\left(\frac{E[\{Y - \mathcal{E}_1(a_1)\}^2 \mid H_1, A_1 = a_1]}{\omega_1(H_1, a_1)}\right)$$

$$\leq \frac{E\left(E[\{Y - \mathcal{E}_1(a_1)\}^2 \mid H_1, A_1 = a_1]\right)}{\min_{h_1} \omega_1(h_1, a_1)}$$

$$= \frac{E\left\{E\left([Y^*\{a_1, \mu_2(H_2)\} - \mathcal{E}_1(a_1)]^2 \mid H_1\right)\right\}}{\min_{h_1} \omega_1(h_1, a_1)} = \frac{\text{var}[Y^*\{a_1, \mu_2(H_2)\}]}{\min_{h_1} \omega_1(h_1, a_1)},$$

where the first equality in the last line follows by manipulations as in

Murphy et al. (2001). Thus, from (9.24), an upper bound on $\sigma^2_{a_1,a_1'}$ is

$$\tilde{\sigma}^2_{a_1,a_1'} = \frac{\text{var}[Y^*\{a_1,\mu_2(H_2)\}]}{\min_{h_1}\omega_1(h_1,a_1)} + \frac{\text{var}[Y^*\{a_1',\mu_2(H_2)\}]}{\min_{h_1}\omega_1(h_1,a_1')}.$$

The analyst can specify $\text{var}[Y^*\{a_1,\mu_2(H_2)\}]$ and $\text{var}[Y^*\{a_1',\mu_2(H_2)\}]$, where it may be reasonable to assume these variances are the same for a_1 and a_1'; and as in Section 9.3, substitute $\tilde{\sigma}_{a_1,a_1'}$ in the sample size formulæ above to obtain a conservative sample size calculation.

Alternatively, the sample size calculation can be based on specification of the standardized effect size $e = \delta/\sigma_{a_1,a_1'}$, which, as in Illustrative SMART Example 2 in Section 9.3.2, may be smaller than the commonly used Cohen's d.

9.4.3 Marginalizing with Respect to Standard of Care

We now consider sample size to ensure that a test of $\mathsf{H}_0 : \mathcal{E}_2(a_1) = \mathcal{E}_2(a_1')$ versus $\mathsf{H}_1 : \mathcal{E}_2(a_1) \neq \mathcal{E}_2(a_1')$ for given $a_1, a_1' \in \mathcal{A}_1$ has the desired power provided that $|\mathcal{E}_2(a_1) - \mathcal{E}_2(a_1')| \geq \delta$. As above, the process $\mu_2(h_2)$ has probability distribution reflecting assignment of stage-two treatment options under the standard of care in the population. Typically, this probability distribution is unknown but could be estimated from historical data or elicited from domain science experts; the sample size calculation obviously will be predicated on the quality of these estimated or elicited propensities. In the following derivation, this distribution is assumed fixed and known.

Under these conditions, from (9.23) and defining

$$W_\mu(a_1) = \frac{\text{I}(A_1 = a_1)\,\omega_{\mu,2}(H_2, A_2)}{\omega_1(H_1, A_1)\,\omega_2(H_2, A_2)},$$

an estimator for $\mathcal{E}_2(a_1)$ is given by

$$\widehat{\mathcal{E}}_2(a_1) = \left\{\sum_{i=1}^n W_{\mu,i}(a_1)\right\}^{-1} \sum_{i=1}^n W_{\mu,i}(a_1)Y_i,$$

where the subscript i on $W_\mu(a_1)$ denotes evaluation at (H_{2i}, A_{2i}); and define $\widehat{\mathcal{E}}_2(a_1')$ similarly. With $T_n = \widehat{\mathcal{E}}_2(a_1) - \widehat{\mathcal{E}}_2(a_1')$, appealing as before to the general theory of M-estimation in Section 2.5 and using $E\{W_\mu(a_1)Y\} = \mathcal{E}_2(a_1)$ and $E\{W_\mu(a_1)\} = 1$ from above, it can be shown that $n^{1/2}[T_n - \{\mathcal{E}_2(a_1) - \mathcal{E}_2(a_1')\}] \xrightarrow{D} \mathcal{N}(0, \sigma^2_{a_1,a_1'})$, where now

$$\sigma^2_{a_1,a_1'} = E\big([W_\mu(a_1)\{Y - \mathcal{E}_2(a_1)\}]^2\big) + E\big([W_\mu(a_1')\{Y - \mathcal{E}_2(a_1')\}]^2\big),$$

which can be estimated by the obvious sample analog plug-in estimator $\widehat{\sigma}^2_{a_1,a'_1}$, say. By the same manipulations as above, for a test that rejects H_0 when $n^{1/2}T_n/\widehat{\sigma}_{a_1,a'_1} > z_{1-\alpha/2}$ to have approximate power $(1-\beta) \times 100\%$ to detect $|\mathcal{E}_2(a_1)-\mathcal{E}_2(a'_1)| \geq \delta$, n should be chosen as the smallest integer for which $\Phi(-z_{1-\alpha/2}-n^{1/2}\delta/\sigma_{a_1,a'_1})+\Phi(-z_{1-\alpha/2}+n^{1/2}\delta/\sigma_{a_1,a'_1}) \geq 1-\beta$. The sample size calculation can be based on the standardized effect size $\delta/\sigma_{a_1,a'_1}$ analogous to the preceding results.

9.4.4 Maximizing over the Second Stage

Sizing a study to test $\mathsf{H}_0 : \mathcal{E}_3(a_1) = \mathcal{E}_3(a'_1)$ is more complicated than the cases we have seen thus far because the maximization operation leads to nonstandard asymptotic behavior of the test statistic under the null hypothesis. Before proceeding with this section, the reader may wish to review the first two sections of Chapter 10, which provide an introduction to the challenges of inference when nonsmooth functionals such as the maximization operation are involved.

For simplicity, we consider the situation where there are two embedded regimes that begin with treatment $a_1 \in \mathcal{A}_1$, denoted $e^{a_1}_1$ and $e^{a_1}_2$; and two embedded regimes that begin with $a'_1 \in \mathcal{A}_1$, denoted $e^{a'_1}_1$ and $e^{a'_1}_2$. Clearly, the regimes that assign a_1 at the first stage are nonoverlapping with those assigning a'_1. The general case is discussed briefly at the end of this section.

For any a_1, let $\mathcal{V}^{a_1} = \{\mathcal{V}(e^{a_1}_1), \mathcal{V}(e^{a_1}_2)\}^T = (\mathcal{V}^{a_1}_1, \mathcal{V}^{a_1}_2)$ be the vector comprising the values of regimes $e^{a'_1}_1$ and $e^{a'_1}_2$, and let $\widehat{\mathcal{V}}^{a_1} = \{\widehat{\mathcal{V}}(e^{a_1}_1), \widehat{\mathcal{V}}(e^{a_1}_2)\}^T$ be the corresponding vector of inverse probability weighted estimators (9.12) for the indicated regimes. Define j^{a_1} to be an element of $\arg\max_{j=1,2} \mathcal{V}(e^{a_1}_j) = \arg\max_{j=1,2} \mathcal{V}^{a_1}_j$. Because the estimators $\widehat{\mathcal{V}}^{a_1}$ and $\widehat{\mathcal{V}}^{a'_1}$ correspond to nonoverlapping regimes, they are based on disjoint groups of subjects and thus are independent, although their components may be correlated. Using the general theory of M-estimation, it is straightforward that

$$n^{1/2}(\widehat{\mathcal{V}}^{a_1} - \mathcal{V}^{a_1}) \xrightarrow{D} \mathbb{Z}^{a_1}, \quad \mathbb{Z}^{a_1} \sim \mathcal{N}(0, \Sigma^{a_1})$$

for (2×2) covariance matrix Σ^{a_1}, and similarly for $n^{1/2}(\widehat{\mathcal{V}}^{a'_1} - \mathcal{V}^{a'_1})$. In the following development, we take Σ^{a_1} and $\Sigma^{a'_1}$ to be known. As in the preceding cases, for sample size calculation one would either specify these matrices or estimate them from historical data.

Define the test statistic

$$T_n = \max\left\{\widehat{\mathcal{V}}(e^{a_1}_1), \widehat{\mathcal{V}}(e^{a_1}_2)\right\} - \max\left\{\widehat{\mathcal{V}}(e^{a'_1}_1), \widehat{\mathcal{V}}(e^{a'_1}_2)\right\}.$$

To characterize the limiting distribution of T_n under H_0, we consider four cases:

(C1) $\mathcal{V}(e_1^{a_1}) \neq \mathcal{V}(e_2^{a_1})$ and $\mathcal{V}(e_1^{a_1'}) \neq \mathcal{V}(e_2^{a_1'})$ in which case

$$
n^{1/2} T_n = n^{1/2} \left[\max \left\{ \widehat{\mathcal{V}}(e_1^{a_1}), \widehat{\mathcal{V}}(e_2^{a_1}) \right\} - \max \left\{ \widehat{\mathcal{V}}(e_1^{a_1'}), \widehat{\mathcal{V}}(e_2^{a_1'}) \right\} \right]
$$

$$
= n^{1/2} \left[\max \left\{ \widehat{\mathcal{V}}(e_1^{a_1}) - \mathcal{V}(e_{j^{a_1}}^{a_1}), \widehat{\mathcal{V}}(e_2^{a_1}) - \mathcal{V}(e_{j^{a_1}}^{a_1}) \right\} \right.
$$

$$
\left. - \max \left\{ \widehat{\mathcal{V}}(e_1^{a_1'}) - \mathcal{V}(e_{j^{a_1'}}^{a_1'}), \widehat{\mathcal{V}}(e_2^{a_1'}) - \mathcal{V}(e_{j^{a_1'}}^{a_1'}) \right\} \right]
$$

$$
= n^{1/2} \left\{ \widehat{\mathcal{V}}(e_{j^{a_1}}^{a_1}) - \mathcal{V}(e_{j^{a_1}}^{a_1}) \right\} - n^{1/2} \left\{ \widehat{\mathcal{V}}(e_{j^{a_1'}}^{a_1'}) - \mathcal{V}(e_{j^{a_1'}}^{a_1'}) \right\} + o_P(1)
$$

$$
\xrightarrow{D} \mathbb{Z}_{j^{a_1}}^{a_1} - \mathbb{Z}_{j^{a_1'}}^{a_1'},
$$

where we have used $\mathcal{V}(e_{j^{a_1}}^{a_1}) = \mathcal{V}(e_{j^{a_1'}}^{a_1'})$, which follows from H_0.

(C2) $\mathcal{V}(e_1^{a_1}) = \mathcal{V}(e_2^{a_1})$ and $\mathcal{V}(e_1^{a_1'}) \neq \mathcal{V}(e_2^{a_1'})$, in which case

$$
n^{1/2} T_n = n^{1/2} \max \left[\left\{ \widehat{\mathcal{V}}(e_1^{a_1}) - \mathcal{V}(e_1^{a_1}) \right\}, \left\{ \widehat{\mathcal{V}}(e_2^{a_1}) - \mathcal{V}(e_2^{a_1}) \right\} \right]
$$

$$
- n^{1/2} \left\{ \widehat{\mathcal{V}}(e_{j^{a_1'}}^{a_1'}) - \mathcal{V}(e_{j^{a_1'}}^{a_1'}) \right\} + o_P(1)
$$

$$
\xrightarrow{D} \max(\mathbb{Z}_1^{a_1}, \mathbb{Z}_2^{a_1}) - \mathbb{Z}_{j^{a_1'}}^{a_1'},
$$

where we have used $\mathcal{V}(e_1^{a_1}) = \mathcal{V}(e_2^{a_1}) = \mathcal{V}(e_{j^{a_1'}}^{a_1'})$.

(C3) $\mathcal{V}(e_1^{a_1}) \neq \mathcal{V}(e_2^{a_1})$ and $\mathcal{V}(e_1^{a_1'}) = \mathcal{V}(e_2^{a_1'})$, in which case

$$
n^{1/2} T_n = n^{1/2} \left\{ \widehat{\mathcal{V}}(e_{j^{a_1}}^{a_1}) - \mathcal{V}(e_{j^{a_1}}^{a_1}) \right\}
$$

$$
- n^{1/2} \max \left[\left\{ \widehat{\mathcal{V}}(e_1^{a_1'}) - \mathcal{V}(e_1^{a_1'}) \right\}, \left\{ \widehat{\mathcal{V}}(e_2^{a_1'}) - \mathcal{V}(e_2^{a_1'}) \right\} \right] + o_P(1)
$$

$$
\xrightarrow{D} \mathbb{Z}_{j^{a_1}}^{a_1} - \max(\mathbb{Z}_1^{a_1'}, \mathbb{Z}_2^{a_1'}),
$$

where we have used $\mathcal{V}(e_{j^{a_1}}^{a_1}) = \mathcal{V}(e_1^{a_1'}) = \mathcal{V}(e_2^{a_1'})$.

(C4) $\mathcal{V}(e_1^{a_1}) = \mathcal{V}(e_2^{a_1})$ and $\mathcal{V}(e_1^{a_1'}) = \mathcal{V}(e_2^{a_1'})$, in which case

$$
n^{1/2} T_n = n^{1/2} \max \left[\left\{ \widehat{\mathcal{V}}(e_1^{a_1}) - \mathcal{V}(e_1^{a_1}) \right\}, \left\{ \widehat{\mathcal{V}}(e_2^{a_1}) - \mathcal{V}(e_2^{a_1}) \right\} \right]
$$

$$
- n^{1/2} \max \left[\left\{ \widehat{\mathcal{V}}(e_1^{a_1'}) - \mathcal{V}(e_1^{a_1'}) \right\}, \left\{ \widehat{\mathcal{V}}(e_2^{a_1'}) - \mathcal{V}(e_2^{a_1'}) \right\} \right]
$$

$$
\xrightarrow{D} \max(\mathbb{Z}_1^{a_1}, \mathbb{Z}_2^{a_1}) - \max(\mathbb{Z}_1^{a_1'}, \mathbb{Z}_2^{a_1'}).
$$

Inspection of (C1)–(C4) shows that the limiting distribution of the test statistic under the null can vary widely according to the values of the marginal mean outcomes (values) $\mathcal{V}(e_1^{a_1})$, $\mathcal{V}(e_2^{a_1})$, $\mathcal{V}(e_1^{a_1'})$, and $\mathcal{V}(e_2^{a_1'})$. Furthermore, it is not possible to identify which of the above four cases holds using the observed data; e.g., the means can be infinitesimally different but not equal. Thus, constructing an exact test is difficult without additional (strong) assumptions (Laber et al., 2014c; McKeague and Qian, 2015; Zhang and Laber, 2015).

We take the point of view that a conservative test is preferable to a liberal one and therefore construct a test using upper and lower bounds on the limiting distribution of $n^{1/2}T_n$. We consider tests of the form "reject H_0 if $n^{1/2}T_n < c_1$ or $n^{1/2}T_n > c_2$." Given error level $\alpha \in (0,1)$, we choose c_1 to be the $(\alpha/2) \times 100$ percentile from a distribution that is stochastically smaller than the limiting distribution of $n^{1/2}T_n$; similarly, we choose c_2 to be the $(1 - \alpha/2) \times 100$ percentile of a distribution that is stochastically larger than the limiting distribution of $n^{1/2}T_n$.

It can be seen that the limiting distribution of $n^{1/2}T_n$ is stochastically larger than that of $\mathbb{Z}_{j^{a_1}}^{a_1} - \max(\mathbb{Z}_1^{a_1'}, \mathbb{Z}_2^{a_1'})$. However, j^{a_1} is not known, so we take c_1 to be the minimum of the $(\alpha/2) \times 100$ percentiles of $\mathbb{Z}_1^{a_1} - \max(\mathbb{Z}_1^{a_1'}, \mathbb{Z}_2^{a_1'})$ and $\mathbb{Z}_2^{a_1} - \max(\mathbb{Z}_1^{a_1'}, \mathbb{Z}_2^{a_1'})$. Because Σ^{a_1} and $\Sigma^{a_1'}$ are assumed to be known, c_1 can be computed through simulation. Similarly, it can be seen that the asymptotic distribution of $n^{1/2}T_n$ is stochastically smaller than that of $\max(\mathbb{Z}_1^{a_1}, \mathbb{Z}_2^{a_1}) - \mathbb{Z}_{j^{a_1'}}^{a_1'}$, and we set c_2 to be the maximum of the $(1 - \alpha/2) \times 100$ percentiles of $\max(\mathbb{Z}_1^{a_1}, \mathbb{Z}_2^{a_1}) - \mathbb{Z}_1^{a_1'}$ and $\max(\mathbb{Z}_1^{a_1}, \mathbb{Z}_2^{a_1}) - \mathbb{Z}_2^{a_1'}$. As with the calculation of c_1, because Σ^{a_1} and $\Sigma^{a_1'}$ are known, c_2 can be computed through simulation.

The asymptotic distribution of $n^{1/2}T_n$ is also nonstandard under the alternative hypothesis. Consequently, we construct our sample size procedure using a lower bound on the power $P(n^{1/2}T_n < c_1) + P(n^{1/2}T_n > c_2)$. Suppose first that $\mathcal{V}_{j^{a_1}}^{a_1} - \mathcal{V}_{j^{a_1'}}^{a_1'} < -\delta$. In this case, $P(n^{1/2}T_n \le c_1)$ is equal to

$$P\left[n^{1/2} \max\left\{ \widehat{\mathcal{V}}(e_1^{a_1}), \widehat{\mathcal{V}}(e_2^{a_1}) \right\} - n^{1/2} \max\left\{ \widehat{\mathcal{V}}(e_1^{a_1'}), \widehat{\mathcal{V}}(e_2^{a_1'}) \right\} < c_1 \right]$$

$$= P\left(\max\left[n^{1/2}\left\{ \widehat{\mathcal{V}}(e_1^{a_1}) - \mathcal{V}_{j^{a_1}}^{a_1} \right\}, n^{1/2}\left\{ \widehat{\mathcal{V}}(e_2^{a_1}) - \mathcal{V}_{j^{a_1}}^{a_1} \right\} \right] \right.$$

$$\left. - \max\left[n^{1/2}\left\{ \widehat{\mathcal{V}}(e_1^{a_1'}) - \mathcal{V}_{j^{a_1'}}^{a_1'} \right\}, n^{1/2}\left\{ \widehat{\mathcal{V}}(e_2^{a_1'}) - \mathcal{V}_{j^{a_1'}}^{a_1'} \right\} \right] \le c_1 + n^{1/2}\delta \right);$$

which, using arguments similar to those above, can be seen to be bounded below by $P\{\mathbb{Z}_{j^{a_1}}^{a_1} - \max(\mathbb{Z}_1^{a_1'}, \mathbb{Z}_2^{a_1'}) \le c_1 + n^{1/2}\delta\} + o_P(1)$. This expression in turn is bounded below by $\mathcal{L}(n, \delta) + o_P(1)$, where

$$\mathcal{L}(n;\delta) = \min\left[P\left\{\mathbb{Z}_1^{a_1} - \max(\mathbb{Z}_1^{a_1'}, \mathbb{Z}_2^{a_1'}) \le c_1 + n^{1/2}\delta\right\},\right.$$
$$\left. P\left\{\mathbb{Z}_2^{a_1} - \max(\mathbb{Z}_1^{a_1'}, \mathbb{Z}_2^{a_1'}) \le c_1 + n^{1/2}\delta\right\}\right].$$

Now suppose that $\mathcal{V}_{j^{a_1}}^{a_1} - \mathcal{V}_{j^{a_1'}}^{a_1'} \ge \delta$. Here, $P\left(n^{1/2}T_n > c_2\right)$ is equal to

$$P\left[n^{1/2}\max\left\{\widehat{\mathcal{V}}(e_1^{a_1}), \widehat{\mathcal{V}}(e_2^{a_1})\right\} - n^{1/2}\max\left\{\widehat{\mathcal{V}}(e_1^{a_1'}), \widehat{\mathcal{V}}(e_2^{a_1'})\right\} > c_2\right]$$
$$= P\left(\max\left[n^{1/2}\left\{\widehat{\mathcal{V}}(e_1^{a_1}) - \mathcal{V}_{j^{a_1}}^{a_1}\right\}, n^{1/2}\left\{\widehat{\mathcal{V}}(e_2^{a_1}) - \mathcal{V}_{j^{a_1}}^{a_1}\right\}\right]\right.$$
$$\left. -\max\left[n^{1/2}\left\{\widehat{\mathcal{V}}(e_1^{a_1'}) - \mathcal{V}_{j^{a_1'}}^{a_1'}\right\}, n^{1/2}\left\{\widehat{\mathcal{V}}(e_2^{a_1'}) - \mathcal{V}_{j^{a_1'}}^{a_1'}\right\}\right] \ge c_2 - n^{1/2}\delta\right);$$

which is bounded below by $P\{\max\left(\mathbb{Z}_1^{a_1}, \mathbb{Z}_2^{a_1}\right) - \mathbb{Z}_{j^{a_1'}}^{a_1'} > c_2 - n^{1/2}\delta\} + o_P(1)$; which, in turn, is bounded below by $\mathcal{U}(n,\delta) + o_P(1)$, where

$$\mathcal{U}(n,\delta) = \min\left[P\left\{\max\left(\mathbb{Z}_1^{a_1}, \mathbb{Z}_2^{a_1}\right) - \mathbb{Z}_1^{a_1'} > c_2 - n^{1/2}\delta\right\},\right.$$
$$\left. P\left\{\max\left(\mathbb{Z}_1^{a_1}, \mathbb{Z}_2^{a_1}\right) - \mathbb{Z}_2^{a_1'} > c_2 - n^{1/2}\delta\right\}\right].$$

To ensure $(1 - \beta) \times 100\%$ power, one can choose the smallest integer n such that $\min\{\mathcal{L}(n,\delta), \mathcal{U}(n,\delta)\} \ge 1 - \beta$.

The preceding arguments can be extended to the setting of more than two initial treatments and more than two embedded regimes per initial treatment. However, as we have seen, the limiting distribution of $n^{1/2}T_n$ depends on the configuration of the marginal mean outcomes under each of the embedded regimes and the number of possible configurations is $O(2^{L-1}m)$, where m is the number of initial treatments under consideration, and L is the number of embedded regimes per initial treatment. Thus, the number of parameters that must be specified can be large. Furthermore, because the sample size is based on bounds reflecting the worst possible configuration of the marginal means, it can become excessively conservative. This conservatism can be mitigated if one imposes more structure on the values of the regimes via parametric modeling.

9.5   Power and Sample Size for Optimal Treatment Regimes

In the context of a SMART, estimation of an optimal treatment regime typically is considered a secondary and hypothesis-generating analysis. Consequently, estimation of an optimal regime is not factored into sample size calculations (Murphy, 2005). Furthermore, although it is widely believed that sizing a SMART to ensure high-quality estimation of an optimal treatment regime requires a larger sample size than, say, to compare two nonoverlapping embedded regimes, there is little empirical or theoretical evidence to support (or refute) this belief. However, interest in precision medicine has prompted increasing consideration of estimation of an optimal regime as a primary analysis for a SMART (Laber et al., 2016), highlighting the need for development of principled sample size procedures for this objective.

In this section, we derive sample size formulæ for a SMART that ensure (i) sufficient power to detect a clinically meaningful difference in the mean marginal outcomes (values) under an optimal treatment regime and under some comparator treatment strategy, such as standard of care in the population; and (ii) the value under the estimated optimal regime is within a prespecified tolerance of that under a true optimal regime with high probability (see below for mathematically precise statements).

We focus here for simplicity on sizing a two-stage SMART with two treatment options that are feasible for all individuals at each stage. For convenience in deriving the results, we code the options at each stage as $-1, 1$, so that $\mathcal{A}_k = \{-1, 1\}$, $k = 1, 2$, where of course the options need not be the same at each stage. We also assume that the intended randomization probabilities are $\omega_k(h_k, a_k) = P(A_k = a_k | H_k = h_k) = 1/2$, $k = 1, 2$. Extension to more than two options at each stage; unequal randomization probabilities; and dependence of the randomization probabilities on h_k, as in the case of response status, is straightforward although requires substantially more complicated notation. Throughout this section, we continue to assume that SUTVA (6.16), the SRA (6.17), the positivity assumption (6.23) hold, where the last two conditions hold by design in a SMART.

We first state formally the operating characteristics that we seek to guarantee for an estimated optimal treatment regime. Denote by $\mathbb{D}_n$ the observed data from a sample of size n; namely, $(X_{1i}, A_{1i}, X_{2i}, A_{2i}, Y_i)$, $i = 1, \ldots, n$. Write $\widehat{d}$ to denote an estimator for an optimal treatment regime $d^{opt} \in \mathcal{D}$ based on $\mathbb{D}_n$; specific estimators will be described below. Write $\mathcal{V}(\widehat{d})$ to denote the marginal mean outcome (value) if the estimated optimal regime $\widehat{d}$ were to be used to select treatment for future patients; as discussed in Section 10.3.2, $\mathcal{V}(\widehat{d}) = E\{Y^*(\widehat{d}) | \mathbb{D}_n\}$ is referred to as the conditional value. Let $B_0 > 0$, α, β, λ, ϵ, and $\zeta \in (0, 1)$ be constants. We wish to choose n so that

(P1) there exists an α-level test of $\mathsf{H}_0 : \mathcal{V}(d^{opt}) \leq B_0$ based on $\widehat{d}$ that has power at least $(1-\beta) \times 100\% + o(1)$ provided that $\mathcal{V}(d^{opt}) \geq B_0 + \lambda$;

(P2) the marginal mean outcome (value) under the estimated optimal regime is within ϵ of the value of an optimal regime with probability at least $1 - \zeta + o(1)$; i.e.,

$$P\{\mathcal{V}(\widehat{d}) \geq \mathcal{V}(d^{opt}) - \epsilon\} \geq 1 - \zeta + o(1).$$

Condition (P1) ensures that there is sufficient power to compare the value of an optimal treatment regime with the mean outcome in the population under a comparator treatment strategy; e.g., standard of care. If B_0 is the marginal mean outcome under standard of care, then, under the null hypothesis $\mathsf{H}_0 : \mathcal{V}(d^{opt}) \leq B_0$, there is no benefit to tailoring treatment recommendations in this patient population using the available patient characteristics and treatment options. However, rejecting this null does not necessarily ensure that the estimated optimal regime is of high quality. Condition (P2) ensures that the estimated optimal regime yields a nearly optimal marginal mean outcome (close to the value achieved by a true optimal regime) with high probability. Thus, together, (P1) and (P2) ensure that the estimated optimal regime will improve patient outcomes relative to standard of care with high probability.

In the following two sections, we discuss sample size procedures that guarantee the criteria (P1) and (P2). A significant challenge in deriving such procedures is that (P1) and (P2) involve $\mathcal{V}(d^{opt})$ which, as noted in previous chapters and demonstrated in Chapter 10, is a nonsmooth functional of the underlying generative data model. Thus, standard large sample methods for inference, including the bootstrap or series approximations, cannot be applied without modification or strong assumptions (Chakraborty et al., 2010; Moodie and Richardson, 2010; Chakraborty et al., 2014b,a; Laber et al., 2014c; Song et al., 2015). The sample size procedure in Section 9.5.1 is predicated on assumptions that are sufficiently strong to render it possible to appeal to standard inferential approaches. That in Section 9.5.2 is derived under much weaker conditions; however, as might be expected, the price for this generality is conservatism of the resulting sample size procedure. The derivation makes use of developments presented in Chapter 10 for inference involving nonsmooth functionals, so that this section is more technical. Accordingly, readers of Section 9.5.2 should review Chapter 10 first. Full details on these methods, including proofs of results, are available in Rose et al. (2019) and the associated supplementary materials.

9.5.1 Normality-based Sample Size Procedure

The sample size procedure we now discuss imposes parametric structure on several components of the generative data model such that it is possible to construct a regular, asymptotically normal estimator of $\mathcal{V}(d^{opt})$ that is amenable to closed form sample size formulæ. The relevance of these parametric assumptions depends on the specific application area. Although the sample size formulæ do not depend on the availability of pilot or historical data, such data could be used to evaluate the plausibility of the assumptions.

The parametric structure is intended to be consistent with Q-learning based on a linear model at the second decision point; Q-learning is covered in detail in Sections 5.7.1 and 7.4.1. Specifically, we assume that the true generative distribution of the data satisfies the following conditions.

(AN1) $Q_2(h_2, a_2) = E(Y|H_2 = h_2, A_2 = a_2) = \tilde{h}_{21}^T \beta_{21,0} + a_2 \tilde{h}_{22}^T \beta_{22,0}$, where $\tilde{h}_{21}$ and $\tilde{h}_{22}$ are vectors of known features constructed from h_2 that may include polynomial terms or nonlinear basis functions involving components of h_2, and $\beta_{21,0}$ and $\beta_{22,0}$ are unknown values characterizing the true $Q_2(h_2, a_2)$.

(AN2) $E(\tilde{H}_{21}^T \beta_{21,0}|H_1 = h_1, A_1 = a_1) = \tilde{h}_{11}^T \xi_{11,0} + a_1 \tilde{h}_{12}^T \xi_{12,0}$, where $\tilde{h}_{11}$ and $\tilde{h}_{12}$ are vectors of known features constructed from h_1, and $\xi_{11,0}$ and $\xi_{12,0}$ are unknown values characterizing this expectation.

(AN3) $\tilde{H}_{22}^T \beta_{22,0} = \tilde{H}_{13}^T \varpi_{13,0} + A_1 \tilde{H}_{14}^T \varpi_{14,0} + \tau_0 Z$, where $\tilde{h}_{13}$ and $\tilde{h}_{14}$ are vectors of known features of h_1, Z is a standard normal random variable that is independent of (H_1, A_1), $\tau_0 > 0$, and $\varpi_{13,0}$ and $\varpi_{14,0}$ are unknown values.

(AN4) $(\tilde{H}_{11}^T \xi_{11,0}, \tilde{H}_{12}^T \xi_{12,0}, \tilde{H}_{13,0}^T \varpi_{13,0}, \tilde{H}_{14}^T \varpi_{14,0})^T$ is multivariate normal with unknown mean ω_0 (4×1) and covariance matrix Ω_0 (4×4).

Assumptions (AN1)–(AN3) are similar to those used in interactive Q-learning (IQ-learning), a variant of g-computation that is based on location-scale models (Laber et al., 2014a; Linn et al., 2017), discussed further in Sections 10.3 and 10.4. However, (AN4) is a stronger condition than required by most Q-learning or IQ-learning procedures, which are not predicated on distributional assumptions on the first-stage history. The joint normality in (AN4) can be replaced or weakened, albeit at the potential cost of more complex expressions.

Under (AN1)–(AN3), using the definition of $Q_1(h_1, a_1)$ as in (5.74) and (5.81) and by calculations similar to those used to derive (5.104), the first-stage Q-function satisfies

$$Q_1(h_1, a_1) = E\left\{ \max_{a_2 \in \mathcal{A}_2} Q_2(h_2, a_2)|H_1 = h_1, A_1 = a_1 \right\}$$

$$= E\{\tilde{H}_{21}^T \beta_{21,0} + |\tilde{H}_{22}^T \beta_{22,0}| \,|H_1 = h_1, A_1 = a_1\}$$

$$= \tilde{h}_{11}^T \xi_{11,0} + a_1 \tilde{h}_{12}^T \xi_{12,0}$$

$$+ (2\pi\tau_0^2)^{-1/2} \int |\tilde{h}_{13}^T \varpi_{13,0} + a_1 \tilde{h}_{14}^T \varpi_{14,0} + z| \, \exp\{-z^2/(2\tau_0^2)\} \, dz$$

$$= \widetilde{h}_{11}^T \xi_{11,0} + a_1 \widetilde{h}_{12}^T \xi_{12,0} + \frac{2\tau_0}{(2\pi)^{1/2}} \exp\left\{ -\frac{(\widetilde{h}_{13}^T \varpi_{13,0} + a_1 \widetilde{h}_{14}^T \varpi_{14})^2}{2\tau_0^2} \right\}$$

$$+ (\widetilde{h}_{13}^T \varpi_{13,0} + a_1 \widetilde{h}_{14}^T \varpi_{14,0}) \left[1 - 2\Phi\left\{ -\frac{(\widetilde{h}_{13}^T \varpi_{13,0} + a_1 \widetilde{h}_{14}^T \varpi_{14,0})}{\tau_0} \right\} \right],$$

where the second and third equalities follow from the structure in (AN1)–(AN3), and the final equality is obtained from the form of the mean of a folded normal distribution; i.e., if $W \sim \mathcal{N}(\mu, \varsigma^2)$, then

$$E\{|W|\} = (2\pi)^{-1/2} \int |\mu + \varsigma w| \exp(-w^2/2) \, dw$$

$$= \frac{2\varsigma}{(2\pi)^{1/2}} \exp\left(-\frac{\mu^2}{2\varsigma^2} \right) + \mu\{1 - 2\Phi(-\mu/\varsigma)\}.$$

Define $\theta_1 = (\xi_{11}^T, \xi_{12}^T, \varpi_{13}^T, \varpi_{14}^T)^T$, let $\beta_1 = (\theta_1^T, \tau)^T$, and let

$$Q_1(h_1, a_1; \beta_1) = \widetilde{h}_{11}^T \xi_{11} + a_1 \widetilde{h}_{12}^T \xi_{12}$$

$$+ \frac{2\tau}{(2\pi)^{1/2}} \exp\left\{ -\frac{(\widetilde{h}_{13}^T \varpi_{13} + a_1 \widetilde{h}_{14}^T \varpi_{14})^2}{2\tau^2} \right\} \qquad (9.25)$$

$$+ (\widetilde{h}_{13}^T \varpi_{13} + a_1 \widetilde{h}_{14}^T \varpi_{14}) \left[1 - 2\Phi\left\{ -\frac{(\widetilde{h}_{13}^T \varpi_{13} + a_1 \widetilde{h}_{14}^T \varpi_{14})}{\tau} \right\} \right],$$

so that $Q_1(h_1, a_1) = Q_1(h_1, a_1; \beta_{1,0})$, where $\beta_{1,0} = (\theta_{1,0}^T, \tau_0)^T = (\xi_{11,0}^T, \xi_{12,0}^T, \varpi_{1,0}^T, \varpi_{14,0}^T, \tau_0)^T$.

From (5.77), (5.84), and (7.47), recall that

$$\mathcal{V}(d^{opt}) = E\{V_1(H_1)\} = E\left\{ \max_{a_1 \in \mathcal{A}_1} Q_1(H_1, a_1) \right\}.$$

We now use this characterization and (AN4) to obtain a closed form expression for $\mathcal{V}(d^{opt})$ and an associated estimator for $\mathcal{V}(d^{opt})$ that is regular and asymptotically normal and thus amenable to familiar sample size calculations.

To streamline notation, define

$$g(v) = \max_{\rho \in \{-1,1\}} \left(v_1 + \rho v_2 + \frac{1}{(2\pi)^{1/2}} \exp\left\{ \frac{-(v_3 + \rho v_4)^2}{2} \right\} \right.$$

$$\left. + (v_3 + \rho v_4) \left[1 - 2\Phi\{-(v_3 + \rho v_4)\} \right] \right), \qquad (9.26)$$

so that if $W(h_1; \theta_1) = (\widetilde{h}_{11}^T \xi_{11}, \widetilde{h}_{12}^T \xi_{12}, \widetilde{h}_{13}^T \varpi_{13}, \widetilde{h}_{14}^T \varpi_{14})^T$, then

$$\max_{a_1 \in \mathcal{A}_1} Q_1(H_1, a_1) = \tau_0 g\{W(H_1; \theta_{1,0})/\tau_0\}.$$

For any $(p \times p)$ symmetric matrix A, let $\text{vech}(A)$ be the $p(p+1)/2$ vector obtained by concatenating the rows of the upper triangular portion of A (equivalently the columns of the lower triangular portion) (the vector-half operator, Henderson and Searle, 1979), so containing the distinct elements of A. Let $\varphi(v; \omega, \Omega)$ denote the density of a multivariate normal distribution with mean ω and covariance matrix Ω, and define

$$\nu\{\tau, \omega, \text{vech}(\Omega)\} = \int \tau\, g(v/\tau)\, \varphi(v; \omega, \Omega)\, dv.$$

With these definitions and under (AN1)–(AN4), it follows that $\mathcal{V}(d^{opt})$ is the smooth function of τ_0, ω_0, and Ω_0 given by

$$\mathcal{V}(d^{opt}) = \nu\{\tau_0, \omega_0, \text{vech}(\Omega_0)\} = \int \tau_0\, g(v/\tau_0)\, \varphi(v; \omega_0, \Omega_0)\, dv; \quad (9.27)$$

this result follows immediately from the characterization of $\mathcal{V}(d^{opt})$ above. This suggests that an estimator $\widehat{\mathcal{V}}(d^{opt})$, say, for $\mathcal{V}(d^{opt})$ can be obtained by substitution of suitable estimators $\widehat{\tau}$, $\widehat{\omega}$, and $\widehat{\Omega}$ for τ_0, ω_0, and Ω_0, respectively, in (9.27); that is, $\widehat{\mathcal{V}}(d^{opt}) = \nu\{\widehat{\tau}, \widehat{\omega}, \text{vech}(\widehat{\Omega})\}$. Provided that the estimators $\widehat{\tau}$, $\widehat{\omega}$, and $\widehat{\Omega}$ satisfy

$$n^{1/2}\big[\{\widehat{\tau}, \widehat{\omega}^T, \text{vech}(\widehat{\Omega})^T\}^T - \{\tau_0, \omega_0^T, \text{vech}(\Omega_0)^T\}^T\big] \xrightarrow{D} \mathcal{N}(0, \Sigma_0) \quad (9.28)$$

for some covariance matrix Σ_0 (15×15), because (9.27) is a smooth function of τ_0, ω_0, and Ω_0, under regularity conditions, a standard Taylor series (delta method) argument can be used to show that

$$n^{1/2}\{\widehat{\mathcal{V}}(d^{opt}) - \mathcal{V}(d^{opt})\} \xrightarrow{D} \mathcal{N}(0, \sigma_0^2),$$
$$\sigma_0^2 = [\nabla\nu\{\tau_0, \omega_0, \text{vech}(\Omega_0)\}]^T\, \Sigma_0\, [\nabla\nu\{\tau_0, \omega_0, \text{vech}(\Omega_0)\}], \quad (9.29)$$

and $\nabla\nu\{\tau_0, \omega_0, \text{vech}(\Omega_0)\}$ is the (15×1) vector of partial derivatives of $\nu\{\tau, \omega, \text{vech}(\Omega)\}$ with respect to $\{\tau, \omega^T, \text{vech}(\Omega)^T\}^T$ evaluated at τ_0, ω_0, and Ω_0. These developments can be exploited to derive sample size formulæ satisfying (P1) and (P2) as follows.

To obtain estimators for τ_0, ω_0, and Ω_0, we focus on least squares estimation techniques. Define $Q_2(h_2, a_2; \beta_2) = \widetilde{h}_{21}^T \beta_{21} + a_2 \widetilde{h}_{22}^T \beta_{22}$, $\beta_2 = (\beta_{21}^T, \beta_{22}^T)^T$. Then a natural estimator for $\beta_{2,0} = (\beta_{21,0}^T, \beta_{22,0}^T)^T$ in (AN1) is the OLS estimator $\widehat{\beta}_2 = (\widehat{\beta}_{21}^T, \widehat{\beta}_{22}^T)^T$ for β_2 in the model $Q_2(h_2, a_2; \beta_2)$, minimizing in β_2

$$\sum_{i=1}^{n}\{Y_i - Q_2(H_{2i}, A_{2i}; \beta_2)\}^2.$$

Based on (AN2), an estimator $\widehat{\xi}_1 = (\widehat{\xi}_{11}^T, \widehat{\xi}_{12}^T)^T$ for $\xi_{1,0} = (\xi_{11,0}^T, \xi_{12,0}^T)^T$

can be found by forming "pseudo outcomes" $\widetilde{H}_{21,i}^T \widehat{\beta}_{21}$ and minimizing in $\xi_1 = (\xi_{11}^T, \xi_{12}^T)^T$

$$\sum_{i=1}^{n} \left\{ \widetilde{H}_{21,i}^T \widehat{\beta}_{21} - \widetilde{H}_{11,i}^T \xi_{11} - A_{1i} \widetilde{H}_{12,i}^T \xi_{12} \right\}^2.$$

Similarly, from (AN3), $\varpi_{1,0} = (\varpi_{13,0}^T, \varpi_{14,0}^T)^T$ can be estimated by $\widehat{\varpi}_1 = (\widehat{\varpi}_{13}^T, \widehat{\varpi}_{14}^T)^T$ minimizing in $\varpi_1 = (\varpi_{13}^T, \varpi_{14}^T)^T$

$$\sum_{i=1}^{n} \left\{ \widetilde{H}_{22,i}^T \widehat{\beta}_{22} - \widetilde{H}_{13,i}^T \varpi_{13} - A_{1i} \widetilde{H}_{14,i}^T \varpi_{14} \right\}^2,$$

and an obvious estimator for τ_0^2 is then

$$\widehat{\tau}^2 = n^{-1} \sum_{i=1}^{n} \left\{ \widetilde{H}_{22,i}^T \widehat{\beta}_{22} - \widetilde{H}_{13,i}^T \widehat{\varpi}_{13} - A_{1i} \widetilde{H}_{14,i}^T \widehat{\varpi}_{14} \right\}^2.$$

Then, letting $\widehat{\theta}_1 = (\widehat{\xi}_{11}^T, \widehat{\xi}_{12}^T, \widehat{\varpi}_{13}^T, \widehat{\varpi}_{14}^T)^T$, natural estimators for ω_0 and Ω_0 are the sample average $\widehat{\omega} = n^{-1} \sum_{i=1}^{n} W(H_{1i}; \widehat{\theta}_1)$, and sample covariance matrix

$$\widehat{\Omega} = n^{-1} \sum_{i=1}^{n} \{W(H_{1i}; \widehat{\theta}_1) - \widehat{\omega}\}\{W(H_{1i}; \widehat{\theta}_1) - \widehat{\omega}\}^T.$$

The theory of M-estimation in Section 2.5 applied to the stacked estimating equations corresponding to the above estimators can then be used to conclude the result in (9.28) and to deduce the form of Σ_0, which depends on $\beta_{2,0}, \xi_{1,0}, \varpi_{1,0}$, and so on. Letting $\widehat{\Sigma}$ be the estimator for Σ_0 obtained by substitution of the corresponding estimators, from (9.29), a consistent estimator for σ_0^2 can be obtained as

$$\widehat{\sigma}^2 = [\nabla \nu \{\widehat{\tau}, \widehat{\omega}, \text{vech}(\widehat{\Omega})\}]^T \, \widehat{\Sigma} \, [\nabla \nu \{\widehat{\tau}, \widehat{\omega}, \text{vech}(\widehat{\Omega})\}].$$

It follows from (9.29) that

$$n^{1/2} \{\widehat{\mathcal{V}}(d^{opt}) - \mathcal{V}(d^{opt})\}/\widehat{\sigma} \xrightarrow{D} \mathcal{N}(0, 1). \tag{9.30}$$

From (9.30), the test of $\mathsf{H}_0 : \mathcal{V}(d^{opt}) \leq B_0$ that rejects when $n^{1/2} \{\widehat{\mathcal{V}}(d^{opt}) - B_0\}/\widehat{\sigma} \geq z_{1-\alpha}$ has type I error probability $\alpha + o(1)$ under H_0 and power of at least $\Phi(-z_{1-\alpha} + n^{1/2}\lambda/\sigma_0) + o(1)$ provided that $\mathcal{V}(d^{opt}) \geq B_0 + \lambda$. Thus, to ensure power of $(1 - \beta) \times 100\%$, one should choose n so that this quantity is $\geq 1 - \beta$, so that taking

$$n = \frac{\sigma_0^2 (z_{1-\alpha} + z_{1-\beta})^2}{\lambda^2}$$

satisfies (P1) asymptotically. This formula involves the standardized effect size λ/σ_0, so that sample size determination can be based on a posited value for this quantity.

From above, the estimated second-stage Q-function is $Q_2(h_2, a_2; \widehat{\beta}_2)$, and the corresponding estimated optimal second-stage decision rule is $\widehat{d}_2(h_2) = \arg\max_{a_2 \in \mathcal{A}_2} Q_2(h_2, a_2; \widehat{\beta}_2)$. Similarly, an estimator for $Q_1(h_1, a_1)$ is given by $Q_1(h_1, a_1; \widehat{\beta}_1)$, where $\widehat{\beta}_1 = (\widehat{\theta}_1^T, \widehat{\tau}^T)^T$, and the estimated optimal first-stage decision rule is $\widehat{d}_1(h_1) = \arg\max_{a_1 \in \mathcal{A}_1} Q_1(h_1, a_1; \widehat{\beta}_1)$. As in Sections 3.5.2 and 7.4.2, let $\Delta Q_k = C_k(H_k) = Q_k(H_k, 1) - Q_k(H_k, -1)$ and $\Delta \widehat{Q}_k = \widehat{C}_k(H_k) = Q_k(H_k, 1; \widehat{\beta}_k) - Q_k(H_k, -1; \widehat{\beta}_k)$, $k = 1, 2$. To select n so that (P2) also holds, assume further that

(AN5) ΔQ_k and $\Delta \widehat{Q}_k$ are sub-Gaussian, so have distributions with tails that decay more rapidly than those of a normal distribution, $k = 1, 2$.

(AN6) there exist M and $\kappa > 0$ such that $P\left\{|\widetilde{H}_{22}^T \beta_{22,0}| \le \epsilon\right\} \le M\epsilon^\kappa$ as $\epsilon \to 0$.

The preceding assumptions are relatively mild; e.g., (AN5) and (AN6) are satisfied if the histories and outcome are normally distributed. The following result characterizes the concentration of the marginal mean outcome (value) under $\widehat{d}$ about that of d^{opt}, which can subsequently be used to choose a sample size n that satisfies (P2). Recall that we continue to take SUTVA, the SRA, and the positivity assumption to hold.

Lemma 9.5.1. *Assume (AN1)–(AN4), regularity conditions such that (9.28) holds, and (AN5)–(AN6). Then there exist L and $\gamma > 0$ such that*

$$|\mathcal{V}(\widehat{d}) - \mathcal{V}(d^{opt})| \le Ln^{-\gamma}|\widehat{\mathcal{V}}(d^{opt}) - \mathcal{V}(d^{opt})| + o_p(1/n^{1/2}).$$

Corollary 9.5.2. *Assume (AN1)–(AN4), regularity conditions such that (9.28) holds, and (AN5)–(AN6). Then setting*

$$n = \left\lceil \left(\frac{z_{1-\zeta}\,\sigma_0}{\epsilon}\right)^2 \right\rceil, \tag{9.31}$$

satisfies (P2), where $\lceil x \rceil$ is the smallest integer greater than or equal to x.

See Rose et al. (2019) for details and proofs.

Summarizing, (P1) is satisfied by the test based on rejecting H_0 when $n^{1/2}\{\widehat{\mathcal{V}}(d^{opt}) - B_0\}/\widehat{\sigma} \ge z_{1-\alpha}$, and choosing n as in (9.31) guarantees (P2). To implement this sample size procedure in practice, then, one must specify σ_0^2. This can be based on historical data or data from a pilot study if these are available; if not, as a surrogate for σ_0^2, one can use a posited value for the variance of Y under the comparator strategy; e.g., standard of care. See Rose et al. (2019) for justification and discussion.

9.5.2 Projection-based Sample Size Procedure

The second sample size procedure we now present does not impose parametric structure on the underlying generative model, nor does it assume that the analysis model is correct. However, without these assumptions, the sampling distribution of the estimated marginal mean outcome (value) need not be regular or asymptotically normal, and the estimated optimal regime need not concentrate about d^{opt}. Consequently, the resulting sample size procedure is more complex. As noted above, the derivation makes use of material in Chapter 10, which the reader should review before proceeding. In what follows, we adopt the alternative notation defined in the remark at the end of the introductory section of Chapter 10; namely, for an i.i.d. sample $Z_1, \ldots, Z_n$ drawn from unknown distribution P, we write $Pf(Z)$ to denote $\int f(z)\,dP(z)$ and $\mathbb{P}_n f(Z) = n^{-1} \sum_{i=1}^{n} f(Z_i)$, and we add a subscript n to estimators to emphasize the size of the sample used to construct them. We also use $\rightsquigarrow$ to denote convergence in distribution. See Chapter 10 for further details.

We assume that estimation and inference will be based on Q-learning with posited (possibly misspecified) parametric linear models for the Q-functions. For $k = 1, 2$, let $Q_k(h_k, a_k; \beta_k) = \tilde{h}_{k1}^T \beta_{k1} + a_k \tilde{h}_{k2}^T \beta_{k2}$ denote the working model for $Q_k(h_k, a_k)$, where $\tilde{h}_{k1}$ and $\tilde{h}_{k2}$ are vectors of known features constructed from h_k, and $\beta_k = (\beta_{k1}^T, \beta_{k2}^T)^T$ are unknown parameters. Suppose that Q-learning is implemented using OLS at each stage to estimate β_k, $k = 1, 2$, yielding estimators $\widehat{\beta}_{2,n} = \arg\min_{\beta_2} \mathbb{P}_n \{Y - Q_2(H_2, A_2; \beta_2)\}^2$ and

$$\widehat{\beta}_{1,n} = \arg\min_{\beta_1} \mathbb{P}_n \left\{ \max_{a_2 \in \mathcal{A}_2} Q_2(H_2, a_2; \widehat{\beta}_2) - Q_1(H_1, A_1; \beta_1) \right\}^2,$$

so that the estimated optimal regime is $\widehat{d}_n = (\widehat{d}_{1,n}, \widehat{d}_{2,n})$, where

$$\widehat{d}_{k,n}(h_k) = \arg\max_{a_k \in \mathcal{A}_k} Q_k(h_k, a_k; \widehat{\beta}_{k,n}), \quad k = 1, 2,$$

and we suppress the subscript "Q" for brevity.

Because we do not assume that the Q-function models are correctly specified, we consider (P1) and (P2) in terms of the asymptotic analog of $\widehat{d}_n$. That is, as in Sections 10.3.1 and 10.4.1, let $\beta_2^* = \arg\min_{\beta_2} P\{Y - Q_2(H_2, A_2; \beta_2)\}^2$ and

$$\beta_1^* = \arg\min_{\beta_1} P \left\{ \max_{a_2 \in \mathcal{A}_2} Q_2(H_2, a_2; \beta_2^*) - Q_1(H_1, A_1; \beta_1) \right\}^2.$$

Define $d_*^{opt} = (d_{1,*}^{opt}, d_{2,*}^{opt})$ such that

$$d_{k,*}^{opt} = \arg\max_{a_k \in \mathcal{A}_k} Q_k(h_k, a_k; \beta_k^*), \quad k = 1, 2.$$

Our goal is to derive a sample size procedure that ensures (P1) and (P2) hold when d^{opt} is replaced by d_*^{opt}.

As discussed in Chapter 10, $\mathcal{V}(d_*^{opt})$ is not a smooth functional of the underlying generative data model, so it is not possible to develop a sample size procedure based on standard asymptotic normal approximations as in the preceding section. Accordingly, to obtain a sample size procedure addressing (P1), we invert a projection confidence interval for $\mathcal{V}(d_*^{opt})$, which provides asymptotically correct coverage even if the Q-functions are misspecified, so that the resulting sample size procedure is robust to such misspecification. This projection interval is analogous to those presented in Chapter 10.

Let $B_k = (\tilde{H}_{k1}^T, A_k \tilde{H}_{k2}^T)^T$, $k = 1, 2$; and let $p_k = \dim(B_k)$. For $k = 2$, define

$$\widehat{\mathfrak{W}}_{2,n} = \{\mathbb{P}_n B_2 B_2^T\}^{-1} \mathbb{P}_n (Y - B_2^T \widehat{\beta}_{2,n})^2 B_2 B_2^T \{\mathbb{P}_n B_2 B_2^T\}^{-1}.$$

Let $\chi_{u,r}$ be the $u \times 100$ percentile of the chi-square distribution with r degrees of freedom. It follows that

$$\mathfrak{F}_{2,n,1-\epsilon} = \left\{ \beta_2 : n(\beta_2 - \widehat{\beta}_{2,n})^T \widehat{\mathfrak{W}}_{2,n}^{-1} (\beta_2 - \widehat{\beta}_{2,n}) \le \chi_{1-\epsilon, p_2} \right\}$$

is a $(1 - \epsilon) \times 100\%$ confidence region for β_2^*. For each β_2 define

$$\beta_1^*(\beta_2) = \arg\min_{\beta_1} P \left\{ \max_{a_2} Q_2(H_2, a_2; \beta_2) - Q_1(H_1, A_1; \beta_1) \right\}^2,$$

so that $\beta_1^*(\beta_2)$ is the population parameter indexing the first-stage Q-function if the second-stage Q-function is $Q_2(h_2, a_2; \beta_2)$; thus, $\beta_1^* = \beta_1^*(\beta_2^*)$. Furthermore, for each β_2, define

$$\widehat{\beta}_{1,n}(\beta_2) = \arg\min_{\beta_1} \mathbb{P}_n \left\{ \max_{a_2} Q_2(H_2, a_2; \beta_2) - Q_1(H_1, A_1; \beta_1) \right\}^2$$

to be the least squares estimator for $\beta_1^*(\beta_2)$, and, for each β_2, define

$$\mathfrak{W}_{1,n}(\beta_2) = \{\mathbb{P}_n B_1 B_1^T\}^{-1} \mathbb{P}_n \Big[B_1 B_1^T$$
$$\times \left\{ \max_{a_2} Q_2(H_2, a_2; \beta_2) - B_1^T \widehat{\beta}_{1,n}(\beta_2) \right\}^2 \Big] \{\mathbb{P}_n B_1 B_1^T\}^{-1}.$$

A $(1 - \epsilon) \times 100\%$ Wald-type confidence region for $\beta_1^*(\beta_2)$ is thus

$$\mathfrak{F}_{1,n,1-\epsilon}(\beta_2)$$
$$= \left[\beta_1 : n\{\beta_1 - \widehat{\beta}_{1,n}(\beta_2)\}^T\widehat{\mathfrak{W}}_{1,n}^{-1}(\beta_2)\{\beta_1 - \widehat{\beta}_{1,n}(\beta_2)\} \leq \chi_{1-\epsilon,p_1}\right].$$

For any $\epsilon_1, \epsilon_2 \in (0,1)$ such that $\vartheta = \epsilon_1 + \epsilon_2 \leq 1$, it follows that a $(1 - \vartheta) \times 100\%$ projection region for (β_1^*, β_2^*) is

$$\Xi_{n,1-\vartheta} = \{(\beta_1, \beta_2) : \beta_2 \in \mathfrak{F}_{2,n,1-\epsilon_2}, \beta_1 \in \mathfrak{F}_{1,n,1-\epsilon_1}(\beta_2)\}.$$

For any β_1, β_2, write $\mathcal{V}^Q(\beta_1, \beta_2)$ to denote the value of regime $d = (d_1, d_2)$, where $d_k(h_k) = \arg\max_{a_k \in \mathcal{A}_k} Q_k(h_k, a_k; \beta_k)$, $k = 1, 2$; and this notation emphasizes the dependence of d on the Q-functions and β_1, β_2. Let $\vartheta_1, \vartheta_2 \in (0,1)$ be such that $\vartheta_1 + \vartheta_2 \leq 1$. To obtain a projection interval for $\mathcal{V}(d_*^{opt})$, we first construct a pointwise $(1 - \vartheta_2) \times 100\%$ confidence interval for $\mathcal{V}^Q(\beta_1, \beta_2)$ for each (β_1, β_2) and then take a union of these intervals over $\Xi_{n,1-\vartheta_1}$. Thus, because $\mathcal{V}(d_*^{opt}) = \mathcal{V}(\beta_1^*, \beta_2^*)$, if $(\beta_1^*, \beta_2^*) \in \Xi_{n,1-\vartheta_1}$ then this union will contain $\mathcal{V}(d_*^{opt})$ with probability at least $1 - \vartheta_2$.

For each (β_1, β_2) define

$$\varrho(\beta_1, \beta_2) = 4YI(A_1\widetilde{H}_{12}^T\beta_{12} > 0)I(A_2\widetilde{H}_{22}^T\beta_{22} > 0)$$
$$+ 2\left\{I(A_1\widetilde{H}_{12}^T\beta_{12} \leq 0) - (1/2)\right\}\max_{a_1 \in \mathcal{A}_1} Q_1(H_1, a_1; \beta_1)$$
$$+ 4I(A_1\widetilde{H}_{12}^T\beta_{12} > 0)\left\{I(A_2\widetilde{H}_{22}^T\beta_{22} \leq 0) - (1/2)\right\}\max_{a_2 \in \mathcal{A}_2} Q_2(H_2, a_2; \beta_2),$$

so that $\mathcal{V}^Q(\beta_1, \beta_2) = P\varrho(\beta_1, \beta_2)$, and thus $\widehat{\mathcal{V}}_n^Q(\beta_1, \beta_2) = \mathbb{P}_n\varrho(\beta_1, \beta_2)$ is a plug-in estimator for $\mathcal{V}^Q(\beta_1, \beta_2)$. It can be verified that $\widehat{\mathcal{V}}_n^Q(\widehat{\beta}_{1,n}, \widehat{\beta}_{2,n})$ is an augmented inverse probability weighted estimator for $\mathcal{V}(d_*^{opt})$ of the form in (7.102).

For each fixed (β_1, β_2) such that $P\varrho^2(\beta_1, \beta_2) < \infty$, it follows that

$$n^{1/2}\{\widehat{\mathcal{V}}_n^Q(\beta_1, \beta_2) - \mathcal{V}^Q(\beta_1, \beta_2)\} = n^{1/2}(\mathbb{P}_n - P)\varrho(\beta_1, \beta_2)$$
$$\leadsto \mathcal{N}\left[0, P\{\varrho(\beta_1, \beta_2) - P\varrho(\beta_1, \beta_2)\}^2\right].$$

Thus, for $\vartheta_1, \vartheta_2 \in (0,1)$ satisfying $\vartheta_1 + \vartheta_2 = \alpha$, a $(1 - \alpha) \times 100\%$ confidence region for $\mathcal{V}(d_*^{opt})$ is formed by taking a union of one-sided confidence sets for $\mathcal{V}^Q(\beta_1, \beta_2)$ over $\Xi_{n,1-\vartheta_1}$. That is, letting

$$\mathcal{B}_{n,1-\vartheta_2}(\beta_1, \beta_2) = \widehat{\mathcal{V}}_n^Q(\beta_1, \beta_2) - \frac{z_{1-\vartheta_2}\left[\mathbb{P}_n\{\varrho(\beta_1, \beta_2) - \mathbb{P}_n\varrho(\beta_1, \beta_2)\}^2\right]^{1/2}}{n^{1/2}},$$

$$\bigcup_{(\beta_1,\beta_2)\in\Xi_{n,1-\vartheta_1}} \left\{\mathcal{B}_{n,1-\vartheta_2}(\beta_1, \beta_2), \infty\right\} = \left\{\inf_{(\beta_1,\beta_2)\in\Xi_{n,1-\vartheta_1}} \mathcal{B}_{n,1-\vartheta_2}(\beta_1, \beta_2), \infty\right\}.$$

Thus, an asymptotic α-level test of $H_0 : \mathcal{V}(d_*^{opt}) \leq B_0$ against the one-sided alternative $H_1 : \mathcal{V}(d_*^{opt}) > B_0$ rejects when

$$\inf_{(\beta_1,\beta_2)\in\Xi_{n,1-\vartheta_1}} \mathcal{B}_{n,1-\vartheta_2}(\beta_1,\beta_2) \geq B_0.$$

To see that this test attains nominal type I error under the null hypothesis, write

$$P\left\{\inf_{(\beta_1,\beta_2)\in\Xi_{n,1-\vartheta_1}} \mathcal{B}_{n,1-\vartheta_2}(\beta_1,\beta_2) \geq B_0\right\}$$

$$\leq P\left\{\inf_{(\beta_1,\beta_2)\in\Xi_{n,1-\vartheta_1}} \mathcal{B}_{n,1-\vartheta_2}(\beta_1,\beta_2) \geq \mathcal{V}(d_*^{opt})\right\}$$

$$\leq P\left\{\mathcal{B}_{n,1-\vartheta_2}(\beta_1^*,\beta_2^*) \geq \mathcal{V}(d_*^{opt})\right\} + \vartheta_1 + o(1)$$

$$= P\left(\frac{n^{1/2}\{\widehat{\mathcal{V}}_n^Q(\beta_1^*,\beta_2^*) - \mathcal{V}^Q(\beta_1^*,\beta_2^*)\}}{\left[\mathbb{P}_n\{\varrho(\beta_1^*,\beta_2^*) - \mathbb{P}_n\varrho(\beta_1^*,\beta_2^*)\}^2\right]^{1/2}} \geq z_{1-\vartheta_2}\right) + \vartheta_1 + o(1)$$

$$= \vartheta_2 + \vartheta_1 + o(1),$$

where the first inequality follows from the assumption that $\mathcal{V}(d_*^{opt}) \leq B_0$. The second inequality follows from partitioning the probability according to whether or not $(\beta_1^*,\beta_2^*) \in \Xi_{n,1-\vartheta_1}$; using $P\{(\beta_1^*,\beta_2^*) \in \Xi_{n,1-\vartheta_1}\} \geq 1 - \vartheta_1 + o(1)$ to bound the probability on the partition where $(\beta_1^*,\beta_2^*) \notin \Xi_{n,1-\vartheta_1}$; and by replacing the infimum over $\Xi_{n,1-\vartheta_1}$ with a single point in the set on the partition where $(\beta_1^*,\beta_2^*) \in \Xi_{n,1-\vartheta_1}$.

The power of this test is

$$P\left\{\inf_{(\beta_1,\beta_2)\in\Xi_{n,1-\vartheta_1}} \mathcal{B}_{n,1-\vartheta_2}(\beta_1,\beta_2) \geq B_0\right\}$$

$$= P\left\{\inf_{(\beta_1,\beta_2)\in\Xi_{n,1-\vartheta_1}} \left(\frac{n^{1/2}\left\{\widehat{\mathcal{V}}_n^Q(\beta_1,\beta_2) - \mathcal{V}^Q(\beta_1,\beta_2)\right\}}{\left[\mathbb{P}_n\{\varrho(\beta_1,\beta_2) - \mathbb{P}_n\varrho(\beta_1,\beta_2)\}^2\right]^{1/2}}\right.\right.$$

$$\left.\left. + \frac{n^{1/2}\left\{\mathcal{V}^Q(\beta_1,\beta_2) - B_0\right\}}{\left[\mathbb{P}_n\{\varrho(\beta_1,\beta_2) - \mathbb{P}_n\varrho(\beta_1,\beta_2)\}^2\right]^{1/2}}\right) \geq z_{1-\vartheta_2}\right\} \qquad (9.32)$$

$$\geq P\left\{\inf_{(\beta_1,\beta_2)\in\Xi_{n,1-\vartheta_1}} \left(\frac{n^{1/2}\left\{\widehat{\mathcal{V}}_n^Q(\beta_1,\beta_2) - \mathcal{V}^Q(\beta_1,\beta_2)\right\}}{\left[\mathbb{P}_n\{\varrho(\beta_1,\beta_2) - \mathbb{P}_n\varrho(\beta_1,\beta_2)\}^2\right]^{1/2}}\right.\right.$$

$$\left.\left. + \frac{\min\left[n^{1/2}\left\{\mathcal{V}^Q(\beta_1,\beta_2) - B_0\right\}, n^{1/2}\lambda\right]}{\left[\mathbb{P}_n\{\varrho(\beta_1,\beta_2) - \mathbb{P}_n\varrho(\beta_1,\beta_2)\}^2\right]^{1/2}}\right) \geq z_{1-\vartheta_2}\right\},$$

where the minimum taken in the last inequality plays the role of substituting the smallest allowable difference under the condition $\mathcal{V}(d_*^{opt}) - B_0 \geq \lambda$ in place of the actual effect size in a standard test. The distribution of the test statistic is complex, and it is not clear how to factor the preceding probability into terms involving the treatment effect, $\mathcal{V}^Q(\beta_1^*, \beta_2^*) - B_0$, and terms whose asymptotic behavior can be approximated in a closed form. Accordingly, we use the bootstrap with oversampling to estimate the power as a function of the sample size; this function can then be inverted to size a study so as to ensure that (P1) holds. We now sketch an argument showing that this same bootstrap procedure can also be used to ensure that (P2) holds.

We assume that pilot data $\mathbb{D}_0$ are available, comprising i.i.d. $(X_{1i}, A_{1i}, X_{2i}, A_{2i}, Y)$, $i = 1, \ldots, n_0$, from P. The bootstrap procedure described below is used to select a sample size $n \geq n_0$ such that one or both the conditions (P1) and (P2) hold. We make the following assumptions.

(PR1) $PY^2 \|B_2\|^2 < \infty$, and $P\|B_1\|^2 \|B_2\|^2 < \infty$.

(PR2) $PB_1 B_1^T$ and $PB_2 B_2^T$ are positive definite.

(PR3) $\inf_{(\beta_1, \beta_2) \in \Theta} P\left\{ \varrho(\beta_1, \beta_2) - P\varrho(\beta_1, \beta_2) \right\}^2 > 0$;

(PR4) The classes $\mathcal{F}_1 = \left\{ \varrho(\beta_1, \beta_2) : (\beta_1, \beta_2) \in \Theta \right\}$ and $\mathcal{F}_2 = \left\{ \varrho^2(\beta_1, \beta_2) : (\beta_1, \beta_2) \in \Theta \right\}$ are Donsker (van der Vaart and Wellner, 1996; Kosorok, 2007).

(PR5) $P\varrho(\beta_1, \beta_2)$ is uniformly continuous in a neighborhood of (β_1^*, β_2^*).

These assumptions are relatively mild and are analogous to those used in the context of asymptotic analyses of Q-learning with linear models (Laber et al., 2014c). The assumption (PR4) can be relaxed, although at the expense of more complex proofs; see Rose et al. (2019) for more general theoretical results.

Let $\mathbb{P}_{n,n_0}^{(b)}$ denote the bootstrap empirical distribution corresponding to a resample of size n drawn with replacement from $\mathbb{D}_0$. For any functional $Z_{n_0} = g(P, \mathbb{P}_{n_0})$, let $Z_{n,n_0}^{(b)} = g\left\{ \mathbb{P}_{n_0}, \mathbb{P}_{n,n_0}^{(b)} \right\}$. Let P_B denote the probability measure associated with bootstrap resampling conditional on the pilot data $\mathbb{D}_0$. The bootstrap estimator of the power (9.32) is

$$P_B \left\{ \inf_{(\beta_1, \beta_2) \in \Xi_{n_0, n, 1-\vartheta_1}^{(b)}} \left(\frac{n^{1/2} \left\{ \widehat{\mathcal{V}}_{n,n_0}^{Q(b)}(\beta_1, \beta_2) - \widehat{\mathcal{V}}_{n_0}^Q(\beta_1, \beta_2) \right\}}{\left[\mathbb{P}_{n,n_0}^{(b)} \left\{ \varrho(\beta_1, \beta_2) - \mathbb{P}_{n,n_0}^{(b)} \varrho(\beta_1, \beta_2) \right\}^2 \right]^{1/2}} \right. \right.$$

$$+ \frac{\min \left[n^{1/2} \left\{ \widehat{\mathcal{V}}_{n_0}^Q(\beta_1, \beta_2) - B_0 \right\}, n^{1/2}\lambda \right]}{\left[\mathbb{P}_{n,n_0}^{(b)} \left\{ \varrho(\beta_1, \beta_2) - \mathbb{P}_{n,n_0}^{(b)} \varrho(\beta_1, \beta_2) \right\}^2 \right]^{1/2}} \Bigg) \geq z_{1-\vartheta_2} \Bigg\},$$

which can be computed to arbitrary precision using Monte Carlo methods. The smallest integer n for which the bootstrap estimated power exceeds $1 - \beta$ is the estimated required sample size.

The following result characterizes the asymptotic behavior of the bootstrap estimated power. As above, we continue to take SUTVA, the SRA, and the positivity assumption to hold.

Theorem 9.5.3. *Assume (PR1)–(PR4). Let $\vartheta_1 \in (0,1)$ be fixed, and let $\varkappa$, L be arbitrary. Define*

$$\mathcal{J}_{n,n_0}^{(b)}(\beta_1, \beta_2) = \frac{n^{1/2} \left\{ \widehat{\mathcal{V}}_{n,n_0}^{(b)}(\beta_1, \beta_2) - \widehat{\mathcal{V}}_{n_0}(\beta_1, \beta_2) \right\}}{\left[\mathbb{P}_{n,n_0}^{(b)} \left\{ \varrho(\beta_1, \beta_2) - \mathbb{P}_{n,n_0}^{(b)} \varrho(\beta_1, \beta_2) \right\}^2 \right]^{1/2}}$$

and

$$\mathcal{J}_n(\beta_1, \beta_2) = \frac{n^{1/2} \left\{ \widehat{\mathcal{V}}_n(\beta_1, \beta_2) - \mathcal{V}^Q(\beta_1, \beta_2) \right\}}{\left[\mathbb{P}_n \left\{ \varrho(\beta_1, \beta_2) - \mathbb{P}_n \varrho(\beta_1, \beta_2) \right\}^2 \right]^{1/2}}.$$

Then

$$\lim_{n,n_0 \to \infty} P \Bigg[\sup_{|v| \leq L} \Bigg| P_B \Bigg\{ \inf_{(\beta_1, \beta_2) \in \Xi_{n_0, n, 1-\vartheta_1}^{(b)}} \mathcal{J}_{n,n_0}^{(b)}(\beta_1, \beta_2) \geq v \Bigg\}$$

$$- P \Bigg\{ \inf_{(\beta_1, \beta_2) \in \Xi_{n, 1-\vartheta_1}} \mathcal{J}_n(\beta_1, \beta_2) \geq v \Bigg\} \Bigg| > \varkappa \Bigg] = 0.$$

The preceding result does not include the term

$$\frac{n^{1/2} \left\{ \widehat{\mathcal{V}}_n^Q(\beta_1, \beta_2) - B_0 \right\}}{\left[\mathbb{P}_n \left\{ \varrho(\beta_1, \beta_2) - \mathbb{P}_n \varrho(\beta_1, \beta_2) \right\}^2 \right]^{1/2}}$$

or its bootstrap analog, as these terms diverge to positive infinity under the alternative provided that $\mathcal{V}^Q(\beta_1, \beta_2)$ is bounded away from B_0 for all (β_1, β_2) in a sufficiently small neighborhood of (β_1^*, β_2^*); see Rose et al. (2019) for additional technical results, including those under local alternatives.

To select a sample size that ensures (P2), we use the following bound. Let $(\tilde{\beta}_{1,n}, \tilde{\beta}_{2,n}) \in \Xi_{n,1-\vartheta_1}$ satisfy $\widehat{\mathcal{V}}_n^Q(\beta_1^*, \beta_2^*) \leq \widehat{\mathcal{V}}_n^Q(\tilde{\beta}_{1,n}, \tilde{\beta}_{2,n}) + o_P(1/n^{1/2})$. Then

$$P\left[\mathcal{V}^Q(\tilde{\beta}_{1,n}, \tilde{\beta}_{2,n}) \geq \mathcal{V}^Q(d_*^{opt})\right.$$

$$+ \inf_{(\beta_1,\beta_2) \in \Xi_{n,1-\vartheta_1}} \left\{\widehat{\mathcal{V}}_n^Q(\beta_1, \beta_2) - \mathcal{V}^Q(\beta_1, \beta_2)\right\}$$

$$- \sup_{(\beta_1,\beta_2) \in \Xi_{n,1-\vartheta_1}} \left\{\widehat{\mathcal{V}}_n^Q(\beta_1, \beta_2) - \mathcal{V}^Q(\beta_1, \beta_2)\right\}\right]$$

$$\geq 1 - \vartheta_1 + o(1).$$

Let $\mathfrak{Q}_{n,1-\vartheta_2,1-\vartheta_1}$ be the $(1-\vartheta_2) \times 100$ percentile of

$$\inf_{(\beta_1,\beta_2) \in \Xi_{n,1-\vartheta_1}} \left\{\widehat{\mathcal{V}}_n^Q(\beta_1, \beta_2) - \mathcal{V}^Q(\beta_1, \beta_2)\right\}$$

$$- \sup_{(\beta_1,\beta_2) \in \Xi_{n,1-\vartheta_1}} \left\{\widehat{\mathcal{V}}_n^Q(\beta_1, \beta_2) - \mathcal{V}^Q(\beta_1, \beta_2)\right\}.$$

Then, provided that $\vartheta_1 + \vartheta_2 \leq \zeta$, setting

$$n = \left\lceil \left(\mathfrak{Q}_{n,1-\vartheta_2,1-\vartheta_1}/\epsilon\right)^2 \right\rceil$$

satisfies (P2). In practice, $\mathfrak{Q}_{n,1-\vartheta_2,1-\vartheta_1}$ is not known; it can be estimated using the bootstrap, so that

$$n = \left\lceil \left(\mathfrak{Q}_{n,1-\vartheta_2,1-\vartheta_1}^{(b)}/\epsilon\right)^2 \right\rceil.$$

See Rose et al. (2019) for further details and proofs.

Remark. Rose et al. (2019) present an extensive suite of simulation studies to evaluate the performance of the normality-based sample size procedure in Section 9.5.1 and the project-based procedure discussed here under a range of conditions. Performance is measured in terms of the criteria (P1) and (P2) and on the basis of the sample size required to estimate and/or evaluate a optimal regime relative to that relative to compare fixed/embedded regimes. Interestingly, and perhaps surprisingly, under the normality-based procedure, the sample size required to guarantee (P1) and (P2) when the underlying model is correctly specified can be considerably smaller than that required to identify an optimal fixed, embedded regime from among those in the SMART provided that a high-quality estimator for σ^2 is available and the true difference between the values attained by an optimal regime and an optimal fixed regime among those embedded in the trial is reasonably large. See Rose et al. (2019) for further discussion of evaluation of performance and implications for practice.

9.6   Extensions and Further Reading

In this chapter, we have presented an overview of fundamental principles and methods for the design and analysis of SMARTs. There is a robust literature on SMARTs; in addition to the references already cited, we provide a nonexhaustive list here. Introductory articles focused on practitioners include Lei et al. (2011), Almirall et al. (2012a), Nahum-Shani et al. (2012a), Almirall et al. (2014), and Kidwell (2014). See Oetting et al. (2011), Almirall et al. (2012b), Nahum-Shani et al. (2012b), and Collins et al. (2014), and Wallace et al. (2016) for accounts of design and analysis methodology.

As interest in conducting SMARTs continues to increase, new methodological developments will be necessary. In principle, SMARTs can be generalized in essentially all of the same ways as a standard k-arm randomized clinical trial, albeit with additional complications due to the sequential randomization. We comment briefly on some key issues for which nontrivial extensions of the methodology discussed in this chapter are required.

In Sections 9.3 and 9.4, we have reviewed both standard and more advanced approaches to sizing a SMART based on comparisons among treatment options at a given stage or on comparisons among embedded regimes, while Section 9.5 proposes methods for sample size determination when estimation of an optimal regime is the primary focus. Additional criteria are discussed by Oetting et al. (2011). Depending on the domain context, there may be alternative criteria for which sample size procedures must be developed.

As with conventional randomized clinical trials, dropout and more generally missing data pose a recurring challenge. In the context of a SMART, dropout complicates standard analyses because subjects who drop out do not reach the entire sequence of decision points. There is relatively little literature on methodology for handling missing information in a SMART. Shortreed et al. (2014) propose a multiple imputation strategy that enables principled analysis under the assumption that missingness is at random. Under these conditions, an alternative approach is to implement inverse probability weighting by the probability of dropout, analogous to the inverse probability of censoring weighting used in Sections 8.3.3 and 8.3.5, in the spirit of Robins et al. (1995). Liu et al. (2017) propose a stage-wise enrichment design for two-stage SMARTs that may address problems of attrition after the first stage.

As with conventional clinical trials with a single point of randomization, there are compelling reasons to consider adaptive randomization in a SMART. In a standard adaptively randomized clinical trial, the randomization probabilities are updated as information from previous participants accumulates on the relative benefits of the treatment options under study (Berry and Fristedt, 1985). In an adaptively randomized trial, the randomization probabilities must balance the estimated benefit to a subject being assigned a particular treatment option against the information gained to be from this assignment and the potential benefit of this information to future participants. That is, there is a tradeoff between efficiency of inferences and ethical considerations, as it is well known that the most efficient design randomizes subjects among the treatment options under study with equal probabilities, but this may not be ethical if preliminary results suggest that some options are less beneficial than others. Development of adaptive randomization strategies for SMARTs involves further complications, again owing to the sequential randomization. As discussed in Section 9.2.4, a SMART can be represented as either a sequence of possibly outcome-dependent randomizations or as a single randomization among the design's embedded regimes; accordingly, adaptive randomization strategies can be developed based on either perspective. See Cheung et al. (2015) for a proposed approach of the former type based on Q-learning and Lin et al. (2019) for an example of the latter.

Chapter 10

Statistical Inference

10.1 Introduction

Statistical analyses of treatment regimes can be motivated by a wide range of scientific objectives. These include: (i) identifying key tailoring variables; i.e., patient characteristics that are necessary for making high-quality treatment recommendations; (ii) evaluating the performance of a true optimal treatment regime; i.e., quantifying the potential benefits of using an optimal regime to treat the patient population in a given disease or disorder context; (iii) evaluating the performance of an estimated optimal regime; i.e., quantifying the benefits of applying a regime estimated using observed data in hand; and (iv) comparing the performance of two or more fixed, given regimes or two or more estimated regimes. When using observed data to address these objectives, measures of statistical uncertainty are required. In this chapter, we quantify uncertainty primarily through confidence sets for the quantity; i.e., estimand, of interest, although we also touch on hypothesis testing.

A standard approach to constructing confidence sets is through an asymptotic approximation to the sampling distribution of an estimator for the targeted estimand. For example, to compare two fixed, given regimes d and $\tilde{d}$, we might choose a level $\alpha \in (0,1)$; construct a $(1 - \alpha) \times 100\%$ confidence interval for the difference in their values, $\Delta(d, \tilde{d}) = \mathcal{V}(d) - \mathcal{V}(\tilde{d})$; and conclude that the regimes have different values if the interval does not contain zero. Define $\widehat{\Delta}_n(d, \tilde{d}) = \widehat{\mathcal{V}}_n(d) - \widehat{\mathcal{V}}_n(\tilde{d})$, where $\widehat{\mathcal{V}}_n(d)$ is an estimator for the value $\mathcal{V}(d)$ of a given regime d, such as the simple or augmented inverse probability weighted estimators (3.24) or (3.30) for a single decision problem. Here, the subscript n emphasizes the dependence of the estimator on the sample size. A confidence set for $\Delta(d, \tilde{d})$ can be constructed using the asymptotic distribution of $n^{1/2}\{\widehat{\Delta}_n(d, \tilde{d}) - \Delta(d, \tilde{d})\}$, which, from the discussion in Section 3.3, is often a normal distribution following from the theory of M-estimation reviewed in Section 2.5. For example, letting $\ell_{\alpha/2}$ and $u_{1-\alpha/2}$ denote the $(\alpha/2) \times 100$ and $(1 - \alpha/2) \times 100$ percentiles of this asymptotic distribution, $[\widehat{\Delta}_n(d, \tilde{d}) - u_{1-\alpha/2}n^{-1/2}, \ \widehat{\Delta}_n(d, \tilde{d}) - \ell_{\alpha/2}n^{-1/2}]$ is a valid asymptotic $(1 - \alpha) \times 100\%$ confidence set.

Unfortunately, the preceding approach fails for many estimands of interest in the context of treatment regimes. The reason for this is that these estimands are nonsmooth functionals of the underlying generative distribution. A consequence of this nonsmoothness is that there are no regular; i.e., locally uniformly convergent (defined formally below), or asymptotically unbiased estimators for these estimands (van der Vaart, 1991; Hirano and Porter, 2012). Thus, any estimator we might use for one of these estimands need not converge uniformly over local neighborhoods of the targeted estimand. The practical implication (of this seemingly technical issue) is that standard asymptotic methods for approximating the sampling distribution of a nonregular estimator, such as normal approximations or the bootstrap, can be quite poor, and consequently inference based on these approximations may not be reliable. The phenomenon of nonregularity of estimators for the value of an optimal regime is demonstrated in simple special cases in the context of a single decision in Sections 3.5.1 and 3.5.3.

Several proposed approaches to constructing valid confidence sets for nonsmooth estimands in the context of treatment regimes have been proposed in the literature. These include subsampling (Chakraborty et al., 2014a,b), projection sets (Robins, 2004), bounding (Laber and Murphy, 2011; Laber et al., 2014c), and regularization (Chakraborty et al., 2010; Moodie and Richardson, 2010; Song et al., 2015; Goldberg et al., 2013). However, there is no established consensus regarding which of these methods is best. Projection sets and bounding approaches have strong theoretical guarantees of performance, but can be cumbersome to implement and may overestimate uncertainty. Subsampling is simple to implement and enjoys some theoretical guarantees, but can be highly sensitive to the choice of tuning parameters. Regularization can improve the empirical performance of bootstrap confidence intervals in some settings; however, it does not guarantee correct coverage and can induce unbounded asymptotic bias (Laber et al., 2014c).

This chapter concerns asymptotic behavior under violation of smoothness assumptions that are assumed as a matter of course in most asymptotic analyses, where by "asymptotic" we mean that the size n of the sample of observed data grows large; i.e., $n \to \infty$. Not surprisingly, the nature of this material makes this chapter admittedly more technical than the rest of the book. Accordingly, readers may approach this chapter in different ways depending on their backgrounds. Because the material involves asymptotic theoretical results, the presentation assumes that all readers are comfortable with standard large sample theory concepts such as stochastic convergence and order in probability. To introduce all readers to the salient features of inference for nonsmooth functionals, which may be unfamiliar to most, the chapter begins in Section 10.2 with a review of these features through an illustrative example, that of constructing confidence intervals for the component-wise maximum of a mean vector. This simple example allows us to examine both the implications of nonsmoothness and the implementation of methods for constructing confidence sets.

For the reader whose main objective is to achieve a basic appreciation of the challenges involved in statistical inference for treatment regimes, coverage of this section, along with Section 10.3.1 and the introduction to Section 10.3.2 in Section 10.3, which focus on the single decision problem, may be sufficient. This reader may also wish to review Section 10.4.1, which extends some of the material in Section 10.3.1 to the multiple decision case and thus demonstrates the additional challenges involved. In approaching all of this material, this reader may wish to downplay study of the details in favor of focusing on the "big picture" implications.

A reader whose goal is a deep understanding of the theoretical underpinnings will wish to study all of the above and all of Section 10.3 and Section 10.4. It may be beneficial to read this material first at a higher level to attain an overarching perspective, skipping derivations and proofs, followed by a subsequent reading focused on the details.

Remark. Throughout this chapter, we use alternative notation so as to match the literature on inference for treatment regimes and to make the required expressions more compact. In particular, we use so-called operator notation; e.g., for an i.i.d. sample $Z_1, \ldots, Z_n$ drawn from fixed but unknown distribution P, we write $Pf(Z)$ to denote $\int f(z) \, dP(z)$ and $\mathbb{P}_n f(Z) = n^{-1} \sum_{i=1}^{n} f(Z_i)$. If $\widehat{\theta} \in \Theta$ is a random variable constructed from the sample $Z_1, \ldots, Z_n$ and f is a parametric function indexed by $\theta \in \Theta$, then $Pf(Z; \widehat{\theta}) = \int f(z; \widehat{\theta}) dP(z)$ and $\mathbb{P}_n f(Z; \widehat{\theta}) = n^{-1} \sum_{i=1}^{n} f(Z_i; \widehat{\theta})$, so that the expectation is only with respect to the distribution P (or $\mathbb{P}_n$) and not uncertainty in $\widehat{\theta}$. In contrast, we use the more typical expectation operator, E, to denote expectation over all sources of uncertainty. We write $\rightsquigarrow$ to denote convergence in distribution and often add a subscript to indicate the size of the sample used to construct an estimator, as for $\widehat{\mathcal{V}}_n(d)$ above. Thus, for example, we write $\overline{Z}_n = \mathbb{P}_n Z$, so that $n^{1/2}(\mathbb{P}_n - P)Z = n^{1/2}(\overline{Z}_n - \mu_0)$ for $\mu_0 = PZ$. For a function f, we often write $x \mapsto f(x)$ to indicate that $f(x)$ is the image of x under the mapping f. We also make use of the nabla operator to streamline expressions; e.g., for parameter ζ and real-valued $f(\cdot; \zeta)$, $\nabla_\zeta f(\cdot; \zeta^*)$ is the vector $\partial f(\cdot; \zeta)/\partial \zeta$ of partial derivatives with respect to the components of ζ (the gradient) evaluated at ζ^*.

10.2   Nonsmoothness and Statistical Inference

As noted above, in this section, we demonstrate the challenges of inference for nonsmooth functionals through the simple illustrative example of constructing confidence intervals for the component-wise maximum of a mean vector. For this demonstration, suppose that the observed data are $X_1, \ldots, X_n$, which comprise n i.i.d. copies of a random vector $X \in \mathbb{R}^p$ drawn from an unknown distribution P. Let $\mu_0 = PX = (\mu_{0,1}, \ldots, \mu_{0,p})^T$ denote the mean of X, and define

$$\theta_0 = \bigvee_{j=1}^{p} \mu_{0,j} = \max(\mu_{0,1}, \ldots, \mu_{0,p})$$

to be the component-wise maximum of μ_0. We consider the problem of constructing a confidence interval for θ_0, where, to avoid the trivial case, we assume $p \geq 2$. To see why this estimand is of interest in the context of treatment regimes, consider a single decision problem in which there are no patient covariates and there are p treatment options. Let $\mu_{0,j}$ denote the mean (expected) outcome under treatment option j. An optimal regime assigns all patients to $\arg\max_j \mu_{0,j}$, and the value of an optimal regime is $\theta_0 = \bigvee_{j=1}^{p} \mu_{0,j}$.

Define $\widehat{\mu}_n = \mathbb{P}_n X = n^{-1} \sum_{i=1}^{n} X_i = (\widehat{\mu}_{n,1}, \ldots, \widehat{\mu}_{n,p})^T$, and let $\widehat{\theta}_n = \bigvee_{j=1}^{p} \widehat{\mu}_{n,j}$. A standard (fixed alternatives) asymptotic confidence set for θ_0 is based on the limiting distribution of $n^{1/2}(\widehat{\theta}_n - \theta_0)$. For any $\nu \in \mathbb{R}^p$, define the set

$$\mathfrak{U}(\nu) = \arg\max_j \nu_j; \tag{10.1}$$

note that $\mathfrak{U}(\nu)$ in (10.1) may contain more than one element if more than one component of ν achieves the component-wise maximum.

The following result characterizes the limiting distribution of $n^{1/2}(\widehat{\theta}_n - \theta_0)$.

Lemma 10.2.1. *Assume regularity conditions ensuring that $n^{1/2}(\mathbb{P}_n - P)X$ is asymptotically normal with mean zero and covariance matrix Σ. Then*

$$n^{1/2}(\widehat{\theta}_n - \theta_0) \rightsquigarrow \bigvee_{j \in \mathfrak{U}(\mu_0)} Z_j,$$

where $Z \sim \mathcal{N}(0, \Sigma)$.

Proof. Let $\mathcal{E}_n$ denote $\mathrm{I}\{\max_{k \notin \mathfrak{U}(\mu_0)} \widehat{\mu}_{n,k} \geq \max_{j \in \mathfrak{U}(\mu_0)} \widehat{\mu}_{n,j}\}$. Then $\mathcal{E}_n = o_P(1)$. Write

$$n^{1/2}(\widehat{\theta}_n - \theta_0) = \bigvee_{j \in \mathfrak{U}(\mu_0)} n^{1/2}(\widehat{\mu}_{n,j} - \theta_0)$$

$$+ \left\{ \bigvee_{k \notin \mathfrak{U}(\mu_0)} n^{1/2}(\widehat{\mu}_{n,k} - \theta_0) - \bigvee_{j \in \mathfrak{U}(\mu_0)} n^{1/2}(\widehat{\mu}_{n,j} - \theta_0) \right\} \mathcal{E}_n.$$

Because $\mu_{0,j} = \theta_0$ for all $j \in \mathfrak{U}(\mu_0)$, the first term on the right-hand side converges to the desired limit by the continuous mapping theorem (e.g., van der Vaart, 2000, Theorem 2.3; see Section 3.5.1). The second term is bounded below by zero and is bounded above by

$$\left\{ \bigvee_{k \notin \mathfrak{U}(\mu_0)} n^{1/2}(\widehat{\mu}_{n,k} - \mu_{0,k}) - \bigvee_{j \in \mathfrak{U}(\mu_0)} n^{1/2}(\widehat{\mu}_{n,j} - \theta_0) \right\} \mathcal{E}_n$$

$$\leq 2 \bigvee_{j=1}^{p} \left| n^{1/2}(\widehat{\mu}_{n,j} - \mu_{0,j}) \right| \mathcal{E}_n = o_P(1),$$

where the inequality follows from replacing θ_0 with $\mu_{0,k}$ for each $k \notin \mathfrak{U}(\mu_0)$, using $\mu_{0,j} = \theta_0$ for all $j \in \mathfrak{U}(\mu_0)$, and applying the triangle inequality. □

Lemma 10.2.1 shows that the limiting distribution of $n^{1/2}(\widehat{\theta}_n - \theta_0)$ depends abruptly on μ_0; e.g., if $\mu_0 = (0,0)^T$ and $\Sigma = I_2$, then the limiting distribution of $n^{1/2}(\widehat{\theta}_n - \theta_0)$ is the maximum of two independent standard normals, whereas if $\mu_0 = (0, \epsilon)$ for *any* $\epsilon > 0$, say $\epsilon = 10^{-15}$, the limiting distribution is standard normal! Thus, the limiting distribution of $n^{1/2}(\widehat{\theta}_n - \theta_0)$ depends only on the submatrix of Σ corresponding to elements in $\mathfrak{U}(\mu_0)$ and not the gaps between elements in μ_0 and θ_0. However, the finite sample distribution of $n^{1/2}(\widehat{\theta}_n - \theta_0)$ can depend critically on these gaps. For example, consider the case where $X \sim \mathcal{N}(\mu_0, I_p)$, where I_p is a $(p \times p)$ identity matrix, and μ_0 has a unique maximizer $\mu_{0,1}$, say. As in Chapter 3, let $\Phi(\cdot)$ denote the cumulative distribution function of a standard normal random variable. In this setting, it can be shown that $P\{n^{1/2}(\widehat{\theta}_n - \theta_0) \leq t\} = \Phi(t) \prod_{j=2}^{p} \Phi\{t + n^{1/2}(\theta_0 - \mu_{0,j})\}$. If some of the gaps, $\theta_0 - \mu_{0,j}$ $j = 2,\ldots,p$, are small relative to $n^{1/2}$, then $P\{n^{1/2}(\widehat{\theta}_n - \theta_0) \leq t\}$ can be quite far from its limiting value $\Phi(t)$. Figure 10.1 compares the finite sample distribution of $n^{1/2}(\widehat{\theta}_n - \theta_0)$ with its limiting distribution as a function of the gaps $\theta_0 - \mu_{0,j}$ for $j \in \mathfrak{U}(\mu_0)$. As anticipated by Lemma 10.2.1, an asymptotic approximation performs poorly when these gaps are small.

Intuitively, the asymptotic approximation is poor because it fails to capture uncertainty about the set $\mathfrak{U}(\mu_0)$. In finite samples, this set is unknown, and, as shown in Figure 10.1, unless there is a unique and well-separated maximizer, uncertainty about this set can have a profound impact on the finite sample distribution of $n^{1/2}(\widehat{\theta}_n - \theta_0)$. However, in the asymptotic framework used in Lemma 10.2.1, there is no uncertainty about $\mathfrak{U}(\mu_0)$ because as $n \to \infty$ the power to test $H_{0,j} : \mu_{0,j} \in \mathfrak{U}(\mu_0)$ goes to one. Thus, there is mismatch between this asymptotic framework and the finite sample behavior of the estimator.

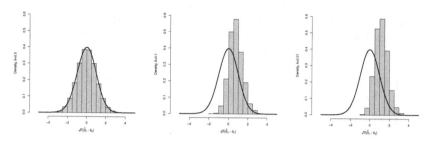

Figure 10.1 *Quality of an asymptotic normal approximation to the sampling distribution of $\widehat{\theta}_n$ when there is a unique maximizer. The histogram shows the true sampling distribution of $n^{1/2}(\widehat{\theta}_n - \theta_0)$ for $n = 100$ when $X_1, \ldots, X_n$ are i.i.d. $\mathcal{N}(\mu, I_6)$, with $\mu_1 = 2$ and $\mu_j = 2 - \delta$ for $j = 2, \ldots, 6$. From left to right, the values of δ are 0.5, 0.1, and 0.01. The solid line denotes the density of the limiting distribution of $n^{1/2}(\widehat{\theta}_n - \theta_0)$, which is standard normal in all cases considered. The quality of the normal approximation becomes increasingly poor as the value of δ shrinks toward zero.*

Accordingly, an asymptotic framework that faithfully captures uncertainty about the set $\mathfrak{U}(\mu_0)$ is required. Local or moving parameter asymptotics are such a framework. In a local asymptotic framework, the true generative model is allowed to change with the sample size so that asymptotic approximations retain key features of the finite sample distribution. In our illustrative example, we ensure that uncertainty about the set $\mathfrak{U}(\mu_0)$ persists even as the sample size grows by allowing the gaps $\theta_0 - \max_{j \notin \mathfrak{U}(\mu_0)} \mu_{0,j}$ to shrink toward zero as n increases.

Suppose that for each n the observed data are $X_{n,1} \ldots, X_{n,n}$, which comprise n i.i.d. copies of $X \in \mathbb{R}^p$ drawn from an unknown distribution P_n. Thus, the underlying generative distribution changes as a function of the sample size (see Chapter 3.10 of van der Vaart and Wellner, 1996). A generative model of this type is said to form a triangular array, as it can be visualized as stacking vectors of increasing length to form a triangle, as shown in Figure 10.2. Let $\mu_{0,n} = P_n X = (\mu_{0,n,1}, \ldots, \mu_{0,n,p})^T$ and $\theta_{0,n} = \bigvee_{j=1}^p \mu_{0,n,j}$ be the analogs of μ_0 and θ_0 under P_n. Assume that

$$\mu_{0,n} = \mu_0 + sn^{-1/2},$$

where $s \in \mathbb{R}^p$ is a fixed vector referred to as a local parameter. In addition, assume that $n^{1/2}(\mathbb{P}_n - P_n)X$ is asymptotically normal with mean zero and covariance matrix Σ, where now $\mathbb{P}_n X = n^{-1} \sum_{i=1}^n X_{n,i}$. As we now observe, the limiting behavior of $n^{1/2}(\widehat{\theta}_n - \theta_{0,n})$ under P_n anticipates the mismatch between the finite sample and asymptotic approximation

Observations					Distribution
$X_{1,1}$					P_1
$X_{2,1}$	$X_{2,2}$				P_2
$X_{3,1}$	$X_{3,2}$	$X_{3,3}$			P_3
$X_{4,1}$	$X_{4,2}$	$X_{4,3}$	$X_{4,4}$		P_4
$\vdots$	$\vdots$	$\vdots$	$\vdots$	$\ddots$	$\vdots$

Figure 10.2 *Schematic for the triangular array* $\{X_{n,i}\}_{i=1}^n$, *where* $X_{n,1}, \ldots, X_{n,n}$ *are drawn i.i.d. from* P_n *for each* n.

depicted in Figure 10.1. The following is an analog of Lemma 10.2.1 under a local asymptotic framework.

Lemma 10.2.2. *Let* $s \in \mathbb{R}^p$ *be fixed. Assume that for each* n *we observe* $\{X_{n,i}\}_{i=1}^n$, *drawn i.i.d. from* P_n, *which satisfy (i)* $P_n X = \mu_0 + sn^{-1/2}$, *and (ii)* $n^{1/2}(\mathbb{P}_n - P_n)X \rightsquigarrow \mathcal{N}(0, \Sigma)$. *Then, under* P_n,

$$n^{1/2}(\widehat{\theta}_n - \theta_{0,n}) \rightsquigarrow \bigvee_{j \in \mathfrak{U}(\mu_0)} \{Z_j + s_j\} - \bigvee_{j \in \mathfrak{U}(\mu_0)} s_j,$$

where $Z \sim \mathcal{N}(0, \Sigma)$.

Proof. Let $\mathcal{E}_n$ be as defined in the proof of Lemma 10.2.1. Then $\mathcal{E}_n = o_{P_n}(1)$. Thus, for n sufficiently large so that $\bigvee_{j=1}^p \mu_{0,n,j} = \bigvee_{j \in \mathfrak{U}(\mu_0)} \mu_{0,n,j}$,

$$n^{1/2}(\widehat{\theta}_n - \theta_{0,n}) = n^{1/2}\left(\bigvee_{j \in \mathfrak{U}(\mu_0)} \widehat{\mu}_{n,j} - \bigvee_{j \in \mathfrak{U}(\mu_0)} \mu_{0,n,j}\right)$$

$$+ n^{1/2}\left(\bigvee_{j \notin \mathfrak{U}(\mu_0)} \widehat{\mu}_{n,j} - \bigvee_{k \in \mathfrak{U}(\mu_0)} \widehat{\mu}_{n,k}\right) \mathcal{E}_n.$$

The preceding expression is equal to

$$\bigvee_{j \in \mathfrak{U}(\mu_0)} \left\{n^{1/2}(\widehat{\mu}_{n,j} - \mu_{0,n,j}) + s_j\right\} - \bigvee_{j \in \mathfrak{U}(\mu_0)} s_j$$

$$+ n^{1/2}\left(\bigvee_{j \notin \mathfrak{U}(\mu_0)} \widehat{\mu}_{n,j} - \bigvee_{k \in \mathfrak{U}(\mu_0)} \widehat{\mu}_{n,k}\right) \mathcal{E}_n.$$

The result follows from the continuous mapping theorem provided we can show that the last term in the foregoing expression is $o_{P_n}(1)$. To see that this condition holds, write

$$0 \le n^{1/2} \left(\bigvee_{j \notin \mathfrak{U}(\mu_0)} \widehat{\mu}_{n,j} - \bigvee_{k \in \mathfrak{U}(\mu_0)} \widehat{\mu}_{n,k} \right) \mathcal{E}_n \le \left[\bigvee_{j \notin \mathfrak{U}(\mu_0)} n^{1/2} \left(\widehat{\mu}_{n,j} - \mu_{0,n,j} \right) \right.$$

$$\left. - \bigvee_{k \in \mathfrak{U}(\mu_0)} \left\{ n^{1/2} \left(\widehat{\mu}_{n,k} - \mu_{0,n,k} \right) - \left(\max_{j \in \mathfrak{U}(\mu_0)} s_j - s_k \right) \right\} \right] \mathcal{E}_n,$$

where the rightmost term is bounded above by $2\{ \bigvee_{j=1}^{p} |n^{1/2}(\widehat{\mu}_{n,j} - \mu_{0,n,j})| + \max_{j,k} |s_j - s_k| \} \mathcal{E}_n = o_{P_n}(1)$. □

Lemma 10.2.2 demonstrates that the sampling distribution of $\widehat{\theta}_n$ is sensitive to $n^{-1/2}$-perturbations of the underlying generative model. When the limiting distribution of a centered and scaled estimator such as $n^{1/2}(\widehat{\theta}_n - \theta_{0,n})$ depends on a $n^{-1/2}$-perturbation of the generative distribution, it is said to be nonregular (Tsiatis, 2006, Chapter 3). However, the problem is not a consequence of a poor choice of estimator, $\widehat{\theta}_n$, but rather the nonsmoothness of the θ_0 as a functional of P (Hirano and Porter, 2012). Indeed, as mentioned at the beginning of this chapter, no regular estimator for θ_0 exists, so the problem of nonregularity cannot be avoided through the choice of a clever estimator.

Confidence Sets for the Maximum of a Mean Vector

The focus of this chapter is on asymptotically valid confidence sets for nonsmooth functionals arising the context of treatment regimes. As a preview for this material, we briefly illustrate the methods that will be developed in detail later in this chapter to construct confidence sets for θ_0.

The simplest, asymptotically correct confidence set for θ_0 is a projection set. Let $\alpha \in (0,1)$ denote the desired error level; e.g., $\alpha = 0.05$ corresponds to a 95% confidence set. Let $\zeta_{n,1-\alpha}$ denote a $(1-\alpha) \times 100\%$ confidence set for μ_0, such as a Wald-type confidence set

$$\zeta_{n,1-\alpha} = \{ \mu \in \mathbb{R}^p : n(\widehat{\mu}_n - \mu)^T \widehat{\Sigma}_n^{-1} (\widehat{\mu}_n - \mu) \le \chi^2_{p,1-\alpha} \},$$

where $\widehat{\Sigma}_n = \mathbb{P}_n (X - \widehat{\mu}_n)(X - \widehat{\mu}_n)^T$, and $\chi^2_{p,1-\alpha}$ is the $(1-\alpha) \times 100$ percentile of a χ^2-distribution with p degrees of freedom. The projection confidence set

$$\Gamma_{n,1-\alpha} = \left\{ \theta \in \mathbb{R} : \theta = \bigvee_{j=1}^{p} \mu_j \text{ for some } \mu \in \zeta_{n,1-\alpha} \right\} \tag{10.2}$$

is a valid confidence interval for θ_0. To see this, write

$$P\left(\theta_0 \notin \Gamma_{n,1-\alpha}\right) = P\left(\theta_0 \notin \Gamma_{n,1-\alpha}, \, \mu_0 \notin \zeta_{n,1-\alpha}\right)$$
$$+ P\left(\theta_0 \notin \Gamma_{n,1-\alpha}, \, \mu_0 \in \zeta_{n,1-\alpha}\right),$$

where the second term on the right-hand side of the above display is zero. Thus, $P\left(\theta_0 \notin \Gamma_{n,1-\alpha}\right) \leq P\left(\mu_0 \notin \zeta_{n,1-\alpha}\right) \leq \alpha + o(1)$.

Projection sets can be applied when the functional of interest can be written as a nonsmooth function of a smooth functional; e.g., the component-wise maximum of a mean. We demonstrate shortly that constructing projection sets becomes more complex as we consider functionals that arise in the study of multiple decision treatment regimes. Furthermore, in these settings, projection sets can become extremely conservative (Laber et al., 2014c); later in this chapter, we derive adaptive projection sets that use pretesting to reduce conservatism.

An alternative approach to constructing confidence sets for nonsmooth functionals is to bound the functional of interest between two smooth functionals and then apply standard inference methods to the bounds; e.g., the bootstrap or a series approximation. Confidence sets constructed in this way are called adaptive confidence sets (Laber and Murphy, 2011; Laber et al., 2014c; McKeague and Qian, 2015). Because we are interested in the limiting distribution of the bounds, they are typically constructed to contain the centered and scaled estimator; in our illustrative example, we thus construct bounds on $n^{1/2}(\widehat{\theta}_n - \theta_0)$.

Let $\{\tau_n\}_{n \geq 1}$ be a sequence of positive constants satisfying $\tau_n \to \infty$ and $\tau_n = o(n^{1/2})$ as $n \to \infty$, and let $\widehat{\sigma}_{j,k}^2$ denote an estimator for $n \operatorname{var}(\widehat{\mu}_{n,j} - \widehat{\mu}_{n,k})$. Define $\widehat{\mathfrak{U}}_n(\mu_0) = \{j : \max_k n^{1/2}(\widehat{\mu}_{n,k} - \widehat{\mu}_{n,j})/\widehat{\sigma}_{j,k} \leq \tau_n\}$, and let $\widehat{\mathcal{S}}_n(\mu_0) = \{s \in \mathbb{R}^p : s_j = \mu_{0,j} \text{ if } j \notin \widehat{\mathfrak{U}}_n(\mu_0)\}$. Then

$$\widehat{U}_n = \sup_{s \in \widehat{\mathcal{S}}_n(\mu_0)} n^{1/2} \left\{ \bigvee_{j=1}^p \left(\widehat{\mu}_{n,j} - \mu_{0,j} + s_j\right) - \bigvee_{j=1}^p s_j \right\}$$

is an upper bound on $n^{1/2}(\widehat{\theta}_n - \theta_0)$, as $\mu_0 \in \widehat{\mathcal{S}}_n(\mu_0)$. A lower bound, $\widehat{L}_n$, can be constructed by replacing the supremum with an infimum in the above expression. These bounds can be viewed as taking the sup (inf) over all $n^{-1/2}$-perturbations of $n^{1/2}(\widehat{\mu}_{n,j} - \mu_{0,j})$ for all $j = 1, \ldots, p$ in which there is insufficient evidence to reject the hypothesis $j \in \mathfrak{U}(\mu_0)$. From this perspective, $\widehat{\mathfrak{U}}_n(\mu_0)$ is a conservative estimator for $\mathfrak{U}(\mu_0)$; and, for each $j \in \mathfrak{U}(\mu_0)$, we have written $n^{1/2}\widehat{\mu}_{n,j} = n^{1/2}(\widehat{\mu}_{n,j} - \mu_{0,j}) + n^{1/2}\mu_{0,j}$ as the sum of a regular, asymptotically normal term and an unknown parameter. If we consider a local parameter sequence such that $\mu_{0,n,j} = \theta_0 + s_j n^{-1/2}$ for each $j \in \widehat{\mathfrak{U}}_n(\mu_0)$, then

$$n^{1/2} \left(\bigvee_{j \in \widehat{\mathfrak{U}}_n(\mu_0)} \widehat{\mu}_{n,j} - \bigvee_{j \in \widehat{\mathfrak{U}}_n(\mu_0)} \mu_{0,n,j} \right)$$

$$= n^{1/2} \left\{ \bigvee_{j \in \widehat{\mathfrak{U}}_n(\mu_0)} \widehat{\mu}_{n,j} - \bigvee_{j \in \widehat{\mathfrak{U}}_n(\mu_0)} \left(\theta_0 + s_j n^{-1/2} \right) \right\}$$

$$= n^{1/2} \left\{ \bigvee_{j \in \widehat{\mathfrak{U}}_n(\mu_0)} \left(\widehat{\mu}_{n,j} - \theta_0 \right) - \bigvee_{j \in \widehat{\mathfrak{U}}_n(\mu_0)} s_j n^{-1/2} \right\}$$

$$= n^{1/2} \left\{ \bigvee_{j \in \widehat{\mathfrak{U}}_n(\mu_0)} \left(\widehat{\mu}_{n,j} - \mu_{0,n,j} + s_j n^{-1/2} \right) - \bigvee_{j \in \widehat{\mathfrak{U}}_n(\mu_0)} s_j n^{-1/2} \right\}.$$

Taking a sup over all $s_j \in \mathbb{R}$ and leaving the arguments to the maximum unchanged for $j \notin \widehat{\mathfrak{U}}_n(\mu_0)$ leads to $\widehat{U}_n$.

It can be shown that, under mild regularity conditions, both $\widehat{L}_n$ and $\widehat{U}_n$ are regular and can be consistently bootstrapped (proofs of similar results are in Laber et al. (2014c); see also Section 10.4). A bootstrap confidence interval for θ_0 based on these bounds can be constructed as follows. Let $\widehat{u}_{n,1-\alpha/2}^{(b)}$ denote the upper $(1 - \alpha/2) \times 100$ percentile of the bootstrap distribution of $\widehat{U}_n$, and let $\widehat{\ell}_{n,\alpha/2}^{(b)}$ denote the lower $(\alpha/2) \times 100$ percentile of the bootstrap distribution of $\widehat{L}_n$. In application, the percentiles $\widehat{u}_{n,1-\alpha/2}^{(b)}$ and $\widehat{\ell}_{n,\alpha/2}^{(b)}$ can be approximated by drawing a large number of samples of size n with replacement from the observed data set, computing the upper and lower bounds on each resampled data set, and then setting $\widehat{u}_{n,1-\alpha/2}$ to be the $(1 - \alpha/2) \times 100$ sample percentile of the upper bounds computed on these resampled data sets and setting $\widehat{\ell}_{n,\alpha/2}$ to be the $(\alpha/2) \times 100$ sample percentile of the lower bounds. Then

$$\left[\widehat{\theta}_n - \widehat{u}_{n,1-\alpha/2}^{(b)} n^{-1/2}, \widehat{\theta}_n - \widehat{\ell}_{n,\alpha/2}^{(b)} n^{-1/2} \right] \tag{10.3}$$

is a valid (asymptotic) $(1 - \alpha) \times 100\%$ confidence interval for θ_0.

Both the adaptive confidence set (10.3) and the projection interval (10.2) involve solving nonconvex optimization problems and thus, analogous to the discussion in Section 4.2.2, are potentially nontrivial to implement for $p \geq 2$. A computationally simpler approach to form an asymptotically correct confidence set for θ_0 is to use a resampling method designed to deal with nonsmooth functionals. The m-out-of-n bootstrap is the canonical subsampling approach for nonsmooth functionals (Bretagnolle, 1983; Shao, 1994; Bickel and Sakov, 2008). The m-out-of-n bootstrap uses bootstrap resampling with a resample size of $m_n = o(n)$. The basic idea is that $n^{-1/2}$-perturbations will be negligible relative to the $m_n^{-1/2}$-perturbations of an estimator constructed from a sample of size m_n. Let $\widehat{\mu}_{m_n,j}^{(b)}$ denote the bootstrap estimator for $\mu_{0,j}$ based on resample size m_n for each $j = 1, \ldots, p$, and assume that, in addition to $m_n = o(n)$, $m_n \to \infty$ as $n \to \infty$. We characterize the large sample behavior of the m-out-of-n bootstrap estimator with an informal asymptotic analysis of the behavior of $\widehat{\theta}_{m_n}^{(b)}$, the bootstrap estimator for θ_0 based on resample size m_n.

It can be shown (Arcones and Giné, 1989) that $m_n^{1/2}(\widehat{\mu}_{m_n}^{(b)} - \widehat{\mu}_n)$ converges in distribution, conditional on the observed data, to a normal random vector with mean zero and covariance matrix Σ. Thus,

$$m_n^{1/2}(\widehat{\theta}_{m_n}^{(b)} - \widehat{\theta}_n) = m_n^{1/2}\left(\bigvee_{j=1}^{p} \widehat{\mu}_{n,j}^{(b)} - \bigvee_{j=1}^{p} \widehat{\mu}_{n,j} \right)$$

$$= \bigvee_{j=1}^{p} \left\{ m_n^{1/2}(\widehat{\mu}_{n,j}^{(b)} - \widehat{\mu}_{n,j}) + \left(\frac{m_n}{n}\right)^{1/2} n^{1/2}(\widehat{\mu}_{n,j} - \mu_{0,j}) + m_n^{1/2}\mu_{0,j} \right\}$$

$$- \bigvee_{j=1}^{p} \left\{ \left(\frac{m_n}{n}\right)^{1/2} n^{1/2}(\widehat{\mu}_{n,j} - \mu_{0,j}) + m_n^{1/2}\mu_{0,j} \right\}$$

$$= \bigvee_{j=1}^{p} \left\{ m_n^{1/2}(\widehat{\mu}_{n,j}^{(b)} - \widehat{\mu}_{n,j}) + m_n^{1/2}(\mu_{0,j} - \theta_0) + o_P(1) \right\}$$

$$- \bigvee_{j=1}^{p} \left\{ m_n^{1/2}(\mu_{0,j} - \theta_0) + o_P(1) \right\}$$

$$\approx \bigvee_{j \in \mathfrak{U}(\mu_0)} \left\{ m_n^{1/2}(\widehat{\mu}_{m_n,j}^{(b)} - \widehat{\mu}_{n,j}) \right\},$$

where we have used $(m_n/n)^{1/2} = o(1)$, $n^{1/2}(\widehat{\mu}_{n,j} - \mu_{n,j})$ is bounded in probability, and $\mu_{0,j} - \theta_0$ is negative for $j \notin \mathfrak{U}(\mu_0)$ and zero otherwise. Finally,

$$\bigvee_{j \in \mathfrak{U}(\mu_0)} \left\{ m_n^{1/2}\left(\widehat{\mu}_{m_n,j}^{(b)} - \widehat{\mu}_{n,j}\right) \right\} \rightsquigarrow \bigvee_{j \in \mathfrak{U}(\mu_0)} Z_j$$

conditional on the data, for $Z \sim \mathcal{N}(0, \Sigma)$, which matches the limiting distribution given in Lemma 10.2.1. Thus, the m-out-of-n bootstrap estimator converges to the correct limiting distribution even though it depends on the unknown set $\mathfrak{U}(\mu_0)$.

10.3 Inference for Single Decision Regimes

As in (3.5), assume that the observed data are i.i.d. (X_{1i}, A_{1i}, Y_i), $i = 1, \ldots, n$, where $X_1 \in \mathbb{R}^{p_{X_1}}$ denotes baseline information; A_1 is the treatment option in $\mathcal{A}_1$ actually received by individual i, and $Y \in \mathbb{R}$ is the observed outcome, coded so that larger values are preferred. For consistency with the literature, throughout this section, we take $\mathcal{A}_1$ to comprise two treatment options coded as -1 and 1; i.e., $\mathcal{A}_1 = \{-1, 1\}$ as in the discussion of outcome weighted learning (OWL) in Section 4.3. With $H_1 = X_1$ denoting history at baseline and potential outcomes redefined in the obvious way as $Y^*(1)$ and $Y^*(-1)$, we assume throughout that suitably modified versions of SUTVA (3.6), the no unmeasured confounders assumption (3.7), and the positivity assumption (3.8) hold.

For regime d, we write the corresponding decision rule d_1 analogous to (4.33) as $d_1(h_1) = \text{sign}\{f_1(h_1)\}$, where $f_1(h_1)$ is a decision function. Except in our discussion of g-computation later in this section, we restrict attention to regimes d with linear decision rules, so regimes for which the decision function characterizing the rule is linear in a finite-dimensional parameter η_1; i.e., $f_1(h_1; \eta_1) = \widetilde{h}_1^T \eta_1$, where $\widetilde{h}_1$ is a vector of known features constructed from h_1 that may include polynomial terms or other nonlinear basis functions involving components of h_1 and thus

$$d_1(h_1; \eta_1) = \text{sign}(\widetilde{h}_1^T \eta_1); \tag{10.4}$$

often, we take $\widetilde{h}_1 = h_1$ for simplicity, but results hold more generally.

10.3.1   Inference on Model Parameters

Q-learning

As discussed in Section 3.5.1, regression-based estimation of an optimal regime, referred to more generally as Q-learning, involves positing a model for the true regression relationship $Q_1(h_1, a_1) = E(Y|H_1 = h_1, A_1 = a_1)$, the so-called Q-function. For a parametric Q-function model, inference on the parameters is often of primary interest, as, in many settings, inference on these parameters can be translated directly into a clinical context; e.g., a test that a particular parameter is zero might correspond to a test of no treatment effect.

Suppose we posit a linear model for the Q-function of the form

$$Q_1(h_1, a_1) = \widetilde{h}_{11}^T \beta_{11} + a_1 \widetilde{h}_{12}^T \beta_{12}, \quad \beta_1 = (\beta_{11}^T, \beta_{12}^T)^T,$$

similar to (5.102), where $\widetilde{h}_{11}$ and $\widetilde{h}_{12}$ are known features constructed from h_1, and $\dim(\beta_1) = p_1$. Analogous to the discussion at the beginning of Section 3.5.3, this model induces a class of regimes with rules of the form $d_1(h_1; \beta_1) = \text{sign}(\widetilde{h}_{12}^T \beta_{12})$, as in (10.4).

Define

$$\beta_1^* = \arg\min_{\beta_1} P\{Y - Q_1(H_1, A_1; \beta_1)\}^2,$$

and let $\widehat{\beta}_{1,n} = \arg\min_{\beta_1} \mathbb{P}_n\{Y - Q_1(H_1, A_1; \beta_1)\}^2$ denote the OLS estimator for β_1^*. For fixed $c \in \mathbb{R}^{p_1}$, we wish to construct an asymptotically valid confidence set for $c^T\beta_1^*$. For example, if c is the jth vector in a standard basis for $\mathbb{R}^p$, then $c^T\beta_1^*$ is the jth element of β_1; alternatively, if $c = (\tilde{h}_{11}^T, \tilde{h}_{12}^T)^T$ then $c^T\beta_1^* = Q_1(h_1, 1; \beta_1^*)$. Here, we do not assume that the above working model for the Q-function is correctly specified; however, if this does not hold, it can be difficult to interpret $c^T\beta_1^*$ in a domain context. If the model is correctly specified, β_1^* is the true value of β_1 as defined in Section 2.4.

The estimator $\widehat{\beta}_{1,n}$ is constructed using OLS and is thereby regular and asymptotically normal under minimal assumptions, as discussed in the review of M-estimation in Section 2.5. For completeness, we demonstrate this result more generally here. Let $B_1 = (\tilde{H}_{11}^T, A_1 \tilde{H}_{12}^T)^T$. Assume that $\Sigma_{Q_1} = PB_1B_1^T$ and $\Omega_{Q_1} = P(Y - B_1^T\beta_1^*)^2 B_1 B_1^T$ are finite and strictly positive definite and that $P\|B_1Y\|^2$ is finite. Then, assuming that $\mathbb{P}_n B_1 B_1^T$ is invertible,

$$
\begin{aligned}
n^{1/2}(\widehat{\beta}_{1,n} - \beta_1^*) &= n^{1/2}(\mathbb{P}_n B_1 B_1^T)^{-1}(\mathbb{P}_n - P)B_1(Y - B_1^T\beta_1^*) \\
&= n^{1/2}(PB_1B_1^T)^{-1}(\mathbb{P}_n - P)B_1(Y - B_1^T\beta_1^*) + o_P(1) \\
&\rightsquigarrow \mathcal{N}(0, \Sigma_{Q_1}^{-1}\Omega_{Q_1}\Sigma_{Q_1}^{-1}).
\end{aligned}
$$

Thus, $c^T n^{1/2}(\widehat{\beta}_{1,n} - \beta_1^*) \rightsquigarrow \mathcal{N}(0, c^T\Sigma_{Q_1}^{-1}\Omega_{Q_1}\Sigma_{Q_1}^{-1}c)$. Letting $\widehat{\Sigma}_{Q_1,n} = \mathbb{P}_n B_1 B_1^T$ and $\widehat{\Omega}_{Q_1,n} = \mathbb{P}_n(Y - B_1^T\widehat{\beta}_{1,n})^2 B_1 B_1^T$, a $(1-\alpha) \times 100\%$ confidence interval for $c^T\beta_1^*$ is then

$$
c^T\widehat{\beta}_{1,n} \pm z_{1-\alpha/2}\{c^T\widehat{\Sigma}_{Q_1,n}^{-1}\widehat{\Omega}_{Q_1,n}\widehat{\Sigma}_{Q_1,n}^{-1}c/n\}^{1/2},
$$

where $z_{1-\alpha/2}$ is the $(1-\alpha/2) \times 100$ percentile of the standard normal distribution.

This result verifies that standard asymptotic approaches based on a normal approximation can be used to construct a confidence set for parameters indexing the Q-function in a single decision problem. More generally, any inference procedure that applies in the context of OLS should be portable to single stage Q-learning. We show in subsequent sections that this is not true for multiple decision problems.

g-Computation

Q-learning in a single decision problem is equivalent to regression modeling and estimation and is therefore amenable to standard model checking, diagnostics, and validation. This is appealing, as regression modeling is familiar to quantitative researchers and implemented in standard software. However, Q-learning focuses on estimation of conditional means, so may not be appropriate for estimating other functionals of the distribution of the outcome distribution; e.g., a prediction interval for the outcome given patient covariates and treatment or the variance of the outcome under an optimal regime (Lizotte and Tahmasebi, 2017).

In contrast, as noted in the multiple decision context in Section 5.4, the g-computation algorithm allows estimation of essentially any functional of the outcome distribution under any regime. However, this comes at the price of additional modeling of conditional densities of the outcome and covariates; in Section 5.5.1, we discuss g-computation in the context of fully parametric models for the required densities, although more flexible models are also possible; see Robins (2004).

In a single decision problem, g-computation involves modeling of the conditional density of Y given $X_1 = x_1$ and $A_1 = a_1$, and interest may focus on functionals of this conditional distribution, including but not limited to the Q-function. Here, we consider a flexible model for this conditional distribution based on mean-variance models (Laber et al., 2014a; Linn et al., 2017). Namely, we assume that the conditional distribution of Y given $X_1 = x_1$ and $A_1 = a_1$ has density of the form

$$p_{Y|X_1,A_1}(y|x_1,a_1;\zeta_1) = \frac{1}{\sigma(x_1;\zeta_{13})}k\left\{\frac{y - \mu(x_1,\zeta_{11}) - a_1 g(x_1,\zeta_{12})}{\sigma(x_1;\zeta_{13})}\right\},$$
$$(10.5)$$

where k is an unspecified density that is symmetric about zero and does not depend on x_1 or a_1; and μ, g, and σ are real-valued functions known up to parameter vector $\zeta_1 = (\zeta_{11}^T, \zeta_{12}^T, \zeta_{13}^T)^T$. Fitting of the model (10.5) thus involves estimation of ζ_1 and k. Assume that μ, g, and σ are continuously differentiable in their parameters for each fixed x_1. Let $\zeta_{1,0} = (\zeta_{11,0}^T, \zeta_{12,0}^T, \zeta_{13,0}^T)^T$ and k_0 denote the parameter values and density function corresponding to the true conditional distribution of Y given X_1 and A_1. We consider the problem of constructing confidence sets for $c^T\zeta_{1,0}$, where $c \in \mathbb{R}^{\dim(\zeta_1)}$, and for the Q-function $Q_1(x_1, a_1)$ at fixed values x_1 and a_1. We also consider the problem of constructing a prediction interval for Y given $X_1 = x_1$ and $A_1 = a_1$; i.e., a random interval $[\widehat{L}_n, \widehat{U}_n]$ so that $P(\widehat{L}_n \le Y \le \widehat{U}_n | X_1 = x_1, A_1 = a_1) \ge 1 - \alpha$, where $\alpha \in (0, 1)$ is prespecified error level.

An estimator for the density k is not needed to construct a confidence interval for $c^T\zeta_{1,0}$; we consider this case first. As in Section 2.5, define the estimating function

$$M(X_1, A_1, Y; \zeta_1)$$

$$= \begin{pmatrix} \dfrac{1}{\sigma(X_1;\zeta_{13})}\{Y - \mu(X_1,\zeta_{11}) - A_1 g(X_1,\zeta_{12})\}\nabla_{\zeta_{11}}\mu(X_1,\zeta_{11}) \\[2ex] \dfrac{1}{\sigma(X_1;\zeta_{13})}\{Y - \mu(X_1,\zeta_{11}) - A_1 g(X_1,\zeta_{12})\}\nabla_{\zeta_{12}}g(X_1,\zeta_{12}) \\[2ex] [\{Y - \mu(X_1,\zeta_{11}) - A_1 g(X_1,\zeta_{12})\}^2 - \sigma^2(X_1,\zeta_{13})]\nabla_{\zeta_{13}}\sigma^2(X_1,\zeta_{13}) \end{pmatrix},$$

and let $\widehat{\zeta}_{1,n}$ denote a solution to the stacked estimating equations

$\mathbb{P}_n M(X_1, A_1, Y; \varsigma_1) = 0$. As discussed in Section 2.5, under standard regularity conditions, as in (2.39) and (2.40), it follows that $n^{1/2}(\widehat{\varsigma}_{1,n} - \varsigma_{1,0}) \rightsquigarrow \mathcal{N}(0, \Sigma)$, where

$$\Sigma = \{P\nabla_{\varsigma_1} M(X_1, A_1, Y; \varsigma_{1,0})\}^{-1}$$
$$\times \{PM(X_1 A_1, Y; \varsigma_{1,0}) M(X_1, A_1, Y; \varsigma_{1,0})^T\}$$
$$\times \{P\nabla_{\varsigma_1} M(X_1, A_1, Y; \varsigma_{1,0})\}^{-T}.$$

Thus, $c^T n^{1/2}(\widehat{\varsigma}_{1,n} - \varsigma_{1,0}) \rightsquigarrow \mathcal{N}(0, c^T \Sigma c)$; and

$$c^T \widehat{\varsigma}_{1,n} \pm z_{1-\alpha/2}(c^T \widehat{\Sigma}_n c/n)^{1/2}$$

is a valid asymptotic $(1 - \alpha) \times 100\%$ confidence set for $c^T \varsigma_{1,0}$, where

$$\widehat{\Sigma}_n = \{\mathbb{P}_n \nabla_{\varsigma_1} M(X_1, A_1, Y; \widehat{\varsigma}_{1,n})\}^{-1}$$
$$\times \{\mathbb{P}_n M(X_1, A_1, Y; \widehat{\varsigma}_{1,n}) M(X_1, A_1, Y; \widehat{\varsigma}_{1n})^T\}$$
$$\times \{\mathbb{P}_n \nabla_{\varsigma_1} M(X_1, A_1, Y; \widehat{\varsigma}_{1,n})\}^{-T}$$

is the plug-in estimator for Σ, analogous to (2.41) and (2.42).

Given the preceding asymptotic results, it is straightforward to construct a confidence set for $Q_1(x_1, a_1)$ using the delta method. If the posited model is correctly specified, then $Q_1(x_1, a_1) = Q_1(x_1, a_1; \varsigma_{1,0}) = \mu(x, ; \varsigma_{11,0}) + ag(x; \varsigma_{12,0})$; thus, because μ and g are continuously differentiable, $Q_1(x_1, a_1; \widehat{\varsigma}_{1,n}) - Q_1(x_1, a_1; \varsigma_{1,0}) = \nabla_{\varsigma_1} Q_1^T(x_1, a_1; \varsigma_{1,0})(\widehat{\varsigma}_{1,n} - \varsigma_{1,0}) + o_P(n^{-1/2})$, and a $(1 - \alpha) \times 100\%$ confidence set for $Q_1(x_1, a_1)$ is

$$Q_1(x_1, a_1; \widehat{\varsigma}_{1,n})$$
$$\pm z_{1-\alpha/2}\{\nabla_{\varsigma_1} Q_1(x_1, a_1; \widehat{\varsigma}_{1,n})^T \widehat{\Sigma}_n \nabla_{\varsigma_1} Q_1(x_1, a_1; \widehat{\varsigma}_{1,n})/n\}^{1/2}.$$

Let $F(y|x_1, a_1) = P(Y \leq y|X_1 = x_1, A_1 = a_1)$ denote the cumulative distribution function of the distribution of Y given $X_1 = x_1$ and $A_1 = a_1$. To construct a $(1 - \alpha) \times 100\%$ conditional prediction interval for Y, we construct an estimator $\widehat{F}_n(y|x_1, a_1)$ for $F(y|x_1, a_1)$ and subsequently obtain

$$\widehat{L}_{n,\alpha/2} = \inf\{\tau \in \mathbb{R} : \widehat{F}_n(\tau|x_1, a_1) \geq \alpha/2\},$$
$$\widehat{U}_{n,1-\alpha/2} = \sup\{\tau \in \mathbb{R} : \widehat{F}_n(\tau|x_1, a_1) \geq 1 - \alpha/2\}.$$
(10.6)

Write

$$F(y|x_1, a_1) = \int \frac{I\{\omega \leq y\}}{\sigma(x_1; \varsigma_{13,0})} k_0 \left\{\frac{\omega - \mu(x_1; \varsigma_{11,0}) - ag(x_1; \varsigma_{12,0})}{\sigma(x_1; \varsigma_{13,0})}\right\} d\omega,$$

which, after a change of variables, is expressed equivalently as

$$\int I\left\{\sigma(x_1; \zeta_{13,0})\epsilon + \mu(x_1; \zeta_{11,0}) + a_1 g(x_1; \zeta_{12,0}) \le y\right\} k_0(\epsilon)\, d\epsilon.$$

Letting $\widehat{k}_n$ be an estimator for k_0, the plug-in estimator for $F(y|x_1, a_1)$ is

$$\widehat{F}_n(y|x_1, a_1)$$
$$= \int I\left\{\sigma(x_1; \widehat{\zeta}_{13,n})\epsilon + \mu(x_1; \widehat{\zeta}_{11,n}) + a_1 g(x_1; \widehat{\zeta}_{12,n}) \le y\right\} \widehat{k}_n(\epsilon)\, d\epsilon.$$

Provided that k_n converges pointwise in probability to k; i.e., $k_n(u) \xrightarrow{p} k(u)$ for each fixed $u \in \mathbb{R}$, it is straightforward to show that $\widehat{F}_n(y|x_1, a_1) \xrightarrow{p} F_y(y|x_1, a_1)$ for each fixed $y \in \mathbb{R}$.

Lemma 10.3.1. *Let x_1 and a_1 be fixed. Assume that as $n \to \infty$: (i) $\widehat{\zeta}_{1,n} \xrightarrow{p} \zeta_{1,0}$; (ii) for each n, the estimator $\widehat{k}_n$ is a proper density, and $\widehat{k}_n(u) \xrightarrow{p} k_0(u)$ for each fixed $u \in \mathbb{R}$; (iii) the function $\zeta_1 \mapsto \{\mu(x_1; \zeta_{11}), g(x_1, \zeta_{12}), \sigma(x_1; \zeta_{13})\}$ is continuous for ζ_1 in a neighborhood of $\zeta_{1,0}$; (iv) $\sigma(x_1; \zeta_{13}) \ge \delta$ for some $\delta > 0$ for all ζ_{13} in a neighborhood of $\zeta_{13,0}$; and (v) the cumulative distribution function of ϵ is continuous. Then $\sup_y |\widehat{F}_n(y|x_1, a_1) - F(y|x_1, a_1)| \xrightarrow{p} 0$.*

Proof. Pointwise convergence of $\widehat{k}_n$ to k_0 in probability implies that $\int |\widehat{k}_n(\epsilon) - k_0(\epsilon)|\, d\epsilon \xrightarrow{p} 0$ (e.g.; Scheffé, 1947; Glick, 1974). Let F_ϵ denote the cumulative distribution function of ϵ. Then

$$\widehat{F}_n(y|x_1, a_1) = F_\epsilon\left\{\frac{y - \mu(x_1; \widehat{\zeta}_{11,n}) - a_1 g(x_1; \widehat{\zeta}_{12,n})}{\sigma(x_1; \widehat{\zeta}_{13,n})}\right\}$$
$$+ \int I\{\sigma(x_1; \widehat{\zeta}_{13,n})\epsilon + \mu(x_1; \widehat{\zeta}_{11,n}) + a_1 g(x_1; \widehat{\zeta}_{12,n}) \le y\}\{\widehat{k}_n(\epsilon) - k_0(\epsilon)\}\, d\epsilon.$$

The second term on the right-hand side is bounded in magnitude by $\int |\widehat{k}_n(\epsilon) - k_0(\epsilon)|\, d\epsilon$, which does not depend on y and converges to zero in probability. Thus, it is sufficient to show that

$$\sup_{y \in \mathbb{R}} \left| F_\epsilon\left\{\frac{y - \mu(x_1; \widehat{\zeta}_{11,n}) - a_1 g(x_1; \zeta_{12,n})}{\sigma(x_1; \widehat{\zeta}_{13,n})}\right\} \right.$$
$$\left. - F_\epsilon\left\{\frac{y - \mu(x_1; \zeta_{11,0}) - a_1 g(x_1; \zeta_{12,0})}{\sigma(x_1; \zeta_{13,0})}\right\} \right|$$

converges to zero in probability. However, this follows immediately, as pointwise convergence in probability of a sequence of (random) cumulative distribution functions implies uniform convergence. $\square$

Corollary 10.3.2. *Assume the conditions of Lemma 10.3.1. Let $\alpha \in (0,1)$ be fixed, and define $L_{\alpha/2}$ and $U_{1-\alpha/2}$ to be the $(\alpha/2) \times 100$ and $(1 - \alpha/2) \times 100$ percentiles of the distribution of Y given $X_1 = x_1$ and $A_1 = a_1$. Then $(\widehat{L}_{n,\alpha/2}, \widehat{U}_{n,1-\alpha/2})$, where $\widehat{L}_{n,\alpha/2}$ and $\widehat{U}_{n,1-\alpha/2}$ are defined in (10.6), converges in probability to $(L_{\alpha/2}, U_{1-\alpha/2})$. Thus,*

$$P\left(\widehat{L}_{n,\alpha/2} \leq Y \leq \widehat{U}_{n,1-\alpha/2}|X_1 = x_1, A_1 = a_1\right) \geq 1 - \alpha + o(1).$$

The preceding result shows that g-computation can be used to construct asymptotically valid $(1 - \alpha) \times 100\%$ prediction intervals for the outcome given patient covariates and treatment. The interval $[\widehat{L}_{n,\alpha/2}, \widehat{U}_{n,1-\alpha/2}]$ is a plug-in estimator and does not account for uncertainty in $\widehat{\zeta}_{1,n}$ or $\widehat{k}_n$. A consequence is that this interval may not deliver nominal coverage with small samples. One solution is to estimate the coverage of the prediction interval using resampling and then to recalibrate the interval to improve coverage; e.g., by choosing endpoints $\widehat{L}_{n,\alpha'/2}$ and $\widehat{U}_{n,1-\alpha'/2}$, where α' is a data-driven error level that may be smaller than the target error level α (Beran, 1990; Hall et al., 1999).

Outcome Weighted Learning

As discussed in Section 4.3, there are numerous variants of outcome weighted learning in the literature (OWL, see Zhao et al., 2012, 2015a, 2019; Chen et al., 2016; Zhou et al., 2017; Liu et al., 2018, and references therein). To simplify our developments and to emphasize the salient features of inference for OWL, we focus on the original formulation that is proposed in Zhao et al. (2012) and is discussed in Section 4.3. This version assumes a constant propensity π_1 that satisfies

$$\pi_1 = P(A_1 = 1|H_1) = P(A_1 = -1|H_1) = 1/2 \tag{10.7}$$

almost surely and linear decision functions of the form $f_1(h_1; \eta_1) = h_1^T \eta_1$, where $\dim(\eta_1) = p_1$. Under these conditions, from (4.34), OWL is based on minimizing the weighted classification error

$$\mathbb{P}_n\left[\frac{Y}{A_1/2 + (1 - A_1)/2}\mathrm{I}\{A_1 \neq \mathrm{sign}(H_1^T \eta_1)\}\right] \tag{10.8}$$
$$= 2\mathbb{P}_n Y\mathrm{I}\{A_1 \, \mathrm{sign}\left(H_1^T \eta_1\right) \leq 0\},$$

where the 0-1 loss function $\mathrm{I}\{A_1 \neq \mathrm{sign}(H_1^T \eta_1)\}$ is replaced by a convex surrogate; that is, OWL is based on a convex relaxation of (10.8). Let $\mathcal{D}_\eta$ denote the space of regimes with linear decision rules.

Thus, an optimal regime d_η^{opt} in the class $\mathcal{D}_\eta$ has the form $d_1^{opt}(h_1; \eta_1^{opt}) = \mathrm{sign}(h_1^T \eta_1^{opt})$, where η^{opt} (scaled to have norm one for identifiability) satisfies

$$
\begin{aligned}
\eta_1^{opt} &= \arg\min_{\eta_1\,:\,\|\eta_1\|=1} 2PYI\{A_1\text{sign}\left(H_1^T\eta_1\right)\le 0\} \\[4pt]
&= \arg\min_{\eta_1\,:\,\|\eta_1\|=1} P\Big[YI\{A_1\text{sign}\left(H_1^T\eta_1\right)\le 0\}I(Y>0) \\
&\qquad\qquad +YI\{A_1\text{sign}\left(H_1^T\eta_1\right)\le 0\}I(Y\le 0)\Big] \\[4pt]
&= \arg\min_{\eta_1\,:\,\|\eta_1\|=1} P\Big(YI\{A_1\text{sign}\left(H_1^T\eta_1\right)\le 0\}I(Y>0) \\
&\qquad\qquad +Y[1-I\{A_1\text{sign}\left(H_1^T\eta_1\right)>0\}]I(Y\le 0)\Big) \\[4pt]
&= \arg\min_{\eta_1\,:\,\|\eta_1\|=1} P\Big[YI\{A_1\text{sign}\left(H_1^T\eta_1\right)\le 0\}I(Y>0) \\
&\qquad\qquad -YI\{A_1\text{sign}\left(H_1^T\eta_1\right)>0\}I(Y\le 0)\Big] \qquad (10.9) \\[4pt]
&= \arg\min_{\eta_1\,:\,\|\eta_1\|=1} P|Y|I\{\text{sign}(Y)A_1\text{sign}\left(H_1^T\eta_1\right)\le 0\}. \quad (10.10)
\end{aligned}
$$

Here, we have used $a_1\,\text{sign}(h_1^T\eta_1)\in\{-1,1\}$ for all h_1, a_1, and η_1; and (10.9) follows because $YI(Y\le 0)$ does not depend on η_1. The final expression (10.10) is often "simplified" to

$$
\eta_1^{opt}=\arg\min_{\eta_1\,:\,\|\eta_1\|=1} P|Y|I\{\text{sign}(Y)A_1H_1^T\eta_1\le 0\}, \qquad (10.11)
$$

which is tantamount to ignoring the case $H_1^T\eta_1=0$, as algebra shows that if one codes $\text{sign}(0)=-1$, then

$$
\begin{aligned}
P|Y|I\{\text{sign}(Y)A_1\text{sign}\left(H_1^T\eta_1\right)\le 0\}&-P|Y|I\{\text{sign}(Y)A_1H_1^T\eta_1\le 0\}\\
&= -P|Y|I\{-\text{sign}(Y)A_1>0\}I(H_1^T\eta_1=0).
\end{aligned}
$$

Nevertheless, it is common either to assume that this term is negligible or to ignore it, so that estimators are based on (10.11). Note that (10.11) can be written as

$$
\eta_1^{opt}=\arg\min_{\eta_1\,:\,\|\eta_1\|=1} P|Y|\ell_{0\text{-}1}\{\text{sign}(Y)A_1H_1^T\eta_1\},
$$

where $\ell_{0\text{-}1}(x)=I(x\le 0)$ is the (nonconvex) 0-1 loss function of (4.26).

Define $W=\text{sign}(Y)A_1H_1$. For the purpose of developing methods for inference, we consider estimators of the form $\widehat{\eta}_{1,n}=\arg\min_{\eta_1\in\mathbb{R}^{p_1}}\mathbb{P}_n|Y|\ell(W^T\eta_1)$, where $\ell:\mathbb{R}\to\mathbb{R}$ is a convex loss function serving as a surrogate for the nonconvex 0-1 loss in (10.11). In

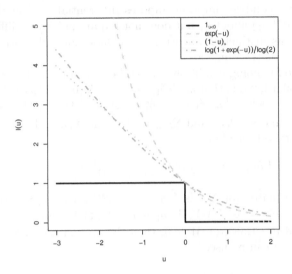

Figure 10.3 *Examples of convex surrogates, $\ell(u)$, for the 0-1 loss function $I(u \leq 0)$: (i) exponential, $\ell(u) = \exp(-u)$; (ii) hinge, $\ell(u) = (1-u)_+$; and (iii) logistic, $\ell(u) = \log\{1 + \exp(-u)\}/\log(2)$, where we have divided by $\log(2)$ to align the surrogates at $u = 0$.*

the original formulation of OWL in Zhao et al. (2012), the authors take $\ell(x) = (1 - x)_+ = \max(0, x)$, the hinge loss function given in (4.35); however, there are many other choices for this loss function, such as the logistic loss $\ell(x) = \log\{1 + \exp(-x)\}$ and the exponential loss $\ell(x) = \exp(-x)$. Figure 10.3 displays several loss functions. There is some preliminary evidence that using smooth; i.e., differentiable, loss functions leads to superior performance as compared to the hinge loss in some contexts (Zhao et al., 2019; Jiang et al., 2019).

Define $\eta_1^* = \arg\min_{\eta_1 \in \mathbb{R}^{p_1}} P|Y|\ell(W^T \eta_1)$; as noted in Section 4.3, by virtue of substitution of the convex surrogate loss function $\ell(\cdot)$ for the 0-1 loss, η_1^{opt} and η_1^* need not coincide. We consider the problem of constructing confidence sets for $c^T \eta_1^*$, where $c \in \mathbb{R}^{p_1}$ is fixed. Because $|y|\ell(w^T \eta_1)$ is the composition of a linear and convex function, it is convex in η_1 for each (y, w). This simplifies both computation and asymptotic arguments (Haberman, 1989; Niemiro, 1992; Hjort and Pollard, 2011). Assume that: (i) η_1^* exists and is unique; and (ii) $|y|\ell\{w^T(\eta_1^* + \delta)\} - |y|\ell(w^T\eta_1^*) = S(y, w; \eta_1^*)^T\delta + R(y, w, \delta; \eta_1^*)$, where $PS(Y, W; \eta_1^*) = 0$, $\Sigma_O = PS(Y, W; \eta_1^*)S(Y, W; \eta_1^*)^T$ is finite, and $PR(Y, W, \delta; \eta_1^*) = (1/2)\delta^T\Omega_O\delta + o(\|\delta\|^2)$ for some positive definite matrix Ω_O. The first assumption ensures that the inference problem is well-defined. The second assumption imposes differentiability on the map $\eta_1 \mapsto P|Y|\ell(W^T\eta_1)$ about η_1^* but does not require pointwise differentiability of ℓ. This distinction allows us to include non-differentiable loss functions such as the hinge loss.

Under the foregoing conditions, it can be shown (e.g., Theorem 2 of Hjort and Pollard, 2011) that $n^{1/2}(\widehat{\eta}_{1,n}-\eta_1^*) \rightsquigarrow \mathcal{N}(0,\Omega_O^{-1}\Sigma_O\Omega_O^{-1})$. Thus, for any fixed $c \in \mathbb{R}^{p_1}$, $c^T n^{1/2}(\widehat{\eta}_{1,n} - \eta_1^*) \rightsquigarrow \mathcal{N}(0,c^T\Omega_O^{-1}\Sigma_O\Omega_O^{-1}c)$. Given consistent estimators $\widehat{\Omega}_{O,n}$ and $\widehat{\Sigma}_{O,n}$ for Ω_O and Σ_O, a $(1-\alpha)\times 100\%$ confidence interval for $c^T\eta_1^*$ is

$$c^T\widehat{\eta}_{1,n} \pm z_{1-\alpha/2}(c^T\widehat{\Omega}_{O,n}^{-1}\widehat{\Sigma}_{O,n}\widehat{\Omega}_{O,n}^{-1}c/n)^{1/2}.$$

A natural estimator for Σ_O is $\widehat{\Sigma}_{O,n} = \mathbb{P}_n S(Y,W;\widehat{\eta}_{1,n})S(Y,W;\widehat{\eta}_{1,n})$. If $PR(Y,W,\delta;\eta_1^*) = \delta^T P\Lambda(Y,W;\eta_1^*)\delta + o(\|\delta\|^2)$ for some continuous, matrix-valued function $\Lambda(Y,W;\eta_1)$, then the plug-in estimator $\widehat{\Omega}_{O,n} = \mathbb{P}_n\Lambda(Y,W;\widehat{\eta}_{1,n})$ can be used.

Example: Exponential Loss

Suppose that $\ell(x) = \exp(-x)$. Because $\ell(x)$ is strictly convex, η_1^* exists and is unique, excepting degenerate cases, e.g., if $W^T\eta_1^* > 0$ with probability one. A Taylor series expansion of $|y|\ell\{w^T(\eta_1^* + \delta)\}$ about $|y|\ell(w^T\eta_1^*)$ yields

$$|y|\exp\left\{w^T(\eta_1^* + \delta)\right\} - |y|\exp\left(w^T\eta_1^*\right) = -|y|\exp(-w^T\eta_1^*)w^T\delta +$$
$$\frac{|y|}{2}\delta^T\exp\left(-w^T\eta_1^*\right)ww^T\delta + \frac{|y|}{2}\delta^T\left\{\exp\left(-w^T\widetilde{\eta}_1\right) - \exp\left(-w^T\eta_1^*\right)\right\}ww^T\delta,$$

where $\widetilde{\eta}_1$ is an intermediate point between η_1^* and $\eta_1^* + \delta$. Matching terms in this expansion with those used in the sufficient conditions for asymptotic normality yields $S(Y,W;\eta_1^*) = -|Y|\exp(-W^T\eta_1^*)W$ and $R(Y,W;\eta_1^*) = (|Y|/2)\delta^T\exp(-W^T\eta_1^*)WW^T\delta + (|Y|/2)\delta^T\{\exp(-W^T\widetilde{\eta}_1) - \exp(-W^T\eta_1^*)\}WW^T\delta$. The conditions required for asymptotic normality hold, provided that $\Omega_O = P|Y|\exp(-W^T\eta_1^*)WW^T$ is positive definite and that $P\sup_{\|\nu-\eta_1^*\|\le\delta}|Y|\exp(W^T\nu)\|W\|^2 < \infty$ for sufficiently small δ.

Example: Hinge Loss

Suppose that $\ell(x) = (1-x)_+$. To simplify the required derivations, assume that

$$\begin{pmatrix} Y \\ W \end{pmatrix} \sim \mathcal{N}\left\{\begin{pmatrix} \mu_Y \\ \mu_W \end{pmatrix}, \begin{pmatrix} \Gamma_Y & \Gamma_{Y,W} \\ \Gamma_{W,Y} & \Gamma_W \end{pmatrix}\right\}.$$

This assumption is not essential, see Hjort and Pollard (2011). Excepting degenerate cases, it can be shown that $P|Y|\ell(W^T\eta_1)$ is strictly convex in η_1 so that η_1^* exists and is unique. Assume that η_1^* is not identically zero and that the covariance matrix of $(Y, W)^T$ is strictly positive definite. Because $\ell(x)$ is not differentiable, we cannot apply a Taylor series argument directly to $\ell(x)$ to verify the requisite expansion holds. Instead, we apply a Taylor series expansion to the expectation of $|Y|\ell(W^T\eta_1)$. Choose $S(y, w; \eta_1^*) = -|y|I\{1 - w^T\eta_1^* \geq 0\}w$ to be a subgradient of $|y|\ell(w^T\eta_1)$ evaluated at η_1^*; thus, $PS(Y, W; \eta_1^*) = 0$. The remainder term, $R(y, w; \eta_1^*) = |y|\ell\{w^T(\eta_1^* + \delta)\} - |y|\ell(w^T\eta_1^*) - S(y, w; \eta_1^*)^T\delta$, is thus

$$R(y, w; \eta_1^*) = |y|\{1 - w^T(\eta_1^* + \delta)\}_+ - |y|(1 - w^T\eta_1^*)_+$$
$$+ |y|I(1 - w^T\eta_1^* \geq 0)w^T\delta,$$

and $PR(Y, W; \eta_1^*) = P[|Y|\{1 - W^T(\eta_1^* + \delta)\}_+ - |Y|(1 - W^T\eta_1^*)_+]$. For each η_1 in a neighborhood of η_1^*, let $\phi(y, v; \eta_1)$ denote the bivariate normal density corresponding to the joint distribution of $(Y, W^T\eta_1)^T$; $\phi(y, v; \eta_1)$ is twice continuously differentiable in η_1 in a neighborhood of η_1^*. Thus, $PR(Y, W; \eta_1^*) = \int |y|(1 - v)_+ \phi(y, v; \eta_1^* + \delta)\, dy\, dv - \int |y|(1 - v)_+ \phi(y, v; \eta_1^*)\, dy\, dv$ and, after a Taylor series approximation, is equivalently expressed as

$$\frac{1}{2}\delta^T\left\{\int |y|(1 - v)_+\nabla^2_{\eta_1}\phi(y, v; \eta_1^*)\, dy\, dv\right\}\delta$$
$$+ \frac{1}{2}\delta^T\left[\int |y|(1 - v)_+\{\nabla^2_{\eta_1}\phi(y, v; \widetilde{\eta}_1) - \nabla^2_{\eta_1}\phi(y, v; \eta_1^*)\}\, dy\, dv\right]\delta,$$

where $\widetilde{\eta}_1$ is an intermediate point between $\eta_1^* + \delta$ and η_1^*; and we have used $\int |y|(1 - v)_+\nabla_{\eta_1}\phi(y, v; \eta_1^*)\, dy\, dv = 0$, which follows from interchanging subdifferentiation and integration (Rockafellar and Wets, 2009). Thus, the conditions for asymptotic normality of $n^{1/2}(\widehat{\eta}_{1,n} - \eta_1^*)$ hold with $\Omega_O = \int |y|(1 - v)_+\nabla^2_{\eta_1}\phi(y, v; \eta_1^*)\, dy\, dv$ and $\Sigma_O = PY^2I(1 - W^T\eta_1^* \geq 0)WW^T$.

10.3.2 Inference on the Value

Optimality of a regime is defined through the value; thus, confidence sets for the value of one or more regimes are often of interest. However, in the context of estimating an optimal regime from a finite sample, there are several potential definitions that might be used to measure the "value of a regime."

To illustrate these definitions, suppose that we have an estimated optimal regime $\widehat{d}_n^{opt}$ and its population analog d^*. For example, $\widehat{d}_n^{opt}$ might be characterized by the rule $\widehat{d}_{1,n}^{opt}(h_1; \widehat{\eta}_{1,n})$ that is the map $h_1 \mapsto$ $\text{sign}(h_1^T \widehat{\eta}_{1,n})$ for some estimator $\widehat{\eta}_{1,n}$, and d^* is the map $h_1 \mapsto \text{sign}(h_1^T \eta_1^*)$ where $\widehat{\eta}_{1,n} \xrightarrow{P} \eta_1^*$ for some η_1^*. If one takes the view that the estimated optimal regime will be deployed to make treatment decisions on future patients, then $\mathcal{V}(\widehat{d}_n^{opt}) = E\{Y^*(\widehat{d}_n^{opt}) | \widehat{d}_n^{opt}\}$, also known as the conditional value, may be an appropriate summary measure. Here, $\mathcal{V}(\widehat{d}_n^{opt})$ is the mean outcome if the population were to be treated according to $\widehat{d}_n^{opt}$. If instead one is interested in evaluating the performance of an estimation algorithm in a given problem domain, the average value, $E\{\mathcal{V}(\widehat{d}_n^{opt})\}$, which averages the conditional value over data sets of size n, is a more relevant summary measure (see Chapter 7 in Hastie et al. (2009) for a related discussion). A third potential summary measure is $\mathcal{V}(d^*)$, the value of the estimated optimal regime under an infinite sample. Under the assumption that d^* is an optimal regime (or at least the best one can do given that the class of regimes and estimation algorithm have been fixed), $\mathcal{V}(d^*)$ is an upper bound on the benefit of applying a treatment regime in given problem domain (Laber et al., 2016).

For general $\widehat{d}_n^{opt}$ and its infinite sample analog d^*, the three preceding measures of value, $\mathcal{V}(\widehat{d}_n^{opt})$, $E\{\mathcal{V}(\widehat{d}_n^{opt})\}$, and $\mathcal{V}(d^*)$, correspond to different scientific objectives: (i) evaluate the performance of an estimated optimal regime as if it will be used to make treatment decisions for future patients; (ii) evaluate the performance of an estimation algorithm in a given context; and (iii) assess if an optimal treatment regime is better than an alternative treatment decision strategy, such as standard of care. Given their mathematical definitions, it is perhaps surprising that these three measures need not be equal even in infinite samples.

To see this, consider regimes d_η with rules of the form $d_1(h_1; \eta_1) = \text{sign}(h_1^T \eta_1)$, where we define $\text{sign}(0) = -1$; and suppose $P(A_1 = 1|H_1) = P(A_1 = -1|H_1) = 1/2$ with probability one as in (10.7). Then it is straightforward that $\mathcal{V}(d_\eta) = 2PY\text{I}\{A_1\text{sign}(H_1^T \eta_1) > 0\}$. Suppose that $\widehat{d}_n^{opt}$ has rule $\text{sign}(h_1^T \widehat{\eta}_{1,n})$, where $\widehat{\eta}_{1,n}$ is an estimator for η_1 satisfying $n^{1/2}\widehat{\eta}_{1,n} \rightsquigarrow Z$, and $Z \sim \mathcal{N}(0, \Sigma)$. Thus, $\eta_1^* = 0$, so that d^* is characterized by the rule $d_1(h_1; \eta_1^*) = \text{sign}(h_1^T \eta_1^*) = -1$. Then, under sufficient regularity conditions, it follows that

$$\mathcal{V}(\widehat{d}_n^{opt}) = 2PY\text{I}\{A_1\text{sign}(H_1^T \widehat{\eta}_{1,n}) > 0\}$$
$$= 2PY\text{I}[A_1\text{sign}\{H_1^T n^{1/2}(\widehat{\eta}_{1,n} - \eta_1^*)\} > 0]$$
$$\rightsquigarrow 2PY\text{I}\{A_1\text{sign}(H_1^T Z) > 0\} = U(Z),$$

say. Recall that P denotes expectation with respect to the joint distribution of (H_1, A_1, Y) corresponding to a future patient but not to that of Z, so that $\mathcal{V}(\widehat{d}_n^{opt})$ converges in distribution to a nondegenerate distribution (assuming regularity conditions that support inter-changing the limit and expectation), and $(H_1, A_1, Y) \perp\!\!\!\perp Z$. Using the preceding result, $E\{\mathcal{V}(\widehat{d}_n^{opt})\}$ converges to $E\{U(Z)\}$, where this expectation is with respect to the distribution of Z. It is straightforward that $E\{U(Z)\} = 2PYE[I\{A_1 \text{sign}(H_1^T Z) > 0\}|H_1, A_1, Y] = PY$, as $E[I\{A_1 \text{sign}(H_1^T Z) > 0)|H_1, A_1, Y] = 1/2$ almost surely. It follows that $E\{\mathcal{V}(\widehat{d}_n^{opt})\}$ converges to PY as $n \to \infty$. Finally, $\mathcal{V}(d^*) = E(Y|A_1 = -1)$, as d^* always assigns treatment -1. Thus, $\mathcal{V}(\widehat{d}_n^{opt})$, $E\{\mathcal{V}(\widehat{d}_n^{opt})\}$, and $\mathcal{V}(d^*)$ need not be equal, even asymptotically. In the sequel, we focus on constructing confidence sets for $\mathcal{V}(\widehat{d}_n^{opt})$ and $\mathcal{V}(d^*)$, as these are most commonly of interest in practice; see Laber and Qian (2018) for additional discussion and references.

Remark. The conditional value is a function of the observed data and is therefore a random quantity. Because the conditional value varies across data sets, it may seem more appropriate to call a random set that contains the conditional value with a prespecified probability a prediction set rather than a confidence set. However, because the conditional value also depends on the unknown generative model, it is standard to use the term confidence set (Dawid, 1994; Laber and Murphy, 2011).

In what follows, to streamline expressions, we write $\widehat{d}_n$ to denote an estimator for an optimal regime and often suppress dependence on a finite-dimensional parameter indexing its rule. We continue to take the propensities to be known as in (10.7).

Inference on the Conditional Value Function

The conditional value function is not a smooth functional of the generative distribution. Thus, as discussed in Section 10.2, a local or moving parameter framework is necessary to capture small sample fluctuations in an asymptotic approximation. For a class of functions $\mathcal{F}$, let $l^\infty(\mathcal{F})$ denote the space of real-valued, uniformly bounded functions on $\mathcal{F}$. We assume that the observed data, $(X_{1,n,i}, A_{1,n,i}, Y_{n,i})$, $i = 1, \ldots, n$, form a triangular array drawn from distribution P_n (with $H_{1,n,i} = X_{1,n,i}$ the history at baseline) that satisfies the following conditions.

(A0) The estimated optimal regime $\widehat{d}_n$ is characterized by the rule $\widehat{d}_{1,n}(h_1) = \text{sign}(h_1^T \widehat{\eta}_{1,n})$, indexed by estimated $\widehat{\eta}_{1,n} \in \mathbb{R}^{p_1}$.

(A1) There exists $\eta_{1,n}^* \in \mathbb{R}^{p_1}$ such that $\eta_{1,n}^* = \eta_1^* + sn^{-1/2}$ for some fixed $s \in \mathbb{R}^{p_1}$ and $n^{1/2}(\widehat{\eta}_{1,n} - \eta_{1,n}^*) = n^{1/2}(\mathbb{P}_n - P_n)u(H_1, A_1, Y) + o_{P_n}(1)$, where u does not depend on s, $\sup_n P_n\|u(H_1, A_1, Y)\|^2 < \infty$, and cov $\{u(H_1, A_1, Y)\}$ is strictly positive definite.

(A2) If $\mathcal{F}$ is any uniformly bounded Donsker class and $n^{1/2}(\mathbb{P}_n - P) \rightsquigarrow \mathbb{T}$ in $l^\infty(\mathcal{F})$ under P, then $n^{1/2}(\mathbb{P}_n - P_n) \rightsquigarrow \mathbb{T}$ in $l^\infty(\mathcal{F})$ under P_n.

(A3) $\sup_n P_n \|Y\|^2 < \infty$.

These assumptions are a simplification of those used in Laber and Murphy (2011). Verification of (A1) can be obtained using methods in the preceding section. Assumption (A2) can be verified using tools from empirical processes; see Chapter 3.10 of van der Vaart and Wellner (1996).

From (3.20), $\widehat{\mathcal{V}}_n(\widehat{d}_n) = 2\mathbb{P}_n Y I\{A_1 H_1^T \widehat{\eta}_{1,n} > 0\}$ is the inverse probability weighted estimator for $\mathcal{V}(\widehat{d}_n)$, where it is assumed that $H_1^T \widehat{\eta}_{1,n} = 0$ with probability zero, so that sign$(H_1^T \widehat{\eta}_{1,n})$ has been replaced by $H_1^T \widehat{\eta}_{1,n}$, similar to (10.11). Define $\mathbb{T}$ to be a Brownian Bridge indexed by $\mathbb{R}^{p_1}$ with covariance function

$$\text{cov}\{\mathbb{T}(\eta_1), \mathbb{T}(\eta_1')\} = 4P\Big(\big[Y I\{A_1 H_1^T \eta_1 > 0\} I\{H_1^T \eta_1^* = 0\} -$$
$$PY I\{A_1 H_1^T \eta_1 > 0\} I\{H_1^T \eta_1^* = 0\} \big]$$
$$\times \big[Y I\{A_1 H_1^T \eta_1' > 0\} I\{H_1^T \eta_1^* = 0\} - PY I\{A_1 H_1^T \eta_1' > 0\} I\{H_1^T \eta_1^* = 0\} \big] \Big);$$

let $\mathbb{W} \sim \mathcal{N}\big(0, 4P[Y I\{A_1 H_1^T \eta_1^* > 0\} - PY I\{A_1 H_1^T \eta_1^* > 0\}]^2 \big)$; and let $\mathbb{Z} \sim \mathcal{N}(0, PDD^T)$, where $D = \{u(H_1, A_1, Y) - Pu(H_1, A_1, Y)\}$. Furthermore, define $\mathcal{G}$ to be the class of functions

$$\mathcal{G} = \big[g(H_1, A_1, Y; \delta) = 2Y I\{A_1 H_1^T \eta_1 > 0\} I\{H_1^T \eta_1^* = 0\} : \eta_1 \in \mathbb{R}^{p_1} \big].$$

Because the functions in $\mathcal{G}$ are indexed by $\mathbb{R}^{p_1}$, we view $n^{1/2}(\mathbb{P}_n - P_n)$ as a random element of $l^\infty(\mathbb{R}^{p_1})$.

Lemma 10.3.3. *Assume (A0)–(A3). Then*

$$n^{1/2} \begin{pmatrix} \mathbb{P}_n - P_n \\ \widehat{\eta}_{1,n} - \eta_{1,n}^* \\ (\mathbb{P}_n - P_n)2Y I\{A_1 H_1^T \eta_1^* > 0\} \end{pmatrix} \rightsquigarrow \begin{pmatrix} \mathbb{T} \\ \mathbb{Z} \\ \mathbb{W} \end{pmatrix}$$

in $l^\infty(\mathbb{R}^{p_1}) \times \mathbb{R} \times \mathbb{R}^{p_1}$ *under* P_n. *Furthermore, for any* $\eta_1 \in \mathbb{R}^{p_1}$,

$$\text{cov}\{\mathbb{T}(\eta_1), \mathbb{Z}\} = 2P\Big(\big[Y I\{A_1 H_1^T \eta_1 > 0\} I\{H_1^T \eta_1^* = 0\}$$
$$- PY I\{A_1 H_1^T \eta_1 > 0\} I\{H_1^T \eta_1^* = 0\} u(H_1, A_1, Y) \big]$$
$$\times \{u(H_1, A_1, Y) - Pu(H_1, A_1, Y)\}^T \Big);$$

$$\text{cov}(\mathbb{Z}, \mathbb{W}) = 2P\big[Y I\{A_1 H_1^T \eta_1^* > 0\} u(H_1, A_1, Y)^T$$
$$- PY I\{A_1 H_1^T \eta_1^* > 0\} Pu(H_1, A_1, Y)^T \big];$$

and $\text{cov}\{\mathbb{T}(\eta_1), \mathbb{W}\} = 0.$

Corollary 10.3.4. *Assume (A0)–(A3). Then*

$$n^{1/2}\{\widehat{\mathcal{V}}_n(\widehat{d}_n) - \mathcal{V}(\widehat{d}_n)\} \rightsquigarrow \mathbb{T}(\mathbb{Z} + s) + \mathbb{W}$$

under P_n, where the covariance structure of $(\mathbb{T}, \mathbb{Z}, \mathbb{W})$ is as described in Lemma 10.3.3.

The preceding results are proved in the supplementary material for Laber and Murphy (2011). A full proof of these results is rather technical and relies on tools that are beyond the scope of this book. However, to provide some insight into Corollary 10.3.4, we sketch an outline of the main ideas of the proof. This outline is incomplete and makes extensive use of approximations without formal justification.

Proof. Write $n^{1/2}\{\widehat{\mathcal{V}}_n(\widehat{d}_n) - \mathcal{V}(\widehat{d}_n)\} = n^{1/2}(\mathbb{P}_n - P_n)2Y\mathrm{I}\{A_1 H_1^T \widehat{\eta}_{1,n} > 0\}$, which we decompose into two parts

$$n^{1/2}(\mathbb{P}_n - P_n)2Y\mathrm{I}\{A_1 H_1^T \widehat{\eta}_{1,n} > 0\}\mathrm{I}\{H_1^T \eta_1^* = 0\}$$
$$+ n^{1/2}(\mathbb{P}_n - P_n)2Y\mathrm{I}\{A_1 H_1^T \widehat{\eta}_{1,n} > 0\}\mathrm{I}\{H_1^T \eta_1^* \neq 0\}.$$

The first term in the above expression converges to $\mathbb{T}(\mathbb{Z}+s)$, and the second term converges to $\mathbb{W}$. To see this, write the first term as $n^{1/2}(\mathbb{P}_n - P_n)2Y\mathrm{I}\{A_1 H_1^T(\mathbb{Z}_n + s) > 0\}\mathrm{I}\{H_1^T \eta_1^* = 0\}$, where $\mathbb{Z}_n = n^{1/2}(\widehat{\eta}_{1,n} - \eta_{1,n}^*)$, and write the second term as $n^{1/2}(\mathbb{P}_n - P_n)2Y\mathrm{I}\{A_1 H_1^T \eta_1^* > 0\} + o_{P_n}(1)$. The mapping $\mathfrak{C} : l^\infty(\mathbb{R}^{p_1}) \times \mathbb{R}^{p_1} \times \mathbb{R} \to \mathbb{R}$ given by $\mathfrak{C}(G, v, b) = G(v) + b$ is continuous at $(\mathbb{T}, \mathbb{Z}, \mathbb{W})$ in the sense required by the extended continuous mapping theorem; e.g., see Theorem 7.24 of Kosorok (2007)). Thus, the desired result follows. □

These results show that the limiting distribution of $n^{1/2}\{\widehat{\mathcal{V}}_n(\widehat{d}_n) - \mathcal{V}(\widehat{d}_n)\}$ depends on the local parameter s and thus $\mathcal{V}(\widehat{d}_n)$ is nonregular. The two primary approaches for constructing a valid confidence set for the conditional value under these conditions are bounding and the m-out-of-n bootstrap.

Bound-based Confidence Sets

The limiting distribution stated in Corollary 10.3.4 is informative for constructing upper and lower bounds on $n^{1/2}\{\widehat{\mathcal{V}}_n(\widehat{d}_n) - \mathcal{V}(\widehat{d}_n)\}$. The local parameter s appears in the first term, $\mathbb{T}(\mathbb{Z}+s)$, but not in the second term, $\mathbb{W}$; therefore, tight upper and lower bounds only should affect (at least asymptotically) subjects contributing to this first term. From the heuristic proof following Corollary 10.3.4, it can be seen that these subjects have realized h_1 belonging to the set $\{h_1 \in \mathbb{R}^{p_1} : h_1^T \eta_1^* = 0\}$; i.e., they are on the decision boundary of $d_1^*(h_1) = \text{sign}(h_1^T \eta_1^*)$. However, in finite samples one cannot identify this set, and therefore we (conservatively) apply the bounds using patients who are "near" this decision boundary. It is critical to note, as discussed in the opening of this chapter, that our concern is constructing high-quality asymptotic approximations to the sampling distribution of the conditional value, and thus we need an asymptotic framework that captures a lack of power in detecting the sign of the treatment effect for some patients in finite samples. To retain this lack of power asymptotically, we consider a sequence of generative models such that, *in the limit*, there may be a point mass on the boundary. However, the probability mass on the boundary for any finite sample may well be zero. Thus, as we have seen, the quality of an asymptotic approximation based on a fixed parameter framework and that (perhaps even correctly) assumes that there are no null treatment effects can be extremely poor in finite samples due to a lack of uniformity in convergence.

Let $\widehat{\Sigma}_n$ denote an estimator for the asymptotic covariance matrix of $\widehat{\eta}_{1,n}$. Upper and lower bounds on $n^{1/2}\{\widehat{\mathcal{V}}_n(\widehat{d}_n) - \mathcal{V}(\widehat{d}_n)\}$ are

$$U_n = \sup_{\omega \in \mathbb{R}^{p_1}} n^{1/2}(\mathbb{P}_n - P_n) 2Y \mathrm{I}\left\{A_1 H_1^T \omega > 0\right\} \mathrm{I}\left\{\frac{n(H_1^T \widehat{\eta}_{1,n})^2}{H_1^T \widehat{\Sigma}_n H_1} \leq \tau_n\right\}$$

$$+ n^{1/2}(\mathbb{P}_n - P_n) 2Y \mathrm{I}\left\{A_1 H_1^T \widehat{\eta}_{1,n} > 0\right\} \mathrm{I}\left\{\frac{n(H_1^T \widehat{\eta}_{1,n})^2}{H_1^T \widehat{\Sigma}_n H_1} > \tau_n\right\}, \quad (10.12)$$

$$L_n = \inf_{\omega \in \mathbb{R}^{p_1}} n^{1/2}(\mathbb{P}_n - P_n) 2Y \mathrm{I}\left\{A_1 H_1^T \omega > 0\right\} \mathrm{I}\left\{\frac{n(H_1^T \widehat{\eta}_{1,n})^2}{H_1^T \widehat{\Sigma}_n H_1} \leq \tau_n\right\}$$

$$+ n^{1/2}(\mathbb{P}_n - P_n) 2Y \mathrm{I}\left\{A_1 H_1^T \widehat{\eta}_{1,n} > 0\right\} \mathrm{I}\left\{\frac{n(H_1^T \widehat{\eta}_{1,n})^2}{H_1^T \widehat{\Sigma}_n H_1} > \tau_n\right\},$$

$$(10.13)$$

where τ_n is a tuning parameter that satisfies $\tau_n \to \infty$ and $\tau_n = o(n)$ as $n \to \infty$. The intuition behind these bounds is as follows. Patients are partitioned into two groups according to whether or not the test statistic $n(h_1^T \widehat{\eta}_{1,n})^2/(h_1^T \widehat{\Sigma}_n h_1)$ exceeds critical value τ_n. This test statistic can be viewed as testing the null hypothesis $\mathsf{H}_0 : h_1^T \eta_1^* = 0$ for each h_1. When the test statistic is large and this null is rejected, the patient is categorized as being far from the decision boundary $\{h_1 \in \mathbb{R}^{p_1} : h_1^T \eta_1^* = 0\}$; otherwise, the patient is categorized as being too close to distinguish from being on the boundary. Among subjects close to the boundary, we take a supremum (infimum) over all local perturbations of the generative model. To verify that U_n and L_n bracket $n^{1/2}\{\widehat{\mathcal{V}}_n(\widehat{d}_n) - \mathcal{V}(\widehat{d}_n)\}$, replace ω with $\mathbb{Z}_n + s$ in (10.12) and (10.13).

We discuss properties of the upper bound with the understanding that equivalent results hold for the lower bound. The sup used to construct the upper bound has a smoothing effect, which makes it regular. Furthermore, because the sup is over local perturbations, it can be shown that this bound is smallest in the sense that any other regular upper bound would have to be at least as large asymptotically. These results are summarized in the following theorem, which is proved in Laber and Murphy (2011).

Theorem 10.3.5. *Assume (A0)–(A3). Then, under P_n,*

$$(L_n, U_n) \rightsquigarrow \left\{ \inf_{\omega \in \mathbb{R}^{p_1}} \mathbb{T}(\omega) + \mathbb{W}, \ \sup_{\omega \in \mathbb{R}^{p_1}} \mathbb{T}(\omega) + \mathbb{W} \right\}.$$

This result cannot be used directly to construct a confidence set for $\mathcal{V}(\widehat{d}_n)$, as the bounds L_n and U_n depend on P_n. To form a confidence set, we approximate the joint distribution of (L_n, U_n) using the bootstrap, as follows.

Let $\mathbb{P}_n^{(b)}$ denote the bootstrap empirical distribution, induced by resampling with replacement. Under $\mathbb{P}_n^{(b)}$, the expectation of a function $f(H_1, A_1, Y)$ is $\mathbb{P}_n^{(b)} f(H_1, A_1, Y) = n^{-1} \sum_{i=1}^{n} W_{n,i} f(H_{1i}, A_{1i}, Y_i)$, where $(W_{n,1}, \ldots, W_{n,n})$ is a draw from a multinomial distribution with n trials, n categories, and success probabilities $(1/n, \ldots, 1/n)$. For a functional $g = g(P, \mathbb{P}_n)$, let $g^{(b)} = g(\mathbb{P}_n, \mathbb{P}_n^{(b)})$ denote its bootstrap analog. The bootstrap upper and lower bounds are

$$U_n^{(b)} = \sup_{\omega \in \mathbb{R}^{p_1}} n^{1/2} (\mathbb{P}_n^{(b)} - \mathbb{P}_n) 2Y \mathbb{I} \left\{ A_1 H_1^T \omega > 0 \right\} \mathbb{I} \left\{ \frac{n(H_1^T \widehat{\eta}_{1,n}^{(b)})^2}{H_1^T \widehat{\Sigma}_n^{(b)} H_1} \leq \tau_n \right\}$$
$$+ n^{1/2} (\mathbb{P}_n^{(b)} - \mathbb{P}_n) 2Y \mathbb{I} \left\{ A_1 H_1^T \widehat{\eta}_{1,n}^{(b)} > 0 \right\} \mathbb{I} \left\{ \frac{n(H_1^T \widehat{\eta}_{1,n}^{(b)})^2}{H_1^T \widehat{\Sigma}_n^{(b)} H_1} > \tau_n \right\},$$

$$(10.14)$$

$$L_n^{(b)} = \inf_{\omega \in \mathbb{R}^{p_1}} n^{1/2} (\mathbb{P}_n^{(b)} - \mathbb{P}_n) 2Y \mathbb{I} \left\{ A_1 H_1^T \omega > 0 \right\} \mathbb{I} \left\{ \frac{n(H_1^T \widehat{\eta}_{1,n}^{(b)})^2}{H_1^T \widehat{\Sigma}_n^{(b)} H_1} \leq \tau_n \right\}$$
$$+ n^{1/2} (\mathbb{P}_n^{(b)} - \mathbb{P}_n) 2Y \mathbb{I} \left\{ A_1 H_1^T \widehat{\eta}_{1,n}^{(b)} > 0 \right\} \mathbb{I} \left\{ \frac{n(H_1^T \widehat{\eta}_{1,n}^{(b)})^2}{H_1^T \widehat{\Sigma}_n^{(b)} H_1} > \tau_n \right\}.$$

$$(10.15)$$

Let $\widehat{\ell}_{n,\alpha/2}^{(b)}$ and $\widehat{u}_{n,1-\alpha/2}^{(b)}$ denote the $(\alpha/2) \times 100$ and $(1 - \alpha/2) \times 100$ percentiles of $L_n^{(b)}$ and $U_n^{(b)}$, respectively. A $(1 - \alpha) \times 100\%$ bootstrap confidence interval based on bounds L_n and U_n is thus

$$\left[\widehat{\mathcal{V}}_n(\widehat{d}_n) - \widehat{u}_{n,1-\alpha/2}^{(b)}/n^{1/2}, \; \widehat{\mathcal{V}}_n(\widehat{d}_n) - \widehat{\ell}_{n,\alpha/2}^{(b)}/n^{1/2}\right].$$

The following result shows that the conditional distribution of $(L_n^{(b)}, U_n^{(b)})$ given the observed data and the (unconditional) distribution of (L_n, U_n) converge to the same limiting distribution. The implication of this result is convergence in probability of the quantiles of each distribution and consequently asymptotically correct coverage of the bootstrap confidence set based on the bounds. Let P_M denote expectation with respect to the randomness induced by sampling with replacement from the observed data, and let $\mathrm{BL}_1(\mathbb{R}^2)$ denote the space of bounded Lipschitz-1 functions on $\mathbb{R}^2$ (Kosorok, 2007). A proof of the following result can be derived from the proof of Theorem 3.3 in Laber and Murphy (2011).

Theorem 10.3.6. *Assume (A0)–(A3) with local parameter $s = 0$ (i.e., fixed asymptotics). In addition, assume that $\widehat{\Sigma}_n^{(b)}$ converges conditionally in probability, given the observed data, to Σ. Then*

$$\sup_{g \in \mathrm{BL}_1(\mathbb{R}^2)} \left| Pg(L_n, U_n) - P_M g(L_n^{(b)}, U_n^{(b)}) \right|$$

converges to zero in probability.

The preceding result ensures asymptotically correct coverage of the bound-based confidence set. However, to construct these bounds requires (C1), an algorithm for computing $L_n^{(b)}$ and $U_n^{(b)}$ for each bootstrap sample, and (C2), a method for choosing the tuning parameter τ_n. We first describe two approaches to (C1) with fixed τ_n and then describe how to tune τ_n adaptively by repeated calls to the algorithm used in (C1).

For conciseness, we focus on algorithms for computing $U_n^{(b)}$; algorithms for computing $L_n^{(b)}$ follow from straightforward modifications. For any $\varpi \in \{-1, 0, \dots, n-1\}^n$, define $\mathcal{I}^{(b)}(\varpi, \tau_n) = \{i \in \{1, \dots, n\} : n(H_{1i}^T \widehat{\eta}_{1,n}^{(b)})^2 \le \tau_n H_{1i}^T \widehat{\Sigma}_n^{(b)} H_{1i}, \varpi_i \ne 0\}$. Computing $U_n^{(b)}$ is equivalent to solving the optimization problem

$$\sup_{\omega \in \mathbb{R}^{p_1}, \theta_1, \dots, \theta_n \in \{0,1\}} \sum_{i \in \mathcal{I}^{(b)}(\varpi, \tau_n)} \varpi_i \theta_i$$

$$\text{such that} \quad \theta_i = 1 \text{ if } A_{1i} H_{1i}^T \omega \ge 0,$$

$$\theta_i = \text{otherwise},$$

where ϖ_i is Y_i times the number of times the patient with index i occurs in the bootstrap sample minus 1. The form of the foregoing optimization characterizes it as a linear mixed integer program (MIP, Wolsey and Nemhauser, 2014). In general, MIPs are NP-hard (Schrijver, 1998); however, they are a well-studied class of problems, and there is a large body of robust and mature software for solving MIPs (IBM ILOG CPLEX, 2019; MOSEK, 2019; Gurobi Optimization, 2019). Algorithms for MIPs can compute the bounds exactly (to machine precision) but may be computationally burdensome, especially in high-dimensional settings.

One approach to reduce the computational burden associated with solving the MIP is to solve a convex relaxation of the original problem. As noted in Section 4.3, this approach has been widely used in classification (Bartlett et al., 2006) and is the basis for OWL. We describe two convex relaxations, both based on replacing the indicator $\mathrm{I}\{A_1 H_1^T \widehat{\eta}_{1,n}^{(b)} > 0\}$ with a smooth surrogate.

The first relaxation uses a sequence of approximations with Gauss-Seidel type updates. Let ϖ_i and $\mathcal{I}^{(b)}(\varpi, \tau_n)$ be as defined above. Then computing the bounds requires finding an element of

$$\arg\sup_{\omega \in \mathbb{R}^{p_1}} \sum_{i \in \mathcal{I}^{(b)}(\varpi, \tau_n)} \varpi_i \mathrm{I}\left\{A_{1i} H_{1i}^T \omega > 0\right\},$$

which some algebra shows to be equivalent to finding an element of

$$\arg\inf_{\omega \in \mathbb{R}^{p_1}} \sum_{i \in \mathcal{I}^{(b)}(\varpi, \tau_n)} |\varpi_i| \mathrm{I}\left\{\mathrm{sign}(\varpi_i) A_{1i} H_{1i}^T \omega \le 0\right\}$$

$$= \arg\inf_{\omega \in \mathbb{R}^{p_1} : \|\omega\|_1 \ge 1} \sum_{i \in \mathcal{I}^{(b)}(\varpi, \tau_n)} \frac{\left\{-\varpi_i A_{1i} H_{1i}^T \omega\right\}_+}{|H_{1i}^T \omega|}, \quad (10.16)$$

where we have used

$$|\varpi_i| \mathrm{I}\{\mathrm{sign}(\varpi_i) A_{1i} H_{1i}^T \omega \le 0\}$$
$$= |\varpi_i| \{-\mathrm{sign}(\varpi_i) A_{1i} H_{1i}^T \omega\}_+ / |\mathrm{sign}(\varpi_i) A_{1i} H_{1i}^T \omega|$$
$$= \{-\varpi_i A_{1i} H_{1i}^T \omega\}_+ / |H_{1i}^T \omega|.$$

The constraint $\|\omega\|_1 \ge 1$ is superfluous; however, this constraint prevents a trivial solution at $\omega \equiv 0$ after the convex relaxation is applied (note that $\omega \equiv 0$ is not a solution to the original problem unless $\varpi_i = 0$ for all i, in which case any $\omega \in \mathbb{R}^{p_1}$ is a solution). Letting $\Gamma(h_1, a_1, \varpi; \omega, \delta) = \{-\varpi a_1 h_1^T \omega\}_+ / |x^T \delta|$, we are interested in computing $\arg\inf_{\omega \in \mathbb{R}^{p_1}} \sum_{i \in \mathcal{I}^{(b)}(\varpi, \tau_n)} \Gamma(H_{1i}, A_{1i}, \varpi_i; \omega, \omega)$. However, for each fixed value of $\delta \in \mathbb{R}^{p_1}$, computing $\arg\inf_{\omega \in \mathbb{R}^{p_1}} \Gamma(H_{1i}, A_{1i}, \varpi_i; \omega, \delta)$ is a linear program and can be solved efficiently even for very large problems. This suggests an iterative Gauss-Seidel updating rule wherein we repeatedly optimize over the first parameter and in each iteration plug-in a current "best guess" for the second parameter. Algorithm 10.1 provides pseudo code for this procedure. The algorithm requires a starting value, $\omega^{(0)}$; a damping factor, $\epsilon \in (0, 1)$; and a tolerance, tol > 0, which dictates the

---

Algorithm 10.1: Gauss-Seidel convex relaxation

Input: $\mathcal{I}^{(b)}(\varpi, \tau_n)$, $\omega^{(0)}$, $\epsilon \in (0, 1)$, $\{H_{1i}, A_{1i}, \varpi_i\}_{i \in \mathcal{I}^{(b)}(\varpi, \tau_n)}$,
     tol > 0

1 Set $k = 0$

2 **do**

3      $\widetilde{\omega} = \arg\inf_{\omega} \sum_{i \in \mathcal{I}^{(b)}(\varpi, \tau_n)} \Gamma\left(H_{1i}, A_{1i}, \varpi_i; \omega, \omega^{(k)}\right)$

4      $\omega^{(k+1)} = \omega^{(k)} + \epsilon\left\{\widetilde{\omega} - \omega^{(k)}\right\}$

5      $k = k + 1$

6 **while** $\|\omega^{(k)} - \omega^{(k-1)}\| >$ *tol*;

   Output: $\omega^{(k)}$

---

stopping criteria for the algorithm. In practice, these parameters must be tuned, and multiple starting values should be considered. A starting place for this tuning is $\omega^{(0)} = \widehat{\eta}_{1,n}^{(b)}$, $\epsilon \in [0.4, 0.6]$, and tol $\approx \epsilon^5$.

An alternative to the iterative Gauss-Seidel algorithm is to solve a single convex relaxation of the original problem. This approach is harder to justify from simple algebraic arguments than the Gauss-Seidel algorithm; however, it is supported by extensive and deep theory (Bartlett et al., 2003, 2006). Let $\ell : \mathbb{R} \to \mathbb{R}$ denote a convex function such as those in Figure 10.3. The relaxed solution is any element of

$$\arg\inf_{\omega \in \mathbb{R}^{p_1}} \sum_{i \in \mathcal{I}^{(b)}(\varpi, \tau_n)} |\varpi_i| \ell\{\text{sign}(\varpi_i) A_{1i} H_{1i}^T \omega\}, \tag{10.17}$$

which is obtained by replacing $\mathrm{I}\left\{\text{sign}(\varpi_i) A_{1i} H_{1i}^T \omega \leq 0\right\}$ for each i in the first term in (10.16) with $\ell\left\{\text{sign}(\varpi_i) A_{1i} H_{1i}^T \omega\right\}$. The objective function in (10.17) is the sum of convex functions and is therefore convex; thus, a minimizer can be computed efficiently using standard methods (Boyd and Vandenberghe, 2004; Bertsekas, 2015).

To illustrate the tradeoff between computational complexity and solution quality, we consider a small simulation experiment. We generate data according to the following generative model: $A_1 \sim$ Uniform $\{-1, 1\}$; $X_1 \sim$ Uniform$[-1, 1]^{p_1}$; $\epsilon \sim \mathcal{N}(0, 1)$; and $Y = A_1(\sum_{j=1}^{p_1} X_{1j} - 1/3)^2 + \epsilon$. For simplicity, assume that the resampling weights are all equal and positive, so that $\varpi_i \propto Y_i$ for all i. For each $p_1 = 5, \ldots, 10$ and for 50 Monte Carlo replications, we generate a data set of size $n = 100$ from the above generative model and approximate $\arg\inf_{\omega \in \mathbb{R}^{p_1}} \sum_{i=1}^{n} |\varpi_i| \mathrm{I}\left\{\text{sign}(\varpi_i) A_{1i} H_{1i}^T \omega \leq 0\right\}$ using the MIP, Gauss-Seidel, and convex relaxation with $\ell(x) = \exp(-x)$. Table 10.1 shows the average value of the objective function after optimization and the run time for each algorithm. The table shows a clear trade-off between solution quality and computation time. MIP uniformly obtains the smallest

p_1	Objective value			Run time (sec.)		
	MIP	GS	Exponential	MIP	GS	Exponential
5	124.7	125.6	141.1	5.55	0.60	0.04
6	136.2	149.3	164.5	6.67	0.90	0.05
7	140.8	158.7	176.0	11.1	0.93	0.06
8	147.1	173.6	194.5	11.1	0.96	0.07
9	152.8	189.5	206.0	13.7	1.4	0.10
10	167.3	211.2	223.4	13.9	1.4	0.13

Table 10.1 *Objective function values and run times for approximating an element of* $\arg\inf_{\omega \in \mathbb{R}^{p_1}} \sum_{i=1}^{n} |\varpi_i| I\{\operatorname{sign}(\varpi_i) A_{1i} H_{1i}^T \omega \leq 0\}$ *using MIP, Gauss-Seidel (GS), and an exponential convex surrogate (Exponential). Results are averaged over 50 Monte Carlo replications.*

average value of the objective function but at the highest computational cost. The convex relaxation has the largest average value but the smallest computational cost. The Gauss-Seidel algorithm occupies a middle ground in terms of solution quality and computation time. It would be interesting, though beyond the scope of this book, to consider such a Gauss-Seidel algorithm as a middle ground between OWL (which uses a convex surrogate) and direct optimization of the value function (as in the MIP).

The foregoing methods assume a fixed value of τ_n. However, the choice of τ_n can have a significant impact on the coverage of the bound-based interval and must be tuned in practice. One approach is to use the double bootstrap (Hall, 1986; Booth and Hall, 1994) to estimate the coverage associated with each value of τ_n within a set of candidate values and then to select the one that is closest to but above nominal level. Algorithm 10.2 shows the double bootstrap procedure for tuning τ_n. This algorithm contains two layers of bootstrap resampling: (L1) an outer layer (lines 4–10) wherein the data are bootstrapped to mimic repeated sampling of training sets of size n from the underlying generative model; and (L2) an inner layer (line 5), wherein the bound-based bootstrap confidence interval is applied to each bootstrap data set constructed in (L1). Thus, if there are M bootstrap resamples in the outer layer and B bootstrap resamples in the inner layer, the bounds must be computed MB times for each candidate value of τ_n. As this can be computationally burdensome, it is common during tuning to choose M and B to be relatively small, e.g., $M = B = 200$; and then, given a selected value of τ_n, to recompute the bootstrap confidence interval with a large number of resamples, e.g., 1000.

Algorithm 10.2: Tuning the critical value τ_n using the double bootstrap

---

Input: $\{(H_{1i}, A_{1i}, Y_i)\}_{i=1}^{n}$, M, $\alpha \in (0, 1)$, $\left\{\tau_n^{(1)}, \ldots, \tau_n^{(L)}\right\}$

1   $\mathcal{V} = \widehat{\mathcal{V}}_n(\widehat{d}_n)$

2   **for** $j = 1, \ldots, L$ **do**

3      $c^{(j)} = 0$

4   **for** $b = 1, \ldots, M$ **do**

5   Draw a sample of size n, say $S_n^{(b)}$, from $\{(H_{1i}, A_{1i}, Y_i)\}_{i=1}^{n}$ with replacement

6   Compute bound-based confidence set, $\zeta_{m_n}^{(b)}$, using sample $S_n^{(b)}$ and critical value $\tau_n^{(j)}$

7   **if** $\mathcal{V} \in \zeta_{m_n}^{(b)}$ **then**

8             $c^{(j)} = c^{(j)} + 1$

9   **end**

10   **end**

11 **end**

12 Set $j^* = \arg\min_{j \,:\, c^{(j)} \geq M(1-\alpha)} c^{(j)}$

Output: Return $\tau_n^{(j^*)}$

---

m-out-of-n Bootstrap Confidence Sets

Bound-based confidence sets are appealing theoretically in the sense that they attempt to address directly instability to local perturbations of the underlying generative model. On the other hand, the local asymptotic theory underpinning these confidence sets is somewhat technical, which makes them less accessible to quantitative researchers without specialized training and more difficult to generalize to new settings. In contrast, the m-out-of-n bootstrap is conceptually and computationally straightforward and serves as a general-purpose tool for constructing confidence sets for nonsmooth functionals (Shao, 1994; Politis et al., 1999; Romano et al., 2012).

Let m_n denote a bootstrap resample size that satisfies $m_n \to \infty$ and $m_n = o(n)$ as $n \to \infty$. For each n, let $\mathbb{P}_{m_n}^{(b)}$ denote the bootstrap empirical measure based on a resample of size m_n; more generally, for any $Z = g(P, \mathbb{P}_n)$ write $Z_{m_n}^{(b)}$ to denote $g(\mathbb{P}_n, \mathbb{P}_{m_n}^{(b)})$. The m-out-of-n bootstrap approximates the sampling distribution of $n^{1/2}\{\widehat{\mathcal{V}}_n(\widehat{d}_n) - \mathcal{V}(\widehat{d}_n)\}$ with the conditional distribution of $m_n^{1/2}\{\widehat{\mathcal{V}}_{m_n}^{(b)}(\widehat{d}_{m_n}^{(b)}) - \widehat{\mathcal{V}}_n(\widehat{d}_{m_n}^{(b)})\}$ given the observed data. For $\alpha \in (0, 1)$, let $\widehat{\ell}_{m_n}$ and $\widehat{u}_{m_n}$ denote the $(\alpha/2) \times 100$

Algorithm 10.3: m-out-of-n bootstrap confidence set for the conditional value

---

Input: m_n, $\{H_{1i}, A_{1i}, Y_i\}_{i=1}^{n}$, M, $\alpha \in (0,1)$

1 **for** $b = 1, \ldots, M$ **do**

2 | Draw a sample of size m_n, say $S_{m_n}^{(b)}$, from $\{H_{1i}, A_{1i}, Y_i\}_{i=1}^{n}$ with replacement

3 | Compute $\widehat{\eta}_{1,m_n}^{(b)}$ on $S_{m_n}^{(b)}$

4 |
$$\Delta_{m_n}^{(b)} = m_n^{1/2}\Big[\sum_{i \in S_{m_n}^{(b)}} Y_i \mathrm{I}\{A_{1i} H_{1i}^T \widehat{\eta}_{1,m_n}^{(b)} > 0\}$$
$$- \sum_{k=1}^{n} Y_k \mathrm{I}\{A_k X_k^T \widehat{\eta}_{1,m_n}^{(b)} > 0\}\Big]$$

5 **end**

6 Relabel so that $\Delta_{m_n}^{(1)} \leq \Delta_{m_n}^{(2)} \leq \cdots \leq \Delta_{m_n}^{(B)}$

7 $\widehat{\ell}_{m_n} = \Delta_{m_n}^{(\lfloor B\alpha/2 \rfloor)}$

8 $\widehat{u}_{m_n} = \Delta_{m_n}^{(\lfloor B(1-\alpha/2) \rfloor)}$

Output: $\left[\widehat{\mathcal{V}}_n(\widehat{d}_n) - \widehat{u}_{m_n} m_n^{-1/2}, \widehat{\mathcal{V}}_n(\widehat{d}_n) - \widehat{\ell}_{m_n} m_n^{-1/2} \right]$

---

and $(1 - \alpha/2) \times 100$ percentiles of $m_n^{1/2}\{\widehat{\mathcal{V}}_{m_n}^{(b)}(\widehat{d}_{m_n}^{(b)}) - \widehat{\mathcal{V}}_n(\widehat{d}_{m_n}^{(b)})\}$. Then

$$\left[\widehat{\mathcal{V}}_n(\widehat{d}_n) - \widehat{u}_{m_n} m_n^{-1/2}, \widehat{\mathcal{V}}_n(\widehat{d}_n) - \widehat{\ell}_{m_n} m_n^{-1/2} \right]$$

is a $(1 - \alpha) \times 100\%$ m-out-of-n bootstrap confidence set for $\mathcal{V}(\widehat{d}_n)$. Algorithm 10.3 provides a schematic for computing this confidence set.

Let $\mathbb{Z}$ be defined as above. To establish consistency of the m-out-of-n bootstrap, in addition to (A0)–(A3) and the asymptotic growth conditions on m_n, we assume (A4) $m_n^{1/2}(\widehat{\eta}_{1,m_n}^{(b)} - \widehat{\eta}_{1,n})$, conditional on the observed data, converges in distribution to $\mathbb{Z}$ in probability. This condition holds under quite general conditions; see Giné and Zinn (1990) and Chapter 3.6 of van der Vaart and Wellner (1996).

Theorem 10.3.7. *Assume (A0)–A4) with local parameter $s = 0$. Let m_n be a sequence of positive integers such that $m_n \to \infty$ and $m_n = o(n)$ as $n \to \infty$. Let P_{M,m_n} denote the expectation induced by sampling m_n observations with replacement from the observed data.*

$$\sup_{g \in \mathrm{BL}_1(\mathbb{R}^{p_1})} \left| Pg(\mathbb{Z}) - P_{M,m_n} g\left\{ m_n^{1/2}(\widehat{\eta}_{1,m_n}^{(b)} - \widehat{\eta}_{1,n}) \right\} \right| \xrightarrow{p} 0.$$

A proof of this result is omitted; however, letting $\mathbb{G}_{mn}^{(b)} = m_n^{1/2}\left(\mathbb{P}_{mn}^{(b)} - \mathbb{P}_n\right)$, the crux of proof is the expansion

$$m_n^{1/2}\left\{\widehat{\mathcal{V}}_{mn}^{(b)}(\widehat{d}_{mn}^{(b)}) - \widehat{\mathcal{V}}_n(\widehat{d}_{mn}^{(b)})\right\} = \mathbb{G}_{mn}^{(b)}Y\mathrm{I}(A_1 H_1^T \widehat{\eta}_{1,mn}^{(b)} > 0)$$

$$= \mathbb{G}_{mn}^{(b)}\left(Y\mathrm{I}\left[A_1 H_1^T\left\{m_n^{1/2}(\widehat{\eta}_{1,mn}^{(b)} - \widehat{\eta}_{1,n})\right.\right.\right.$$

$$\left.\left.\left. +(m_n/n)^{1/2}n^{1/2}\left(\widehat{\eta}_{1,n} - \eta_1^*\right)\right\} > 0\right]\mathrm{I}(H_1^T \eta_1^* = 0)\right)$$

$$+ \mathbb{G}_{mn}^{(b)}Y\mathrm{I}(A_1 H_1^T \widehat{\eta}_{1,mn}^{(b)} > 0)\mathrm{I}\left\{H_1^T \eta_1^* = 0\right\},$$

where $\mathbb{G}_{mn}^{(b)}$, seen as an element of $l^\infty(\mathbb{R}^{p_1})$ via $\eta \mapsto \mathbb{G}_{mn}^{(b)}Y\mathrm{I}\left\{AH_1^T\eta > 0\right\}$ $\mathrm{I}\left\{XT\eta_1^* = 0\right\}$, converges in distribution to $\mathbb{T}$ (van der Vaart and Wellner, 1996, Theorem 3.6.3); and $(m_n/n)^{1/2}n^{1/2}(\widehat{\eta}_{1,n} - \eta_1^*)$ converges to zero in probability.

Application of the m-out-of-n bootstrap confidence interval requires a choice of resample size m_n. The asymptotic conditions $m_n \to \infty$ and $m_n = o(n)$ do not provide guidance on what m_n should be for a given data set. Reducing m_n reduces the amount of information contained in each resample, which in turn makes the conditional distribution of $\widehat{\mathcal{V}}_{mn}^{(b)}(\widehat{d}_{mn}^{(b)})$ more variable. Thus, confidence sets based on resamples of size m_n may be larger and lead to higher coverage as m_n decreases, although this intuition is imperfect, as bias may increase as m_n decreases. Because it is desirable to construct the smallest confidence set that delivers nominal coverage, one approach to choosing m_n is to consider a sequence of decreasing candidate values for m_n and to choose the largest m_n for which the estimated coverage is at or above nominal level. For each candidate resample size m_n, the coverage of the m-out-of-n bootstrap using m_n is estimated using the double bootstrap (Hall, 1986; Booth and Hall, 1994). Algorithm 10.4 displays the double bootstrap tuning procedure as proposed by Chakraborty et al. (2014a,b). Lines 5–11 of this algorithm estimate the coverage of the m-out-of-n bootstrap for resample size m_n, and the algorithm terminates when the estimated coverage is within a prespecified tolerance of nominal coverage or a minimal resample size is reached.

Remark. In practice, the bound-based interval tends to deliver correct, if conservative, coverage across a wide range of generative models, including those engineered to induce a highly unstable sampling distribution. However, these intervals can be computationally expensive and are nontrivial to extend to new domains. In contrast, subsampling based intervals using the m-out-of-n bootstrap are less conservative but can

---

Algorithm 10.4: Tuning the resample size in the m-out-of-n bootstrap using the double bootstrap

Input: m_0, step, $m_{\min}$, $\{(A_{1i}, H_{1i}, Y_i)\}_{i=1}^n$, M, $\alpha \in (0,1)$, tol

1   $m_n = m_0$

2   $V = \widehat{V}_n(\widehat{d}_n)$

3   **do**

4      $c = 0$

5   **for** $b = 1, \ldots, M$ **do**

6   Draw a sample of size n, say $S_n^{(b)}$, from $\{(H_{1i}, A_{1i}, Y_i)\}_{i=1}^n$ with replacement

7   Compute confidence set, $\zeta_{m_n}^{(b)}$, via Alg. (10.3) using sample $S_n^{(b)}$ and resample size m_n

8   **if** $V \in \zeta_{m_n}^{(b)}$ **then**

9 | $c = c + 1$

10   **end**

11   **end**

12      $m_n = m_n - \text{step}$

13 **while** $c/M <= 1 - \alpha - \text{tol}$ *and* $m_n > m_{\min}$;

    Output: Return $m_n + \text{step}$

---

undercover in some settings and can be sensitive to tuning but are trivial to implement and extend to new domains. Our view is that overcoverage is a lesser sin than undercoverage and thus we recommend bound-based intervals, especially in settings where they have been derived and tested.

Value of an Optimal Regime within a Class

For simplicity, we continue to assume that the propensities are known and fixed as in (10.7). To construct a confidence set for $V(d^*)$, where, as previously, d^* is the population analog of $\widehat{d}_n$, first suppose that d^* is known. As noted in Section 3.3, for any fixed regime d, usual estimators for $V(d)$ can be shown to be asymptotically normal under standard conditions. For example, under the conditions here, for fixed d, a natural estimator for $V(d)$ is the inverse probability weighted estimator $\widehat{V}_n(d) = 2\mathbb{P}_n Y I\{A_1 d(H_1) > 0\}$, and $n^{1/2}\{\widehat{V}_n(d) - V(d)\} = 2n^{1/2}(\mathbb{P}_n - P)YI\{A_1 d(H_1) > 0\}$ is regular and asymptotically normal provided Y has a second moment. Thus, either a normal approximation or the bootstrap can be used to construct an approximation to the sampling distribution of $n^{1/2}\{\widehat{V}_n(d) - V(d)\}$ and subsequently to form a confidence set for $V(d)$. For any fixed regime d, let $\zeta_{n,1-\nu}(d)$ denote a $(1 - \nu) \times 100$

percent confidence set for $\mathcal{V}(d)$; i.e., $P\{\mathcal{V}(d) \in \zeta_{n,1-\nu}(d)\} \geq 1 - \nu + o(1)$. Thus, $\zeta_{n,1-\nu}(d^*)$ is a valid $(1 - \nu) \times 100\%$ confidence set for $\mathcal{V}(d^*)$.

Of course, d^* is not known in general; however, suppose that we have an asymptotic confidence set for d^*, say $\mathcal{B}_{n,1-\eta}$, so that $P(d^* \in \mathcal{B}_{n,1-\delta}) \geq 1 - \delta + o(1)$. Then, using arguments presented in the introduction to this chapter, it can be seen that

$$\bigcup_{d \in \mathcal{B}_{n,1-\delta}} \zeta_{n,1-\nu}(d)$$

is a valid asymptotic $(1 - \delta - \nu) \times 100\%$ projection confidence set for $\mathcal{V}(d^*)$. For example, under (A0)–(A3), one can choose

(i) $\zeta_{n,1-\nu}(d) = [\widehat{\mathcal{V}}_n(d) - z_{1-\nu/2}\widehat{\sigma}_n(d)/n^{1/2}, \ \widehat{\mathcal{V}}_n(d) + z_{1-\nu/2}\widehat{\sigma}_n(d)/n^{1/2}]$,

where $\widehat{\sigma}_n^2(d) = \mathbb{P}_n[2Y\mathrm{I}\{A_1 d(H_1) > 0\} - 2\mathbb{P}_n Y\mathrm{I}\{A_1 d(H_1) > 0\}]^2$; and (ii) $\mathcal{B}_{n,1-\delta} = \{d : d_1(h_1) = \mathrm{sign}(h_1^T \eta_1), \eta_1 \in \mathcal{W}_{n,1-\delta}\}$, where for $\eta_1 \in \mathbb{R}^{p_1}$

$$\mathcal{W}_{n,1-\delta} = \{\eta_1 \in \mathbb{R}^{p_1} : n(\eta_1 - \widehat{\eta}_{1,n})^T \widehat{\Sigma}_n^{-1}(\eta_1 - \widehat{\eta}_{1,n}) \leq \chi^2_{p,1-\delta}\}$$

is a $(1 - \delta) \times 100\%$ Wald-type confidence set for η_1^*.

The foregoing projection interval is simple to construct and is valid under local and fixed asymptotic frameworks. However, it can be excessively conservative, especially when many patients have realized history h_1 far from the decision boundary $\{h_1 : h_1^T \eta_1^* = 0\}$ (Laber et al., 2014c). An adaptive projection set attempts to reduce conservatism by applying the projection only to patients with $H_1 = h_1$ such that $h_1^T \eta_1^* \approx 0$. If all the patients are on the decision boundary, the adaptive projection set is equivalent to the projection set, whereas if $|H_1^T \eta_1^*|$ is bounded away from zero with probability one, the adaptive projection set is asymptotically equivalent to a standard percentile bootstrap confidence interval.

Let $\tau_n > 0$ and $\widehat{\Sigma}_n$ be as defined in the bound-based confidence sets above. Write

$$\mathfrak{M}_n(\eta_1, \eta) = 2n^{1/2}\left(\mathbb{P}_n - P\right)Y\mathrm{I}\left\{A_1 H_1^T \eta_1 > 0\right\}\mathrm{I}\left\{\frac{n(H_1^T \eta_1)^2}{H_1^T \widehat{\Sigma}_n H_1} > \tau_n\right\}$$

$$+ 2n^{1/2}\left(\mathbb{P}_n - P\right)Y\mathrm{I}\left\{A_1 H_1^T \eta > 0\right\}\mathrm{I}\left\{\frac{n(H_1^T \eta_1)^2}{H_1^T \widehat{\Sigma}_n H_1} \leq \tau_n\right\}.$$

Then $\mathfrak{M}_n(\eta_1^*, \eta_1^*) = n^{1/2}\{\widehat{\mathcal{V}}_n(\eta_1^*) - \mathcal{V}(\eta_1^*)\}$. We show that $\mathfrak{M}_n(\eta_1, \eta)$ is smooth in its first argument, and thus it is possible to substitute an estimator for η_1^* in the first argument and apply a union over only the second argument. This leads to a significant reduction in conservatism over the standard projection set (Wu, 2015). The following results describe the adaptive projection set and its properties.

Lemma 10.3.8. *Assume (A0)–(A3), $\tau_n \to \infty$, and $\tau_n = o(1)$ as $n \to \infty$. Then $\mathfrak{M}_n(\widehat{\eta}_{1,n}, \eta_1^*) = \mathfrak{M}_n(\eta_1^*, \eta_1^*) + o_{P_n}(1)$.*

Proof. Under the local generative model, $\mathfrak{M}_n(\widehat{\eta}_{1,n}, \eta_1^*) - \mathfrak{M}_n(\eta_1^*, \eta_1^*)$ is

$$2n^{1/2}(\mathbb{P}_n - P_n)Y \operatorname{sign}\left(A_1 H_1^T \eta_{1,n}^*\right) \mathrm{I}\left\{(H_1^T \widehat{\eta}_{1,n})(H_1^T \eta_n^*) < 0\right\}$$
$$\times \mathrm{I}\left\{A_1 H_1^T \widehat{\eta}_{1,n} > 0\right\} \mathrm{I}\left\{\frac{n(H_1^T \widehat{\eta}_{1,n})^2}{H_1^T \widehat{\Sigma}_n H_1} > \tau_n\right\},$$

which is bounded above in magnitude by

$$2n^{1/2}(\mathbb{P}_n + P_n)|Y| \mathrm{I}\left\{(H_1^T \widehat{\eta}_{1,n})(H_1^T \eta_n^*) < 0\right\}$$
$$\times \mathrm{I}\left\{A_1 H_1^T \widehat{\eta}_{1,n} > 0\right\} \mathrm{I}\left\{\frac{n(H_1^T \widehat{\eta}_{1,n})^2}{H_1^T \widehat{\Sigma}_n H_1} > \tau_n\right\}. \tag{10.18}$$

The events $(H_1^T \widehat{\eta}_{1,n})(H_1^T \eta_{1,n}^*) < 0$ and $n(H_1^T \widehat{\eta}_{1,n})^2 > \tau_n H_1^T \widehat{\Sigma}_n H_1$ imply that $\|n^{1/2}(\widehat{\eta}_{1,n} - \eta_{1,n}^*)\| \geq (\tau_n \widehat{\lambda}_{n,\min})^{1/2}$, where $\widehat{\lambda}_{n,\min}$ is the smallest eigenvalue of $\widehat{\Sigma}_n$. Thus, (10.18) is bounded above by $\{(\mathbb{P}_n + P_n)|Y|\} n^{1/2}\mathrm{I}\{\|n^{1/2}(\widehat{\eta}_{1,n} - \eta_{1,n}^*)\| \geq (\tau_n \widehat{\lambda}_{n,\min})^{1/2}\} = o_{P_n}(1)$. $\square$

As above, let $\mathfrak{M}_n^{(b)}(\widehat{\eta}_{1,n}^{(b)}, \eta_1)$ be the bootstrap analog of $\mathfrak{M}_n(\widehat{\eta}_{1,n}, \eta_1)$. The results presented next follow directly.

Lemma 10.3.9. *Assume (A0)–(A3) with $s = 0$, and let $\eta_1 \in \mathbb{R}^{p_1}$ be fixed. Then*

$$\sup_{g \in BL_1(\mathbb{R})} \left| Pg\left\{\mathfrak{M}_n(\widehat{\eta}_{1,n}, \eta_1)\right\} - P_M g\left\{\mathfrak{M}_n^{(b)}(\widehat{\eta}_{1,n}^{(b)}, \eta_1)\right\} \right| \xrightarrow{p} 0.$$

Corollary 10.3.10. *Assume (A0)–(A3) with $s = 0$, and let $\widehat{\ell}_{n,\nu/2}^{(b)}(\eta_1)$ and $\widehat{u}_{n,1-\nu/2}^{(b)}(\eta_1)$ denote the $(\nu/2) \times 100$ and $(1 - \nu/2) \times 100$ percentiles of $\mathfrak{M}_n^{(b)}(\widehat{\eta}_{1,n}^{(b)}, \eta_1)$. Let $\mathcal{W}_{n,1-\delta}$ be defined as above. Then*

$$\bigcup_{\eta_1 \in \mathcal{W}_{n,1-\delta}} \left[\widehat{\ell}_{n,\nu/2}^{(b)}(\eta_1), \widehat{u}_{n,1-\nu/2}^{(b)}(\eta_1)\right]$$

is an asymptotically valid $(1 - \delta - \nu) \times 100\%$ confidence set for $\mathcal{V}(d^*)$.

The preceding result describes the construction of an adaptive projection confidence set and shows that it provides asymptotically correct coverage. However, implementing this interval requires taking the union of bootstrap confidence sets over the ellipsoid $\mathcal{W}_{n,1-\delta}$. The simplest approximation to this union is to sample a large number of points uniformly distributed across $\mathcal{W}_{n,1-\delta}$ (Krauth, 2006; Lange, 2010), say, $\eta_1^{(1)}, \ldots, \eta_1^{(J)}$, and then to compute

$$\bigcup_{j=1}^{J} \left[\widehat{\ell}_{n,\nu/2}(\eta_1^{(j)}), \widehat{u}_{n,1-\nu/2}(\eta_1^{(j)}) \right].$$

Another practical consideration is the choice of tuning parameter τ_n. As in the bound-based confidence set and m-out-of-n bootstrap confidence set, tuning can be done using the double bootstrap.

Value when the Q-function Is Assumed Correctly Specified

If instead one considers regression-based estimation of the value of a regime, if one is willing to assume that the postulated form for the Q-function is correctly specified, this can lead to smaller confidence sets.

We focus on the construction of a confidence set for $\mathcal{V}(d^*)$ assuming a correctly specified linear Q-function so that d^* is equivalent to d^{opt}. Assume that the posited, correctly specified Q-function model is

$$Q_1(h_1, \beta_1; \beta_{1,n}) = h_1^T \beta_{11,n} + a_1 h_1^T \beta_{12,n}, \quad \beta_{1,n} = (\beta_{11,n}^T, \beta_{12,n}^T)^T,$$

and $\beta_{1,0,n} = (\beta_{11,0,n}^T, \beta_{12,0,n}^T)^T \in \mathbb{R}^{p_1 \times p_1}$ denotes the true parameter vector under the local generative distribution P_n. Letting $\widehat{\beta}_{1,n} = (\widehat{\beta}_{11,n}^T, \widehat{\beta}_{12,n}^T)^T$ denote the OLS estimator for $\beta_{1,n}$, an estimator $\widehat{d}_n$ for an optimal regime has estimated rule $\widehat{d}_{1,n}(h_1) = \text{sign}(h_1^T \widehat{\beta}_{1,n})$. Using $\mathcal{V}(d) = E\{Q_1\{H_1, d_1(H_1)\}$ as in (3.14), an estimator for $\mathcal{V}(\widehat{d}_n)$ is $\widetilde{\mathcal{V}}_n(\widehat{d}_n) = \mathbb{P}_n Q_1\{H_1, \widehat{d}_{1,n}(H_1)\} = \mathbb{P}_n H_1^T \widehat{\beta}_{11,n} + \mathbb{P}_n |H_1^T \widehat{\beta}_{12,n}|$. Thus,

$$n^{1/2}\{\widetilde{\mathcal{V}}_n(\widehat{d}_n) - \mathcal{V}(\widehat{d}_n)\} = n^{1/2}(\mathbb{P}_n - P_n)\{H_1^T \widehat{\beta}_{11,n} + |H_1^T \widehat{\beta}_{12,n}|\}.$$

Note that while the absolute value function is not differentiable, it can be shown that $n^{1/2}\{\widetilde{\mathcal{V}}_n(\widehat{d}_n) - \mathcal{V}(\widehat{d}_n)\}$ can be bootstrapped consistently under mild regularity conditions. Thus, we focus on inference for $\mathcal{V}(d^*)$.

To construct a confidence set for $\mathcal{V}(d^*)$, one can use an adaptive projection set. In this setting, for a fixed regime d with rule $d_1(h_1) = \text{sign}(h_1^T \beta_1)$, it can be seen that

$$n^{1/2}\{\widehat{\mathcal{V}}_n(d) - \mathcal{V}(d)\} = n^{1/2}(\mathbb{P}_n - P_n)\{H_1^T \widehat{\beta}_{11,n} + \text{sign}(H_1^T \beta_1)H_1^T \widehat{\beta}_{12,n})\}$$
$$+ P_n H_1^T n^{1/2}(\widehat{\beta}_{11,n} - \beta_{11,0,n}) + P_n \text{sign}(H_1^T \beta_1)H_1^T n^{1/2}(\widehat{\beta}_{12,n} - \beta_{12,0,n}),$$

which is regular and asymptotically normal. To construct an adaptive projection interval, let τ_n and $\widehat{\Sigma}_{12,n}$ be as defined above, and define

$$\mathfrak{M}_n(\beta_1, \beta) = n^{1/2}(\mathbb{P}_n - P_n)\{H_1^T \widehat{\beta}_{11,n} + \text{sign}\left(H_1^T \beta_1\right) H_1^T \widehat{\beta}_{12,n}\}$$

$$+ P_n H_1^T n^{1/2}(\widehat{\beta}_{11,n} - \beta_{11,0,n})$$

$$+ P_n \text{sign}\left(H_1^T \beta_1\right) H_1^T n^{1/2}(\widehat{\beta}_{12,n} - \beta_{12,0,n}) \mathrm{I}\left\{\frac{n(H_1^T \beta_1)^2}{H_1^T \widehat{\Sigma}_{12,n} H_1} > \tau_n\right\}$$

$$+ P_n \text{sign}\left(H_1^T \beta\right) H_1^T n^{1/2}(\widehat{\beta}_{12,n} - \beta_{12,0,n}) \mathrm{I}\left\{\frac{n(H_1^T \beta_1)^2}{H_1^T \widehat{\Sigma}_{12,n} H_1} \leq \tau_n\right\}.$$

Let $\widehat{\ell}_{n,\nu/2}^{(b)}(\beta_1)$ and $\widehat{u}_{n,1-\nu/2}^{(b)}(\beta_1)$ denote the $(\nu/2) \times 100$ and $(1-\nu/2) \times 100$ percentiles of the bootstrap distribution of $\mathfrak{M}_n(\widehat{\beta}_{1,n}, \beta_1)$, and let $\mathcal{W}_{n,1-\eta}$ denote a $(1 - \eta) \times 100\%$ confidence set for $\beta_{1,0}$. An $(1 - \delta - \nu) \times 100\%$ adaptive projection interval for $\mathcal{V}(d^*)$ assuming a linear Q-function is then

$$\bigcup_{\beta_1 \in \mathcal{W}_{n,1-\delta}} \left[\widehat{\ell}_{n,\nu/2}^{(b)}(\beta_1), \widehat{u}_{n,1-\nu/2}^{(b)}(\beta_1)\right].$$

Remark. Throughout this section, we have considered several approaches for constructing confidence sets for estimands of interest in single decision problems. As noted previously, we generally recommend bound-based intervals where it is possible to construct them; such intervals are consistent under local perturbations of the generative models and therefore tend to provide correct coverage in small samples. In a new domain, one can attempt to construct a bound-based interval by deriving the limiting distribution of the (appropriately centered and scaled) estimator under a sequence of local alternatives and then take the sup (inf) over all such sequences to obtain upper (lower) bounds. An alternative, but closely related approach, is to derive a projection confidence set and then to make it adaptive through pretesting. This approach can sometimes be simpler.

10.4 Inference for Multiple Decision Regimes

To introduce methodology for inference for multiple decision regimes, we consider a setting with $K = 2$ stages and two treatment options at each stage, which are feasible for all individuals. Extensions to $K > 2$ and more than two treatment options are generally straightforward; see Laber et al. (2014c) for extensions in Q-learning which can be readily adapted to bounding or adaptive-projection confidence sets.

As in Chapters 5–7, the observed data are as in (5.16) with $K = 2$,

$$(X_{1i}, A_{1i}, X_{2i}, A_{2i}, Y_i), \quad i = 1, \ldots, n,$$

which comprise n i.i.d. trajectories (X_1, A_1, X_2, A_2, Y). Here, $X_1 \in \mathbb{R}^{p_{X_1}}$

denotes baseline covariates; $A_1 \in \mathcal{A}_1 = \{-1, 1\}$ denotes treatment at Decision 1; $X_2 \in \mathbb{R}^{p \times 2}$ denotes patient information ascertained in the intervening period between Decisions 1 and 2; $A_2 \in \mathcal{A}_2 = \{-1, 1\}$ denotes the second-stage treatment; and $Y \in \mathbb{R}$ denotes the outcome, coded so that higher values are preferred. As in (5.15), define the observed histories $H_1 = X_1$ and $H_2 = (X_1, A_1, X_2)$ at Decisions 1 and 2, respectively, so that H_k, $k = 1, 2$, is the information available to inform selection of a treatment option at Decision k. Assume throughout that the identifiability assumptions given in Section 5.3.3 and more formally in Section 6.2.4 hold; namely, with suitably defined potential outcomes, SUTVA (5.17), the SRA in (5.18) and (5.19), and the positivity assumption (5.20) hold with $K = 2$. Under these conditions, we work directly with the data-generating model.

In what follows, we consider selected inference problems, including constructing confidence sets for parameters indexing regimes, confidence sets for the value of a fixed or estimated optimal regime, and additional methods for estimation of an optimal regime. Analogous to (10.4) in the single stage setting, we often consider regimes $d = (d_1, d_2)$ with rules of the general form

$$d_k(h_k; \eta_1) = \text{sign}(\widetilde{h}_k^T \eta_k), \quad k = 1, 2, \qquad (10.19)$$

so involving a decision function linear in a finite-dimensional parameter η_k, where h_k is a vector of known features of h_k.

10.4.1 Q-learning

We first consider the problem of constructing confidence sets for parameters indexing the Q-functions in Q-learning.

Bound-based Confidence Sets

Consider linear working models for the Q-functions of the form

$$Q_k(h_k, a_k; \beta_k) = \widetilde{h}_{k1}^T \beta_{k1} + a_k \widetilde{h}_{k2}^T \beta_{k2}, \quad \beta_k = (\beta_{k1}^T, \beta_{k2}^T)^T, \quad k = 1, 2,$$
$$(10.20)$$

where $\widetilde{h}_{k1}$ and $\widetilde{h}_{k2}$ are known feature vectors constructed from h_k, and $p_k = \dim(\beta_k)$, $k = 1, 2$. The models (10.20) induce a class of regimes with rules of the form

$$d_k(h_k; \beta_k) = \text{sign}(\widetilde{h}_{k2}^T \beta_{k2}), \quad k = 1, 2,$$

analogous to (10.19), indexed by the parameters β_{k2}.

Define $\widehat{\beta}_{2,n} = \arg\min_{\beta_2} \mathbb{P}_n \{Y - Q(H_2, A_2; \beta_2)\}^2$ and

$$\widehat{\beta}_{1,n} = \arg\min_{\beta_1} \mathbb{P}_n \left\{ \max_{a_2 \in \mathcal{A}_2} Q_2(H_2, a_2; \widehat{\beta}_{2,n}) - Q_1(H_1, A_1; \beta_1) \right\}^2 ;$$

here, $\max_{a_2 \in \mathcal{A}_2} Q_2(H_{2i}, a_2; \widehat{\beta}_{2,n})$ is the pseudo outcome $\widetilde{V}_{2i}$ for individual i as in (5.91) with $K = 2$. From Sections 5.7.1 and 7.4.1, Q-learning using OLS results in the estimated optimal regime $\widehat{d}_{Q,n}^{opt} = (\widehat{d}_{Q,1,n}^{opt}, \widehat{d}_{Q,2,n}^{opt})$ as in (5.97), where, from (5.96), the estimated optimal rules are given by

$$\widehat{d}_{Q,k,n}^{opt}(h_k) = d_k^{opt}(h_k; \widehat{\beta}_{k,n}) = \arg\max_{a_k \in \mathcal{A}_k} Q_k(h_k, a_k; \widehat{\beta}_{k,n}), \quad k = 1, 2.$$

Let $\beta_2^* = \arg\min_{\beta_2} P\{Y - Q_2(H_2, A_2; \beta_2)\}^2$ and

$$\beta_1^* = \arg\min_{\beta_1} P \left\{ \max_{a_2 \in \mathcal{A}_2} Q_2(H_2, a_2; \beta_2^*) - Q_1(H_1, A_1; \beta_1) \right\}^2$$

be the population analogs of $\widehat{\beta}_{2,n}$ and $\widehat{\beta}_{1,n}$, respectively. Given constants $c_k \in \mathbb{R}^{p_k}$, the goal is to construct valid asymptotic confidence sets for $c_k^T \beta_k^*$ for $k = 1, 2$. We do not assume that the posited Q-function models are correctly specified; i.e., we do not assume $Q_k(h_k, a_k) = Q_k(h_k, a_k; \beta_k^*)$, $k = 1, 2$. However, it may difficult to attach scientific meaning to these confidence sets otherwise.

Constructing a confidence set for $c_2^T \beta_2^*$ is straightforward, as this is a standard regression modeling task, and the methods from Section 10.3.1 can be applied directly. Define $B_k = (\widetilde{H}_{k1}^T, A_k \widetilde{H}_{k2}^T)^T$, $\Sigma_{Q_k} = P B_k B_k^T$, $k = 1, 2$, and $\Omega_{Q_2} = P(Y - B_2^T \beta_2^*)^2 B_2 B_2^T$. Then it can be shown that $n^{1/2}(\widehat{\beta}_{2,n} - \beta_2^*) \rightsquigarrow \mathcal{N}(0, \Sigma_{Q_2}^{-1} \Omega_{Q_2} \Sigma_{Q_2}^{-1})$. Therefore, given estimators $\widehat{\Sigma}_{Q_2,n}$ and $\widehat{\Omega}_{Q_2,n}$ for Σ_{Q_2} and Ω_{Q_2}, a $(1 - \alpha) \times 100\%$ confidence set for $c_2^T \beta_2^*$ is

$$c_2^T \widehat{\beta}_{2,n} \pm z_{1-\alpha/2} (c_2^T \widehat{\Sigma}_{Q_2,n}^{-1} \widehat{\Omega}_{Q_2,n} \widehat{\Sigma}_{Q_2,n}^{-1} c_2 / n)^{1/2}.$$

Unfortunately, the preceding normal-based approach to constructing a confidence set cannot be applied to construct a confidence set for $c_1^T \beta_1^*$, as estimation of β_1 is based on the pseudo outcomes and thus is not a standard regression problem. Defining $\widehat{\Sigma}_{Q_k,n} = \mathbb{P}_n B_k B_k^T$, $k = 1, 2$,

$$c_1^T n^{1/2}(\widehat{\beta}_{1,n} - \beta_1^*) = c_1^T \widehat{\Sigma}_{Q_1,n}^{-1} n^{1/2} \mathbb{P}_n B_1 \left\{ \max_{a_2 \in \mathcal{A}_2} Q_2(H_2, a_2; \widehat{\beta}_{2,n}) - B_1^T \beta_1^* \right\}.$$

Adding and subtracting $\max_{a_2 \in \mathcal{A}_2} Q_2(H_2, a_2; \beta_2^*) = \widetilde{H}_{21}^T \beta_{21}^* + |\widetilde{H}_{22}^T \beta_{22}^*|$ inside the braces on the right-hand side and rearranging terms yields

$$c_1^T n^{1/2}(\widehat{\beta}_{1,n} - \beta_1^*) = c_1^T \widehat{\Sigma}_{Q_1,n}^{-1} n^{1/2} \mathbb{P}_n B_1 \{ |\widetilde{H}_{22}^T \widehat{\beta}_{22,n}| - |\widetilde{H}_{22}^T \beta_{22}^*| \}$$

$$+ c_1^T \widehat{\Sigma}_{Q_1,n}^{-1} n^{1/2} \mathbb{P}_n B_1 \left\{ \max_{a_2 \in \mathcal{A}_2} Q_2(H_2, a_2; \beta_2^*) - B_1^T \beta_1^* \right\}$$

$$+ c_1^T \widehat{\Sigma}_{Q_1,n}^{-1} (\mathbb{P}_n B_1 \widetilde{H}_{21}^T) n^{1/2}(\widehat{\beta}_{21,n} - \beta_{21}^*).$$

By construction, β_1^* is a solution to

$$PB_1\left\{\max_{a_2\in\mathcal{A}_2} Q_2(H_2, a_2; \beta_2^*) - B_1^T\beta_1^*\right\} = 0;$$

thus,

$$c_1^T n^{1/2}(\widehat{\beta}_{1,n} - \beta_1^*)$$
$$= c_1^T\widehat{\Sigma}_{Q_1,n}^{-1}\mathbb{P}_n B_1\mathbb{U}_n\{n^{1/2}(\widehat{\beta}_{22,n} - \beta_{22}^*), n^{1/2}\beta_{22}^*\} + \mathbb{S}_n, \qquad (10.21)$$

where $\mathbb{U}_n(v, w) = |\widetilde{H}_{22}^T(v + w)| - |\widetilde{H}_{22}^T w|$,

$$\mathbb{S}_n = c_1^T\widehat{\Sigma}_{Q_1,n}^{-1}n^{1/2}(\mathbb{P}_n - P)B_1\left\{\max_{a_2\in\mathcal{A}_2} Q_2(H_2, a_2; \beta_2^*) - B_1^T\beta_1^*\right\}$$
$$+ c_1^T\widehat{\Sigma}_{Q_1,n}^{-1}(\mathbb{P}_n B_1\widetilde{H}_{21}^T)n^{1/2}(\widehat{\beta}_{21,n} - \beta_{21}^*)$$

$$= c_1^T\begin{pmatrix} \widehat{\Sigma}_{Q_1,n}^{-1} & 0 \\ 0 & \widehat{\Sigma}_{Q_1,n}^{-1} \end{pmatrix}$$

$$\times n^{1/2}(\mathbb{P}_n - P)\begin{pmatrix} B_1\{\max_{a_2\in\mathcal{A}_2} Q_2(H_2, a_2; \beta_2^*) - B_1^T\beta_1^*\} \\ (\mathbb{P}_n B_1\widetilde{H}_{21}^T)(I_{p_{21}}, 0_{p_{22}})\widehat{\Sigma}_{Q_2,n}^{-1}B_2(Y - B_2^T\beta_2^*) \end{pmatrix},$$

$p_{2j} = \dim(\beta_{2j})$, $j = 1, 2$, and $0_{p_{22}}$ is a $(p_{21} \times p_{22})$ matrix of zeroes.

The above expression shows that $\mathbb{S}_n$ is regular and asymptotically normal; thus, a bound-based confidence set should only affect the term $c_1^T\widehat{\Sigma}_{Q_1,n}^{-1}\mathbb{P}_n B_1\mathbb{U}_n\{n^{1/2}(\widehat{\beta}_{22,n} - \beta_{22}^*), n^{1/2}\beta_{22}^*\}$. Moreover, if $\widetilde{h}_{22}^T\beta_{22}^*$ is bounded away from zero, then

$$\mathbb{U}_n\{n^{1/2}(\widehat{\beta}_{22,n} - \beta_{22}^*), n^{1/2}\beta_{22}^*\}\big|_{\widetilde{H}_{22}=\widetilde{h}_{22}} = |\widetilde{h}_{22}^T\widehat{\beta}_{22,n}| - |\widetilde{h}_{22}^T\beta_{22}^*|$$
$$\approx \text{sign}(\widetilde{h}_{22}^T\beta_{22}^*)\widetilde{h}_{22}^T(\widehat{\beta}_{22,n} - \beta_{22}^*)$$

is regular and asymptotically normal. Thus, the bound should affect $\mathbb{U}_n\{n^{1/2}(\widehat{\beta}_{22,n} - \beta_{22}^*), n^{1/2}\beta_{22}^*\}$ only through points that are close to the boundary $\widetilde{h}_{22}^T\beta_{22}^* = 0$.

We formalize these notions by using a pretest to partition the observed data into two groups: (G1) those individuals for whom there is insufficient evidence to reject the hypothesis $\widetilde{h}_{22}^T\beta_{22}^* = 0$; and (G2) those for whom there is sufficient evidence to reject this hypothesis. Let $\widehat{T}_n(\widetilde{h}_{22})$ denote a test statistic that diverges to $+\infty$ if $\widetilde{h}_{22}^T\beta_{22}^* \neq 0$ and is bounded in probability otherwise. Hereafter, we assume that $\widehat{T}_n(\widetilde{h}_{22}) = n(\widetilde{h}_{22}^T\widehat{\beta}_{22,n})^2/(\widetilde{h}_{22}^T\widehat{\Sigma}_{22,n}\widetilde{h}_{22})$, where $\widehat{\Sigma}_{22,n}$ is an estimator for Σ_{22}, the asymptotic covariance matrix of $n^{1/2}(\widehat{\beta}_{22,n} - \beta_{22}^*)$. The pretest assigns subjects with $\widehat{T}_n(\widetilde{h}_{22}) \le \lambda_n$ to (G1) and to (G2) otherwise, where λ_n is a sequence of critical values.

From (10.21), with $p_{22} = \dim(\beta_{22})$, an upper bound on $c_1^T n^{1/2}(\widehat{\beta}_{1,n} - \beta_1^*)$ is

$$\mathcal{U}_n = \sup_{\omega \in \mathbb{R}^{p_{22}}} c_1^T \widehat{\Sigma}_{Q_1,n}^{-1} \mathbb{P}_n B_1 \mathbb{U}_n\{n^{1/2}(\widehat{\beta}_{22,n} - \beta_{22}^*), \omega\} \mathrm{I}\{\widehat{T}_n(\widetilde{H}_{22}) \le \lambda_n\}$$
$$+ c_1^T \widehat{\Sigma}_{Q_1,n}^{-1} \mathbb{P}_n B_1 \mathbb{U}_n\{n^{1/2}(\widehat{\beta}_{22,n} - \beta_{22}^*), n^{1/2}\beta_{22}^*\} \mathrm{I}\{\widehat{T}_n(\widetilde{H}_{22}) > \lambda_n\} + \mathbb{S}_n.$$

A lower bound, $\mathcal{L}_n$, is obtained by replacing the sup with an inf. Substituting $\omega = n^{1/2}\beta_{22}^*$ in the above expression confirms that $\mathcal{L}_n \le c_1^T n^{1/2}(\widehat{\beta}_{1,n} - \beta_1^*) \le \mathcal{U}_n$. The sup (inf) used in the bounds has a smoothing effect that makes the bounds regular. To illustrate this smoothing effect, let $\widetilde{h}_{22}$ be fixed, and suppose $h_{22}^T \beta_{22}^* = 0$. Then

$$\mathbb{U}_n\{n^{1/2}(\widehat{\beta}_{22,n} - \beta_{22}^*), n^{1/2}\beta_{22}^*\}\big|_{\widetilde{H}_{22} = \widetilde{h}_{22}}$$
$$= |\widetilde{h}_{22}^T n^{1/2}(\widehat{\beta}_{22,n} - \beta_{22}^*)| \rightsquigarrow |\widetilde{h}_{22}^T \mathbb{Z}_\infty|,$$

where $\mathbb{Z}_\infty \sim \mathcal{N}(0, \widetilde{h}_{22}^T \Sigma_{22} \widetilde{h}_{22})$. If $\widetilde{h}_{22}^T \beta_{22}^* \ne 0$, then

$$\mathbb{U}_n\{n^{1/2}(\widehat{\beta}_{22,n} - \beta_{22}^*), n^{1/2}\beta_{22}^*\}\big|_{\widetilde{H}_{22} = \widetilde{h}_{22}}$$
$$= \mathrm{sign}(\widetilde{h}_{22}^T \beta_{22}^*) n^{1/2}(\widehat{\beta}_{22,n} - \beta_{22}^*) + o_P(1) \rightsquigarrow \mathrm{sign}(\widetilde{h}_{22}^T \beta_{22}^*) \mathbb{Z}_\infty =_D \mathbb{Z}_\infty,$$

where $=_D$ denotes equality in distribution. Thus, the limiting distribution of $\mathbb{U}_n\{n^{1/2}(\widehat{\beta}_{22,n} - \beta_{22}^*), n^{1/2}\beta_{22}^*\}\big|_{\widetilde{H}_{22} = \widetilde{h}_{22}}$ depends abruptly on whether or not $\widetilde{h}_{22}^T \beta_{22}^* = 0$. This abrupt change vanishes after the sup is applied as, regardless of whether or not $\widetilde{h}_{22}^T \beta_{22}^* = 0$,

$$\sup_{\omega \in \mathbb{R}^{p_{22}}} \mathbb{U}_n\{n^{1/2}(\widehat{\beta}_{22,n} - \beta_{22}^*), \omega\}\big|_{\widetilde{H}_{22} = \widetilde{h}_{22}}$$
$$= \sup_{\omega \in \mathbb{R}^{p_{22}}} \left[|\widetilde{h}_{22}^T\{n^{1/2}(\widehat{\beta}_{22} - \beta_{22}^*) + \omega\}| - |\widetilde{h}_{22}^T \omega|\right]$$
$$\rightsquigarrow \sup_{\omega \in \mathbb{R}^{p_{22}}} \left\{|\widetilde{h}_{22}^T(\mathbb{Z}_\infty + \omega)| - |\widetilde{h}_{22}^T \omega|\right\},$$

where we have used the continuous mapping theorem applied to the function $z \mapsto \sup_{\omega \in \mathbb{R}^{p_{22}}}\{|\widetilde{h}_{22}^T(z + \omega)| - |\widetilde{h}_{22}^T \omega|\}$.

The following result characterizes the asymptotic behavior of the bound $\mathcal{U}_n$; results for the lower bound are obtained by identical arguments with the sup replaced by an inf. Define

$$\Omega_{Q_1} = P\left\{\max_{a_2 \in \mathcal{A}_2} Q_2(H_2, a_2) - B_1^T \beta_1^*\right\}^2 B_1 B_1^T.$$

We make the following assumptions.

(Q1) The histories H_2; the B_k, $k = 1, 2$, involving the features; and the outcome satisfy the moment conditions $P\|H_2\|^2\|B_1\|^2 < \infty$ and $PY^2\|B_2\|^2 < \infty$.

(Q2) The matrices Σ_{Q_k} and Ω_{Q_k}, $k = 1, 2$, are strictly positive definite.

(Q3) For any $s \in \mathbb{R}^{p_{22}}$, there exists a sequence of local alternatives P_n such that

$$\int \left\{ n^{1/2} \left(dP_n^{1/2} - dP^{1/2} \right) - (1/2)\varsigma(s)dP^{1/2} \right\}^2 \to 0$$

for some real-valued and measurable function $\varsigma(s)$ such that P_n satisfies: (i) if $\beta_{2,n}^* = \arg\min_{\beta_2} P_n \{Y - Q_2(H_2, A_2; \beta_2)\}^2$, then $\beta_{22,n}^* = \beta_{22}^* + sn^{-1/2} + o(n^{-1/2})$; and (ii) $P_n\|H_2\|^2\|B_1\|^2$, $P_nY^2\|B_2\|^2$ are bounded sequences (see van der Vaart and Wellner, 1996, for a discussion of similar conditions).

(Q4) With probability one, $\lambda_n \to \infty$ and $\lambda_n/n \to 0$ as $n \to \infty$, where λ_n is a sequence of critical values as above.

The sequence of probability measures P_n in assumption (Q3) allows the treatment effects $\tilde{h}_{22}^T \beta_{22,n}^*$ to converge to zero at rate $n^{-1/2}$ when $\tilde{h}_{22}^T \beta_{22}^* = 0$. As discussed in Section 10.2, such moving parameter asymptotics are critical in capturing salient features of the finite sample behavior of nonsmooth functionals like $\widehat{\beta}_1$.

Theorem 10.4.1. *Let $c_1 \in \mathbb{R}^{p_1}$ be a fixed constant, and assume (Q1)–(Q2) and (Q4). Then*

(i) $c_1^T n^{1/2}(\widehat{\beta}_{1,n} - \beta_1^*)$ satisfies

$$c_1^T n^{1/2}(\widehat{\beta}_{1,n} - \beta_1^*) \rightsquigarrow c_1^T \mathbb{S}_\infty + c_1^T \Sigma_{Q_1}^{-1} PB_1|\tilde{H}_{22}^T \mathbb{V}_\infty| I(\tilde{H}_{22}^T \beta_{22}^* = 0)$$
$$+ c_1^T \Sigma_{Q_1}^{-1} PB_1 \tilde{H}_{22}^T \mathbb{V}_\infty I(\tilde{H}_{22}^T \beta_{22}^* \neq 0).$$

(ii) If, for each n, the data-generating model is P_n, which satisfies (Q3), then the limiting distribution of $c_1^T n^{1/2}(\widehat{\beta}_{1,n} - \beta_{1,n}^*)$ is equal to that of

$$c_1^T \mathbb{S}_n + c_1^T \Sigma_{Q_1}^{-1} PB_1 \left\{ \left| \tilde{H}_{22}^T \left(\mathbb{V}_\infty + s \right) \right| - \left| \tilde{H}_{22}^T s \right| \right\} I(\tilde{H}_{22}^T \beta_{22}^* = 0)$$
$$+ c_1^T \Sigma_{Q_1}^{-1} PB_1 \tilde{H}_{22}^T \mathbb{V}_\infty I(\tilde{H}_{22}^T \beta_{22}^* \neq 0). \quad (10.22)$$

(iii) The limiting distribution of $\mathcal{U}_n$ under P or a sequence of distributions P_n that satisfy (Q3) is equal to that of

$$c_1^T \mathbb{S}_\infty + c_1^T \Sigma_{Q_1}^{-1} PB_1 \tilde{H}_{22}^T \mathbb{V}_\infty I \left\{ \tilde{H}_{22}^T \beta_{22}^* \neq 0 \right\}$$

$$+ \sup_{\omega \in \mathbb{R}^{p_{22}}} c_1^T \Sigma_{Q_1}^{-1} P B_1 \left\{ \left| \tilde{H}_{22}^T (\mathbb{V}_\infty + \omega) \right| - \left| \tilde{H}_{22}^T \omega \right| \right\} I \left\{ \tilde{H}_{22}^T \beta_{22}^* = 0 \right\},$$

where $(\mathbb{S}_\infty^T, \mathbb{V}_\infty^T)^T$ is multivariate normal with mean zero.

An expression for the covariance matrix of $(\mathbb{S}_\infty^T, \mathbb{V}_\infty^T)^T$ is given in Laber et al. (2014b), along with the proof of this result. The limiting distribution of $\mathcal{U}_n$ does not depend on the local parameter s and is therefore regular. Furthermore, it can be seen that if $\tilde{H}_{22}^T \beta_{22}^* \neq 0$ with probability one, then the limiting distribution of $\mathcal{U}_n$ is equal to the limiting distribution of $c_1^T n^{1/2} (\widehat{\beta}_{1,n} - \beta_1^*)$; thus, the bound is tight if the treatment effects are bounded away from zero almost surely. If there is a point mass of subjects with zero treatment effect, then the limiting distribution of $\mathcal{U}_n$ is stochastically larger than the limiting distribution of $c_1^T n^{1/2} (\widehat{\beta}_{1,n} - \beta_1^*)$.

Remark. The asymptotic distribution of $\widehat{\beta}_{n,1}$ depends on the local parameter, s, and is therefore nonregular. Nevertheless, one might attempt to estimate the limiting distribution of $c_1^T n^{1/2} (\widehat{\beta}_{1,n} - \beta_{1,n}^*)$ and use this to construct a confidence set for $c_1^T \beta_1^*$. However, it is impossible to construct a consistent estimator for the limiting distribution in (10.22). To see this, let F_s denote the distribution function for (10.22), and let $\widehat{F}_{s,n}$ denote an estimator for this distribution. By construction, P_n is contiguous with respect to P; thus, if $\widehat{F}_{s,n}$ converges to F_s under P_n, it must also converge under P. This is a contradiction, as P contains no information about s.

The bounds $\mathcal{L}_n$ and $\mathcal{U}_n$ depend on P and thus cannot be computed using the observed data. To construct a confidence set for $c_1^T \beta_1^*$, we use the bootstrap. As in Section 10.3.2, for any functional $g = g(P, \mathbb{P}_n)$, its bootstrap analog is denoted $g^{(b)} = g(\mathbb{P}_n, \mathbb{P}_n^{(b)})$. Given $\nu \in (0, 1)$, let $\widehat{\ell}_{n,\nu/2}^{(b)}$ denote the $(\nu/2) \times 100$ percentile of the distribution of $\mathcal{L}_n^{(b)}$ and let $\widehat{u}_{n,1-\nu/2}^{(b)}$ denote the $(1 - \nu/2) \times 100$ percentile of the distribution of $\mathcal{U}_n^{(b)}$. An asymptotic $(1 - \nu) \times 100\%$ confidence interval for $c_1^T \beta_1^*$ is

$$\left[c_1^T \widehat{\beta}_{1,n} - \widehat{u}_{n,1-\nu/2}^{(b)} / n^{1/2}, \; c_1^T \widehat{\beta}_{1,n} - \widehat{\ell}_{n,\nu/2}^{(b)} / n^{1/2} \right].$$

The following result establishes the validity of this confidence interval.

Theorem 10.4.2. *Let $c_1 \in \mathbb{R}^{p_1}$ be fixed. Assume (Q1)–(Q2) and (Q4). Then*

$$\sup_{g \in BL_1(\mathbb{R}^2)} \left| P g \left\{ \mathcal{L}_n, \mathcal{U}_n \right\} - P_M g \left\{ \mathcal{L}_n^{(b)}, \mathcal{U}_n^{(b)} \right\} \right| \xrightarrow{P} 0.$$

Corollary 10.4.3. *Let $c_1 \in \mathbb{R}^{p_1}$ and $\nu \in (0, 1)$ be fixed. Assume (Q1)–(Q2) and (Q4), and let $\widehat{\ell}_{n,\nu/2}^{(b)}$ be the $(\nu/2) \times 100$ percentile of $\mathcal{L}_n^{(b)}$ and*

$\widehat{u}_{n,1-\nu/2}^{(b)}$ be the $(1 - \nu/2) \times 100$ percentile of $\mathcal{U}_n^{(b)}$. Then

$$P_M\left(c_1^T\widehat{\beta}_{1,n} - \widehat{u}_{n,1-\nu/2}^{(b)}/n^{1/2} \leq c_1^T\beta_1^* \leq c_1^T\widehat{\beta}_{1,n} - \widehat{\ell}_{n,\nu/2}^{(b)}/n^{1/2}\right)$$
$$\geq 1 - \nu + o_P(1).$$

Furthermore, if $P(\widetilde{H}_{22}^T\beta_{22}^* = 0) = 0$, then the inequality can be strengthened to equality.

The preceding theorem shows that the bound-based confidence interval delivers nominal coverage asymptotically under moment conditions and a growth condition on the tuning parameter λ_n. In practice, it is recommended that λ_n be tuned using the double bootstrap as in Algorithms 10.2 and 10.4.

Adaptive Projection Intervals

Bound-based confidence intervals sandwich the nonregular functional $c_1^T n^{1/2}(\widehat{\beta}_{1,n} - \beta_1^*)$ between two regular estimators and then apply the bootstrap to these bounds. A closely related approach is to apply the bootstrap to a set of regular functionals to construct a set of confidence intervals, the union of which has high probability of containing $c_1^T\beta_1^*$.

For any $\beta_{22} \in \mathbb{R}^{p_{22}}$ and $c_1 \in \mathbb{R}^{p_1}$, define

$$\widehat{\beta}_{1,n}(\beta_{22})$$
$$= \arg\min_{\beta_1} \mathbb{P}_n\left\{\widetilde{H}_{21}^T\widehat{\beta}_{21} + \text{sign}(\widetilde{H}_{22}^T\beta_{22})\widetilde{H}_{22}^T\widehat{\beta}_{22} - Q_1(H_1, A_1; \beta_1)\right\}^2,$$

and, analogously,

$$\beta_1^*(\beta_{22})$$
$$= \arg\min_{\beta_1} P\left\{\widetilde{H}_{21}^T\beta_{2,0}^* + \text{sign}(\widetilde{H}_{22}^T\beta_{22})\widetilde{H}_{22}^T\beta_{2,1}^* - Q_1(H_1, A_1; \beta_1)\right\}^2,$$

so that $\beta_1^* = \beta_1^*(\beta_{22}^*)$. Regarding β_{22} as fixed,

$$c_1^T n^{1/2}\{\widehat{\beta}_{1,n}(\beta_{22}) - \beta_1^*(\beta_{22})\}$$
$$= c_1^T\widehat{\Sigma}_{Q_1,n}^{-1} n^{1/2}\mathbb{P}_n B_1\{\widetilde{H}_{21}^T\widehat{\beta}_{21} + \text{sign}(\widetilde{H}_{22}^T\beta_{22})\widetilde{H}_{22}^T\widehat{\beta}_{22} - B_1^T\beta_1^*(\beta_{22})\}$$
$$= c_1^T\widehat{\Sigma}_{Q_1,n}^{-1}\left(\mathbb{P}_n B_1\widetilde{H}_{21}^T\right) n^{1/2}(\widehat{\beta}_{21,n} - \beta_{21}^*)$$
$$+ c_1^T\widehat{\Sigma}_{Q_1,n}^{-1}\left\{\mathbb{P}_n B_1\widetilde{H}_{22}^T\text{sign}(\widetilde{H}_{22}^T\beta_{22})\right\} n^{1/2}(\widehat{\beta}_{22,n} - \beta_{22}^*)$$
$$+ c_1^T\widehat{\Sigma}_{Q_1,n}^{-1} n^{1/2}(\mathbb{P}_n - P)B_1\left\{\widetilde{H}_{21}^T\beta_{21}^* + \text{sign}(\widetilde{H}_{22}^T\beta_{22})\widetilde{H}_{22}^T\beta_{22}^*\right\}$$
$$= n^{1/2}(\mathbb{P}_n - P)\Lambda\left(\begin{array}{c}\Sigma_{Q_2}^{-1}B_2(Y - B_2^T\beta_2^*) \\ B_1\left\{\widetilde{H}_{21}^T\beta_{21}^* + \text{sign}(\widetilde{H}_{22}^T\beta_{22})\widetilde{H}_{22}^T\beta_{22}^*\right\}\end{array}\right) + o_P(1),$$

where

$$\Lambda = \begin{pmatrix} c_1^T \Sigma_{Q_1}^{-1} \{ PB_1 \widetilde{H}_{21}^T \} \\ c_1^T \Sigma_{Q_1}^{-1} \left\{ PB_1 \widetilde{H}_{22}^T \mathrm{sign}(\widetilde{H}_{22}^T \beta_{22}) \right\} \\ c_1^T \Sigma_{Q_1}^{-1} \end{pmatrix}^T.$$

Thus, $c_1^T \{ \widehat{\beta}_{1,n}(\beta_{22}) - \beta_1^*(\beta_{22}) \}$ is regular and asymptotically normal, so that a confidence interval for $\beta_1^*(\beta_{22})$ could be constructed using this result.

In practice, it is often easier to construct a confidence interval for $\beta_1^*(\beta_{22})$ using the bootstrap. Given $\nu \in (0,1)$, let $\widehat{\ell}_{n,\nu/2}^{(b)}(\beta_{22})$ and $\widehat{u}_{n,1-\nu/2}^{(b)}(\beta_{22})$ denote the $(\nu/2) \times 100$ and $(1 - \nu/2) \times 100$ percentiles of $c_1^T n^{1/2} \{ \widehat{\beta}_{1,n}^{(b)}(\beta_{22}) - \widehat{\beta}_{1,n}(\beta_{22}) \}$. Then

$$\Gamma_{n,1-\nu}(\beta_{22})$$
$$= \left[c_1^T \widehat{\beta}_{1,n}(\beta_{22}) - \frac{\widehat{u}_{n,1-\nu/2}^{(b)}(\beta_{22})}{n^{1/2}}, \; c_1^T \widehat{\beta}_{1,n}(\beta_{22}) - \frac{\widehat{\ell}_{n,\nu/2}^{(b)}(\beta_{22})}{n^{1/2}} \right]$$

is a $(1 - \nu) \times 100\%$ confidence interval for $c_1^T \beta_1^*(\beta_{22})$. If β_{22}^* were known, then $\Gamma_{n,1-\nu}(\beta_{22}^*)$ would be a valid confidence interval for $c_1^T \beta_1^*(\beta_{22}^*) = c_1^T \beta_1^*$. Of course, β_{22}^* is unknown, but we can construct a confidence interval for it; e.g., given $\alpha \in (0,1)$ a Wald-type $(1-\alpha) \times 100\%$ confidence set for β_{22}^* is

$$\zeta_{n,1-\alpha} = \left\{ \beta_{22} : n(\widehat{\beta}_{22,n} - \beta_{22})^T \widehat{\Sigma}_{22,n}^{-1} (\widehat{\beta}_{22,n} - \beta_{22}) \leq \chi_{\dim(\beta_{22}^*),1-\alpha}^2 \right\}.$$

Then $\bigcup_{\beta_{22} \in \zeta_{n,1-\alpha}} \Gamma_{n,1-\nu}(\beta_{22})$ is a $(1 - \alpha - \nu) \times 100\%$ confidence set for $c_1^T \beta_1^*$.

The preceding projection confidence interval is based on writing $|\widetilde{h}_{22}^T \beta_{22}^*| = \mathrm{sign}(\widetilde{h}_{22}^T \beta_{22}^*) \widetilde{h}_{22}^T \beta_{22}^*$ and then treating only β_{22}^* appearing inside the sign function as a nuisance parameter. This interval tends to be less conservative than a projection interval that treats β_{22}^* in the expression $|\widetilde{h}_{22}^T \beta_{22}^*|$, so in both $\mathrm{sign}(\widetilde{h}_{22}^T \beta_{22}^*)$ and $\widetilde{h}_{22}^* \beta_{22}^*$, as the nuisance parameter. A projection interval of this type is proposed by (Robins, 2004) and discussed by (Laber et al., 2014c).

The bound-based and adaptive projection sets are closely related. If the union $\bigcup_{\beta_{22} \in \zeta_{n,1-\alpha}} \Gamma_{n,1-\nu}(\beta_{22})$ is an interval, then it can be expressed as

$$\left[\inf_{\beta_{22} \in \mathbb{R}^{p_{22}}} \Gamma_{n,1-\nu}(\beta_{22}), \; \sup_{\beta_{22} \in \mathbb{R}^{p_{22}}} \Gamma_{n,1-\nu}(\beta_{22}) \right].$$

Thus, the adaptive projection set can be viewed as being constructed by taking the sup/inf over quantiles of a regular surrogate for $c_1^T n^{1/2}(\widehat{\beta}_{1,n} - \beta_1^*)$, whereas the bound-based interval takes the quantiles of the sup/inf of a regular surrogate. The sup of the quantile process is generally smaller than the quantile of the sup of a process; however, the two are not directly comparable because the underlying surrogate processes are different.

Projection Interval for the Value of an Optimal Regime

If one is willing to assume that the first-stage Q-function is correctly specified, one can use a projection interval to construct a confidence set for the value of an optimal regime. Recall from (5.76) and (5.77) and Section 7.2.3 that $\mathcal{V}(d^{opt}) = E\{\max_{a_1 \in \mathcal{A}_1} Q_1(H_1, a_1)\} = P \max_{a_1 \in \mathcal{A}_1} Q_1(H_1, a_1)$, where d^{opt} is an optimal regime in the class $\mathcal{D}$ of all regimes. Let $Q_1(h_1, a_1; \beta_1)$, $\beta_1 \in \mathbb{R}^{p_1}$ be a posited model for $Q_1(h_1, a_1)$, and further assume that the model is correctly specified, so that there exists $\beta_1^* = \beta_{1,0}$ such that $Q_1(h_1, a_1; \beta_{1,0}) = Q_1(h_1, \beta_1)$ for all h_1 and a_1. For any $\beta_1 \in \mathbb{R}^{p_1}$ such that $E[\{\max_{a_1 \in \mathcal{A}_1} Q_1(H_1, a_1; \beta_1)\}^2] < \infty$, it follows that

$$n^{1/2}(\mathbb{P}_n - P)\left\{\max_{a_1 \in \mathcal{A}_1} Q_1(H_1, a_1; \beta_1)\right\} \rightsquigarrow \mathcal{N}\left\{0, \sigma^2_{Q_1}(\beta_1)\right\},$$

where

$$\sigma^2_{Q_1}(\beta_1) = P\left\{\max_{a_1 \in \mathcal{A}_1} Q_1(H_1, a_1; \beta_1) - P\max_{a_1 \in \mathcal{A}_1} Q_1(H_1, a_1; \beta_1)\right\}^2.$$

Let $\widehat{\sigma}^2_{Q_1}(\beta_1)$ be the plug-in estimator for $\sigma^2_{Q_1}(\beta_1)$ given by $\widehat{\sigma}^2_{Q_1}(\beta_1) = \mathbb{P}_n\{\max_{a_1 \in \mathcal{A}_1} Q_1(H_1, a_1; \beta_1) - \mathbb{P}_n\max_{a_1 \in \mathcal{A}_1} Q_1(H_1, a_1; \beta_1)\}^2$. For any fixed $\beta_1 \in \mathbb{R}^{p_1}$ and $\nu \in (0, 1)$, an asymptotic $(1 - \nu) \times 100\%$ confidence interval for $P\max_{a_1 \in \mathcal{A}_1} Q_1(H_1, a_1; \beta_1)$ is

$$\Gamma_{n,1-\nu}(\beta_1) = \left[\mathbb{P}_n \max_{a_1 \in \mathcal{A}_1} Q_1(H_1, a_1; \beta_1) - \frac{z_{1-\alpha/2}\widehat{\sigma}_{Q_1}(\beta_1)}{n^{1/2}},\right.$$
$$\left.\mathbb{P}_n \max_{a_1 \in \mathcal{A}_1} Q_1(H_1, a_1; \beta_1) + \frac{z_{1-\alpha/2}\widehat{\sigma}_{Q_1}(\beta_1)}{n^{1/2}}\right].$$

In particular, $\Gamma_{n,1-\nu}(\beta_1^*)$ is a $(1 - \nu) \times 100\%$ confidence interval for $\mathcal{V}(d^{opt})$.

In general, $\beta_{1,0}$ is not known. However, given a $(1 - \alpha) \times 100\%$ confidence region for $\beta_{1,0}$, say $\zeta_{n,1-\alpha}$, it follows that $\bigcup_{\beta_1 \in \zeta_{n,1-\alpha}} \Gamma_{1,1-\nu}(\beta_1)$ is an asymptotic $(1 - \alpha - \nu) \times 100\%$ confidence region for $\mathcal{V}(d^{opt})$. The adaptive projection interval procedure described above can be modified to construct a confidence region for $\beta_{1,0}$, i.e., by simply omitting the inner product with the constant vector c_1.

10.4.2 Value Search Estimation with Convex Surrogates

Consider a restricted class of regimes $\mathcal{D}_\eta$ comprising regimes d_η with rules $d_k(h_k; \eta_k)$, $\dim(\eta_k) = p_k$, $k = 1, 2$, indexed by $\eta = (\eta_1^T, \eta_2^T)^T$. We discuss inference on η based on convex relaxations of value or policy search estimators for the value $\mathcal{V}(d_\eta)$.

As in (5.65), write the propensities as

$$\omega_k(h_k, a_k) = p_{A_k|H_k}(a_k|h_k) = P(A_k = a_k|H_k = h_k), \quad k = 1, 2,$$

which for simplicity we take to be known. We focus on a variant of the equivalent representation of the inverse probability weighted estimator (5.107) given in (5.110). Namely, for any function $g : \mathcal{H}_1 \to \mathbb{R}$ and any fixed regime d_η, define

$$\widehat{\mathcal{V}}_n^g(d_\eta) = \mathbb{P}_n\left[\frac{\{Y - g(H_1)\}\mathrm{I}\{A_1 = d_1(H_1; \eta_1)\}\mathrm{I}\{A_2 = d_2(H_2; \eta_2)\}}{\omega_1(H_1, A_1)\omega_2(H_2, A_2)}\right].$$

Note that $E\{\widehat{\mathcal{V}}_n^g(d_\eta)\} = \mathcal{V}(d_\eta) - E\{g(H_1)\}$, so that g does not (asymptotically) affect the argmax of $\widehat{\mathcal{V}}_n^g(d_\eta)$; the role of g is to reduce variability (Laber and Zhao, 2015; Zhou et al., 2017). As emphasized in Sections 5.7.4 and 7.4.3, maximization of any inverse or augmented inverse probability weighted estimator for $\mathcal{V}(d_\eta)$ in η is computationally challenging in all but the simplest settings owing to the nonsmoothness inherent in the indicator functions. Accordingly, as discussed in Section 7.4.5, value search estimation with convex surrogates replaces these indicator functions with convex relaxations, rendering the optimization feasible even in problems with very high-dimensional η.

For definiteness, we focus on the class $\mathcal{D}_\eta$ with linear rules as in (10.19), so with

$$d_k(h_k; \eta_1) = \mathrm{sign}(\widetilde{h}_k^T \eta_k), \quad k = 1, 2,$$

where, as before, $\widetilde{h}_k$ are known features of h_k and $\eta_k \in \mathbb{R}^{p_k}$, $k = 1, 2$. Then it can be seen that

$$\widehat{\mathcal{V}}_n^g(d_\eta) = \mathbb{P}_n\left[\frac{\{Y - g(H_1)\}\mathrm{I}\{\min(A_1\widetilde{H}_1^T\eta_1, A_2\widetilde{H}_2^T\eta_2) > 0\}}{\omega_1(H_1, A_1)\omega_2(H_2, A_2)}\right].$$

Lemma 10.4.4. Let $w \in \mathbb{R}$, $v_1, \eta_1 \in \mathbb{R}^{p_1}$, and $v_2, \eta_2 \in \mathbb{R}^{p_2}$, where $v_k^T \eta_k \neq 0$ for $k = 1, 2$, then

$$w\mathrm{I}\{\min(v_1^T\eta_1, v_2^T\eta_2) > 0\} = |w|I\{\min(v_1^T\eta_1, v_2^T\eta_2) > 0\}I(w > 0)$$

$$+ |w| I\{\min\left(-v_1^T \eta_1, v_2^T \eta_2\right) > 0\} \, I(w < 0)$$
$$- |w| I\{v_2^T \eta_2 > 0\} \, I(w < 0).$$

Proof. Write

$$w \, \mathrm{I}\{\min(v_1^T \eta_1, v_2^T \eta_2) > 0\}$$

$$\begin{aligned}
&= |w| \mathrm{I} \left\{\min\left(v_1^T \eta_1, v_2^T \eta_2\right) > 0\right\} \mathrm{I}(w > 0) \\
&\quad - |w| \mathrm{I} \left\{\min\left(v_1^T \eta_1, v_2^T \eta_2\right) > 0\right\} \mathrm{I}(w < 0) \\
&= |w| \mathrm{I} \left\{\min\left(v_1^T \eta_1, v_2^T \eta_2\right) > 0\right\} \mathrm{I}(w > 0) \\
&\quad - |w| \left(1 - \mathrm{I}\left\{v_1^T \eta_1 < 0\right\}\right) \mathrm{I} \left\{v_2^T \eta_2 > 0\right\} \mathrm{I}(w < 0) \\
&= |w| \mathrm{I} \left\{\min\left(v_1^T \eta_1, v_2^T \eta_2\right) > 0\right\} \mathrm{I}(w > 0) \\
&\quad + |w| \mathrm{I} \left\{-v_1^T \eta_1 > 0\right\} \mathrm{I} \left\{v_2^T \eta_2 > 0\right\} \mathrm{I}(w < 0) \\
&\quad - |w| \mathrm{I} \left\{v_2^T \eta_2 > 0\right\} \mathrm{I}(w < 0).
\end{aligned}$$

$\square$

Applying the lemma with $w = \{y - g(h_1)\} \{\omega_1(h_1, a_1)\omega_2(h_2, a_2)\}^{-1}$ and $v_k = a_2 \tilde{h}_k$, $k = 1, 2$,

$$\begin{aligned}
&\widehat{\mathcal{V}}_n^g(d_\eta) \\
&= \mathbb{P}_n \left[\frac{|Y - g(H_1)| \mathrm{I}\{\min(A_1 \tilde{H}_1^T \eta_1, A_2 \tilde{H}_2^T \eta_2) > 0\} \mathrm{I}\{Y - g(H_1) > 0\}}{\omega_1(H_1, A_1)\omega_2(H_2, A_2)} \right] \\
&\quad + \mathbb{P}_n \left[\frac{|Y - g(H_1)| \mathrm{I}\{\min(-A_1 \tilde{H}_1^T \eta_1, A_2 \tilde{H}_2^T \eta_2) > 0\} \mathrm{I}\{Y - g(H_1) < 0\}}{\omega_1(H_1, A_1)\omega_2(H_2, A_2)} \right] \\
&\quad - \mathbb{P}_n \left\{ \frac{|Y - g(H_1)| \mathrm{I}(A_2 \tilde{H}_2^T \eta_2 > 0) \mathrm{I}\{Y - g(H_1) < 0\}}{\omega_1(H_1, A_1)\omega_2(H_2, A_2)} \right\}.
\end{aligned}$$

Let $\psi_1 : \mathbb{R} \to \mathbb{R}$ be a non-decreasing, concave function that satisfies $\psi_1(z) \leq \mathrm{I}(z > 0)$ for all $z \in \mathbb{R}$, and let $\psi_2 : \mathbb{R} \to \mathbb{R}$ be a concave function that satisfies $\psi_2(z) \leq \mathrm{I}(z < 0)$ for all $z \in \mathbb{R}$; e.g., $\psi_1(z) = \min(z, 1)$, and $\psi_2(z) = \min(-z, 1)$. Let $\psi = (\psi_1, \psi_2)$, and define the convex relaxation

$$\begin{aligned}
&\mathfrak{L}^{g,\psi}(h_2, a_2, y; \eta) \\
&= \frac{|y - g(h_1)| \psi_1\{\min(a_1 \tilde{h}_1^T \eta_1, a_2 \tilde{h}_2^T \eta_2)\} \mathrm{I}\{y - g(h_1) > 0\}}{\omega_1(h_1, a_1)\omega_2(h_2, a_2)} \\
&\quad + \frac{|y - g(h_1)| \psi_1\{\min(-a_1 \tilde{h}_1^T \eta_1, a_2 \tilde{h}_2^T \eta_2)\} \mathrm{I}\{y - g(h_1) < 0\}}{\omega_1(h_1, a_1)\omega_2(h_2, a_2)} \\
&\quad + \frac{|y - g(h_1)| \psi_2(a_2 \tilde{h}_2^T \eta_2) \mathrm{I}\{y - g(h_1) < 0\}}{\omega_1(h_1, a_1)\omega_2(h_2, a_2)}.
\end{aligned}$$

The proof of the following result is omitted for brevity.

Lemma 10.4.5. *Let* $\psi_1 : \mathbb{R} \to \mathbb{R}$ *be non-decreasing and concave, and let* $\psi_2 : \mathbb{R} \to \mathbb{R}$ *be concave. For any fixed* (h_2, a_2, y) *the map* $\eta \mapsto \mathcal{L}^{g,\psi}(h_2, a_2, y; \eta)$ *is concave.*

Define the value (policy) search estimator for η under relaxation ψ as

$$\widehat{\eta}_{1,n}^{g,\psi} = \arg\max_{\eta} \mathbb{P}_n \mathcal{L}^{g,\psi}(H_2, A_2, Y; \eta).$$

Because the objective $\mathbb{P}_n \mathcal{L}^{g,\psi}(H_2, A_2, Y; \eta)$ is concave, this estimator can be computed efficiently even in high-dimensional settings. Moreover, as $\widehat{\eta}_{1,n}^{g,\psi} = \arg\min_{\eta}\{-\mathbb{P}_n \mathcal{L}^{g,\psi}(H_2, A_2, Y; \eta)\}$, where $\arg\max_{\eta} \mathbb{P}_n \mathcal{L}^{g,\psi}(H_2, A_2, Y; \eta)$ is convex, it follows under standard regularity conditions that $\widehat{\eta}_{1,n}^{g,\psi}$ is asymptotically normal.

The preceding discussion takes the function g to be fixed and known. In practice, g must be estimated from the observed data. One possibility is to take the estimator for g to be an estimator for $\max_{a_1 \in \mathcal{A}_1} Q_1(h_1, a_1)$; justification for this choice is as follows. From above, for any regime d, $\widehat{\mathcal{V}}_n^g(d)$ has expectation $\mathcal{V}(d) - Pg(H_1) = E\{Y^*(d) - g(H_1)\}$. Thus, a maximizer of $\widehat{\mathcal{V}}_n^g(d_\eta)$ should be an approximate maximizer of $\mathcal{V}(d_\eta)$. Therefore, a heuristic for choosing g is as the minimizer of $E\{Y^*(d^{opt}) - g(H_1)\}^2$, with the idea that $Y^*(d) - g(H_1)$ will have low variability for d near d^{opt}. This choice corresponds to $g(h_1) = E\{Y^*(d^{opt})|H_1 = h_1\} = \max_{a_1 \in \mathcal{A}_1} Q_1(h_1, a_1)$. Thus, to estimate g in practice, one might apply Q-learning to first construct an estimator $\widehat{Q}_{1,n}(h_1, a_1)$ of $Q_1(h_1, a_1)$ and subsequently set $\widehat{g}_n(h_1) = \max_{a_1 \in \mathcal{A}_1} \widehat{Q}_{1,n}(h_1, a_1)$. The estimator for η is then $\widehat{\eta}_{1,n}^{\widehat{g}_n} = \arg\max_{\eta} \mathbb{P}_n \mathcal{L}^{\widehat{g}_n,\psi}(H_2, A_2, Y; \eta)$. Likewise, if the propensities $\omega_k(h_k, a_k)$ are unknown, fitted models for them can be substituted.

10.4.3   g-Computation

Recall from Sections 5.4 and 6.3 that, for any fixed regime $d = (d_1, d_2)$, any functional of the distribution of $Y^*(d)$ can be expressed in terms of the observed data via the g-computation algorithm. Here, we consider estimation of $P(d, y) = P\{Y^*(d) \leq y\}$ via a variant of g-computation referred to as *interactive Q-learning* (IQ-learning Laber et al. (2014a); Linn et al. (2017)). IQ-learning is based on the decomposition

$$P(d, y)$$
$$= E\left(E\left[P\left\{Y \leq y | H_2, A_2\right\} \Big|_{A_2 = d_2(H_2)} \Big| H_1, A_1 \right] \Big|_{A_1 = d_1(H_1)} \right), \quad (10.23)$$

following from the g-computation algorithm, which suggests modeling the distribution of $Y^*(d)$ by first modeling the conditional distribution of Y given $(H_2, A_2) = (\overline{X}_2, \overline{A}_2)$ and subsequently modeling the conditional distribution of (H_2, A_2) given (H_1, A_1). A major drawback of this approach is that modeling the conditional distribution of (H_2, A_2) is notoriously difficult if the dimension of X_2 and thus H_2 is moderate or large. IQ-learning addresses this challenge by assuming additional structure on the relationship between Y and (H_2, A_2).

Because A_2 is binary, there exist real-valued functions m and c such that

$$E(Y|H_2, A_2) = m(H_2) + A_2 c(H_2).$$

IQ-learning assumes a location-scale outcome model

$$Y = m(H_2) + A_2 c(H_2) + \sigma(H_2, A_2)\epsilon, \tag{10.24}$$

where $\sigma(H_2, A_2)$ is a positive standard deviation function, and ϵ is mean zero and independent of (H_2, A_2). Letting F_ϵ denote distribution function of ϵ, under (10.24), (10.23) is equal to

$$
\begin{aligned}
&E\left(E\left[P\left\{Y \le y|H_2, A_2\right\}\Big|_{A_2=d_2(H_2)}\Big|H_1, A_1\right]\Big|_{A_1=d_1(H_1)}\right) \\
&= E\left\{E\left(F_\epsilon\left[\frac{y - m(H_2) - d_2(H_2)c(H_2)}{\sigma\{H_2, d_2(H_2)\}}\right]\Big|H_1, A_1\right)\Big|_{A_1=d_1(H_1)}\right\} \\
&= \int\int\left[F_\epsilon\left\{\frac{y - v - w}{u}\right\} g_d\left(v, w, u|h_1\right)\, d\nu(v, w, u|h_1)\right] dP(h_1),
\end{aligned}
$$

where $g_d(\cdot|h_1)$ is the conditional density of $[m(H_2), d_2(H_2)c(H_2), \sigma\{H_2, d_2(H_2)\}]$ given $H_1 = h_1$ and $A_1 = d_1(h_1)$, and ν is a dominating measure. Thus, given estimators $\widehat{g}_{d_1,n}$ for g_{d_1} and $\widehat{F}_{\epsilon,n}$ for F_ϵ, the IQ-learning estimator for $P\{Y^*(d) \le y\}$ is

$$\widehat{P}_n^{IQ}(d, y) \triangleq \mathbb{P}_n\int\left[\widehat{F}_{\epsilon,n}\left\{\frac{y - v - w_{d_2}}{u_{d_2}}\right\}\widehat{g}_{d,n}(v, w, u|H_1)d\lambda(v, w, u)\right].$$

Thus, regardless of the dimension of H_2, the IQ-learning estimator comprises a univariate distribution function estimator and a three-dimensional conditional density estimator. Consequently, the IQ-learning formulation is potentially advantageous relative to direct modeling of the distribution of (H_2, A_2) given (H_1, A_1) when the dimension of H_2 is larger than three.

We now present results characterizing the limiting behavior of $\widehat{P}_n^{IQ}(d, y)$ under the following assumptions.

(IQ1) F_ϵ is continuous, and $\widehat{F}_{n,\epsilon}$ is a proper cumulative distribution function that converges pointwise to F_ϵ.

(IQ2) $\int |\widehat{g}_{d,n}(v, w, u|h_1) - g_d(v, w, u|h_1)| \, d\lambda(v, w, u)$ converges to zero in probability for almost all h_1.

(IQ3) $\mathbb{P}_n \int |\widehat{g}_{d_1,n}(v, w_{d_2}, u_{d_2}|h_1) - g_{d_1}(v, w_{d_2}, u_{d_2}|h_1)|$ converges to zero in probability.

Lemma 10.4.6. *Assume (IQ1)–(IQ3), and let d be a fixed regime. Then, $\sup_y |\widehat{P}_n^{\mathrm{IQ}}(y, d) - P(d, y)|$ converges to zero in probability.*

This lemma shows that the map $y \mapsto \widehat{P}_n^{\mathrm{IQ}}(d, y)$ converges in probability to $y \mapsto P(d, y)$ where both maps are viewed as elements of $l^\infty(\mathbb{R})$, the space of uniformly bounded real-valued functions on $\mathbb{R}$. Thus, if $\mathcal{O} : l^\infty(\mathbb{R}) \to \mathbb{R}$ is continuous, then it follows from the continuous mapping theorem that $\mathcal{O}\left\{\widehat{P}_n^{\mathrm{IQ}}(d, \cdot)\right\}$ converges in probability to $\mathcal{O}\left\{P(d, \cdot)\right\}$.

The following corollary applies this result to establish consistency of an estimated quantile.

Corollary 10.4.7. *Assume (IQ1)–(IQ3), and let d be a fixed regime. For any $p \in (0, 1)$ and cumulative distribution function G, write $\mathcal{O}_p(G) = G^-(p) = \inf\{\tau : G(\tau) \geq p\}$. Then, $\mathcal{O}_p\left\{\widehat{P}_n^{\mathrm{IQ}}(d, \cdot)\right\} - \mathcal{O}_p\{P(d, \cdot)\}$ converges to zero in probability.*

The preceding results pertain to a fixed, given regime. We now illustrate how IQ-learning can be used to construct value (policy) search estimators for an optimal regime. Let $\mathcal{D}$ denote a class of regimes of interest, and let $\mathcal{P}$ denote the space of probability distribution functions over Y. In addition, let $F : \mathcal{P} \to \mathbb{R}$ denote a criterion function, so that $F(R)$ measures the "goodness" of the distribution R; e.g., $F(R) = \int y \, dR(y)$ or $F(R) = \inf\{\tau : R(\tau) \geq \alpha\}$ for some fixed $\alpha \in (0, 1)$. Define an optimal regime relative to F within $\mathcal{D}$ as any regime that satisfies $d^{opt} \in \arg\max_{d \in \mathcal{D}} F\{P(d, \cdot)\}$. The IQ-learning estimator for d^{opt} satisfies

$$\widehat{d}_n^{opt} \in \arg\max_{d \in \mathcal{D}} F\left\{\widehat{P}_n^{\mathrm{IQ}}(d, \cdot)\right\}.$$

Neither the argmax used above nor in the definition of d^{opt} need be singleton; i.e., they both represent equivalence classes; thus, a notion of distance between the estimator $\widehat{d}_n^{opt}$ and d^{opt} must reflect the fact that neither may be unique. A natural approach is to endow the class of regimes $\mathcal{D}$ with a pseudo metric that respects this equivalence. For example, it can be shown that the distance $p_F : \mathcal{D} \times \mathcal{D} \to \mathbb{R}$ defined by $(d, d') \mapsto |F\{P(d, \cdot)\} - F\{P(d', \cdot)\}|$ is a pseudo-metric on $\mathcal{D}$. Furthermore, by construction, $p_F(d, d') = 0$ for any $d, d' \in \arg\max_{\widetilde{d} \in \mathcal{D}} F\{P(\widetilde{d}, \cdot)\}$, and $p_F(d, d') > 0$ if $d \in \arg\max_{\widetilde{d} \in \mathcal{D}} F\{P(\widetilde{d}, \cdot)\}$ but $d' \notin \arg\max_{\widetilde{d} \in \mathcal{D}} F\{P(\widetilde{d}, \cdot)\}$.

Given the pseudo metric p_F on $\mathcal{D}$, we can construct the induced metric, m_F, on the quotient space of $\mathcal{D}$. Thus, without loss of generality, we assume that $\mathcal{D}$ is a metric space endowed with the metric m_F; notions like continuity and open sets are defined using this metric. We make the following assumptions, which are standard for establishing consistency of an argmax.

(IQ4) $\mathcal{D}$ is compact.

(IQ5) There exists $d^{opt} \in \mathcal{D}$ such that for any open neighborhood $\mathfrak{N}$ of d^{opt} $F\{P(d^{opt}, \cdot)\} > \sup_{d \in \mathcal{D} \setminus \mathfrak{N}} F\{P(d, \cdot)\}$.

(IQ6) The map $d \mapsto F\{P(d, \cdot)\}$ is upper semicontinuous.

(IQ7) $\sup_{d \in \mathcal{D}} |F\{\widehat{P}_n^{IQ}(d, \cdot)\} - F\{P(d, \cdot)\}|$ converges to zero in probability.

The following result establishes consistency of the IQ-learning estimator.

Theorem 10.4.8. *Assume (IQ4)–(IQ7). Then $d_F(\widehat{d}_n^{opt}, d^{opt})$ converges to zero in probability.*

Generally, (IQ4) and (IQ6) are straightforward to verify, whereas (IQ5) is not and is typically assumed as a matter of course. Verification of (IQ7) must be handled on a case by case basis. Establishing (IQ7) can be simplified if it can be shown that F is Lipschitz with respect to some norm on $\mathcal{P}$. For example, consider the mean functional $F(P) = \int y \, dP(y)$, and suppose that for all $d \in \mathcal{D}$ there exists constant L such that $|Y^*(d)| \leq L$ with probability one. Then

$$|F(P) - F(P')| \leq K \int |dP - dP'| = L\mathrm{Wass}(P, P'),$$

where Wass denotes the Wasserstein metric. Thus, in this case it suffices to show that $\sup_{d \in \mathcal{D}} \mathrm{Wass}\{\widehat{P}_n^{IQ}(d, \cdot), P(d, \cdot)\}$ converges to zero in probability. Working directly with $\widehat{P}_n^{IQ}$ and P is often easier than working with $F\{\widehat{P}(d, \cdot)\}$ and $F\{P(d, \cdot)\}$.

Remark. In some settings, the pseudo metric p_F may be difficult to work with because the relationship between d and $Y^*(d)$ may be complex or poorly understood. If there is additional structure in $\mathcal{D}$, this can sometimes be used to construct a pseudo metric that is easier to work with. Suppose that the class of regimes of interest comprises regimes d with rules of the form

$$d_k(h_k) = \mathrm{sign}\{f_k(h_k)\}, \quad k = 1, 2 \text{ for some } (f_1, f_2) \in \mathcal{F},$$

where $\mathcal{F}$ is a metric space with distance $m_{\mathcal{F}} : \mathcal{F} \times \mathcal{F} \to \mathbb{R}$; e.g., the class of regimes $\mathcal{D}_\eta$ comprising regimes d_η with linear decision functions $f(h_k; \eta_k) = \mathrm{sign}(\tilde{h}_k^T \eta_k)$, $k = 1, 2$, as in (10.19), where $\dim(\eta_k) = p_k$ and $\mathcal{F} = \mathbb{R}^{p_1} \times \mathbb{R}^{p_2}$, equipped with the Euclidean metric. For any $d \in \mathcal{D}$ there exists $f \in \mathcal{F}$ so that $d_k(h_k) = \mathrm{sign}\{f_k(h_k)\}$ for all h_k, $k = 1, 2$;

to make this relationship explicit, write d_f, where f dictates d. Defining $p_{\mathcal{F}} : \mathcal{D} \times \mathcal{D} \to \mathbb{R}$ to be the map $(d_f, d_{f'}) \mapsto e_{\mathcal{F}}(f, f')$, $p_{\mathcal{F}}$ is a pseudometric on $\mathcal{D}$. The challenge is then to establish that convergence in $p_{\mathcal{F}}$ implies convergence in p_F.

10.5 Discussion

We have presented a survey of a select set of inferential methods for estimands of interest in dynamic treatment regimes. Our selection of methods is biased toward those that we have used in our applied work or we feel illustrate key concepts used in the literature. Thus, we hope that this chapter, while incomplete, will provide a sufficient introduction to a rich and active area of research within dynamic treatment regimes. While the approaches described here are rather technical, they are designed to provide statistically rigorous answers to clinical questions that commonly arise in the context of precision medicine. This is aligned with our view that one should let the underlying clinical science guide the development of statistical methods. These clinical questions are (and should be) generally constructed without reference to a specific statistical methodology, but, as we have seen, the correct approach to inference can depend critically on which statistical methods are applied for estimation. We expect inferential methods to become even more complex as machine learning and other nonparametric methods are used to estimate Q-functions and related quantities.

Chapter 11

Additional Topics

As we noted at the outset, this book is meant to provide a comprehensive account of fundamental statistical frameworks and methodology for dynamic treatment regimes and to endow the reader with a strong foundation for further study of the expansive literature on this topic. We believe that the book covers core material essential to these objectives. Accordingly, the book deliberately does not present detailed accounts of ongoing advances and specialized topics. That said, we conclude the book with a summary of our perspective on the future of this area and a brief discussion of some additional topics needing or undergoing development.

At the time of this writing, methodological research on treatment regimes is burgeoning. New approaches to estimation of an optimal treatment regime appear regularly in major journals; such work includes refinement and extension of existing methods, incorporation of deep learning and other artificial intelligence techniques, and methods based on alternative criteria for optimality. It is our conviction that great progress in the treatment of chronic diseases and disorders in particular can be realized if treatment is regarded widely as a holistic sequential decision-making problem rather than as a series of isolated decisions. The continued development of new methodology for discovery of optimal treatment regimes ensures that appropriate tools will be available as this perspective gains traction among domain scientists.

However, we acknowledge that there is an enormous research-practice gap. Although more and more health sciences researchers are embracing this view, the breadth and volume of methodological development is light years ahead of its adoption in practice. It is our experience that even the fundamental approaches reviewed in this book are not being implemented in practice to the extent that they should be, despite broad interest in precision medicine and data-driven decision making. Many in health sciences research continue to think retrospectively; for example, questions on actions that should be taken following the single decision point that is the focus of a conventional randomized clinical trial are often raised after completion of the trial. We encourage readers interested in advancing methodology for treatment regimes to advocate strongly to domain science collaborators for the benefits of thinking sequentially, in a prospective manner, and to emphasize the availability of cutting edge methodological tools to support this endeavor.

We close by mentioning a few additional topics, both methodological and conceptual; by no means is this an exhaustive compilation of such topics. Where appropriate, we cite a few articles to guide the reader to the relevant literature.

Regimes Based on Multiple Competing Outcomes

Throughout this book and indeed in the most of the literature on dynamic treatment regimes, it is assumed that there is a single, scalar health outcome of interest reflecting the benefit of treatment. As we have reviewed at length, an optimal treatment regime is one that maximizes the expected outcome that would be achieved if all patients in the population followed its rules relative to the expected outcome achieved if the population were to follow any other strategy for selecting treatments.

However, in some settings, clinical decision making of necessity must balance multiple and possibly competing outcomes. A notable example is in the treatment of cancer, where the efficacy of often toxic therapies must be weighed against the potential for serious adverse effects. In general, competing outcomes may reflect efficacy, cost of treatment, patient burden, and so on. The challenge of balancing competing outcomes is certainly not unique to sequential decision making, and it is fair to say that there is no consensus on a preferred approach even when interest focuses on a simple comparison of treatment options at a single decision point. When interest focuses on an optimal treatment regime, this challenge is intensified.

As in the vast literature on competing outcomes, a natural approach in this setting is to define a utility function that synthesizes the competing outcomes into a single, composite outcome. In the case of two competing outcomes Y_1 and Y_2, say, $U(y_1, y_2)$ measures the utility of observing $Y_1 = y_1$ and $Y_2 = y_2$ and might be taken to be a convex combination of the two outcomes; i.e., $U(y_1, y_2) = \omega y_1 + (1 - \omega) y_2$. Here, the weights ω are solicited from domain science experts, or might be otherwise specified as assigning values to regions in the (y_1, y_2) plane; see Wang et al. (2012) for an example in the context of treatment regimes. A single or multiple decision optimal regime can then be estimated using the standard methods discussed in this book applied to the observed utilities for each individual. Of course, the challenges of constructing such composite outcomes are well known, and a single such outcome may not account for heterogeneity in patient and clinician preferences. In some settings, it may be possible to estimate the utility function from observational data under the assumption that clinicians implicitly are attempting to maximize a utility measure that reflects the goal of maximizing expected benefit; see Luckett et al. (2019b). Construction of a composite outcome does not directly incorporate patient utilities so may be biased toward those of clinicians. A common approach to eliciting patient utility is to administer a questionnaire designed to measure preferences across different health outcome profiles. Items on the questionnaire are assumed to be linked through a statistical model to a latent utility function, and thus a patient's responses can be used to estimate his utility function. Butler et al. (2018) propose methods for estimation of an optimal treatment regime based on this premise; see also Lin et al. (2019).

The preceding approaches place the competing outcomes on equal footing in the sense that utility functions can place weight preferentially on one or the other of the outcomes. If, say, Y_1 is a measure reflecting efficacy, coded so that larger is better, and Y_2 is cost of treatment, it may not be sensible to minimize cost (maximize negative cost) without regard for efficacy. Here, it may be more appropriate to view Y_1 as the primary outcome of interest and Y_2 as a secondary outcome and define an optimal regime as one that maximizes expected primary outcome subject to a constraint on the secondary outcome. For example, defining $Y_1^*(d)$ and $Y_2^*(d)$ to be the obvious potential outcomes under regime $d \in \mathcal{D}$, given a threshold τ, define d_τ^{opt} to maximize $E\{Y_1^*(d)\}$ such that $E\{Y_2^*(d)\} \geq \tau$. Another approach in this context is to estimate a set-valued treatment regime; that is, a regime that maps patient information to a set of acceptable treatment options, where this set comprises a single option if that option is best across all competing outcomes and otherwise contains all treatment options that are not dominated by another option across all outcomes. See Laber et al. (2014b) and Lizotte and Laber (2016).

Infinite Horizon Decision Problems

Throughout this book, we have focused on the setting in which K key decision points are identified, where K is finite. This formulation is appropriate in a vast range of disease and disorder contexts in which the decision points may correspond to acknowledged milestones in the progression of a disease, to the occurrence of expected events, or to natural evaluation points in clinical practice. In some settings, however, the number of decision points may be very large or infinite. For example, in some mHealth applications, patients may receive multiple interventions per day over the course of many months, as in the case of a messaging application to promote weight loss by encouraging healthy eating and physical activity throughout the day. Weight loss is likely to occur gradually over a long time horizon, so that an optimal treatment regime dictating the timing and content of messages would do so at numerous decision points over this extended period. Similarly, facilitated by the advent of wearable technology, the management of an ongoing condition such as diabetes requires continuing adjustment of treatment in response to the changing status of the patient over an essentially infinite time horizon.

In these and similar contexts, the goal is to estimate an optimal treatment regime that can be applied essentially indefinitely; i.e., over a potentially infinite number of decision points. The observed data available for this enterprise almost certainly traverse only a finite time horizon. Accordingly, additional structure must be assumed to permit extrapolation beyond the time horizon. A standard assumption is that the observed data follow a homogeneous Markov Decision Process (MDP); MDPs are used routinely to model decision processes evolving in discrete time (e.g., Sutton and Barto, 2018). Specifically, write the observed data as

$$(X_{1i}, A_{1i}, \ldots, X_{Ti}.A_{Ti}, X_{T+1,i}), \quad i = 1, \ldots, n,$$

where T (an integer) is the time horizon over which the data were collected, X_t and A_t are the state of patient information and treatment received at time t, and the patient's history to time t is $H_t = (X_1, A_1, \ldots, X_{t-1}, A_{t-1}, X_t)$. It is assumed that the $(X_1, A_1, \ldots, X_T, A_T, X_{T+1})$ is the truncation of the infinite process $(X_1, A_1, \ldots, X_T, A_T, X_{T+1}, \ldots)$, which is Markov and homogeneous, with, for any $t \geq 1$ and set B,

$$P(X_{t+1} \in B|H_t, A_t) = P(X_{t+1} \in B|X_t, A_t),$$

so depending on only the most recent state of information and thus possessing the Markov property. This assumption may be justified based on scientific knowledge, and its plausibility can be evaluated based on the data.

Assume a utility function $y(x_t, a_t, x_{t+1})$ can be specified that captures the momentary utility of being in state $X_t = x_t$, choosing treatment option $A_t = a_t$, and then transitioning to state $X_{t+1} = x_{t+1}$, and let $Y_t = y(X_t, A_t, X_{t+1})$ be the observed utility at time t. A treatment regime in this context is then an infinite sequence of decision rules $d = (d_1, d_2, \ldots)$ such that d_t maps the current state of patient information x_t to an option in the set of options $\mathcal{A}_t$ at time t. Letting $X_t^*(d)$ and $Y_t^*(d)$ be the obvious potential state of patient information and utility at time t under a regime $d \in \mathcal{D}$, where $\mathcal{D}$ is the class of all such regimes, an optimal treatment regime is defined as maximizing the discounted mean potential outcome

$$\mathcal{V}(x, d) = E \left\{ \sum_{t \geq 1} \gamma^{t-1} Y_t^*(d) \middle| X_1 = x \right\}$$

over all x and $d \in \mathcal{D}$, where $\gamma \in [0, 1)$ is a discount factor that balances the tradeoff between immediate and distal utilities. See Ertefaie and Strawderman (2018) and Luckett et al. (2019a) and references therein for details and accounts of methodology for estimation of an optimal regime under these conditions.

A related topic is that of *just-in-time adaptive interventions*, which can be thought of as treatment regimes that exploit the ability to collect data on a patient and deliver interventions in real time that adapt to the immediate state of the patient via smartphones and wearable devices. See Nahum-Shani et al. (2018) for an overview. The *micro-randomized trial* has been proposed as the "gold-standard" study design for this setting; see Klasnja et al. (2015) and Liao et al. (2016).

Variable Selection for Decision Making

A practical challenge in estimation of an optimal treatment regime is development of the required statistical models, in particular the patient information that should be included in these models, as for Q-learning; or determining the form of the dependence of the rules defining a restricted class of regimes on patient information. Identifying the so-called tailoring variables that are critical to include in the rules can be viewed as a problem of variable selection. However, although there is a vast literature on variable selection in regression, these methods are largely focused on minimizing prediction error; that is, identifying variables that are important for high-quality predictions. In the context of treatment regimes, the important variables are those that have a qualitative interaction with treatment and thus are critical for high-quality decision making. Thus, methods that can identify such prescriptive variables and incorporate this selection into the framework of estimation of an optimal treatment regime are an important adjunct to methods for estimation. See Biernot and Moodie (2010), Gunter et al. (2011b), Fan et al. (2016), Zhu et al. (2019), Zhang and Zhang (2018b), and Wallace et al. (2019) for discussion and proposed methods.

Missing Information

As in almost any data analytic setting in the health sciences, dropout and more generally missing data are ubiquitous. As discussed in Section 9.6 in the context of SMARTs, dropout from the trial complicates analysis because participants who drop out do not reach all K decision points. The same is true in the case of subjects in an observational data set. Although some methods for handling such missing information in analysis of treatment regimes are available, cited in Section 9.6, further development and evaluation of approaches, particularly for estimation of an optimal regime in the presence of missing information, is required.

Continuous Treatment

With a few exceptions, we have restricted attention in this book to the setting where there is a finite number of available treatment options at each decision point, which is relevant in a broad range of disease and disorder areas. In some settings, the treatment options may be doses of a drug in a continuous range of candidate doses, as discussed briefly in Section 9.2.3. See Stephens (2015) and Chen et al. (2016) for accounts of methods for estimation of an optimal regime in this case.

Conceptual Challenges

Finally, we note that some of the most significant challenges for the future are not methodological but conceptual and have implications for policy. As interest in evaluation and discovery of treatment regimes becomes more widespread, the question of how to evaluate an experimental treatment option for which evidence shows plays a critical role in an overall treatment regime from a regulatory perspective is inevitable. Likewise, it is likely that regulatory policy will need to be defined for entire treatment regimes that involve treatment options produced by competing industry sponsors. Different stakeholders will undoubtedly focus on different issues. For example, in our experience, a common question for those vested in a particular treatment option is how to characterize the "contribution" of that option to an overall regime. Others may debate the regulatory implications for all treatment options involved in an estimated optimal regime for which strong evidence of superiority over standard of care exists. These and other questions are not statistical methodological questions; rather, they are conceptual and policy questions. As discussion ensues and consensus on how to formulate and address these questions emerges, there will be opportunities for new statistical methods development.

Bibliography

Almirall, D., Compton, S. N., Gunlicks-Stoessel, M., Duan, N., and Murphy, S. A. (2012a). Designing a pilot sequential multiple assignment randomized trial for developing an adaptive treatment strategy. *Statistics in Medicine* **31**, 1887–1902.

Almirall, D., Lizotte, D., and Murphy, S. A. (2012b). SMART design issues and the consideration of opposing outcomes. Discussion of "Evaluation of viable dynamic treatment regimes in a sequentially randomized trial of advanced prostate cancer" by Wang et al. *Journal of the American Statistical Association* **107**, 509–512.

Almirall, D., Nahum-Shani, I., Sherwood, N. E., and Murphy, S. A. (2014). Introduction to SMART designs for the development of adaptive interventions: With application to weight loss research. *Translational Behavioral Medicine* **4**, 260–274.

Andersen, P. K., Borgan, Ø., Gill, R. D., and Keiding, N. (1993). *Statistical Methods Based on Counting Processes*. Springer, New York.

Anstrom, K. J. and Tsiatis, A. A. (2001). Utilizing propensity scores to estimate causal treatment effects with censored time-lagged data. *Biometrics* **57**, 1207–1218.

Arcones, M. A. and Giné, E. (1989). The bootstrap of the mean with arbitrary bootstrap sample size. *Annales de l'IHP Probabilités et Statistiques* **25**, 457–481.

Artman, W. J., Nahum-Shani, I., Wu, T., Mckay, J. R., and Ertefaie, A. (2018). Power analysis in a SMART design: sample size estimation for determining the best embedded dynamic treatment regime. *Biostatistics* in press.

Bai, X., Tsiatis, A. A., Lu, W., and Song, R. (2017). Optimal treatment regimes for survival endpoints using a locally-efficient doubly-robust estimator from a classfication perspective. *Lifetime Data Analysis* **23**, 584–604.

Bai, X., Tsiatis, A. A., and O'Brien, S. M. (2013). Doubly-robust estimators of treatment-specific survival distributions in observational studies with stratified sampling. *Biometrics* **69**, 830–839.

Bartlett, P. L., Jordan, M. I., and McAuliffe, J. D. (2003). Large margin classifiers: Convex loss, low noise, and convergence rates. In *Advances in Neural Information Processing Systems 16 (NIPS 2003)*.

Bartlett, P. L., Jordan, M. I., and McAuliffe, J. D. (2006). Convexity, classification, and risk bounds. *Journal of the American Statistical Association* **101**, 138–156.

Bembom, O. and van der Laan, M. J. (2007). Statistical methods for analyzing sequentially randomized trials. *Journal of the National Cancer Institute* **99**, 1577–1582.

Beran, R. (1990). Calibrating prediction regions. *Journal of the American Statistical Association* **85**, 715–723.

Berry, D. A. and Fristedt, B. (1985). *Bandit Problems: Sequential Allocation of Experiments*. Springer, New York.

Bertsekas, D. P. (2015). *Convex Optimization Algorithms*. Athena Scientific, Belmont, Massachusetts.

Bickel, P. J. and Sakov, A. (2008). On the choice of m in the m out of n bootstrap and confidence bounds for extrema. *Statistica Sinica* **18**, 967–985.

Biernot, P. and Moodie, E. E. M. (2010). A comparison of variable selection approaches for dynamic treatment regimes. *The International Journal of Biostatistics* **6**.

Blatt, D., Murphy, S., and Zhu, J. (2004). A-learning for approximate planning. *Technical Report 04-63, The Methodology Center, Pennsylvania State University* .

Boos, D. D. and Stefanski, L. (2013). *Essential Statistical Inference*. Springer, New York.

Booth, J. G. and Hall, P. (1994). Monte Carlo approximation and the iterated bootstrap. *Biometrika* **81**, 331–340.

Boyd, S. and Vandenberghe, L. (2004). *Convex Optimization*. Cambridge University Press, Cambridge.

Breiman, L. (2001). Random forests. *Machine Learning* **45**, 5–32.

Breiman, L., Freidman, J. H., Olshen, R. A., and Stone, C. J. (1984). *Classification and Regression Trees*. Chapman & Hall/CRC Press, Boca Raton, Florida.

Breslow, N. E. (1972). Discussion of the paper by D. R. Cox. *Journal of the Royal Statistical Society, Series B* **34**, 216–217.

Bretagnolle, J. (1983). Lois limites du bootstrap de certaines fonctionnelles. *Annales de l'IHP Probabilités et Statistiques* **19**, 281–296.

Butler, E. L., Laber, E. B., Davis, S. M., and Kosorok, M. R. (2018). Incorporating patient preferences into estimation of optimal individualized treatment rules. *Biometrics* **74**, 18–26.

Carlin, B. P., Berry, S. M., Lee, J. J., and Müller, P. (2010). *BAyesian Adaptive Methods for Clinical Trials*. Chapman & Hall/CRC Press, Boca Raton, Florida.

Chaffee, P. and van der Laan, M. (2012). Targeted maximum likelihood estimation for dynamic treatment regimes in sequentially randomized controlled trials. *The International Journal of Biostatistics* **8**.

Chakraborty, B., Ghosh, P., Moodie, E. E. M., and Rush, A. J. (2016). Estimating optimal shared-parameter dynamic regimens with application to a multistage depression clinical trial. *Biometrics* **72**, 865–876.

Chakraborty, B., Laber, E. B., and Zhao, Y. (2014a). Inference for optimal dynamic treatment regimes using an adaptive m-out-of-n bootstrap scheme. *Biometrics* **69**, 714–723.

Chakraborty, B., Laber, E. B., and Zhao, Y.-Q. (2014b). Inference about the expected performance of a data-driven dynamic treatment regime. *Clinical Trials* **11**, 408–417.

Chakraborty, B., Murphy, S. A., and Strecher, V. (2010). Inference for non-regular parameters in optimal dynamic treatment regimes. *Statistical Methods in Medical Research* **19**, 317–343.

Chen, G., Zeng, D., and Kosorok, M. R. (2016). Personalized dose finding using outcome weighted learning. *Journal of the American Statistical Association* **111**, 1509–1521.

Chen, P. Y. and Tsiatis, A. A. (2001). Causal inference on the difference of the restricted mean lifetime between two groups. *Biometrics* **57**, 1030–1038.

Cheung, Y. K., Chakraborty, B., and Davidson, K. W. (2015). Sequential multiple assignment randomized trial (SMART) with adaptive randomization for quality improvement in depression treatment program. *Biometrics* **71**, 450–459.

Cohen, J. (1988). *Statistical Power Analysis for the Behavioral Sciences, Second Edition*. L. Erlbaum Associates, Hillsdale, New Jersey.

Collins, L., Murphy, S., and Bierman, K. (2004). A conceptual framework for adaptive preventive interventions. *Prevention Science* **5**, 185–196.

Collins, L. M., Nahum-Shani, I., and Almirall, D. (2014). Optimization of behavioral dynamic treatment regimens based on the sequential, multiple assignment, randomized trial (SMART). *Clinical Trials* **11**, 426–434.

Cortes, C. and Vapnik, V. (1995). Support-vector networks. *Machine Learning* **20,** 273–297.

Cox, D. R. (1972). Regression models and life tables (with discussion). *Journal of the Royal Statistical Society, Series B* **34,** 187–220.

Cox, D. R. (1975). Partial likelihood. *Biometrika* **69,** 269–276.

Dawid, A. P. (1994). Selection paradoxes of Bayesian inference. In *Multivariate Analysis and Its Applications*, pages 211–220. Institute of Mathematical Statistics, Hayward, California.

Dean, A., Morris, M., Stufken, J., and Bingham, D. (2015). *Handbook of Design and Analysis of Experiments.* Chapman & Hall/CRC Press, Boca Raton, Florida.

Diáz, I., Savenkov, O., and Ballman, K. (2018). Targeted learning ensembles for optimal individualized treatment rules with time-to-event outcomes. *Biometrika* **105,** 723–738.

Ertefaie, A. and Strawderman, R. L. (2018). Constructing dynamic treatment regimes over indefinite time horizons. *Biometrika* **105,** 963–977.

Ertefaie, A., Wu, T., Lynch, K. G., and Nahum-Shani, I. (2016). Identifying a set that contains the best dynamic treatment regimes. *Biostatistics* **17,** 135–148.

Fan, A., Lu, W., and Song, R. (2016). Sequential advantage selection for optimal treatment regime. *Annals of Applied Statistics* **10,** 32–53.

Fan, C., Lu, W., Song, R., and Zhou, Y. (2017). Concordance-assisted learning for estimating optimal individualized treatment regimes. *Journal of the Royal Statistical Society, Series B* **79,** 1565–1582.

Fava, M., Rush, A. J., Trivedi, M. H., Nierenberg, A. A., Thase, M. E., Sackeim, H. A., Quitkin, F. M., Wisniewski, S., Lavori, P. W., Rosenbaum, J. F., and Kupfer, D. J. (2003). Background and rationale for the Sequenced Treatment Alternatives to Relieve Depression (STAR*D) study. *Psychiatric Clinics of North America* **26,** 457–494.

Foster, J. C., Taylor, J. M., and Ruberg, S. J. (2011). Subgroup identification from randomized clinical trial data. *Statistics in Medicine* **30,** 2867–2880.

Geng, Y., Zhang, H. H., and Lu, W. (2015). On optimal treatment regimes selection for mean survival time. *Statistics in Medicine* **34,** 1169–1184.

Giné, E. and Zinn, J. (1990). Bootstrapping general empirical measures. *Annals of Probability* **18,** 851–869.

Glick, N. (1974). Consistency conditions for probability estimators and integrals of density estimators. *Utilitas Math* **6**, 61–74.

Goldberg, D. E. (1989). *Genetic Algorithms in Search, Optimization, and Machine Learning*. Addison-Wesley, Reading, Massachusetts.

Goldberg, Y. and Kosorok, M. R. (2012). Q-learning with censored data. *Annals of Statistics* **40**, 529–260.

Goldberg, Y., Song, R., Kosorok, M. R., et al. (2013). Adaptive Q-learning. In *From Probability to Statistics and Back: High-Dimensional Models and Processes–A Festschrift in Honor of Jon A. Wellner*, pages 150–162. Institute of Mathematical Statistics, Hayward, California.

Gunter, L., Chernick, M., and Sun, J. (2011a). A simple method for variable selection in regression with respect to treatment selection. *Pakistan Journal of Statistics and Operation Research* **7**, 363–380.

Gunter, L., Zhu, J., and Murphy, S. A. (2007). Variable selection for optimal decision making. In *Artificial Intelligence in Medicine. AIME 2007. Lecture Notes in Computer Science*, pages 149–154, Berlin Heidelberg. Springer.

Gunter, L., Zhu, J., and Murphy, S. A. (2011b). Variable selection for qualitative interactions. *Statistical Methodology* **8**, 42–55.

Gunter, L., Zhu, J., and Murphy, S. A. (2011c). Variable selection for qualitative interactions in personalized medicine while controlling the family-wise error rate. *Journal of Biopharmaceutical Statistics* **21**, 1063–1078.

Gurobi Optimization (2019). Gurobi Optimizer Reference Manual, Version 8.1. www.gurobi.com/.

Haberman, S. J. (1989). Concavity and estimation. *Annals of Statistics* **17**, 1631–1661.

Hager, R., Tsiatis, A. A., and Davidian, M. (2018). Optimal two-stage dynamic treatment regimes from a classification perspective with censored survival data. *Biometrics* **74**, 1180–1192.

Hall, P. (1986). On the bootstrap and confidence intervals. *Annals of Statistics* **14**, 1431–1452.

Hall, P., Peng, L., and Tajvidi, N. (1999). On prediction intervals based on predictive likelihood or bootstrap methods. *Biometrika* **86**, 871–880.

Hastie, T. J., Tibshirani, R. J., and Friedman, J. H. (2009). *The Elements of Statistical Learning: Data Mining, Inference, and Prediction, Second Edition*. Springer-Verlag, New York.

Henderson, H. V. and Searle, S. (1979). Vec and vech operators for matrices, with some uses in Jacobians and multivariate statistics. *Canadian Journal of Statistics* **7**, 65–81.

Henderson, R., Ansell, P., and Alshibani, D. (2010). Regret-regression for optimal dynamic treatment regimes. *Biometrics* **66**, 1192–1201.

Hernán, M., Brumback, B., and Robins, J. (2000). Marginal structural models to estimate the causal effect of zidovudine on the survival of HIV-positive men. *Epidemiology* **11**, 561–570.

Hernán, M. A., Lanoy, E., Costagliola, D., and Robins, J. M. (2006). Comparison of dynamic treatment regimes via inverse probability weighting. *Basic & Clinical Pharmacology & Toxicology* **98**, 237–242.

Hirano, K. and Porter, J. R. (2012). Impossibility results for nondifferentiable functionals. *Econometrica* **80**, 1769–1790.

Hjort, N. L. and Pollard, D. (2011). Asymptotics for minimisers of convex processes. *arXiv preprint arXiv:1107.3806* .

Horvitz, D. G. and Thompson, D. J. (1952). Generalization of sampling without replacement from a finite universe. *Journal of the American Statistical Association* **47**, 663–685.

Huang, X., Goldberg, Y., and Xu, J. (2019). Multicategory individualized treatment regime using outcome weighted learning. *Biometrics* in press.

Huang, X., Ning, J., and Wahed, A. S. (2014). Optimization of individualized dynamic treatment regimes for recurrent diseases. *Statistics in Medicine* **33**, 2363–2378.

Hudgens, M. G. and Halloran, M. E. (2008). Toward causal inference with interference. *Journal of the American Statistical Association* **103**, 832–842.

IBM ILOG CPLEX (2019). IBM ILOG CPLEX Optimization Studio. www.ibm.com/products/ilog-cplex-optimization-studio.

Jiang, B., Song, R., Li, J., and Zeng, D. (2019). Entropy learning for dynamic treatment regimes. *Statistica Sinica* in press.

Jiang, R., Lu, W., Song, R., and Davidian, M. (2017a). On estimation of optimal treatment regimes for maximizing t-year survival probability. *Journal of the Royal Statistical Society, Series B* **79**, 1165–1185.

Jiang, R., Lu, W., Song, R., Hudgens, M. G., and Napravavnik, S. (2017b). Doubly robust estimation of optimal treatment regimes for survival data with application to an HIV/AIDS study. *Annals of Applied Statistics* **11**, 1763–1786.

Jones, B. and Kenward, M. G. (2014). *Design and Analysis of Cross-*

Over Trials. Chapman & Hall/CRC Press, Boca Raton, Florida.

Kang, C., Janes, H., and Huang, Y. (2014). Combining biomarkers to optimize patient treatment recommendations. *Biometrics* **70**, 695–720.

Karatzoglou, A., Meyer, D., and Hornik, K. (2006). Support vector machines in R. *Journal of Statistical Software* **15**, 1–28.

Kelleher, S. A., Dorfman, C. S., Vilardaga, J. C. P., Majestic, C., Winger, J., Gandhi, V., Nunez, C., Van Denburg, A., Shelby, R. A., Reed, S. D., Murphy, S. A., Davidian, M., Laber, E. B., Kimmick, Gretchen, G., Westbrook, K. W., Abernathy, A. P., and Somers, T. J. (2017). Optimizing delivery of a behavioral pain intervention in cancer patients using a sequential multiple assignment randomized trial (SMART). *Contemporary Clinical Trials* **57**, 51–57.

Kidwell, K. M. (2014). SMART designs in cancer research: Learning from the past, current limitations and looking toward the future. *Clinical Trials* **11**, 445–456.

Kidwell, K. M. and Wahed, A. S. (2013). Weighted log-rank statistic to compare shared-path adaptive treatment strategies. *Biostatistics* **14**, 229–312.

Klasnja, P., Hekler, E. B., Shiffman, S., Boruvka, A., Almirall, D., Tewari, A., and Murphy, S. A. (2015). Microrandomized trials: An experimental design for developing just-in-time adaptive interventions. *Health Psychology* **34**, 1220–1228.

Kosorok, M. R. (2007). *Introduction to Empirical Processes and Semiparametric Inference*. Springer-Verlag, New York.

Krauth, W. (2006). *Statistical Mechanics: Algorithms and Computations*, volume 13. Oxford University Press, Oxford.

Laber, E. and Qian, M. (2018). Generalization error for decision problems. *arXiv preprint arXiv:1812.08696* .

Laber, E. B., Linn, K. A., and Stefanski, L. A. (2014a). Interactive model building for Q-learning. *Biometrika* **101**, 831–847.

Laber, E. B., Lizotte, D. J., and Ferguson, B. (2014b). Set-valued dynamic treatment regimes for competing outcomes. *Biometrics* **70**, 53–61.

Laber, E. B., Lizotte, D. J., Qian, M., Pelham, W. E., and Murphy, S. A. (2014c). Dynamic treatment regimes: Technical challenges and applications. *Electronic Journal of Statistics* **8**, 1225–1271.

Laber, E. B. and Murphy, S. A. (2011). Adaptive confidence intervals for the test error in classification. *Journal of the American Statistical Association* **106**, 904–913.

Laber, E. B. and Zhao, Y. Q. (2015). Tree-based methods for individualized treatment regimes. *Biometrika* **102**, 501–514.

Laber, E. B., Zhao, Y. Q., Regh, T., Davidian, M., Tsiatis, A., Stanford, J. B., Zeng, D., and Kosorok, M. R. (2016). Using pilot data to size a two-arm randomized trial to find a nearly optimal personalized treatment strategy. *Statistics in Medicine* **35**, 1245–1256.

Lange, K. (2010). *Numerical Analysis for Statisticians.* Springer-Verlag, New York.

Lavori, P. W. and Dawson, R. (2000). A design for testing clinical strategies: Biased adaptive within-subject randomization. *Journal of the Royal Statistical Society, Series A* **163**, 29–38.

Lavori, P. W. and Dawson, R. (2004). Dynamic treatment regimes: Practical design considerations. *Clinical Trials* **1**, 9–20.

Lei, H., Nahum-Shani, I., Lynch, K., Oslin, D., and Murphy, S. A. (2011). A SMART design for building individualized treatment sequences. *Annual Review of Clinical Psychology* **8**, 21–48.

Letham, B., Rudin, C., McCormick, T. H., and Madigan, D. (2015). Interpretable classifiers using rules and Bayesian analysis: Building a better stroke prediction model. *Annals of Applied Statistics* **9**, 1350–1371.

Liao, P., Klasnja, P., Tewari, A., and Murphy, S. A. (2016). Sample size calculations for micro-randomized trials in mHealth. *Statistics in Medicine* **35**, 1944–1971.

Lin, R., Thall, P. F., and Yuan, Y. (2019). An adaptive trial design to optimize dose-schedule regimes with delayed outcomes. *Biometrics* in press.

Linn, K. A., Laber, E. B., and Stefanski, L. A. (2017). Interactive Q-learning for quantiles. *Journal of the American Statistical Association* **112**, 638–649.

Lipkovich, I., Dmitrienko, A., Denne, J., and Enas, G. (2011). Subgroup identification based on differential effect search: Recursive partitioning method for establishing response to treatment in patient subpopulations. *Statistics in Medicine* **30**, 2601–2621.

Liu, Y., Wang, Y., Kosorok, M. R., Zhao, Y., and Zeng, D. (2018). Augmented outcome-weighted learning for estimating optimal dynamic treatment regimens. *Statistics in Medicine* **37**, 3776–3788.

Liu, Y., Wang, Y., and Zeng, D. (2017). Sequential multiple assignment randomized trials with enrichment design. *Biometrics* **73**, 378–390.

Lizotte, D. J. and Laber, E. B. (2016). Multi-objective Markov decision processes for data-driven decision support. *Journal of Machine*

Learning Research **17**, 1–28.

Lizotte, D. J. and Tahmasebi, A. (2017). Prediction and tolerance intervals for dynamic treatment regimes. *Statistical Methods in Medical Research* **26**, 1611–1629.

Lou, Z., Shao, J., and Yu, M. (2018). Optimal treatment assignment to maximize expected outcome with multiple treatments. *Biometrics* **74**, 506–516.

Lu, W., Zhang, H. H., and Zeng, D. (2013). Variable selection for optimal treatment decision. *Statistical Methods in Medical Research* **22**, 493–504.

Luckett, D. J., Laber, E. B., Kahkoska, A. R., Maahs, D. M., Mayer-Davis, E., and Kosorok, M. R. (2019a). Estimating dynamic treatment regimes in mobile health using V-learning. *Journal of the American Statistical Association* in press.

Luckett, D. J., Laber, E. B., and Kosorok, M. R. (2019b). Estimation and optimization of composite outcomes. *arXiv preprint arXiv:1711.10581v3* .

Luedtke, A. R. and van der Laan, M. (2016a). Statistical inference for the mean outcome under a possibly non-unique optimal treatment strategy. *Annals of Statistics* **44**, 713–742.

Luedtke, A. R. and van der Laan, M. (2016b). Super-learning of an optimal dynamic treatment rule. *The International Journal of Biostatistics* **12**.

Mark, S. and Robins, J. (1993). Estimating the causal effect of smoking cessation in the presence of confounding factors using a rank preserving structural failure time model. *Statistics in Medicine* **12**, 1605–1628.

Matts, J. P. and Lachin, J. M. (1988). Properties of permuted-block randomization in clinical trials. *Controlled Clinical Trials* **9**, 327–344.

McKeague, I. W. and Qian, M. (2015). An adaptive resampling test for detecting the presence of significant predictors. *Journal of the American Statistical Association* **110**, 1422–1433.

Mebane, W. R. and Sekhon, J. S. (2011). Genetic optimization using derivatives: The rgenoud package for R. *Journal of Statistical Software* **42**, 1–26.

Mi, X., Zou, F., and Zhu, R. (2019). Bagging and deep learning in optimal individualized treatment rules. *Biometrics* in press.

Moodie, E. (2009). Risk factor adjustment in marginal structural model estimation of optimal treatment regimes. *Biometrical Journal* **51**,

774–788.

Moodie, E. and Richardson, T. (2010). Estimating optimal dynamic regimes: Correcting bias under the null. *Scandinavian Journal of Statistics* **37**, 126–146.

Moodie, E. E. M., Dean, N., and Sun, Y. (2014). Q-learning: Flexible learning about useful utilities. *Statistics in Biosciences* **6**, 223–243.

Moodie, E. E. M., Richardson, T. S., and Stephens, D. A. (2007). Demystifying optimal dynamic treatment regimes. *Biometrics* **63**, 447–455.

MOSEK (2019). MOSEK, Version 9.1. www.mosek.com/.

Muessig (2019). AllyQuest Adherence App Intervention for HIV-positive Men Who Have Sex With Men and Transgender Women: PilotTrial (AQ2). Clinical Trials.gov Identifier NCT03916484, https://clinicaltrials.gov/ct2/show/NCT03916484.

Murphy, S. A. (2003). Optimal dynamic treatment regimes (with discussions). *Journal of the Royal Statistical Society, Series B* **65**, 331–366.

Murphy, S. A. (2005). An experimental design for the development of adaptive treatment strategies. *Statistics in Medicine* **24**, 1455–1481.

Murphy, S. A., Lynch, K. G., Oslin, D., Mckay, J. R., and TenHave, T. (2007a). Developing adaptive treatment strategies in substance abuse research. *Drug and Alcohol Dependence* **88**, s24–s30.

Murphy, S. A., Oslin, D., Rush, A. J., and Zhu, J. (2007b). Methodological challenges in constructing effective treatment sequences for chronic psychiatric disorders. *Neuropsychopharmacology* **32**, 257–262.

Murphy, S. A., van der Laan, M. J., Robins, J. M., and CPPRG (2001). Marginal mean models for dynamic regimes. *Journal of the American Statistical Association* **96**, 1410–1423.

Mustanski (2018). A Pragmatic Trial of an Adaptive eHealth HIV Prevention Program for Diverse Adolescent MSM (SMART). ClinicalTrials.gov Identifier NCT03511131, https://clinicaltrials.gov/ct2/show/NCT03511131.

Nahum-Shani, I., Qian, M., Almiral, D., Pelham, W., Gnagy, B., Fabiano, G., Waxmonsky, J., Yu, J., and Murphy, S. A. (2012a). Experimental design and primary data analysis methods for comparing adaptive interventions. *Psychological Methods* **17**, 457–477.

Nahum-Shani, I., Qian, M., Almiral, D., Pelham, W., Gnagy, B., Fabiano, G., Waxmonsky, J., Yu, J., and Murphy, S. A. (2012b). Q-learning: A data analysis method for constructing adaptive interventions. *Psychological Methods* **17**, 478–494.

Nahum-Shani, I., Smith, S. N., Spring, B. J., Collins, L. M., Witkiewitz, K., Tewari, A., and Murphy, S. A. (2018). Just-in-time adaptive interventions (JITAIs) in mobile health: Key components and design principles for ongoing health behavior support. *Annals of Behavioral Medicine* **52**, 446–462.

Neyman, J. (1923). On the application of probability theory to agricultural experiments. Essay in principles. Section 9 (translation published in 1990). *Statistical Science* **5**, 472–480.

Niemiro, W. (1992). Asymptotics for M-estimators defined by convex minimization. *Annals of Statistics* **20**, 1514–1533.

Oetting, A. I., Levy, J. A., Weiss, R. D., and Murphy, S. A. (2011). Statistical methodology for a SMART design in the development of adaptive treatment strategies. In Shrout, P., Shrout, P., Keyes, K., and Ornstein, K., editors, *Causality and Psychopathology: Finding the Determinants of Disorders and their Cures*, pages 179–205, Arlington, VA. American Psychiatric Publishing, Inc.

Orellana, L., Rotnitzky, A., and Robins, J. M. (2010a). Dynamic regime marginal structural mean models for estimation of optimal dynamic treatment regimes, part I: Main content. *The International Journal of Biostatistics* **6**.

Orellana, L., Rotnitzky, A., and Robins, J. M. (2010b). Dynamic regime marginal structural mean models for estimation of optimal dynamic treatment regimes, part II: Proofs and additional results. *The International Journal of Biostatistics* **6**.

Politis, D. N., Romano, J. P., and Wolf, M. (1999). *Subsampling*. Springer-Verlag, New York.

Qian, M. and Murphy, S. (2011). Performance guarantees for individualized treatment rules. *Annals of Statistics* **39**, 1180–1210.

Rich, B., Moodie, E. E., and Stephens, D. A. (2014). Simulating sequential multiple assignment randomized trials to generate optimal personalized warfarin dosing strategies. *Clinical Trials* **11**, 435–444.

Richardson, T. S. and Rotnitzky, A. (2014). Causal etiology of the research of James M. Robins. *Statistical Science* **29**, 459–484.

Rivest, R. L. (1987). Learning decision lists. *Machine Learning* **2**, 229–246.

Robins, J. (1986). A new approach to causal inference in mortality studies with sustained exposure periods: Application to control of the healthy worker survivor effect. *Mathematical Modelling* **7**, 1393–

1512.

Robins, J. (1987). Addendum to: A new approach to causal inference in mortality studies with sustained exposure periods: Application to control of the healthy worker survivor effect. *Computers and Mathematics with Applications* **14**, 923–945.

Robins, J. (1989). The analysis of randomized and nonrandomized AIDS treatment trials using a new approach to causal inference in longitudinal studies. In Sechrest, L., Freeman, H., and Mulley, A., editors, *Health Service Research Methodology: A Focus on AIDS*, pages 113–159, New York. NCHSR, U.S. Public Health Service.

Robins, J. (1993). Information recovery and bias adjustment in proportional hazards regression analysis of randomized trials using surrogate markers. *Proceedings of the Biopharmaceutical Section, American Statistical Association* pages 24–33.

Robins, J. (1997). Causal inference from complex longitudinal data. In Berkane, M., editor, *Latent Variable Modeling and Applications to Causality: Lecture Notes in Statistics*, pages 69–117, New York. Springer-Verlag.

Robins, J. (1999a). Marginal structural models versus structural nested models as tools for causal inference. In Halloran, M. E. and Berry, D., editors, *Statistical Models in Epidemiology, the Environment, and Clinical Trials*, volume 116 of *IMA*, pages 95–134, New York. Springer.

Robins, J. M. (1999b). Association, causation, and marginal structural models. *Synthese* **121**, 151–179.

Robins, J. M. (2004). Optimal structural nested models for optimal sequential decisions. In Lin, D. Y. and Heagerty, P., editors, *Proceedings of the Second Seattle Symposium on Biostatistics*, pages 189–326, New York. Springer.

Robins, J. M., Hernán, M. A., and Brumback, B. (2000). Marginal structural models and causal inference in epidemiology. *Epidemiology* **11**, 550–60.

Robins, J. M., Orellana, L., and Rotnitzky, A. (2008). Estimation and extrapolation of optimal treatment and testing strategies. *Statistics in Medicine* **27**, 4678–4721.

Robins, J. M. and Rotnitzky, A. (1992). Recovery of information and adjustment for dependent censoring using surrogate markers. In Jewell, N., Dietz, K., and Farewell, V., editors, *AIDS Epidemiology–Metholdological Issues*, pages 297–331, Boston. Birkhäuser.

Robins, J. M., Rotnitzky, A., and Zhao, L. P. (1994). Estimation of regression coefficients when some regressors are not always observed. *Journal of the American Statistical Association* **89,** 846–866.

Robins, J. M., Rotnitzky, A., and Zhao, L. P. (1995). Analysis of semiparametric regression models for repeated outcomes in the presence of missing data. *Journal of the American Statistical Association* **90,** 106–121.

Rockafellar, R. T. and Wets, R. J.-B. (2009). *Variational Analysis.* Springer Verlag, Berlin Heidelberg.

Romano, J. P., Shaikh, A. M., et al. (2012). On the uniform asymptotic validity of subsampling and the bootstrap. *Annals of Statistics* **40,** 2798–2822.

Rose, E., Laber, E., Davidian, M., Tsiatis, A., Zhao, Y., and Kosorok, M. (2019). Sample size calculations for SMARTs. *NC State University Department of Statistics Technical Report* **1,** 1–30.

Rosenbaum, P. R. and Rubin, D. B. (1983). The central role of the propensity score in observational studies for causal effects. *Biometrika* **70,** 41–55.

Rosenbaum, P. R. and Rubin, D. B. (1984). Reducing bias in observational studies using subclassification on the propensity score. *Journal of the American Statistical Association* **79,** 516–524.

Rubin, D. and van der Laan, M. (2012). Statistical issues and limitations in personalized medicine research with clinical trials. *International Journal of Biostatistics* **8.**

Rubin, D. B. (1974). Estimating causal effects of treatments in randomized and nonrandomized studies. *Journal of Educational Psychology* **66,** 688–701.

Rubin, D. B. (1978). Bayesian inference for causal effects: The role of randomization. *Annals of Statistics* **6,** 34–58.

Rubin, D. B. (1980). Bias reduction using Mahalanobis-metric matching. *Biometrics* **36,** 293–298.

Rubin, D. B. (2005). Causal inference using potential outcomes. *Journal of the American Statistical Association* **100,** 322–331.

Rush, A., Fava, M., Wisniewski, S., Lavori, P., Trivedi, M., Sackeim, H., Thase, M., Nierenberg, A., Quitkin, F., Kashner, T., Kupfer, D., Rosenbaum, J., Alpert, J., Stewart, J., McGrath, P., Biggs, M., Shores-Wilson, K., Lebowitz, B., Ritz, L., and Niederehe, G. (2004). Sequenced treatment alternatives to relieve depression (STAR*D): Rationale and design. *Controlled Clinical Trials* **25,** 119–142.

Saarela, O., Arjas, E., Stephens, D. A., and Moodie, E. E. M. (2015).

Predictive Bayesian inference and dynamic treatment regimes. *Biometrical Journal* **57**, 941–958.

Scheffé, H. (1947). A useful convergence theorem for probability distributions. *Annals of Mathematical Statistics* **18**, 434–438.

Schrijver, A. (1998). *Theory of Linear and Integer Programming*. John Wiley & Sons, Hoboken, New Jersey.

Schuler, M. S. and Rose, S. (2017). Targeted maximum likelihood estimation for causal inference in observational studies. *American Journal of Epidemiology* **185**, 65–73.

Schulte, P. J., Tsiatis, A. A., Laber, E. B., and Davidian, M. (2014). Robust estimation of optimal dynamic treatment regimes for sequential treatment decisions. *Statistical Science* **29**, 640–661.

Shao, J. (1994). Bootstrap sample size in nonregular cases. *Proceedings of the American Mathematical Society* **122**, 1251–1262.

Shen, J., Wang, L., and Taylor, J. M. G. (2017). Estimation of the optimal regime in treatment of prostate cancer recurrence from observational data using flexible weighting models. *Biometrics* **73**, 635–645.

Shi, C., Song, R., and Lu, W. (2016). Robust learning for optimal treatment decision with np-dimensionality. *Electronic Journal of Statistics* **10**, 2894–2921.

Shortreed, S. M., Laber, E., Stroup, T. S., Pineau, J., and Murphy, S. A. (2014). A multiple imputation strategy for sequential multiple assignment randomized trials. *Statistics in Medicine* **33**, 4202–4214.

Song, R., Luo, S., Zeng, D., Zhang, H. H., Lu, W., and Li, Z. (2017). Semiparametric single-index model for estimating optimal individualized treatment strategy. *Electronic Journal of Statistics* **11**, 364–384.

Song, R., Wang, W., Zeng, D., and Kosorok, M. R. (2015). Penalized Q-learning for dynamic treatment regimens. *Statistica Sinica* **25**, 901–920.

Stefanski, L. A. and Boos, D. D. (2002). The calculus of M-estimation. *The American Statistician* **56**, 29–38.

Stephens, D. A. (2015). G-estimation for dynamic treatment regimes in the longitudinal setting. In Kosorok, M. R. and Moodie, E. E. M., editors, *Adaptive Treatment Strategies in Practice: Planning Trials and Analyzing Data for Personalized Medicine*, pages 89–117, Philadelphia, PA. SIAM.

Su, X., Tsai, C. L., Wang, H., Nickerson, D. M., and Li, B. (2009).

Subgroup analysis via recursive partitioning. *Journal of Machine Learning Research* **10**, 141–158.

Sutton, R. S. and Barto, A. G. (2018). *Reinforcement Learning: An Introduction, Second Edition*. MIT Press, Cambridge.

Swartz, M. S., Perkins, D. O., Stroup, T. S., McEvoy, J. P., Nieri, J. M., and Haal, D. D. (2003). Assessing clinical and functional outcomes in the clinical antipsychotic of intervention effectiveness (CATIE) schizophrenia trial. *Schizophrenia Bulletin* **29**, 33–43.

Tao, Y. and Wang, L. (2017). Adaptive contrast weighted learning for multi-stage multi-treatment decision-making. *Biometrics* **73**, 145–155.

Taylor, J. M. G., Cheng, W., and Foster, J. C. (2015). Reader Reaction to "A robust method for estimating optimal treatment regimes" by Zhang et al. (2012). *Biometrics* **71**, 267–273.

Tchetgen Tchetgen, E. J. and VanderWeele, T. J. (2012). On causal inference in the presence of interference. *Statistical Methods in Medical Research* **21**, 55–75.

Therneau, T., Atkinson, B., and Ripley, B. (2015). Package `rpart`: Recursive partitioning and regression trees. *Available at* `http://cran.us.r-project.org/` .

Tian, L., Alizadeh, A. A., Gentles, A. J., and Tibshirani, R. (2014). A simple method for estimating interactions between a treatment and a large number of covariates. *Journal of the American Statistical Association* **109**, 1517–1532.

Tsiatis, A. A. (2006). *Semiparametric Theory and Missing Data*. Springer-Verlag, New York.

Tsiatis, A. A. (2014). Competing risks: Theory. In *Wiley StatsRef: Statistics Reference Online*. doi: 10.1002/9781118445112.stat05131.

van der Laan, M. J. (2010). Targeted maximum likelihood based causal inference: Part I. *The International Journal of Biostatistics* **6**.

van der Laan, M. J. and Luedtke, A. R. (2015). Targeted learning of the mean outcome under an optimal dynamic treatment rule. *Journal of Causal Inference* **3**, 61–95.

van der Laan, M. J. and Petersen, M. L. (2007a). Causal effect models for realistic individualized treatment and intention to treat rules. *The International Journal of Biostatistics* **3**.

van der Laan, M. J. and Petersen, M. L. (2007b). Statistical learning of origin-specific statically optimal individualized treatment rules. *The International Journal of Biostatistics* **3**.

van der Laan, M. J. and Rose, S. (2018). *Targeted Learning in Data Sci-*

ence: Causal Inference for Complex Longitudinal Studies. Springer, New York.

van der Laan, M. J. and Rubin, D. (2006). Targeted maximum likelihood learning. *The International Journal of Biostatistics* **2**.

van der Vaart, A. (1991). On differentiable functionals. *Annals of Statistics* **19**, 178–204.

van der Vaart, A. W. (2000). *Asymptotic Statistics.* Cambridge University Press, Cambridge.

van der Vaart, A. W. and Wellner, J. A. (1996). *Weak Convergence and Empirical Processes.* Springer, New York.

Vansteelandt, S. and Joffe, M. (2014). Structural nested models and g-estimation: The partially realized promise. *Statistical Science* **29**, 707–731.

Vapnik, V., Golowich, S., and Smola, A. (1997). Support vector regression for function approximation, regression estimation, and signal processing. *Advances in Neural Information Processing Systems* **9**, 281–287.

Wallace, M., Moodie, E. E. M. M., and Stephens, D. A. (2019). Model selection for g-estimation of dynamic treatment regimes. *Biometrics* in press.

Wallace, M. P., Moodie, E. E. M., and Stephens, D. A. (2016). SMART thinking: A review of recent developments in sequential multiple assignment randomized trials. *Current Epidemiology Reports* **3**, 225–232.

Wallace, M. P. and Moodie, E. M. M. (2015). Doubly-robust dynamic treatment regimen estimation via weighted least squares. *Biometrics* **71**, 636–644.

Wallace, M. P., Moodie, E. M. M., and Stephens, D. A. (2015). Model assessment in dynamic treatment regimen estimation via double robustness. *Biometrics* **71**, 636–644.

Wang, L., Rotnitzky, A., Lin, X., Millikan, R., and Thall, P. (2012). Evaluation of viable dynamic treatment regimes in a sequentially randomized trial of advanced prostate cancer. *Journal of the American Statistical Association* **107**, 493–508.

Wang, L., Zhou, Y., Song, R., and Sherwood, B. (2018). Quantile-optimal treatment regimes. *Journal of the American Statistical Association* **113**, 1243–1254.

Watkins, C. J. C. H. and Dayan, P. (1992). Q-learning. *Machine Learning* **8**, 279–292.

Whitehead, J. (1997). *The Design and Analysis of Sequential Clinical*

Trials, Second Edition. John Wiley & Sons, Chichester.

Wolsey, L. A. and Nemhauser, G. L. (2014). *Integer and Combinatorial Optimization*. John Wiley & Sons, Hoboken, New Jersey.

Wu, C. J. and Hamada, M. S. (2011). *Experiments: Planning, Analysis, and Optimization*, volume 552. John Wiley & Sons, Hoboken, New Jersey.

Wu, F. (2015). *Adaptive projection intervals*. PhD thesis, North Carolina State University.

Xu, Y., Müller, P., Wahed, A. S., and Thall, P. F. (2016). Bayesian nonparametric estimation for dynamic treatment regimes with sequential transition times. *Journal of the American Statistical Association* **111**, 921–950.

Xu, Y., Yu, M., Zhao, Y., Li, Q., Wang, S., and Shao, J. (2015). Regularized outcome weighted subgroup identification for differential treatment effects. *Biometrics* **71**, 645–653.

Zajonc, T. (2012). Bayesian inference for dynamic treatment regimes: Mobility, equity, and efficiency in student tracking. *Journal of the American Statistical Association* **107**, 80–92.

Zhang, B., Tsiatis, A., Davidian, M., Zhang, M., and Laber, E. (2012a). Estimating optimal treatment regimes from a classification perspective. *Stat* **1**, 103–114.

Zhang, B., Tsiatis, A. A., Laber, E. B., and Davidian, M. (2012b). A robust method for estimating optimal treatment regimes. *Biometrics* **68**, 1010–1018.

Zhang, B., Tsiatis, A. A., Laber, E. B., and Davidian, M. (2013). Robust estimation of optimal dynamic treatment regimes for sequential treatment decisions. *Biometrika* **100**, 681–694.

Zhang, B. and Zhang, M. (2018a). C-learning: A new classification framework to estimate optimal dynamic treatment regimes. *Biometrics* **74**, 891–899.

Zhang, B. and Zhang, M. (2018b). Variable selection for estimating the optimal treatment regimes in the presence of a large number of covariates. *Amnals of Applied Statistics* **12**, 2335–2358.

Zhang, Y. and Laber, E. B. (2015). Comment on "An adaptive resampling test for detecting the presence of significant predictors" by McKeague and Qian. *Journal of the American Statistical Association* **110**, 1451–1454.

Zhang, Y., Laber, E. B., Davidian, M., and Tsiatis, A. A. (2018). Interpretable dynamic treatment regimes. *Journal of the American Statistical Association* **113**, 1541–1549.

Zhang, Y., Laber, E. B., Tsiatis, A. A., and Davidian, M. (2015). Using decision lists to construct interpretable and parsimonious treatment regimes. *Biometrics* **71**, 895–904.

Zhao, Y., Zeng, D., Laber, E. B., and Kosorok, M. R. (2015a). New statistical learning methods for estimating optimal dynamic treatment regimes. *Journal of the American Statistical Association* **110**, 583–598.

Zhao, Y., Zeng, D., Laber, E. B., Song, R., Yuan, M., and Kosorok, M. R. (2015b). Doubly robust learning for estimating individualized treatment with censored data. *Biometrika* **102**, 151–168.

Zhao, Y., Zeng, D., Rush, A. J., and Kosorok, M. R. (2012). Estimating individual treatment rules using outcome weighted learning. *Journal of the American Statistical Association* **107**, 1106–1118.

Zhao, Y., Zeng, D., Socinski, M. A., and Kosorok, M. R. (2011). Reinforcement learning strategies for clinical trials in nonsmall cell lung cancer. *Biometrics* **67**, 1422–1433.

Zhao, Y.-Q., Laber, E. B., Ning, Y., Sumona, S., and Sands, B. E. (2019). Efficient augmentation and relaxation learning for individuallized treatment rules using observational data. *Journal of Machine Learning Research* **20**, 1–23.

Zhou, X., Mayer-Hamblett, N., Khan, U., and Kosorok, M. R. (2017). Residual weighted learning for estimating individualized treatment rules. *Journal of the American Statistical Association* **112**, 169–187.

Zhu, R., Zhao, Y. Q., Chen, G., Ma, S., and Zhao, H. (2017). Greedy outcome weighted tree learning of optimal personalized treatment rules. *Biometrics* **73**, 391–400.

Zhu, W., Zeng, D., and Song, R. (2019). Proper inference for value function in high-dimensional Q-learning for dynamic treatment regimes. *Journal of the American Statistical Association* **114**, 1404–1417.

Index